Tinnitus: An Issue of Otolaryngology Clinics

Tinnitus: An Issue of Otolaryngology Clinics

Editor: Kimi Brown

AMERICAN
MEDICAL PUBLISHERS
www.americanmedicalpublishers.com

AMERICAN MEDICAL PUBLISHERS
www.americanmedicalpublishers.com

Cataloging-in-Publication Data

Tinnitus : an issue of otolaryngology clinics / edited by Kimi Brown.
p. cm.
Includes bibliographical references and index.
ISBN 979-8-88740-513-1
1. Tinnitus. 2. Tinnitus--Diagnosis. 3. Tinnitus--Treatment. 4. Otolaryngology.
5. Hearing disorders. I. Brown, Kimi.
RF293.8 .T56 2023
617.8--dc23

American Medical Publishers,
41 Flatbush Avenue,
1st Floor, New York,
NY 11217, USA

ISBN 979-8-88740-513-1 (Hardback)

Contents

Preface

Tinnitus is a disorder wherein a person experiences noises such as ringing, hissing, or clicking in one or both ears. This noise is not caused by an external sound. Tinnitus is quite common and generally observed in older adults. The noise experienced may be loud or quiet, continuous or intermittent, and some individuals are unaffected by it. However, other people become highly disturbed by it, especially when they are fatigued or stressed. Tinnitus is generally considered a symptom of underlying health conditions rather than a disorder. The common reasons that lead to this disorder are noise-induced hearing loss, ear infections, disease of the heart or blood vessels, Ménière's disease, brain tumors, inner ear tumors, emotional stress and traumatic brain injury. The degree of hearing loss controls the level of concentration that may result in anxiety and depression in some cases. Acceptance and commitment therapy (ACT) is beneficial in the treatment of tinnitus. This book traces the progress of research on tinnitus and highlights its clinical aspects. It unravels the recent studies related to tinnitus. Those in search of information to further their knowledge will be greatly assisted by this book.

Significant researches are present in this book. Intensive efforts have been employed by authors to make this book an outstanding discourse. This book contains the enlightening chapters which have been written on the basis of significant researches done by the experts.

Finally, I would also like to thank all the members involved in this book for being a team and meeting all the deadlines for the submission of their respective works. I would also like to thank my friends and family for being supportive in my efforts.

Editor

A Mixed-Methods Trial of Broad Band Noise and Nature Sounds for Tinnitus Therapy: Group and Individual Responses Modeled under the Adaptation Level Theory of Tinnitus

Mithila Durai[1,2] *and Grant D. Searchfield*[1,2,3*]

[1] *Eisdell Moore Centre, Section of Audiology, University of Auckland, Auckland, New Zealand,* [2] *Center for Brain Research, University of Auckland, Auckland, New Zealand,* [3] *Brain Research New Zealand, Auckland, New Zealand*

Correspondence:
Grant D. Searchfield
g.searchfield@auckland.ac.nz

Objectives: A randomized cross-over trial in 18 participants tested the hypothesis that nature sounds, with unpredictable temporal characteristics and high valence would yield greater improvement in tinnitus than constant, emotionally neutral broadband noise.

Study Design: The primary outcome measure was the Tinnitus Functional Index (TFI). Secondary measures were: loudness and annoyance ratings, loudness level matches, minimum masking levels, positive and negative emotionality, attention reaction and discrimination time, anxiety, depression and stress. Each sound was administered using MP3 players with earbuds for 8 continuous weeks, with a 3 week wash-out period before crossing over to the other treatment sound. Measurements were undertaken for each arm at sound fitting, 4 and 8 weeks after administration. Qualitative interviews were conducted at each of these appointments.

Results: From a baseline TFI score of 41.3, sound therapy resulted in TFI scores at 8 weeks of 35.6; broadband noise resulted in significantly greater reduction (8.2 points) after 8 weeks of sound therapy use than nature sounds (3.2 points). The positive effect of sound on tinnitus was supported by secondary outcome measures of tinnitus, emotion, attention, and psychological state, but not interviews. Tinnitus loudness level match was higher for BBN at 8 weeks; while there was little change in loudness level matches for nature sounds. There was no change in minimum masking levels following sound therapy administration. Self-reported preference for one sound over another did not correlate with changes in tinnitus.

Conclusions: Modeled under an adaptation level theory framework of tinnitus perception, the results indicate that the introduction of broadband noise shifts internal adaptation level weighting away from the tinnitus signal, reducing tinnitus magnitude. Nature sounds may modify the affective components of tinnitus via a secondary, residual pathway, but this appears to be less important for sound effectiveness. The different rates of adaptation to broadband noise and nature sound by the auditory system may explain the different tinnitus loudness level matches. In addition to group effects there also appears to be a great deal of individual variation. A sound therapy framework based on adaptation level theory is proposed that accounts for individual variation in preference and response to sound.

Clinical Trial Registration: www.anzctr.org.au, identifier #12616000742471.

Keywords: clinical trial, tinnitus, auditory perception, adaptation, psychoacoustics, ecology model, sound therapy

INTRODUCTION

Subjective tinnitus is the involuntary perception of one or more sounds by an individual, in the absence of an external physical source (Henry et al., 2005; Moller, 2006; Kaltenbach, 2011; De Ridder et al., 2014). It is now broadly understood to arise as a result of peripheral lesions in the auditory system resulting in altered cortical input. This triggers compensatory neuroplasticity changes across several overlapping brain networks (Schecklmann et al., 2013a,b; Vanneste et al., 2011, 2013; Husain and Schmidt, 2014). Final tinnitus magnitude is thought to result from differences in personality and activity within auditory, emotion, attention, and memory networks (Searchfield et al., 2012; Searchfield, 2014; Durai et al., 2015). Fifteen to twenty percentage of the tinnitus population experience significant disruption to quality of life (Heller, 2003; Hoffmann and Reed, 2004), manifesting as impaired concentration, problems with hearing, irritation, frustration and annoyance, anxiety, depression, disruption of everyday activities, and disturbed sleep (Davis and El Refaie, 2000; Heller, 2003; Bartels et al., 2010; Malouff et al., 2011). Reports of tinnitus affect vary a great deal from individual to individual, leading to models of tinnitus that include individual psychology and personality as strong contributors (Searchfield et al., 2012; Searchfield, 2014). A failure to account for the heterogeneous nature of tinnitus has likely contributed to the difficulties in identifying useful therapies.

Sound therapy is currently used in several tinnitus treatment paradigms. Sound therapy uses external sounds to modify tinnitus perception and/or reactions to it (Scott et al., 1990; Jastreboff, 1999; Henry et al., 2006; Tyler, 2006; Hoare et al., 2011; Searchfield et al., 2012). Immediate effects are provided by masking (Scott et al., 1990; Tyler, 2006), and long-term changes in tinnitus functional networks have also been observed (Noreña and Eggermont, 2006; Távora-Vieira et al., 2011; Tyler et al., 2012). The potential for tinnitus and external sound to interact exists as both undergo similar auditory processing within the system, including feature extraction, schema formation, and semantic objective formation (Searchfield et al., 2012; Searchfield, 2014). Although categorization of patient characteristics has been used to guide focus of treatments [e.g., hearing aids, counseling, use of sound therapy (Jastreboff, 1998)] and some sound therapies alter the therapeutic sound based on pitch (Stein et al., 2016) and give participants choices about the stimuli, how sound is selected based on individual needs does not appear to be widespread or documented. Sounds used in therapy include broadband noise (BBN), narrow-band noise (either pitch-matched or unmatched to tinnitus), nature sounds or music (Sandlin and Olsson, 1999; Vernon and Meikle, 2000; Folmer and Carroll, 2006). Despite its popularity, there is no consensus as to the most appropriate sound parameters for tinnitus therapy, or if the treatment provides independent benefit over psychological effects (Tyler, 2006; McKenna and Irwin, 2008; Hobson et al., 2010) or hearing aids (Henry et al., 2015). Several recent studies using different types of sound have shown small (Kim et al., 2014) or no significant differences in effect (Barozzi et al., 2016) between different therapy sounds on tinnitus. There is some evidence that dynamic sounds that temporally vary may provide greater benefit for reducing tinnitus symptoms compared to fixed intensity sounds (Vernon and Meikle, 2000; Henry et al., 2004; Davis, 2006; Hann et al., 2008). Customized music and counseling applied via the Neuromonics Tinnitus Treatment for 6 months resulted in greater alleviation of tinnitus symptoms and greater user acceptability than when participants were provided with counseling and BBN, or counseling only (Davis et al., 2008). Schreitmüller et al. (2013) observed that nature sounds, even though they presented with higher dynamics and higher masking thresholds, were accepted more by the listener than white noise. Ocean or wave sounds have recently been introduced by several hearing aid manufacturers in their tinnitus therapy devices (Callaway, 2014; Dos Santos and Powers, 2015).

The reasons why temporally varying sound may be more effective in treating tinnitus in some individuals are unclear. The added therapeutic success of dynamic sounds, particularly sounds relevant to an individual's everyday environment, may be due to the provision of greater informational (central) auditory masking, whereby both therapeutic sound and tinnitus compete for cognitive resources (Kidd et al., 2002). Informational or "central" masking is possible with tinnitus, as the phenomenon is due to central processing itself. Another way in which music or nature sounds can promote relief is by engaging the emotional regions of the brain; as relaxation aids (Davis et al., 2008; Hanley and Davis, 2008). Unpleasant sounds mimicking tinnitus have been found to activate the tinnitus network more strongly than neutral tones (Schlee et al., 2008). Simulation of tinnitus (using an aversive tinnitus-like auditory stimuli) in patients without tinnitus have been shown to activate neural networks comparable to that of tinnitus, including recruitment of the limbic system (Mirz et al., 2000a,b). Differences in processing of pleasant sounds have also been observed between tinnitus

Abbreviations: ALT, Adaptation Level Theory; ANOVA, Analysis of Variance; ANZCTR, Australian New Zealand Clinical Trial Registry; BBN, Broadband Noise; CAB, Comprehensive Attention Battery; DASS, Depression, Anxiety and Stress Scale; EAP, Equal Annoyance Point; ELP, Equal Loudness Point; Hz, Hertz; LLM, Loudness Level Match; MML, Minimum Masking Level; MPQ, Multidimensional Personality Questionnaire; NZ, New Zealand; PANAS, Positive and Negative Affect Scale; TCHQ, Tinnitus Case History Questionnaire; TFI, Tinnitus Functional Index; THQ, Tinnitus Handicap Questionnaire; COSIT, Client Oriented Scale of Improvement for Tinnitus.

patients compared to those without hearing loss or tinnitus (Carpenter-Thompson et al., 2014), as greater activation of the bilateral hippocampus and right insula. It is possible that tinnitus and emotionally negative auditory perceptions from known sources may share similar neural processing networks, which are counteracted by the presence of pleasant stimuli. Short term exposure to emotional stimuli in the auditory modality (but not visual modality) influences ratings of tinnitus: with presentation of more unpleasant sounds resulting in increased tinnitus magnitude (Durai et al., 2017b).

An ecological model (Searchfield, 2014) of tinnitus that incorporates Adaptation Level Theory (ALT; Helson, 1964; Searchfield et al., 2012) has been proposed to account for individual differences in responses to sound therapy, in which a multitude of inherent, and environmental factors interact to determine final tinnitus magnitude. The ALT is based on Helson's (Helson, 1948, 1964) theory, whereby an adaptation level (AL) acts as an internal anchor/reference point used to make sensory magnitude estimations, and this is susceptible to change over time and context (Helson, 1948, 1964; Coren and Ward, 1989). For loud and/or annoying tinnitus, a high internal AL is established—thus the tinnitus is perceived as being of high magnitude. The final AL magnitude estimates of tinnitus, as well as distress judgements, are derived by interactions between the focal component (tinnitus), contextual component (any background noise or applied sounds), and various residual components (individual cognitive and behavioral characteristics such as personality traits, memory, and past experiences, emotion, etc.) (Searchfield et al., 2012; Searchfield, 2014; Durai et al., 2015). The ALT model of tinnitus predicts that BBN and sounds that fluctuate or are emotive (such as nature sounds in our soundscape) should both affect tinnitus positively but through different mechanisms. Variables affecting the success of different sounds might include individual-specific top-down processing related to personality, memory, prediction, attention, and emotion as well as bottom up processes related to primitive auditory analysis such as contrast (Searchfield et al., 2012). Up until this study there have been no controlled trials to test sound therapy based on the ALT model. The presence of several influencing factors on tinnitus-external sound interactions might account for individual success (or lack of success) with sound therapy. A successful sound therapy is not one that affects tinnitus alone; it must be comfortable as well. Testing different parameters and individual preferences of sound therapy are therefore significant in strengthening support for, and improving, sound therapy effectiveness (Barros Suzuki et al., 2016).

We hypothesized that nature sounds would affect top-down processing, and this, along with positive effects on emotion would result in greater reduction in tinnitus magnitude than BBN, that would primarily affect bottom-up processing. Barozzi et al. (2016) found that nature and BBN resulted in similar reductions of the Tinnitus Handicap Questionnaire (THQ) following 6 months of administration, but they did not explore individual characteristics and mechanism of benefit relative to study outcomes. An experimental study piloting some of the methods employed here (Durai et al., unpublished manuscript) found that 30 min administration of unpredictable surf-like sound resulted in significantly lower tinnitus loudness than a predictable surf sound. A 2 week feasibility trial found greater number of participants preferred the unpredictable surf sound (Durai et al., unpublished manuscript). The effects of other contributory factors (e.g., greater relaxation to one sound over the other, different emotions evoked by the two sounds, anticipation) were not controlled for in that short-term trial. A longer-term clinical trial comparing BBN and nature sounds measuring various individual residuals (e.g., emotion, attention) was deemed critical to understand sound therapy effects.

METHODS

This study was approved by the University of Auckland Human Participants Ethics Committee. All participants gave written informed consent in accordance with the Declaration of Helsinki. This trial was retrospectively registered on Australian New Zealand Clinical Trials Registry (ANZCTR; Trial #12616000742471).

Trial Design

A randomized controlled, cross-over study design using mixed (qualitative and quantitative) methods was employed. Repeated outcome measures were obtained at three time points: baseline when the sound was first fitted, 4 weeks after administration, and 8 weeks after administration for both BBN and nature sound therapies. There was a 3 week wash-out period in between the two conditions. The outcome measures taken at each appointment and time-frame protocol for data collection are presented in **Table 1** and **Figure 1**, respectively.

Participants

The inclusion criteria were: adults aged between 18 and 69 years residing in the Auckland region (NZ), constant tinnitus and a minimum weighted score of 21 on the Tinnitus Functional Index (TFI; this cut-off score is calculated based on convergent validity results between TFI mean scores and response levels of a tinnitus global severity item; a score of 21 delineates individuals who consider their tinnitus as problematic from those who do not view tinnitus as a problem; Meikle et al., 2012), normal middle ear function, and a maximum of a moderate degree of hearing loss (<70 dB loss on average across frequencies). A participant information sheet was provided to participants that outlined the background and aims of the trial and details of measurements to be taken at various appointments.

Initial Assessments

Following a comprehensive case history [Tinnitus Case History Questionnaire; TCHQ; (Langguth et al., 2007)], a hearing assessment was conducted in a sound treated room (ISO 8253-1:2010). Pure tone audiometry (0.25–16 kHz, Carhart and Jerger, 1959) was undertaken using a GSI-61 two-channel audiometer and TDH-50P headphones or E.A.RTONE 3A insert earphones and Sennheiser HDA-200 high-frequency headphones. Tympanometry was undertaken

TABLE 1 | Outcome measurements taken at the different time points of the trial.

	1st baseline + 1st sound fitting	4 week follow-up	8 week follow-up	2nd baseline + 2nd sound fitting	4 week follow-up	8 week follow-up
Quantitative questionnaires	TFI	TFI	TFI	TFI	TFI	TFI
	Tinnitus loudness rating (1–10)	Tinnitus loudness rating (1–10)	Tinnitus loudness rating (1–10)	Tinnitus loudness rating (1–10)	Tinnitus loudness rating (1–10)	Tinnitus loudness rating (1–10)
	Tinnitus annoyance rating (1–10)	Tinnitus annoyance rating (1–10)	Tinnitus annoyance rating (1–10)	Tinnitus annoyance rating (1–10)	Tinnitus annoyance rating (1–10)	Tinnitus annoyance rating (1–10)
	PANAS	PANAS	PANAS	PANAS	PANAS	PANAS
	DASS	DASS	DASS	DASS	DASS	DASS
Psychoacoustic measurements	LLM MML	LLM MML	LLM MML	LLM MML	LLM MML	LLM MML
Attention measurements	CAB		CAB	CAB		CAB
Qualitative		Qualitative interview schedule	Qualitative interview schedule		Qualitative interview schedule	Qualitative interview schedule

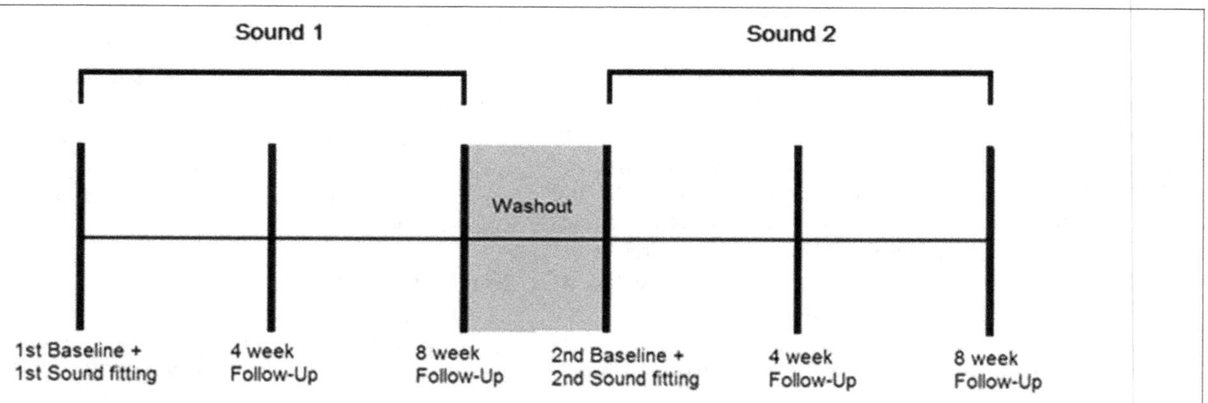

FIGURE 1 | Protocol for data collection. Multiple outcome measurements were taken at the following time points: 1st sound fitting (Baseline), and 4 and 8 weeks after first fitting while the sound was being used. A washout period of 3 weeks followed in which no sound was administered. Multiple outcome measurements were then taken at the following time points: 2st sound fitting (Baseline), and 4 and 8 weeks after second fitting while the sound was being used.

using a GSI Immittance audiometer to check middle-ear function. Tinnitus pitch match was carried out using tinnitus testing software (The University of Auckland) using high frequency circumaural headphones (Sennheiser HDA-200). Tinnitus pitch match was assessed throughout the test frequency range of 0.25–16 kHz using a two-alternative forced-choice (2AFC) method. Each tone was presented at a sensation level of 15 dB SL. Pitch match was then compared to tones one octave above and below to rule out octave confusion. The measurement was repeated until two repeatable responses were obtained. The Multidimensional Personality Questionnaire (MPQ; Tellegen, 1982) was also administered at the initial appointment to measure levels of individual personality traits.

Interventions

Sound Therapy Stimuli

Broadband noise (BBN) was generated using Audacity 2.1.2. (A.2.1.2., 2016). The natural sounds were Surf, Cicadas/Farm Sounds and Rain sounds directly recorded from the natural setting by the researchers using a Roland R-05 WAV/MP3 Recorder with CS-10 EM binaural ear level microphones and edited to 30 min duration using Audacity 2.1.2. software (A.2.1.2., 2016). All stimuli were adjusted for sound level such that the long-term average loudness (dB SPL) was equivalent. The detailed acoustic parameters and spectrum of each sound stimulus are provided in Appendix A in Supplementary Material. Each sound therapy was administered for 8 weeks each via a Philips ViBE SA4VBE08KF/97 4GB MP3 Player and Panasonic

RP-HJE290GUK Premium Black Earphones with a Budloks Earphone Sports Grip earpiece attached for secure retention within the ear. Participants were instructed to listen to the sound therapy for a minimum of 1 h per day.

Tinnitus Loudness and Annoyance Functions and Selection of Nature Sound

BBN and the three nature sounds were played for 2 min each (in randomized order) at the participants desired comfort level. At the end of each sound, participants were asked to rate the sound on a scale of 1–10, with 1 corresponding to a highly negative and/or unpleasant sound and 10 corresponding to highly positive and/or pleasant sound.

BBN and the three nature sounds again were played (in randomized order) to participants at increasing sound levels: from the threshold at which the sound was first heard to the minimum masking level (MML) where the sound first masked the individual's tinnitus. Tinnitus annoyance, tinnitus loudness ratings and noise annoyance ratings (on a scale of low 1–10 high) were undertaken at fixed sound level intervals from 0 dB SL to MML. Participants were also asked to judge the relative loudness of tinnitus and noise on a scale of 1–10 as each sound was increased in sound level, with 1 corresponding with the nature noise being not audible (tinnitus is only audible) and 10 being tinnitus is not audible (fully masked by the sound).

At the end of the task, participants selected which nature sound stimuli they preferred to use in the trial, and this was administered as the Nature sound intervention. Participants were also asked the following questions:

1. Why did you select this particular sound?
2. What kind of feelings (if any) does this sound elicit?

The average valence rating, Equal Loudness Level (the sound level where the combined tinnitus and noise loudness rating given to a noise level was 5, indicating that both tinnitus and noise were of equal perceived loudness) and Equal Annoyance Level (the sound level tinnitus at which annoyance rating functions and noise annoyance rating functions intersect, indicating that both tinnitus and noise are of equal perceived annoyance) of all participants were calculated and recorded for BBN and each environmental sound.

The MP3 volume was initially set for BBN and the nature sound to be one step (10%) below Equal Loudness Level, and if participants preferred it to be slightly higher or lower due to comfort reasons, the sounds were further adjusted accordingly. The final sound set was therefore at an audibility where sound interfered with tinnitus perception but that was also comfortable for the user.

Outcomes

Assessments: Questionnaires for Clinical Evaluation

The Tinnitus Functional Index (TFI; Meikle et al., 2012) was the primary outcome measure, in addition, the following outcome questionnaires were used: Tinnitus Loudness Rating (scale of 1–10), Tinnitus Annoyance Rating (scale of 1–10), Positive and Negative Affect Schedule (PANAS; Tellegen, 1982; Watson et al., 1988), and the Depression, Anxiety and Stress Scale (DASS Scale; Lovibond and Lovibond, 1995). The TFI (Meikle et al., 2012) is a recently developed questionnaire and assesses both severity of tinnitus and its impact on life over eight diverse subscales of intrusiveness, sense of control, cognitive, sleep, auditory, relaxation, quality of life, and emotional. TFI shows high responsiveness to treatment-related change and has been validated as an intake questionnaire with good test-retest reliability in the NZ population (Chandra et al., 2014). Tinnitus loudness ratings were made on a 10-point rating scale where 1 corresponded to a very quiet and 10 with extremely loud. Annoyance ratings were made on a similar scale with one being very low in distress and/or annoyance and 10 being extremely high in distress and/or annoyance. PANAS measures the extent to which positive and negative emotional states are experienced by an individual over the period of the past week. The DASS scale measures levels of affective symptoms.

Assessments: Psychoacoustic Tinnitus Characteristics

Tinnitus psychoacoustic outcomes were measured using tinnitus testing software (The University of Auckland) using high frequency circumaural headphones (Sennheiser HDA-200). Loudness level matching (LLM) was obtained using the pitch-matched stimulus sound at 30 dB above the threshold level and decreasing it slowly in 2 dB steps until the participant stated it was same loudness as their tinnitus. This was repeated three times, and the average of the last two runs was taken. This was subtracted from the threshold level to obtain a level match in dB SL. Minimum masking level (in dB SL) was obtained using a narrow-band noise (NBN) stimulus of 1/3 octave width, raising it from the threshold level until the participant reported that the tinnitus was no longer audible. This procedure was repeated three times, and the average level was calculated. This was subtracted from the threshold level to give the MML match in dB SL.

Assessments: Attention

The Comprehensive Attention Battery (CAB®; Rodenbough, 2003) was used to behaviorally measure individual attention and concentration ability. The CAB is a reliable computer supervised test battery and can be repeated before and after intervention administration to assess for any resulting change. The Discrimination Reaction Time Task (measuring focused attention) and Reaction Time Task (measuring alertness needed for general cognitive task performance; Zomeren and Brouwer, 1994) were utilized in this trial from the CAB series of tests, as in previous studies these domains showed the greatest interaction with tinnitus (Wise, 2012). Focused attention requires attention to be directed toward one aspect of sensory information while excluding others, and is analogous to selective attention (Eysenck and Keane, 2015). Alertness consists of three components: (1) Expectancy, (2) Orientation to various stimuli, and (3) Readiness to produce a motor output. Decreased Reaction Time Task or Discrimination Reaction Time Task scores over time can therefore indicate loss of concentration or increased cognitive load, or inability to focus attention selectively, which can result if tinnitus is increased in magnitude.

For the Reaction Time Task, a gray square was presented in the middle of an otherwise dark/black computer screen. The visual assessment required the participant to respond as soon as possible (touching the square) when it quickly changed to a green color. The presentation lasted 200 ms and occurred after a time delay randomly varying from 1 to 4 s (1000–4000 ms).

For the Discrimination Reaction Time Task, the visual task involved watching a gray square presented in the center of a dark/black computer screen. Random visual presentations of three different colored squares occurred: red, blue or green. Participants were required to touch the square as soon as possible, registering their response, if the square changed to the target color (red) while ignoring non-target colors (blue or green). The target presentations lasted 200 ms, interspersed with 1800 ms time delays. In the auditory task condition, random auditory presentations (spoken) occurred of three different color words: Red, blue, or green. Participants responded whenever they heard the target color word (green) and ignored verbalizations of non-target color words (red or blue). Word presentation lasted ~300 ms. In the mixed visual and auditory condition, participants heard verbal instructions "The Target Is" followed by either: (1) The gray square changing in color to indicate a visual target, or (2) An auditory presentation (spoken) denoting an auditory target, color word. Whenever the target was seen or heard (depending on whether the target given was visual or auditory in nature), the participant was required to press the square as quickly as possible. While anticipating the indicated target, participants experienced randomized presentation of visual and auditory non-targets; spoken color words or visually presented color changes for the gray square. Targets were altered seven times during the assessment. The tasks resulted in assessment of pure visual reaction time (50 stimuli), pure auditory reaction time (50 stimuli), and visual and auditory reaction time (100 stimuli).

Assessments: Qualitative Interviews

At each follow-up appointment and at the end of the trial all participants were interviewed, and the interviews were digitally recorded, transcribed, and responses coded into themes (Gale et al., 2013). The interview schedule for each follow-up appointment was as follows:

1. How often did you use sounds stimuli?
2. In which particular environments did you find yourself using the sounds?
3. How is the quality of the intervention sound?
4. How you feel the sound is interacting with your tinnitus?
5. Has the quality (characteristics of your tinnitus such as the pitch, duration, fluctuation, etc.) of your tinnitus changed over the last month? If yes, how?

Additional questions asked during the final end-of-trial interview were:

6. Which of the two stimuli (BBN or nature) did you prefer the most? Why?
7. Will you be willing to wear this device as a form of tinnitus management for the next 6 months? Why or why not?
8. How can each of the sound stimuli be improved and why would this be an improvement?
9. Any other comments?

Sample Size

A power analysis indicated that 21 participants would need to enter this two-treatment crossover study. The probability was 80% that the study will detect a treatment difference at a two-sided 0.05 significance level, if the true difference between treatments was 13.0 units on the TFI. This is based on the assumption that the standard deviation of the difference in the TFI is 20.

Randomization

The order of sound presentation for participants (Order 1 = BBN then Nature OR Order 2 = Nature then BBN) was decided using an online, free True Random Number Generator (https://www.random.org/). There were no significant differences in personality trait scores between participants placed in Order 1 compared to Order 2. Throughout the trial the same researcher tested all participants. The only blinding applied was participants were not shown the results of their tinnitus outcome measures at the different time points until the end of the trial. Blinding to intervention type could not be provided due to the distinct perceptual sound characteristics of the two sound stimuli. No tinnitus counseling was provided; participants had their hearing tests and tinnitus results explained, and instructions were provided on use of the MP3 player and how to set volume relative to their tinnitus. The nature sound trialed was that chosen by the user.

Statistical Methods

A 2 × 3 repeated-measures Analysis of Variance (ANOVA) was used to examine changes in outcome measures between the two sound types (BBN, natures sounds) at the three time points (baseline, 4 weeks of intervention and 8 weeks of intervention). All assumptions were tested for all outcomes for each independent variable to see if they were met before running ANOVA. In cases where a significant main effect was observed, Bonferroni *post-hoc* tests were administered.

For outcome measures where there was no group effect for intervention observed at 8 weeks, further bivariate correlation and ANOVA analyses of changes in outcome measures (8 weeks-baseline) was conducted in order to explore whether age, gender, and degree of hearing loss [categorized as slight, mild, moderate, moderately severe, severe, or profound (Clark, 1981) based on average of 3000, 4000, and 6000 Hz hearing thresholds bilaterally] effects were present.

In order to extract potential converging information of the different outcome measures and identify key factors influencing the effect of sound therapy administration on tinnitus over time, a Principal Component Analysis (PCA) was conducted. Changes in all outcome measures (regardless of BBN or Nature sounds) between 8 weeks and baseline as well as baseline measures of personality were included. All components with Eigenvalue >1 were extracted. Following inspection of data and the scree plot, a decision was made regarding the final number of components to be included in rotational analysis with Direct Oblimin rotation. Correlations about 0.5 were criterion used to define and load key variables to respective components and construct dimensions.

The framework method (Gale et al., 2013) was used to analyse the qualitative interviews, consisting of five steps: familiarization, identification of a thematic framework, indexing, charting, and mapping and interpretation. Familiarization involved careful listening to the digital recordings and transcribing, and re-reading the transcription. Common themes were identified in the transcripts, and in the charting phase, the data was rearranged according to theme. In the mapping and interpretative stages, the charted data was compared, and contrasted to identify patterns within the data. Quotations from participants and their thematic analysis were included in the results following standard practice in qualitative methodology (Rossman and Wilson, 1985; Onwuegbuzie and Leech, 2005).

RESULTS

Participants Flow and Baseline Data

Thirty-one participants from the University of Auckland Tinnitus Research Volunteer Database expressed interest in the trial; seven participants did not meet the criteria or were excluded for other reasons (one participant was administered the intervention sounds but the data was excluded from final analysis due to a too low baseline TFI score; removed due to basement effects). The data from 24 participants (8 females, 16 males, mean age = 56.31, range 37–65) was taken for the final trial (**Figure 2**). Eighteen participants (7 female, 11 male, mean age = 60.63, range 38–65) completed the trial, retention was 76%. Three participants were lost to follow-up (did not respond to emails, attend follow-up appointments and/or did not finish trialing both sounds) and three participants had early termination. Early termination of trial refers to cases where participants voluntarily expressed they wanted to stop the trial between the 4 and 8 week appointment period for one or both of the Intervention sounds, but still attended follow-up appointments.

The average baseline outcome measures of participants at the start of the trial is provided in **Table 2** (individual baseline outcome measures are provided in Appendix B in Supplementary Material). The mean Tinnitus Functional Index (TFI) score of participants was 41.5 (*SD* = 15.5). All participants had experienced chronic bothersome tinnitus for a minimum of 4 years with an average length of time since tinnitus onset of 17.5 years (*SD* = 12.2, ranging from 4 to 45 years). Thirty-nine percent of participants described tinnitus quality as cricket sounds, 39% as tonal and 22% as noise. Measured tinnitus pitch ranged from 800 to 15,750 Hz, and there was no clustering observed around any particular pitch match. Fifty percent of participants had not used any form of tinnitus treatment in the past, 25% had tried one treatment and 25% had tried more than one treatment. Three out of the 18 participants (17%) wore pairs of hearing aids. When asked whether loud sounds tended to make their tinnitus worse, 42% responded that it did exacerbate it, 32% responded no and

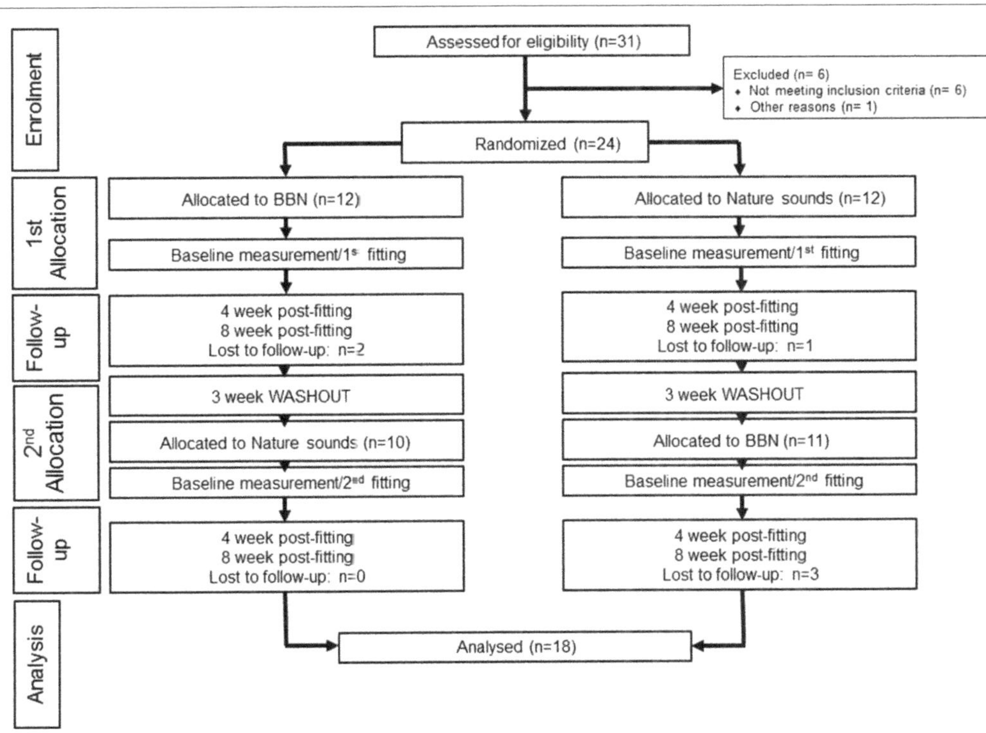

FIGURE 2 | CONSORT flow diagram of participants.

TABLE 2 | Average baseline characteristics of participants as measured at the start of the trial.

		Order 1	Order 2
Demographics	Gender	Five female, four male	Two female, six male
	Age	59.3 (9.6)	56.6 (7.7)
Tinnitus characteristics	Duration (Years)	18.2 (15.5)	14 (8.5)
	Loudness rating (1–10)	6.2 (1.5)	7 (0.8)
	Annoyance rating (1–10)	5.7 (2.2)	5.6 (1.2)
	Total TFI score (weighted)	38.6 (12.5)	47.4 (17)
	LLM	3 (4)	4.8 (4.5)
	MML	6 (6)	7.4 (6.4)
Emotional/ psychological	Positive emotionality	34.2 (6)	34.1 (6.7)
	Negative emotionality	16.2 (5.4)	16.5 (6.7)
	Anxiety	5 (6.4)	4.6 (5.7)
	Depression	3.1 (4)	2.9 (3.6)
	Stress	6.8 (5)	7.1 (7.7)
Personality traits	Stress reaction	7.6 (2.1)	6.3 (4.9)
	Social closeness	5.1 (2.5)	6.1 (2.8)
	Self-control	14.4 (3.1)	13.4 (3.1)
	Alienation	1.1 (1.2)	1.5 (1.5)

Values inside brackets in columns represent one standard deviation. Order 1, BBN then Nature as order of intervention presentation for participants. Order 2, Nature then BBN as order of intervention presentation for participants.

26% did not know. Forty-two percent of participants felt that their tinnitus was reduced by music or by certain types of nature sounds (such as the noise of a waterfall, running shower water, etc.) and the remaining 58% did not know.

Loudness and Annoyance Functions for Sound Therapy Stimuli and Tinnitus

All the sounds resulted in decreased tinnitus loudness and annoyance, and increases in sound loudness and annoyance occurred as noise level was raised (**Figures 3, 4**). The average ratings for sound therapy stimuli at MML are provided in **Table 3**. When the sounds were ranked based on average rating changes with noise level increases, Rain was ranked #1 (equal) for tinnitus loudness decline, #4 (equal) for sound loudness growth, #1 (equal) for tinnitus annoyance decline, and #2 (equal) for sound annoyance growth. Cicadas was ranked as #1 (equal) in tinnitus loudness decline, #4 (equal) for sound loudness growth, #1 (equal) for tinnitus annoyance decline, and #1 for sound annoyance growth. Surf was ranked #4 for tinnitus loudness decline, #1 for sound loudness growth, #4 for tinnitus annoyance decline and #2 (equal) for sound annoyance growth. BBN was ranked #1 (equal) for tinnitus loudness decline, #1 for sound loudness growth, #1 (equal) for tinnitus annoyance decline, and #4 for sound annoyance growth. The Equal Loudness Level ranking was: Rain/BBN > Cicadas > Surf. The Equal Annoyance Level ranking was: Surf > Rain > Cicadas > BBN.

Selection of Nature Sound

Eleven out of the 18 participants (61%) selected the Rain sound to be used in the trial, and key reasons were that it was soothing and interacted more with tinnitus. Five participants selected the Surf sound (28%) while two selected Cicadas (11%).ain had the highest valence rating (most pleasant) by participants, followed by the Surf and Cicadas respectively. BBN was the least pleasant of all the sounds (**Figure 5**). All participants except one (who expressed neutral feelings) reported the nature sound was pleasant, soothing, relaxing and elicited happy feelings.

Intervention Outcomes: Tinnitus Measures

There was a significant main effect of sound therapy time on TFI scores, with a 5.7 point decrease in TFI scores at 8 weeks compared to baseline [$F_{(2, 28)} = 4.144, p < 0.05$; **Figure 6**]. There was a significant effect of sound types at 8 weeks [$F_{(1, 28)} = 6.875, p < 0.05$], with BBN sound administration resulting in a mean 8.2 point decrease in scores, while nature sounds resulted in a 3.2 point decrease. The small change in TFI in response to the nature sounds at 4 weeks (4.2 point decrease) was not statistically significant. There were no significant difference in tinnitus measures between before the washout (8 week follow-up appointment for the first sound) and immediately after the washout (sound fitting appointment for the second sound). There was also no effect of order: the degree of change in tinnitus outcome measures was not significantly different between the first and second sound administered.

There was no difference in loudness or annoyance ratings following sound therapy at 4 weeks compared to baseline. At 8 weeks the loudness ratings were 13% lower than at baseline irrespective of the BBN or nature sound condition [$F_{(2, 28)} = 1.551, p < 0.05$; **Figure 7**]. At 8 weeks, annoyance ratings were 25% lower than at baseline irrespective of BBN or nature sound condition [$F_{(2, 28)} = 2.815, p < 0.05$]. There was no significant difference in tinnitus loudness ratings and annoyance ratings between BBN or nature sound conditions at either 4 or 8 weeks.

There was a significant effect of sound type on psychoacoustic loudness level matches at 8 weeks [$F_{(1, 28)} = 3.134, p < 0.05$], with BBN sound administration resulting in a greater mean increase in loudness level match (2.6 dB increase in LLM) while nature sounds had slight increase (0.47 dB increase in LLM; **Figure 8**). There was no significant difference between BBN or nature sound conditions at 4 weeks. There was no significant main effect of sound therapy time on tinnitus minimum masking levels between baseline and 4 weeks or baseline and 8 weeks. There was no significant change in minimum masking levels between 4 weeks and baseline. There was no significant difference between minimum masking levels with sound types at either 4 or 8 weeks.

Intervention Outcomes: Psychological Measures

There was a significant effect of sound therapy time on PANAS positive emotionality scores [$F_{(2, 28)} = 2.210, p < 0.05$] with lower levels reported 8 weeks compared to baseline (1.4 points; **Figure 9**). There was no significant difference between sound types on positive emotionality scores at either 4 or 8 weeks.

There was a very small but significant effect of sound therapy time on negative emotionality scores [$F_{(2, 28)} = 1.247, p < 0.05$], with an increase in scores at 8 weeks compared to baseline (0.2 points). There was no change in negative emotionality scores

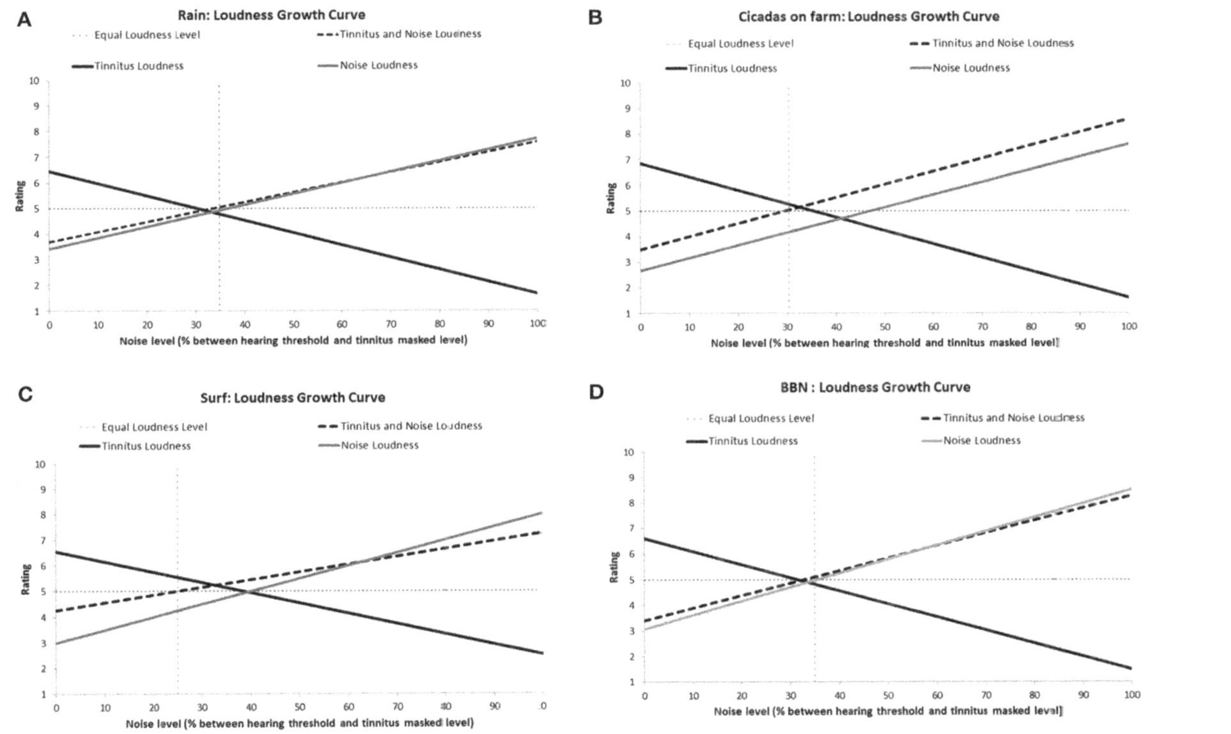

FIGURE 3 | Loudness ratings growth curves for each therapy sound [Rain (A), Cicadas on farm **(B)**, Surf **(C)**, BBN **(D)**] as a function of noise level (% between hearing threshold and minimum masking level for tinnitus). Loudness functions show decreases in tinnitus loudness (solid black line), increases in sound loudness (solid gray line), and increases in combined tinnitus and sound loudness as a function of sound level (dashed line). The Equal Loudness Level (vertical dashed line) defines the sound level at which both tinnitus and sound were of equal perceived loudness (tinnitus and sound loudness rating = 5).

between 4 weeks and baseline. There was no significant difference between sound types on negative emotionality scores at either 4 or 8 weeks.

There was a significant effect of sound therapy time on all outcomes measures of anxiety, depression and stress (**Figure 10**). Reduced anxiety scores were observed between 4 weeks and baseline (0.3 points), and 8 weeks and baseline (1.1 points) [$F_{(2, 28)} = 3.721$, $p < 0.05$]; reduced depression scores were observed between 4 weeks and baseline (0.6 points), and 8 weeks and baseline (1.4 points) [$F_{(2, 28)} = 2.44$, $p < 0.05$]; stress scores were increased between 4 weeks and baseline (2.3 points), and decreased between 8 weeks and baseline (1.1 points) [$F_{(2, 28)} = 3.01$, $p < 0.05$].

There were no significant effects of sound therapy time or sound type on either attention reaction response times or attention discrimination response times.

Principal Component Analysis

The Kaiser-Meyer-Olkin measure (KMO) verified the sampling adequacy for the analysis (KMO = 0.62). Bartlett's test of sphericity indicated that inter-measure correlations were sufficiently large for PCA ($p < 0.001$). The majority (87.5%) of variation in outcome variables following sound therapy administration over time were accounted for by changes in tinnitus impact on life (27%), tinnitus perceptual characteristics (9%), stress reduction/relaxation (21%), changes in positive mood (16%), and changes in negative mood (14%). This was a satisfactory amount of variation. The individual correlations/strength of loadings of each intervention outcome measure on to each principle component is provided in **Table 4**.

Correlations and Differences of Age, Gender, and Hearing Loss on Outcome Measures

The effects of age, gender, or hearing loss on outcome measure changes were investigated. Participants with mild hearing loss had a decrease in LLM (5.7 dB SL), while those with moderately severe hearing loss showed a slight increase in LLM (0.83 dB SL) between baseline and 8 weeks [$F_{(3, 15)} = 2.32$, $p < 0.05$]. During administration of BBN and natures sounds, significant differences by gender were present for negative emotionality [$F_{(1, 15)} = 6.393$, $p < 0.05$]; females displayed an increase in scores between baseline and 4 weeks (2.4 point increase), while males had a decrease in scores between baseline and 4 weeks (4.4 point decrease). Significant differences by gender were present for depression [$F_{(1, 15)} = 3.096, p < 0.05$], anxiety [$F_{(1, 15)} = 5.532, p < 0.05$], and stress [$F_{(1, 15)} = 6.37, p < 0.05$]. Females had a slight increase in depression scores (0.52 points) and anxiety scores (0.82 points) between baseline and 4 weeks; males had a decrease in depression scores (3.35 points) and anxiety scores (2.09 points)

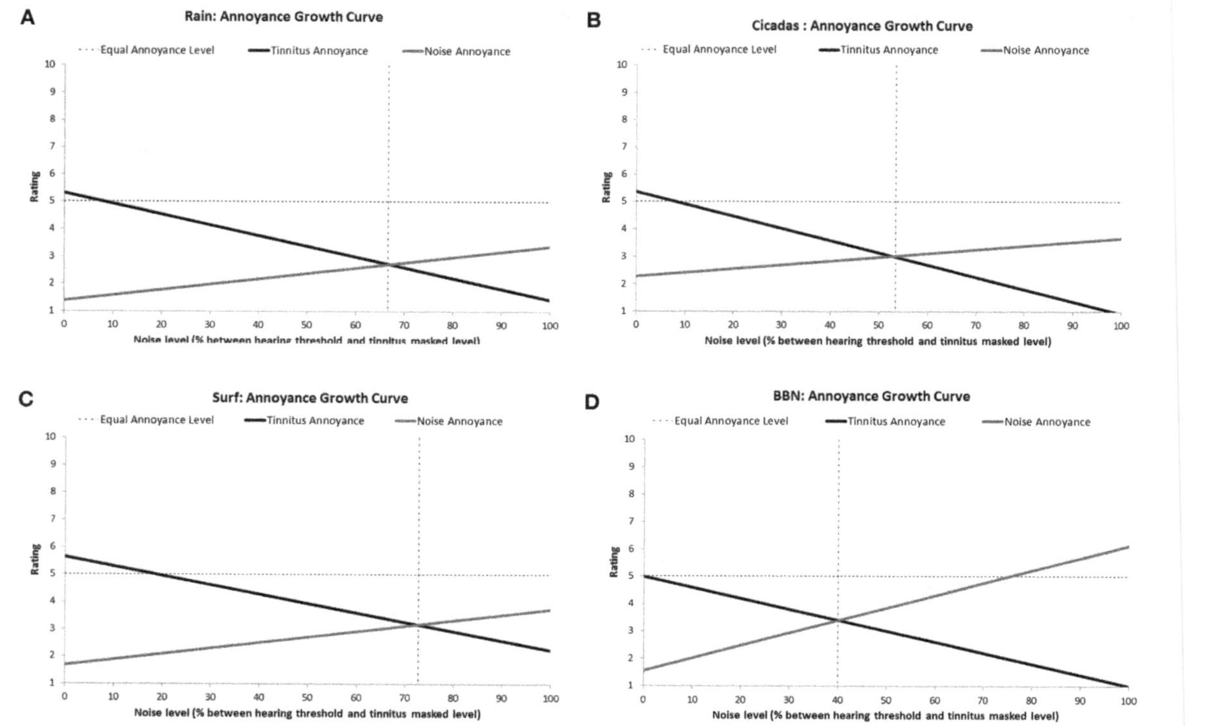

FIGURE 4 | Annoyance ratings growth curves of each therapy sound [Rain (A), Cicadas on Farm **(B)**, Surf **(C)**, BBN **(D)**] as a function of noise level (% between hearing threshold and minimum masking level for tinnitus]. Annoyance functions show decreases in tinnitus annoyance (solid black line) and increases in sound annoyance (solid gray line) as a function of sound level. The equal annoyance point (vertical dashed line) defines the sound level at which both tinnitus and sounds were of equal perceived annoyance (point of intersection between tinnitus annoyance and sound annoyance functions).

TABLE 3 | Ratings on a scale of 1–10 of tinnitus and sound loudness and annoyance at the MML of tinnitus.

Rating at MML (on scale of 1–10)	Rain	Cicadas	Surf	BBN
Tinnitus loudness	2 (2=)	2 (2=)	3 (4)	1 (1)
Noise loudness	8 (1=)	8 (1=)	8 (1=)	9 (4)
Tinnitus annoyance	1 (1=)	1 (1=)	2 (4)	1 (1=)
Sound annoyance	3 (1)	4 (2=)	4 (2=)	6 (4)

For example, BBN at MML was rated as being louder and more annoying than other sounds; however, the administration of BBN at this level also resulted in one of the lowest tinnitus loudness and annoyance ratings. The number in brackets represents ranking from 1 (best on measure for sound therapy) to 4 (worst on measure for sound therapy).

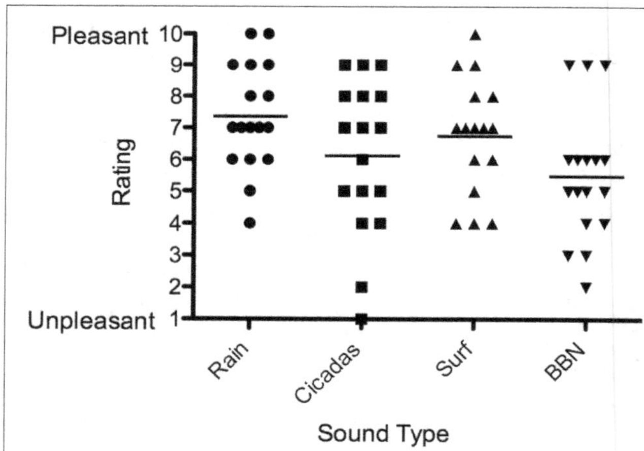

FIGURE 5 | Valence ratings of sound therapy stimuli [Rain (circles), Cicadas on Farm (squares), Surf (triangles), BBN (inverted triangles)] by participants. Horizontal lines represent average valence ratings for each sound stimulus.

for the same time period. Females had an increase in stress scores (2.96 points) between baseline and 8 weeks; males had a decrease in stress scores (2.42 points) for the same time period.

Individual Differences

For all outcome measures where there were no effects of sound types after 8 weeks of trial, individual results were explored in a descriptive manner for any patterns (**Figure 11**). Overall, there was a considerably large amount of individual variability present in responses to sound therapy.

A greater number of participants seemed to experience a decrease in tinnitus loudness ratings at 8 weeks compared to baseline (than an increase or no change); this was slightly more likely to occur during administration of nature sound than BBN. For those who experienced an increase in tinnitus loudness rating with the presence of sound, this was most likely to occur regardless of whether BBN or nature sound was administered. Likewise more participants seemed to experience a decrease in

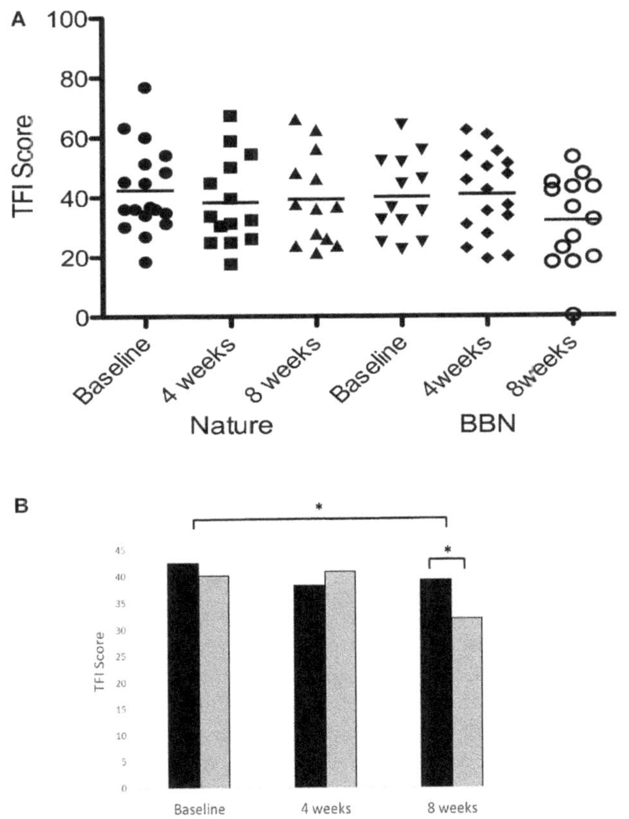

FIGURE 6 | (A) Individual TFI scores of participants at baseline, at 4 weeks follow-up and at 8 weeks follow-up following administration of BBN and nature sound stimuli. Horizontal lines represent average TFI scores. **(B)** Average TFI scores of participants at baseline (filled circles for nature sounds; inverted triangles for BBN), at 4 weeks follow-up (squares for nature sounds; diamonds for BBN) and at 8 weeks follow-up (triangles for nature sounds; open circles for BBN) following administration of BBN (black) and nature (gray) sound stimuli. The significant difference is indicated by $^*p < 0.05$. Error bars represent ± one standard error.

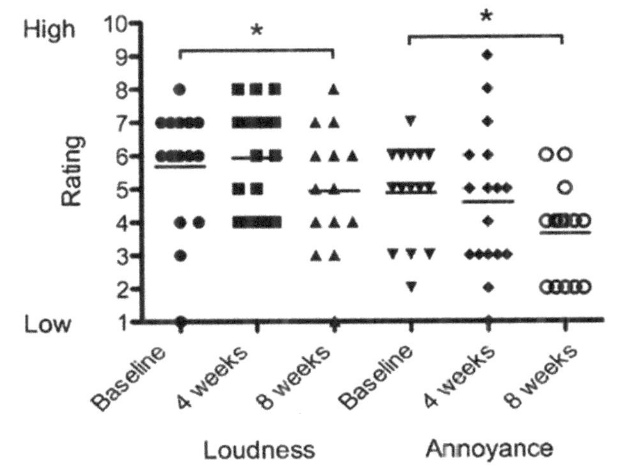

FIGURE 7 | Tinnitus loudness ratings (on a scale of 1–10, where 1 corresponded with very quiet tinnitus and 10 with extremely loud tinnitus) and annoyance ratings (on a scale of 1–10, where 1 corresponded low in distress and/or annoyance and 10 with extremely high distress) of participants at baseline (filled circles for loudness ratings; inverted triangles for annoyance ratings), at 4 weeks follow-up (squares for loudness ratings; diamonds for annoyance ratings) and at 8 weeks follow-up (triangles for loudness ratings; open circles for annoyance ratings). Significant differences are indicated by $^*p < 0.05$. Horizontal lines represent average rating scores.

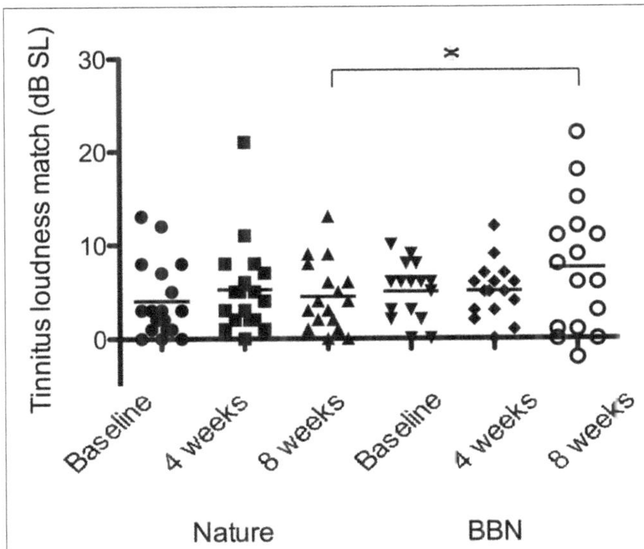

FIGURE 8 | Average LLMs (in dB SL) at baseline (filled circles for nature sounds; inverted triangles for BBN), at 4 weeks follow-up (squares for nature sounds; diamonds for BBN) and at 8 weeks follow-up (triangles for nature sounds; open circles for BBN) following administration of BBN (black) and nature (gray) sound stimuli. Horizontal lines represent average tinnitus loudness matches (in dB SL). Significant differences are indicated by $^*p < 0.05$. Error bars represent ± one standard error.

tinnitus annoyance ratings at 8 weeks compared to baseline (than an increase or no change); however this was more likely to occur during administration of BBN sound. For those who experienced an increase in tinnitus loudness rating with the presence of sound, this was most likely to occur for a specific sound type (either BBN or nature sound, but not both).

More participants seemed to experience a decrease in MML and anxiety scores at 8 weeks compared to baseline; for both these outcome measures, a decrease was more likely to occur during administration of BBN than nature sound. For negative emotionality, positive emotionality, depression, stress, attention reaction, and discrimination response time scores, individuals were roughly equally distributed by whether there was an increase, a decrease, or no change between 8 weeks and baseline. One participant had a significant decrease in depression scores under the BBN condition; the decrease in depression scores seemed to be considerably less for nature sound administered to the same individual. Another participant had a considerable decrease in depression scores with nature sound; BBN however led to an increase in depression scores in the same person.

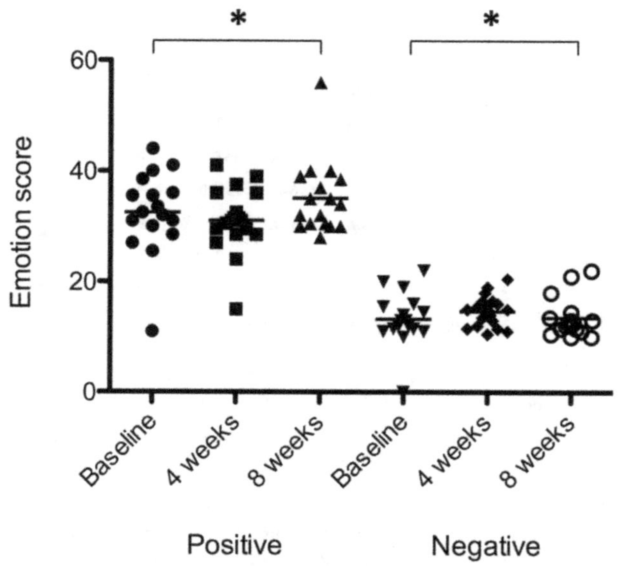

FIGURE 9 | Positive emotionality and negative emotionality scores at baseline (filled circles for positive emotionality; inverted triangles for negative emotionality), at 4 weeks follow-up (squares for positive emotionality; diamonds for negative emotionality) and at 8 weeks follow-up (triangles for positive emotionality; open circles for negative emotionality). Horizontal lines represent average scores. Significant differences are indicated by $^{*}p < 0.05$.

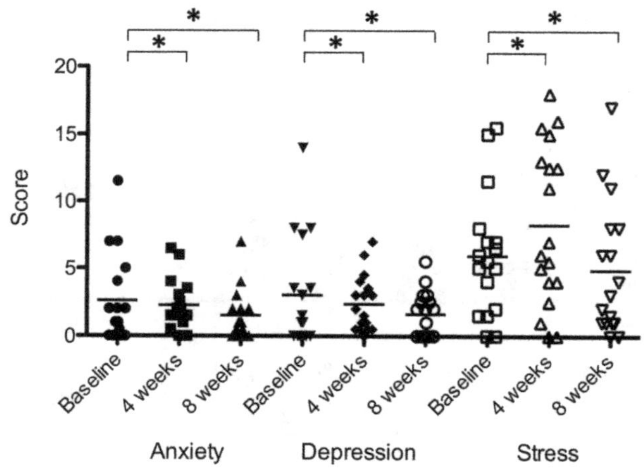

FIGURE 10 | Anxiety, depression, and stress scores of participants at baseline (filled circles for anxiety; inverted triangles for depression; open squares for stress), at 4 weeks follow-up (squares for anxiety; diamonds for depression; open triangles for stress) and at 8 weeks follow-up (triangles for anxiety; unfilled circles for depression; open inverted triangles for stress). Horizontal lines represent average scores. Significant differences are indicated by $^{*}p < 0.05$.

Intervention Outcomes: Qualitative Reports

Following qualitative analysis using the framework method, certain key areas emerged with regards to the sound trial. Common threads identified during the qualitative interviews are outlined below (relevant excerpts are included in Appendix C in Supplementary Material).

Hours and Environments of Use

Most participants used both sounds for the minimum amount required each day and reported usage ranged from 0.5 to 1.5 h for BBN. The nature sounds were listened to for longer periods of time: nine participants reported consistently using the nature sound for 2 h or more. One participant used the sounds at work (7 h/day). If participants were involved in engaging activities, they often let the sounds run on. The vast majority of participants used the sounds in more than one environment: 48% in quiet, usually in the evenings or in bed reading, 26% working on quiet tasks around the house, garden or in the car, and 26% at the office or doing computer work. A few participants reported experimenting with the sounds in some situations with extra sound such as TV, radio, while having conversations, or in traffic noise. The use of sounds in the presence of noise did not make the tinnitus worse.

Early Termination of Trial

For 17% of participants (three participants), the trial had to be terminated early due to significant exacerbation of tinnitus. In two out of the three cases, termination occurred during administration of BBN sound. The reason for variation was a specific life event (death of brother-in-law, disruption to sleep activity) and an incident (workplace incident exposure to loud noise). The third case terminated during nature sound administration, as they had disruption to sleep activity and did not observe any benefit.

Effectiveness of Intervention Sounds at 4 Weeks

At 4 weeks 42% of participants reported experiencing a worsening of tinnitus with both sounds. Among those who reported no change in tinnitus (39%), a slightly higher proportion reported this during administration of BBN than nature sound. In contrast, slightly more participants (19%) obtained tinnitus relief with nature sound compared to BBN. Six participants felt tinnitus was exacerbated with BBN sound and nine participants with nature sound. For some participants the increase in tinnitus was not observed while the sound was playing, but immediately, or shortly, after the sound was stopped. There was no noticeable change in tinnitus for six participants listening to BBN sound and five participants listening to nature sound.

Effectiveness of Intervention Sounds at 8 weeks

At 8 weeks 52% of participants did not perceive any change. A lack of perceived change was more prevalent following administration of the nature sound than the BBN. The group that had benefit (13% of participants) was almost three times more likely to benefit from BBN than nature sounds. However, BBN was also reported more likely to make tinnitus became worse (34%). There were no statistically significant underlying differences in baseline outcome measures (e.g., baseline TFI score, LLM, etc.) or demographic factors (e.g., age, gender, etc.) between participant groups who reported benefit, no change or worse tinnitus at 8 weeks follow-up.

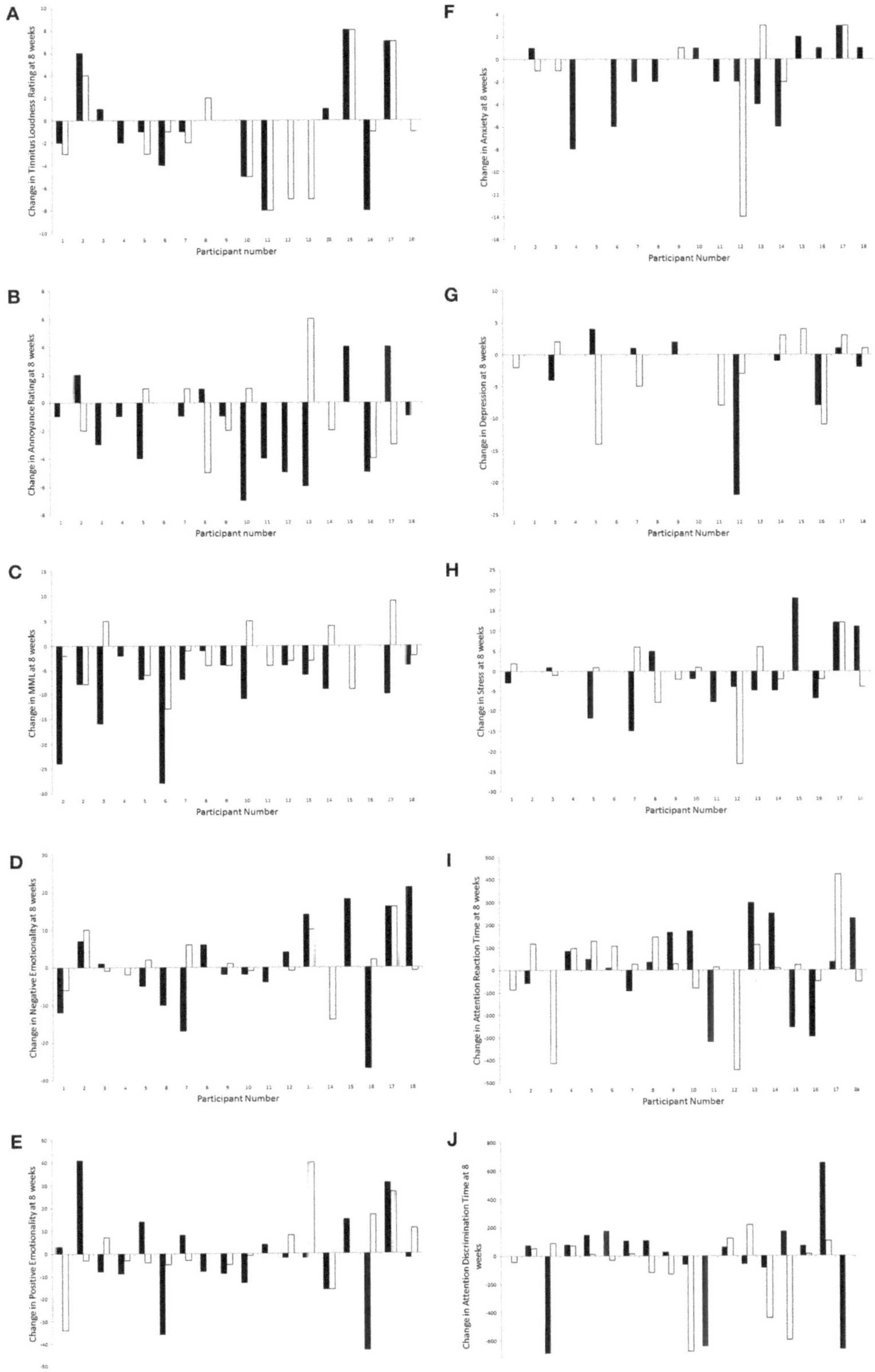

FIGURE 11 | Changes in outcome measures [(A), tinnitus loudness ratings; **(B)**, tinnitus annoyance ratings; **(C)**, MML; **(D)**, negative emotionality; **(E)**, positive emotionality; **(F)**, anxiety; **(G)**, depression; **(H)**, stress; **(I)**, attention reaction time; **(J)**, attention discrimination time] for each participant following administration of BBN (black) and nature (white) sound stimuli.

TABLE 4 | Principal components analysis (with direct oblimin rotation) loadings of intervention study outcomes.

	Tinnitus		Psychological			h^2
	Component 1	Component 2	Component 3	Component 4	Component 5	
	Tinnitus influence—impact on life	Tinnitus—perceptual characteristics	Stress reduction/relaxation	Positive mood	Negative mood	
TFI total score	**0.787**	**0.608**	0.076	0.027	0.003	0.995
Tinnitus loudness ratings	−0.493	**0.860**	0.075	0.005	−0.050	0.990
Tinnitus annoyance ratings	**0.984**	0.010	−0.052	−0.053	−0.085	0.982
Tinnitus loudness level match	**0.984**	0.010	−0.052	−0.053	−0.085	0.982
Tinnitus minimum masking level	0.134	**0.967**	0.047	−0.031	−0.115	0.969
Positive emotionality	−0.032	0.083	−0.310	**0.898**	0.039	0.912
Negative emotionality	0.118	0.112	−0.032	−0.318	**0.788**	0.750
Depression	−0.050	0.109	**0.601**	**−0.730**	−0.017	0.905
Anxiety	−0.171	0.053	**0.887**	−0.102	0.142	0.850
Stress	0.091	−0.037	**0.856**	−0.270	0.282	0.896
Attention reaction response times	**−0.547**	0.061	**0.584**	−0.278	−0.397	0.879
Attention discriminatory response times	−0.074	−0.447	0.258	**0.685**	−0.246	0.803
Personality: stress reaction	0.073	−0.027	**−0.730**	−0.041	**0.558**	0.853
Personality: self-control	−0.044	0.326	−0.252	**0.636**	0.481	0.808
Personality: social closeness	−0.083	−0.258	0.211	0.390	**0.773**	0.869
Personality: alienation	0.168	0.080	−0.072	−0.066	**−0.713**	0.552
% of variance explained by each factor	0.27	0.09	0.21	0.16	0.14	0.875

Eigen-value > 1 criteria applied. Correlations above 0.5 and total variance explained by principal components are presented in bold.

Preference of Intervention Sound at 8 weeks

Preference for one sound was asked, regardless of its interaction pattern with tinnitus. Of the 18 participants, only three (26%) did not have any preference. Thirty-two percent of participants preferred the BBN and a slightly higher 42% preferred the nature sound. Chi-squared tests showed that participants were not significantly more likely to choose any one of BBN, nature sound, or no preference as a response than the other. Nature sounds were reported as relaxing and had a distracting element to them that had a psychological benefit. BBN sound was described as interacting better with the tinnitus, and led to a noticeable difference in tinnitus. Among those who preferred BBN, the nature sound was commonly described as the more pleasant sound, but BBN was more efficient for treatment. In contrast, others did not like the distracting effect of the nature sound and found attention was directed toward the tinnitus instead. Participants also mentioned that they initially conceptualized BBN to be less pleasant to listen to, but discovered that it was more tolerable than they had imagined. There were no significant differences in hearing observable by sound preference; those with poorer hearing on average were less likely to have a preference although this was not statistically significant.

Long-Term Use of Sound Device for Tinnitus Management

Nine (half of total) participants were interested in continuing using the device for long-term tinnitus management and believed their tinnitus would change as a result. There was roughly equal split as to whether participants wanted to listen to BBN or nature sound over time. Two participants were interested in continuing sound therapy but did not believe their tinnitus would change. Eight participants were not interested in continuing, predominantly because there was either (1) no benefit, (2) tinnitus became louder in volume as a result of sound therapy, and/or (3) sounds made them more aware of their tinnitus as discussed previously.

Quality of Intervention Sounds

There were no concerns regarding the sound quality of both s from the majority of participants; however one participant felt their volume control increased dramatically from one step to another for the BBN.

Relationship between Intervention Outcomes and Qualitative Reports

No trends were observed when grouping participant's tinnitus quantitative intervention outcome measures (loudness rating, annoyance rating, and LLM of tinnitus) by whether participants reported benefit or not from sound. There were also no observable trends when grouping by participant preference for an intervention sound.

DISCUSSION

The administration of sound therapy led to reduction in tinnitus over 8 weeks. This effect was largely due to BBN sound therapy which resulted in a 8.2 point reduction of TFI scores (Meikle et al., 2012); this was significantly different to the 3.2 point reduction following 8 weeks of Nature sound administration. The TFI reflects impact of tinnitus on quality of life (Meikle et al., 2012). Both the TFI changes were not large enough to meet one suggested clinical criterion for meaningful reduction in TFI outcome scores [a 13-point reduction (Meikle et al., 2012)] but BBN did if a different criteria of 7–8 point change (Folmer et al., 2015) was applied. For most participants sound resulted in small but significant changes in secondary outcome measures of tinnitus (reduced loudness rating scale and reduced annoyance rating scale) and psychologically related measures (increased positive emotionality, reduced anxiety, reduced depression, and reduced stress). Unlike response to rating scales, the loudness level matches increased for BBN, while there was minimal increase for loudness level matches for Nature sounds between baseline and 8 weeks follow-up. There was no significant change in MML matches following sound therapy administration. For BBN, while there was a slight decrease in loudness level matches for nature sound between baseline and 8 weeks follow-up. The results showed large individual preferences.

In this study participants played the sounds for 1–1.5 h/day, which is less than many tinnitus treatment paradigms suggest (e.g., Neuromonics Tinnitus Treatment and Tinnitus Retraining Therapy recommend 6–8 h use; Davis et al., 2008; Hanley and Davis, 2008). The time frame (8 weeks) of administration was also less than the 6 months or greater suggested by these treatments. The degree of change observed with sound may be different if used for longer periods of time per day or administered over a longer time frame (e.g., individual responses might converge or diverge over a greater amount of time).

Individual Effects (Age, Gender, Hearing Loss)

There were some interesting differences observed in gender and hearing loss with regards to some of the changes in outcome measures (Hunter and Gillen, 2009). For the psychological outcomes of negative emotionality, depression, anxiety and stress, females had an initial worsening of symptoms between baseline and 4 weeks, while males had a decrease. LLMs significantly decreased over 8 weeks among individuals with mild hearing loss (by 6 points) while those with moderately severe hearing loss actually had an increase in LLM (by slightly <1 point). The introduction of sound therapy was most beneficial in cases of mild deafferentation and/or auditory pathway damage. This may be interpreted in two ways: the tinnitus characteristics of those with lower levels of deafferentation may be more driven by attentional and psychological variables, such that new sound provides attention diversion and relief translating into lower tinnitus loudness measurements, or in instances of severe damage/deafferentation to the hearing system, sound therapy is not able to reach the appropriate cortical regions to elicit any changes, even when set a comfortable and audible listening level (Schaette et al., 2010). This has implications clinically when setting levels for sound therapy, especially when user-set. The counter to increasing levels to create greater tinnitus interaction is that if the level is set too high, there is a risk of triggering negative emotion and discomfort to the sound itself (Scott et al., 1990; Searchfield, 2014); thereby also preventing any AL shifts (Searchfield et al., 2012).

Individual Effects (Personality Traits)

The four personality traits examined in this study have been associated with tinnitus perception and distress. Tinnitus sufferers displaying higher levels of stress reaction, lower social closeness, lower self-control, and higher alienation than individuals with hearing loss (but not tinnitus; Rizzardo et al., 1998; Scott and Lindberg, 2000; Sirois et al., 2006; Welch and Dawes, 2008; Bartels et al., 2010; Durai et al., 2015; Durai and Searchfield, 2016). In this study, personality traits of self-control and social closeness were significantly negatively correlated, and social closeness and alienation were positively correlated. This is similar to previous findings applying the MPQ to tinnitus groups (Durai et al., 2017a). Females in this study had greater levels of social closeness than males. Males in this study had higher alienation than females. Welch and Dawes (2008) observed an elevation in alienation scores among men in their general population sample of 32-year-olds. Males also displayed higher emotional suppression scores than females in the study by Durai and Searchfield (Durai et al., 2017b). Thus, underlying personality differences appear to exist between males and females who experience tinnitus.

Participants with moderate hearing loss also had significantly higher self-control scores than those with severe hearing loss. Both genetic and environmental factors interact to create an individual's personality (Bouchard and Loehlin, 2001; Specht et al., 2011). Some of the personality traits identified in this study, such as stress reaction and social closeness, are difficult to change (Welch and Dawes, 2008). If any change is possible, it will be gradual and dependent on the age of the individual—absolute level changes have been reported to be more pronounced during adolescence and the elderly years of life, due to biological maturation, social expectations and conditioning processes (Costa and McRae, 1992; Costa and McCrae, 2006; Roberts et al., 2006; Corr and Matthews, 2009).

Personality differences can add to the heterogeneity presented in tinnitus, although this has been given little attention. It may be valuable to attempt to understand this contributory factor further by incorporating personality into assessment and for sub grouping to see how it shapes tinnitus perception, distress, and emotional response.

Attention Effects

Attention (focused attention and general alertness; Zomeren and Brouwer, 1994) was the only measurement dimension that did not change over the 8 weeks. However, there were significant correlations present between changes in reaction time task attention scores and changes in MML and stress scores at 8 weeks. At 8 weeks, changes in discrimination time task attention scores significantly correlated with changes in TFI, depression, and anxiety scores. This suggests a complex interaction between attention, cognitive, and psychological affect, tinnitus perceptual characteristics and tinnitus impact on life, as suggested in the ecological model of tinnitus (Searchfield, 2014).

Interpretation under the Adaptation Level Theory

Under the ALT model, the "presence of sound effect" (decrease in tinnitus outcomes after administration of either sound therapy stimuli) suggests a shifting of internal AL steadily away from the tinnitus and towards background noise stimulus (**Figure 12**). This may occur due to component weighting shifts and attention diversion. Increased positive psychological benefits may also create a facilitating residual effect, which also shifts AL. It is possible that characteristics of specific sound stimuli may work by placing greater emphasis on altering one pathway than another (e.g., BBN has been reported to aid in attention diversion; nature sounds were reported as eliciting high valence emotions). Durai et al. (2015) explored the possibility that tinnitus distress and loudness may be underlined by different perceptual and decision making processes that can be represented by two distinct adaptation levels. An AL can exist for any sensory modality, but also within each modality (Helson, 1948, 1964; Coren and Ward, 1989; Masuyama, 1994). The AL for distress might be more prone to contextual and indirect psychological influences, given the complexity of non-auditory region involvement such as the emotional, arousal, attention, and memory networks (Zenner et al., 2006; Jastreboff, 2007; De Ridder et al., 2011; Kaltenbach, 2011). De Ridder et al. (2014) have outlined a "tinnitus core" sub-network within the brain. It has been suggested that the minimal set of brain areas that needs to be simultaneously active in order for tinnitus to be consciously perceived. Affective components of tinnitus are represented by additional and overlapping networks. There is a possibility that tinnitus signal AL weighting decreases via the direct pathway toward external sound (involvement of core networks) while the affective component decreases occur via a residual pathway.

It is postulated that high levels of stress reaction, low social closeness, low self-control and high alienation may act as "maladaptive" personality residuals under this framework, diverting attention and auditory processing resources toward the tinnitus, thus increasing its AL weighting. The subsequent co-activation of various sub networks encoding tinnitus characteristics in the cortex with increased awareness/salience might then potentially explain the relationship between personality trait and psychoacoustic tinnitus characteristics (De Ridder et al., 2014, 2015). The relationship of attention within ALT is complex and it is difficult to determine weighting changes directly, due to the overlapping nature of networks possibly involved.

ALT stresses the active interaction between an individual experiencing tinnitus, cognition and their environment (both the immediate surroundings and broader factors, including their culture, beliefs, work, and social environment). The influence of

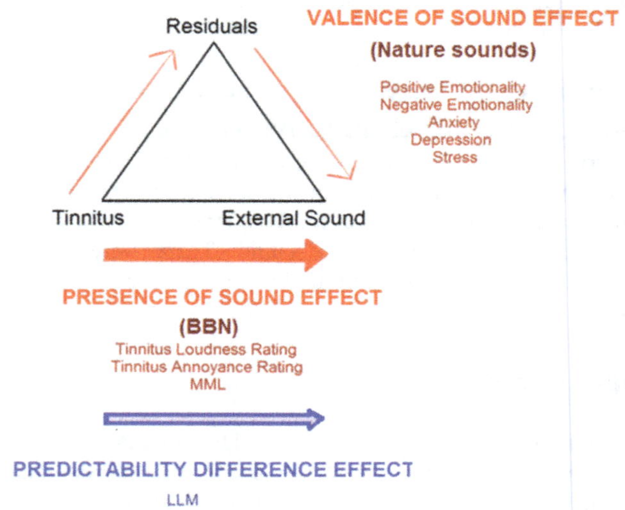

FIGURE 12 | Conceptualization of current study findings under an adaptation level theory (ALT) framework for tinnitus perception (Schecklmann et al., 2013b). Tinnitus is envisaged as a sensory stimulus with an existing internal adaptation level (AL) which acts as a reference point for all tinnitus-related judgments and is able to be manipulated by context and time. A high tinnitus AL results in tinnitus that is judged by the sufferer as being of high magnitude and/or eliciting high distress. Three key components set the final AL: (1) the focal component/stimuli being attended to (tinnitus), (2) background stimuli, as well as (3) residuals (various psychological and cognitive individual influences, including emotion, personality, past experiences, arousal, and level of prediction elicited by sound stimuli). The "presence of sound effect" (red arrows) illustrates steady shifts in AL away from the tinnitus and toward sound therapy stimuli, which can occur by directly increasing the weighting placed on external sound, via attention, and auditory streaming shifts. A valence of sound effect increases weighting placed on external sound via the residual pathway. The latter occurs as external sounds provide psychological relief from tinnitus and can counteract tinnitus-related negative emotions, anxiety, stress, and depression, thereby creating a facilitating residual effect which reduces tinnitus severity. The "predictability difference effect" (blue arrow) illustrates a potential difference between BBN and nature sounds in terms of the amount of prediction errors elicited; this may also influence the degree of adaptation each sound undergoes over time. Shifts in AL away from tinnitus toward external sound would discontinue upon adaptation of the auditory system to the external sound itself. Auditory system adaptation to BBN and natural sound therapy may occur at different rates. Adaptation to BBN occurs sometime between 4 and 8 weeks after the first introduction of the sound, leading to the need to increase the sound level required to match tinnitus in Loudness Level Matching. There may be small but immediate valence effects, but nature sounds due to their intermittent nature may take longer to reach peak adaptation, such that at 8 weeks no change in Loudness Level Matching may be observed.

the environment and health factors was evident in qualitative reports by participants, e.g., "Still feeling sick from flu, not feeling well at all, so not sure how accurate tinnitus perception might be," "Stressed at work, because in my view I feel tinnitus is stress or noise related, so hear it more." The physical location as well as time of day can alter the magnitude of tinnitus. Overall the success of sound appears to be partially related to individual influences, which interact to determine final tinnitus magnitude and its impact. It is not yet possible clinically to prescribe sounds that are tailored to an individual's tinnitus with confidence that they are the best sounds. However, the use of the rating functions described in this study may assist selection of sound type for therapy.

Factors Influencing Sound Therapy Effect on Tinnitus

Two components relating to sound therapy effects on tinnitus were interpreted, influencing impact of life such as presence, distress, and reactions to tinnitus (encompassing TFI scores, annoyance ratings, and LLMs) in addition to altering perceptual tinnitus characteristics such as subjective loudness and maskability (TFI scores, loudness ratings, and MML). However, we also cannot rule out placebo effects on either the qualitative or quantitative results, in scenarios where placebo effects are relevant, choice over treatment can increase these effects (Geers and Rose, 2011) which may account for qualitative preferences for the nature sounds, but does not account for the greater effects on the TFI with the BBN sound. TFI scores were the only variable which loaded onto both components of impact of life and perceptual characteristics. This is in line with one of the aims of the TFI, which is to comprehensively cover the broad range of symptoms associated with tinnitus severity (Meikle et al., 2012).

Based on the pattern of results it was also reasoned that three residuals of sound therapy effects on tinnitus were stress reduction/relaxation, and positive mood and negative mood. Under broad classification, the components map well onto the ALT model explanation of tinnitus-related and residual psychology-related effects of sound therapy discussed. The discrepancy in mood change (both positive and negative) in relation to sound therapy administration is interesting. Negative Emotionality and the personality trait of Social Closeness loaded strongly positively on the negative mood dimension, while Alienation as a personality trait loaded strongly negatively. In contrast, strong negative loadings of Stress Reaction on Stress reduction/relaxation and Self Control moderately positively loaded on positive mood. One possible interpretation is that stress and self-control are indices for discerning subgroups of individuals with exacerbated tinnitus following sound therapy. The sequence of events resulting in increased tinnitus may follow the indirect residual pathway (driven by an increase in negative affect) and the presence of certain underlying personality trait levels (e.g., social closeness, stress reaction) may determine the extent to which this pathway occurs and the magnitude of shifts in weighting toward tinnitus. However, this is only speculation and further research is needed in this regard.

Attention reaction response times loaded moderately negatively on tinnitus impact of life and moderately positively on stress reduction/relaxation. Attention discriminatory response times loaded moderately positively on positive mood. One possible explanation for this observation is that decreased tinnitus impact and increased psychological well-being in general may be related to increased attentional response times. Various studies suggest that reaction time is shorter under conditions of physiological stress (Desiderato, 1964; Ohmura et al., 2009).

Sound Adaptation as a Confound

The loudness level match is commonly used to psychoacoustically measure changes in tinnitus; however its interpretation in cases where external sound is administered for long periods of time can be difficult. Discrepancies between subjective loudness rating scores and loudness level match measures have been observed in the past, and termed the tinnitus loudness paradox (Penner, 1986; Henry and Meikle, 1996; Searchfield et al., 2012). Interpreted under ALT, the loudness paradox arises because subjective loudness judgments estimate the current tinnitus AL: it is made in a sound proof booth with no contextual noise stimuli (Penner, 1986; Henry and Meikle, 1996). In contrast, the objective match is made when an external test stimulus is introduced and the individual has to match it with the existing tinnitus AL. If the AL is initially set high, the matching sound level does not have to be increased as much before it is perceived as being of equal loudness as the tinnitus. However, if the matching sound undergoes adaptation to sound over time it would appear quieter, and would therefore have to be raised in order to match the intensity of tinnitus loudness (which undergoes slower adaptation; Searchfield et al., 2012; Durai et al., 2015). The auditory system may adjust to sound therapy stimuli over time; this would eventually stop further AL shifts and/or result in shifts back toward tinnitus.

It is highly likely that adaptation to the intervention sound may confound the interpretation of loudness level matches in this study. Underlying neural changes can occur through gain control, or adjustment of input-output sound functions of auditory neurons (Marks and Arieh, 2006; Robinson and McAlpine, 2009). Studies have observed stimulus-specific adaptation effects at all levels of the auditory system from early auditory encoding (Marks and Arieh, 2006) to the auditory cortex (Robinson and McAlpine, 2009; Rabinowitz et al., 2011). Adaptation of the auditory system to BBN and nature sounds may occur at different rates. Because BBN is a predictable sound, it may be adapted to at a faster rate, and lead to an increase when an external sound is used to match tinnitus in loudness level matching. Unpredictable natural sounds are adapted to more slowly; therefore no change in loudness level match is obtained.

It is possible that intermittent tinnitus masking may not appear to alter tinnitus due to auditory continuity effects (Näätänen et al., 2001) whereby the brain "fills in the gap' where masking sound is applied and tinnitus appears as a continuous percept. This learning effect involves several networks in the brain that overlap with that of tinnitus, including the limbic structures, basal ganglia, and prefrontal cortex (Hassler, 1978).

Davis et al. (2007) observed more consistent benefit over 12 months if Neuromonics Tinnitus Treatment involved masking of tinnitus for the first 2 months followed by intermittent perception of tinnitus compared to where there is intermittent perception of tinnitus throughout treatment. It may be useful to run future trials in which the temporal structure of sounds are changed often to maintain novelty and prevent sound adaptation, continuity illusion, and facilitate AL shifts toward external sound (Schreitmüller et al., 2013).

Clinical Implications and Sub Grouping of Tinnitus Characteristics

Participants often demonstrated a clear preference for one nature sound over the others in the initial selection task; mostly Rain (highest valence ratings by participants and reported as having greater interaction with tinnitus, possibly due to its broad frequency spectrum, and more consistent nature) over Surf or Cicadas. Similar loudness and annoyance growth curves for tinnitus and interactions between all sounds (nature and BBN) were present with increasing volume levels. However, BBN had higher sound annoyance rating at tinnitus masking level than all three nature sounds. BBN sound therapy has been recommended (Jastreboff and Hazell, 2004) as it is proposed to be more easily tolerated, neutral in nature, and better for facilitating habituation than tones or NBN (Jastreboff, 1999; Jastreboff and Hazell, 2004). The results of this study would agree with these suggestions, although we believe the process of tinnitus adaptation is more complex than habituation (Searchfield et al., 2012). Also, considering the BBN had a stronger effect on adaptation level while nature sounds influence residual emotion pathways, and nature sounds are more accepted (Schreitmüller et al., 2013), another clinical application would be the combing the two sounds or staging their use.

Sixteen percent of the participants experienced an exacerbation of tinnitus sufficient enough to terminate the trial early; however, this was mainly due to external situational factors or incidents. It was not possible to identify any characteristics (e.g., personality trait, age, gender, duration of tinnitus, other tinnitus variables) which isolated these individuals from others in the study. From the qualitative reports at 4 weeks after administration, there were subgroups in self-reported response to sound therapy: 42% had worsening of tinnitus, 39% no change, and 19% obtained relief. Moreover, at 8 weeks after administration, there was variation in responses: 52% had worsening, 34% had no change, and 13% had relief from sounds. The number of participants reporting benefit was lower than anticipated based on hearing aid (Folmer and Carroll, 2006; Hobson et al., 2010; Searchfield et al., 2010) and tinnitus aid (Bauer and Brozoski, 2011; Barozzi et al., 2016) studies. This may, at least in part, be due to mode of sound delivery. MP3 players and earbuds were used as a lower cost intervention than tinnitus aids. Improvements in implementation of MP3 players from a previous study were made based on participant reports (Durai et al., unpublished manuscript); an easier user interface was implemented by switching from Apple iPod shuffles to the Philips ViBE MP3 Player (with more accessible manual controls) and use of retaining hooks with the earbuds. However, even these improvements resulted in less use than hearing aids. Patient reports suggest the MP3 players were used 1–1.5 h per day, significantly less than that usually recommended for sound therapy using ear-level devices (6–8 h per day; Jastreboff, 1999; Jastreboff and Jastreboff, 2000). The sounds also did not compensate for hearing loss. Threshold adjusted noise (Searchfield et al., 2002) is implemented in several tinnitus aids (e.g., Siemens, Phonak, Oticon). The flat frequency response we used may have led to less interaction with tinnitus in the region of hearing loss, but would be similar for both the intervention sounds. Tinnitus aids can use sound in a number of ways through inbuilt sounds or by streaming sounds (Searchfield, 2016). A future trial should build on the findings in sound selection described here using tinnitus aids streaming sounds that are downloaded to tablet computers or smartphones, e.g., from hearing aid manufacturers Apps (e.g., Tinnitus Balance App, https://www.phonak.com/us/en/support/apps.html) or independent online sources (e.g., TinnitusTunes, http://www.tinnitustunes.com). Another factor to consider is the long duration of tinnitus (mean time since onset was 17 years) among participants in this study. Tinnitus neural networks tend to change as tinnitus duration increases (Schlee et al., 2009; Vanneste et al., 2011) which may impose limitations on brain plasticity and the extent of change triggered by the presence of sound.

Interestingly, there was no correlation between the reported effects of sound or preference of sound and the intervention outcomes measured in this clinical trial. These findings highlight that qualitative and quantitative measures do not always clinically equate. Melin et al. (1987) observed similar discrepancies in their study in which hearing aids were fit to individuals with tinnitus for 6 weeks. The results were explained in terms of demand characteristics: when asked during interviews, subjects may tend to exaggerate (or underestimate) the ability of the intervention to change tinnitus, while the scaling may not be as sensitive to these effects. The extent of this reporting bias might differ between numerical rating scales and qualitative interviews. The inclusion of systematic qualitative methods in sound therapy treatment paradigms may be more advantageous than quantitative measures in identifying shifts in environmental factors or significant change in factors outside of the individual which can influence tinnitus (Malterud, 2001), such as individual health or stress determinants (e.g., changes in tinnitus characteristics present as a result of illness, as reported in this trial) or to identify concerns which arise (e.g., situational factors which may result in discontinuation of sound, as reported in this trial).

Subgroups have been identified among tinnitus sufferers, which vary based on pathophysiology, perceptual features, co-morbid conditions, and how they respond to specific treatments (Stouffer and Tyler, 1990; Lockwood et al., 2002; Heller, 2003; Tyler et al., 2008). The results support the existence of different classes of tinnitus, and the ALT may eventually be most supported as a framework for only a particular tinnitus subgroup. Both auditory and non-auditory residual factors may shift the AL more readily among such individuals. Moreover, age, gender, hearing loss, personality traits, and duration of sound therapy may all (hypothetically) be factors which can help delineate individuals.

The measures used in this study were selected based on validity and usefulness from past pilot studies. It is acknowledged that there are other standardized measures available such as the Clinical Global Impression Scale (Busner and Targum, 2007) and the COSIT (Dillon et al., 1997; Searchfield, 2016) for measuring perceived improvement of tinnitus. In this trial tinnitus counseling was deliberately not provided. Current tinnitus treatment paradigms such as Tinnitus Activities Treatment (Tyler et al., 2007) and Tinnitus Retraining Therapy (Jastreboff and Jastreboff, 2000; Jastreboff and Hazell, 2004; Jastreboff, 2007) use sound therapy alongside counseling of some form. Some trials of these therapies have been criticized (Sandlin and Olsson, 1999; McKenna and Irwin, 2008) as the benefits of sound therapy, over and above counseling, have not been determined. The results reported here are independent of counseling but it is strongly advocated that the use of sound clinically should be in addition to (not instead of) counseling. Sound therapy involves more than passive exposure to sound (Bauer and Brozoski, 2008; Davis et al., 2008), and participants need to be informed of this, and counseled also about how to use the sound. For some of the participants sound therapy ended up diverting attention toward the tinnitus instead. Individually tailoring sound therapy and counseling to target different components of the ALT would be expected to demonstrate an additive effect in shifting AL weighting away from tinnitus if administered together, than if each was administered in isolation. Attention training (Searchfield et al., 2007; Wise, 2012; Wise et al., 2016) might enhance adaptation to tinnitus through the presence of sound effect, while psychoeducation (or mindfulness or Cognitive Behavioral Therapy; Sweetow, 1984, 1986; Martinez-Devesa et al., 2010) might increase tinnitus adaptation through the valence sound effect.

CONCLUSIONS

Overall, the presence of sound had a positive effect on the TFI; after 8 weeks of administration, sound therapy with BBN resulted in a greater reduction of TFI than nature sound. The positive effect of sound on tinnitus was supported by secondary tinnitus and psychological-related outcome measures, but not interviews. BBN and nature sounds did not differ significantly on secondary outcome measures of tinnitus, emotion, attention, and psychological state after 8 weeks of administration. Interpreted under an ALT framework, internal AL weighting shifts away from the tinnitus signal and toward the sound therapy stimuli may occur, via a direct pathway toward external sound (involvement of core networks) while the affective component of tinnitus decreases via the residual pathway. The auditory system may adjust to sound therapy stimuli over time; this may eventually stop further AL shifts and result in shifts back toward tinnitus. It such cases predictable BBN might undergo loudness adaptation at a faster rate than unpredictable nature sounds.

This study provides further evidence for the heterogeneous nature of tinnitus. ALT appears to provide a framework for sound selection that could be applied to improve future sound-therapies. In this study, the selection of sound therapy stimuli by individuals was found to be, at least in part, governed by certain characteristics of the stimuli itself. Within a clinical setting, it is important to understand individual variation and that each person presents with different needs. Individual preferences were shown within this study that might be applied to improve outcomes if known apriori. It may be beneficial to have a wide range of sounds available in the clinic. The results of the Principal Component Analysis and ALT model interpretation are both compatible with an ecological framework of tinnitus, a multitude of factors (e.g., attention and personality, characteristics of and preference for sound stimuli) appeared to determine the magnitude and experience of tinnitus at any one time. Regular qualitative assessments will allow for a more comprehensive picture to be obtained regarding various factors influencing sound success. Selecting sounds based on the ALT model would involve weighing treatment sound stimuli and sound levels based on sound valence ratings, tinnitus and sound loudness and annoyance (dependent on the individual's profile at a particular point in time) as well as alternating presentation of sounds that evoke positive feelings (through the valence sound effect) and sounds with high interaction with tinnitus (for a presence of sound effect) over time, dependent on the individual's profile at a particular point in time. Trials of sound therapy selection based on Adaptation Level Therapy are needed.

ETHICS STATEMENT

Fifty individuals were invited by email invitations sent out to randomly selected members on the University of Auckland Tinnitus Research Volunteer Database (372 people from throughout New Zealand, majority from within Auckland). These are individuals with debilitating tinnitus who are interested in volunteering for tinnitus studies and clinical trials related to tinnitus relief. The inclusion criteria were: adults aged between 18 and 69 years residing in the Auckland region (NZ), constant tinnitus, and a minimum score of 38 on Tinnitus Functional Index (TFI), normal middle ear function, and a maximum of a moderate degree of hearing loss (<70 dB loss on average across frequencies). All subjects gave written informed consent in accordance with the Declaration of Helsinki. Participants read the Participant Information Sheet which listed any risks, benefits and layout of the trial as well as contact details. If participants were interested in continuing, a consent form was signed at the start of the trial.

AUTHOR CONTRIBUTIONS

MD was involved in manuscript preparation, collection of environmental sound recordings, development of sound therapy stimuli, sound therapy administration, data collection, and analysis. GS was involved in manuscript preparation, collection of environmental sound recordings, advise in development of sound therapy, and study design.

FUNDING

The author(s) disclosed receipt of the following financial support for the research, authorship, and/or publication of this article: Deafness Research Foundation New Zealand.

REFERENCES

A.2.1.2. (2016). Audacity: Free Audio Editor and Recorder.

Barozzi, S., Del Bo, L., Crocetti, A., Dyrlund, O., Passoni, S., Zolin, A., et al. (2016). A comparison of nature and technical sounds for tinnitus therapy. *Acta Acustica United Acustica* 102, 540–546. doi: 10.3813/AAA.918971

Barros Suzuki, F. A., Suzuki, F. A., Yonamine, F. K., Onishi, E. T., and Penido, N. O. (2016). Effectiveness of sound therapy in patients with tinnitus resistant to previous treatments: importance of adjustments. *Braz. J. Otorhinolaryngol.* 82, 297–303. doi: 10.1016/j.bjorl.2015.05.009

Bartels, H., Middel, B., Pedersen, S. S., Staal, M. J., and Albers, F. W. (2010). The distressed (Type D) personality is independently associated with tinnitus: a case-control study. *Psychosomatics* 51, 29–38. doi: 10.1176/appi.psy.51.1.29

Bauer, C. A., and Brozoski, T. J. (2008). "Tinnitus: theories mechanisms and treatments," in *Auditory Trauma, Protection, and Repair, Springer Handbook of Auditory Research*, eds J. Schacht, A. N. Popper, and R. R. Fay (New York, NY: Springer), 101–129.

Bauer, C. A., and Brozoski, T. J. (2011). Effect of tinnitus retraining therapy on the loudness and annoyance of tinnitus: a controlled trial. *Ear Hear.* 32, 145–155. doi: 10.1097/AUD.0b013e3181f5374f

Bouchard, T. Jr., and Loehlin, J. (2001). Genes, evolution, and personality. *Behav. Genet.* 31, 243–273. doi: 10.1023/A:1012294324713

Busner, J., and Targum, S. D. (2007). The clinical global impressions scale: applying a research tool in clinical practice. *Psychiatry (Edgmont)* 4, 28–37.

Callaway, S. L. (2014). *The Oticon Approach to Care of the Tinnitus Patient [Pamphlet]*. Oticon.

Carhart, R., and Jerger, J. (1959). Preferred methods for clinical determination of pure-tone thresholds. *J. Speech Hear. Res.* 24, 330–345. doi: 10.1044/jshd.2404.330

Carpenter-Thompson, J. R., Kwaku, A., Schmidt, S. A., Dolcosa, F., and Husain, F. T. (2014). Alterations of the emotional processing system may underlie preserved rapid reaction time in tinnitus. *Brain Res.* 1567, 28–41. doi: 10.1016/j.brainres.2014.04.024

Chandra, N., Lee, A., and Searchfield, G. D. (2014). "Validation of the Tinnitus Functional Index in New Zealand," in *8th International TRI Tinnitus Conference* (Auckland), 31.

Clark, J. G. (1981). Uses and abuses of hearing loss classification. *ASHA* 23, 493–500.

Coren, S., and Ward, L. M. (1989). *Sensation and Perception*. New York, NY: Harcourt Brace Jovanovich.

Corr, P. J., and Matthews, G. (2009). *The Cambridge Handbook of Personality Psychology*. New York, NY: Cambridge University Press.

Costa, P. T., and McRae, R. R. (1992). *Revised NEO Personality Inventory (NEO-PI-R) and NEO Five-Factor Inventory (NEO-FFI) Professional Manual.* Odessa, FL: Psychological Assessment Resources, Inc.

Costa, P. T., and McCrae, R. R. (2006). Age changes in personality and their origins: comment on Roberts, Walton, and Viechtbauer (2006). *Psychol. Bull.* 132, 26–28. doi: 10.1037/0033-2909.132.1.26

Davis, A., and El Refaie, A. (2000). "Epidemiology of tinnitus," in *Tinnitus Handbook*, ed R. S. Tyler (San Diego, CA: Singular Publishing), 1–23.

Davis, P. B. (2006). "Music and the acoustic desensitization protocol for tinnitus," in *Tinnitus Treatment: Clinical Protocols*, ed R. S. Tyler (New York, NY: Thieme), 146–160.

Davis, P. B., Paki, B., and Hanley, P. J. (2007). The neuromonics tinnitus treatment: third clinical trial. *Ear Hear.* 28, 242–259. doi: 10.1097/AUD.0b013e3180312619

Davis, P. B., Wilde, R. A., Steed, L. G., and Hanley, P. J. (2008). Treatment of tinnitus with a customized acoustic neural stimulus: a controlled clinical study. *ENT J.* 87, 330–339.

De Ridder, D., Congedo, M., and Vanneste, S. (2015). The neural correlates of subjectively perceived and passively matched loudness perception in auditory phantom perception. *Brain Behav.* 5:e00331. doi: 10.1002/brb3.331

De Ridder, D., Elgoyhen, A. B., Romo, R., and Langguth, B. (2011). Phantom percepts: tinnitus and pain as persisting aversive memory networks. *Proc. Natl. Acad. Sci. U.S.A.* 108, 8075–8080. doi: 10.1073/pnas.1018466108

De Ridder, D., Vanneste, S., Weisz, N., Londero, A., and Schlee, W. (2014). An integrative model of auditory phantom perception: tinnitus as a unified percept of interacting separable subnetworks. *Neurosci. Biobehav. Rev.* 44, 16–32. doi: 10.1016/j.neubiorev.2013.03.021

Desiderato, O. (1964). Generalization of conditioned suppression. *J. Comp. Physiol. Psychol.* 57, 434–437. doi: 10.1037/h0047275

Dillon, H., James, A., and Ginis, J. (1997). The Client Oriented Scale of Improvement (COSI) and its relationship to several other measures of benefit and satisfaction provided by hearing aids. *J. Am. Acad. Audiol.* 8, 27–43.

Dos Santos, G. M., and Powers, L. (2015). *Tinnitus: The Siemens Package [Pamphlet]*. Erlangen: Sivantos.

Durai, M., and Searchfield, G. D. (2016). Anxiety and depression, personality traits relevant to tinnitus: a scoping review. *Int. J. Audiol.* 55, 605–615. doi: 10.1080/14992027.2016.1198966

Durai, M., O'Keeffe, M. G., and Searchfield, G. D. (2017a). The personality profile of tinnitus sufferers and a non-tinnitus control group. *J. Am. Acad. Audiol.* doi: 10.3766/jaaa.15103. [Epub ahead of print].

Durai, M., O'Keeffe, M. G., and Searchfield, G. D. (2017b). Examining the short term effects of emotion under an adaptation level theory model of tinnitus perception. *Hear. Res.* 345, 23–29. doi: 10.1016/j.heares.2016.12.013

Durai, M., Searchfield, G. D., and Kobayashi, K. (2015). A preliminary examination of the roles of contextual stimuli and personality traits under the adaptation level theory model of tinnitus. *Acta Acustica United Acustica* 101, 543–555. doi: 10.3813/AAA.918851

Eysenck, M. W., and Keane, M. T. (2015). *Cognitive Psychology: A Student's Handbook*. New York, NY: Psychology Press.

Folmer, R. L., and Carroll, J. R. (2006). Long-term effectiveness of ear-level devices for tinnitus. *Otolaryngol. Head Neck Surg.* 134, 132–137. doi: 10.1016/j.otohns.2005.09.030

Folmer, R. L., Theodoroff, S. M., Casiana, L., Shi, Y., Griest, S., and Vachhani, J. (2015). Repetitive transcranial magnetic stimulation treatment for chronic tinnitus: a randomized clinical trial. *JAMA Otolaryngol. Head Neck Surg.* 141, 716–722. doi: 10.1001/jamaoto.2015.1219

Gale, N. K., Heath, G., Cameron, E., Rashid, S., and Redwood, S. (2013). Using the framework method for the analysis of qualitative data in multi-disciplinary health research. *BMC Med. Res. Methodol.* 13:117. doi: 10.1186/1471-2288-13-117

Geers, A., and Rose, J. (2011). Treatment choice and placebo expectation effects. *Soc. Personal. Psychol. Compass* 5, 734–750. doi: 10.1111/j.1751-9004.2011.00385.x

Hanley, P. J., and Davis, P. B. (2008). Treatment of tinnitus with a customized, dynamic acoustic neural stimulus: underlying principles and clinical efficacy. *Trends Amplif.* 12, 210–222. doi: 10.1177/1084713808319942

Hann, D., Searchfield, G. D., Sanders, M., and Wise, K. (2008). Strategies for the selection of music in the short-term management of mild tinnitus. *Aust. N.Z. J. Audiol.* 30, 129–140. doi: 10.1375/audi.30.2.129

Hassler, R. (1978). Striatal control of locomotion, intentional actions and of integrating and perceptive activity. *J. Neurol. Sci.* 36, 187–224. doi: 10.1016/0022-510X(78)90082-5

Heller, A. J. (2003). Classification and epidemiology of tinnitus. *Otolaryngol. Clin. North Am.* 36, 239–248. doi: 10.1016/S0030-6665(02)00160-3

Helson, H. (1948). Adaptation level as a basis for a quantitative theory of frames of reference. *Psychol. Rev.* 55, 297–313. doi: 10.1037/h0056721

Helson, H. (1964). *Adaptation Level Theory*. New York, NY: Harper and Row.

Henry, J. A., and Meikle, M. A. (1996). "Loudness recruitment only partially explains the small size of tinnitus loudness matches," in *Proceedings of the Fifth International Tinnitus Seminar*, eds G. E. Reichand and J. A. Vernon (Portland: American Tinnitus Association), 148–157.

Henry, J. A., Dennis, K. C., and Schechter, M. A. (2005). General review of tinnitus: prevalence, mechanisms, effects, and management. *J. Speech Lang. Hear. Res.* 48, 1204–1235. doi: 10.1044/1092-4388(2005/084)

Henry, J. A., Frederick, M., Sell, S., Griest, S., and Abrams, H. B. (2015). Validation of a novel combination hearing aid and tinnitus therapy device. *Ear Hear.* 36, 42–52. doi: 10.1097/AUD.0000000000000093

Henry, J. A., Rheinsburg, B., and Zaugg, T. (2004). Comparison of custom sounds for achieving tinnitus relief. *J. Am. Acad. Audiol.* 15, 585–598. doi: 10.3766/jaaa.15.8.6

Henry, J. A., Schechter, M. A., Zaugg, T. L., Griest, S., Jastreboff, P. J., Vernon, J. A., et al. (2006). Outcomes of clinical trial: tinnitus masking versus tinnitus retraining therapy. *J. Am. Acad. Audiol.* 17, 104–132. doi: 10.3766/jaaa.17.2.4

Hoare, D. J., Kowalkowski, V. L., Kang, S., and Hall, D. A. (2011). Systematic review and meta-analyses of randomized controlled trials examining tinnitus management. *Laryngoscope* 121, 1555–1564. doi: 10.1002/lary.21825

Hobson, J., Chisholm, E., and El Refaie, A. (2010). Sound therapy (masking) in the management of tinnitus in adults. *Cochrane Database Syst. Rev.* CD006371. doi: 10.1002/14651858.CD006371.pub2

Hoffmann, H. J., and Reed, G. W. (2004). "Epidemiology of tinnitus," in *Tinnitus. Theory and Management*, ed J. B. Snow (Hamilton: B.C. Decker), 16–41.

Hunter, I. R., and Gillen, M. C. (2009). Stress coping mechanisms in elderly adults an initial study of recreational and other coping behaviors in nursing home patients. *Adultspan J.* 8, 43–53. doi: 10.1002/j.2161-0029.2009.tb00056.x

Husain, F. T., and Schmidt, S. A. (2014). Using resting state functional connectivity to unravel networks of tinnitus. *Hear. Res.* 307, 153–162. doi: 10.1016/j.heares.2013.07.010

Jastreboff, P. J. (1998). "Tinnitus; the method of," in *Current Therapy in Otolaryngology Head and Neck Surgery*, ed G. A. Gates (St. Louis, MO: Mosby), 90–95.

Jastreboff, P. J. (1999). "Optimal sound use in TRT - Theory and practice," in *Proceedings of the Sixth International Tinnitus Seminar*, ed J. W. P. Hazell (London: Ed Hazell Publishing THC), 491–494.

Jastreboff, P. J. (2007). Tinnitus retraining therapy. *Prog. Brain Res.* 166, 415–423. doi: 10.1016/S0079-6123(07)66040-3

Jastreboff, P. J., and Hazell, J. W. P. (2004). *Tinnitus Retraining Therapy: Implementing the Neurophysiological Model.* Cambridge: Cambridge University Press.

Jastreboff, P. J., and Jastreboff, M. M. (2000). Tinnitus Retraining Therapy (TRT) as a method for treatment of tinnitus and hyperacusis patients. *J. Am. Acad. Audiol.* 11, 162–177.

Kaltenbach, J. A. (2011). Tinnitus: models and mechanisms. *Hear. Res.* 276, 52–60. doi: 10.1016/j.heares.2010.12.003

Kidd, G., Mason, C. R., and Arbogast, T. L. (2002). Similarity, uncertainty, and masking in the identification of nonspeech auditory patterns. *J. Acoust. Soc. Am.* 111, 1367–1376. doi: 10.1121/1.1448342

Kim, B. J., Chung, S. W., Jung, J. Y., and Suh, M. W. (2014). Effect of different sounds on the treatment outcome of tinnitus retraining therapy. *Clin. Exp. Otorhinolaryngol.* 7, 87–93. doi: 10.3342/ceo.2014.7.2.87

Langguth, B., Goodey, R., Azevedo, A., Bjorne, A., Cacace, A., Crocetti, A., et al. (2007). Consensus for tinnitus patient assessment and treatment outcome measurement: tinnitus research initiative meeting, Regensburg, July 2006. *Prog. Brain Res.* 166, 525–536. doi: 10.1016/S0079-6123(07)66050-6

Lockwood, A. H., Salvi, R. J., and Burkard, R. F. (2002). Tinnitus. *N.Engl. J. Med.* 347, 904–910. doi: 10.1056/NEJMra013395

Lovibond, S. H., and Lovibond, P. F. (1995). *Manual for the Depression Anxiety Stress Scales.* Sydney: Psychology Foundation.

Malouff, J. M., Schutte, N. S., and Zucker, L. A. (2011). Tinnitus-related distress: a review of recent findings. *Curr. Psychiatry Rep.* 13, 31–36. doi: 10.1007/s11920-010-0163-1

Malterud, K. (2001). The art and science of clinical knowledge: evidence beyond measures and numbers. *Lancet* 358, 397–400. doi: 10.1016/S0140-6736(01)05548-9

Marks, L. E., and Arieh, Y. (2006). Differential effects of stimulus context in sensory processing. *Eur. Rev. Appl. Psychol. Rev.* 56, 213–221. doi: 10.1016/j.erap.2005.09.009

Martinez-Devesa, P., Perera, R., Theodoulou, M., and Waddell, A. (2010). Cognitive behavioural therapy for tinnitus. *Cochrane Database Syst. Rev.* CD005233. doi: 10.1002/14651858.cd005233.pub3

Masuyama, E. (1994). Application of adaptation level theory to human experiment on temperature sensation. *Jpn. J. Erg.* 30, 201–208. doi: 10.5100/jje.30.201

McKenna, L., and Irwin, R. (2008). Sound therapy for tinnitus sacred cow or idol worship?: an investigation of the evidence. *Audiol. Med.* 6, 16–24. doi: 10.1080/16513860801899389

Meikle, M. B., Henry, J. A., Griest, S. E., Stewart, B. J., Abrams, H. B., McArdle, R., et al. (2012). The tinnitus functional index: development of a new clinical measure for chronic, intrusive tinnitus. *Ear Hear.* 33, 153. doi: 10.1097/AUD.0b013e31822f67c0

Melin, L., Scott, B., Lindberg, P., and Lyttkens, L. (1987). Hearing aids and tinnitus -an experimental group study. *Br. J. Audiol.* 21, 91–97. doi: 10.3109/03005368709077782

Mirz, F., Gjedde, A., Ishizu, K., and Pedersen, C. B. (2000a). Cortical networks subserving the perception of tinnitus – a PET study. *Acta Otolaryngol. Suppl.* 543, 241–243. doi: 10.1080/000164800454503

Mirz, F., Gjedde, A., Sodkilde-Jrgensen, H., and Pedersen, C. B. (2000b). Functional brain imaging of tinnitus-like perception induced by aversive auditory stimuli. *Neuroreport* 11, 633–637. doi: 10.1097/00001756-200002280-00039

Moller, A. R. (2006). *Hearing: Anatomy, Physiology, and Disorders of the Auditory System.* Boston, MA: Academic Press.

Näätänen, R., Tervaniemi, M., Sussman, E., Paavilainen, P., and Winkler, I. (2001). 'Primitive intelligence' in the auditory cortex. *Trends Neurosci.* 24, 283–288. doi: 10.1016/S0166-2236(00)01790-2

Noreña, A. J., and Eggermont, J. J. (2006). Enriched acoustic environment after noise trauma abolishes neural signs of tinnitus. *Neuroreport* 17, 559–563. doi: 10.1097/00001756-200604240-00001

Ohmura, Y., Yamaguchi, T., Futami, Y., Togashi, H., Izumi, T., Matsumoto, M., et al. (2009). Corticotropin releasing factor enhances attentional function as assessed by the five-choice serial reaction time task in rats. *Behav. Brain Res.* 198, 429–433. doi: 10.1016/j.bbr.2008.11.025

Onwuegbuzie, A. J., and Leech, N. L. (2005). On Becoming a pragmatic researcher: the importance of combining quantitative and qualitative research methodologies. *Int. J. Soc. Res. Methodol.* 8, 375–387. doi: 10.1080/13645570500402447

Penner, M. J. (1986). Magnitude estimation and the "paradoxical" loudness of tinnitus. *J. Speech Hear. Res.* 29, 407–412. doi: 10.1044/jshr.2903.407

Rabinowitz, N. C., Willmore, B. D., Schnupp, J. W., and King, A. J. (2011). Contrast gain control in auditory cortex. *Neuron* 70, 1178–1191. doi: 10.1016/j.neuron.2011.04.030

Rizzardo, R., Savastano, M., Maron, M. B., Mangialaio, M., and Salvadori, L. (1998). Psychological distress in patients with tinnitus. *J. Otolaryngol.* 27, 21–25.

Roberts, B. W., Walton, K. E., and Viechtbauer, W. (2006). Patterns of mean-level change in personality traits across the life course: a meta-analysis of longitudinal studies. *Psychol. Bull.* 132, 1–25. doi: 10.1037/0033-2909.132.1.1

Robinson, B. L., and McAlpine, D. (2009). Gain control mechanisms in the auditory pathway. *Curr. Opin. Neurobiol.* 19, 402–407. doi: 10.1016/j.conb.2009.07.006

Rodenbough, J. R. (2003). *Comprehensive Attention Battery® (Version 5.0).* Greensboro, NC: Neuropsych Works, Inc.

Rossman, G. B., and Wilson, B. L. (1985). Numbers and words: combining quantitative and qualitative methods in a single large-scale evaluation study. *Eval. Rev.* 9, 627–643. doi: 10.1177/0193841X8500900505

Sandlin, R. E., and Olsson, R. J. (1999). Evaluation and selection of maskers and other devices used in the treatment of tinnitus and hyperacusis. *Trends Amplif.* 4, 6–26. doi: 10.1177/108471389900400102

Schaette, R., Konig, O., Hornig, D., Gross, M, and Kempter, R. (2010). Acoustic stimulation treatments against tinnitus could be most effective when tinnitus pitch is within the stimulated frequency range. *Hear. Res.* 269, 95–101. doi: 10.1016/j.heares.2010.06.022

Schecklmann, M., Landgrebe, M., Poeppl, T. B., Kreuzer, P., Männer, P., Marienhagen, J., et al. (2013a). Neural correlates of tinnitus duration and distress: a positron emission tomography study. *Hum. Brain Mapp.* 34, 233–240. doi: 10.1002/hbm.21426

Schecklmann, M., Lehner, A., Poeppl, T. B., Kreuzer, P. M., Rupprecht, R., Rackl, J., et al. (2013b). Auditory cortex is implicated in tinnitus distress: a voxel-based morphometry study. *Brain Struct. Funct.* 218, 1061–1070. doi: 10.1007/s00429-013-0520-z

Schlee, W., Hartmann, T., Langguth, B., and Weisz, N. (2009). Abnormal resting-state cortical coupling in chronic tinnitus. *BNC Neurosci.* 10:11. doi: 10.1186/1471-2202-10-11

Schlee, W., Weisz, N., Bertrand, O., Hartmann, T., and Elbert, T. (2008). Using auditory steady state responses to outline the functional connectivity in the tinnitus brain *PLoS ONE* 8:e3720. doi: 10.1371/annotation/c71826c3-da07-42e8-a563-bde0257a0845

Schreitmüller, S., von Wedel, H., Walger, M., and Meister, H. (2013). Untersuchungen von Rauschsignalen für die akustische Tinnitustherapie [Effect of dynamics on acceptance and concealment effect]. *HNO* 61, 38–45. doi: 10.1007/s00106-012-2642-7

Scott, B., and Lindberg, P. (2000). Psychological profile and somatic complaints between help-seeking and non-help-seeking tinnitus subjects. *Psychosomatics* 41, 347–352. doi: 10.1176/appi.psy.41.4.347

Scott, B., Lindberg, P., Lyttkens, L., and Melin, L. (1990). Predictors of tinnitus discomfort, adaptation and subjective loudness. *Br. J. Audiol.* 24, 51–62. doi: 10.3109/03005369009077842

Searchfield, G. D. (2014). Tinnitus What and Where: An Ecological Framework. *Front. Neurol.* 5:271. doi: 10.3389/fneur.2014.00271

Searchfield, G. D. (2016). "Hearing aids for tinnitus," in *Tinnitus: Clinical and Research Perspectives*, eds D. M. Baguley and M. Fagelson (San Diego, CA: Plural Publishing, Inc.).

Searchfield, G. D., Kaur, M., and Martin, W. H. (2010). Hearing aids as an adjunct to counseling: tinnitus patients who choose amplification do better than those who don't. *Int. J. Audiol.* 49, 574–579. doi: 10.3109/14992021003777267

Searchfield, G. D., Kobayashi, K., and Sanders, M. (2012). An adaptation level theory of tinnitus audibility. *Front. Syst. Neurosci.* 6:46. doi: 10.3389/fnsys.2012.00046

Searchfield, G. D., Morrison-Low, J., and Wise, K. (2007). Object identification and attention training for treating tinnitus. *Prog. Brain Res.* 166, 441–460. doi: 10.1016/S0079-6123(07)66043-9

Searchfield, G. D., Warr, A. A., Kuklinski, J. V., and Purdy, S. C. (2002). "Digital instruments for tinnitus:mixing point identification and threshold-adjusted noise," in *Proceedings of the Seventh International Tinnitus Seminar*, ed R. Patuzzi (Perth, WA: The University of Western Australia), 191–195.

Sirois, F. M., Davis, C. G., and Morgan, M. S. (2006). "Learning to live with what you can't rise above": control beliefs, symptom control, and adjustment to tinnitus. *Health Psychol.* 25, 119–123. doi: 10.1037/0278-6133.25.1.119

Specht, J., Egloff, B., and Schmukle, S. C. (2011). Stability and change of personality across the life course: the impact of age and major life events on mean-level and rank-order stability of the Big Five. *J. Pers. Soc. Psychol.* 101, 862–882. doi: 10.1037/a0024950

Stein, A., Wunderlich, R., Lau, P., Engell, A., Wollbrink, A., Shaykevich, A., et al. (2016). Clinical trial on tonal tinnitus with tailor-made notched music training. *BMC Neurol.* 16:38. doi: 10.1186/s12883-016-0558-7

Stouffer, J. L., and Tyler, R. S. (1990). Characterization of tinnitus by tinnitus patients. *J. Speech Hear. Disord.* 55, 439–453. doi: 10.1044/jshd.5503.439

Sweetow, R. W. (1984). Cognitive behavioral modification in tinnitus management. *Hear. Instrum.* 35, 14–18.

Sweetow, R. W. (1986). Cognitive aspects of tinnitus-patient management. *Ear Hear.* 7, 390–396. doi: 10.1097/00003446-198612000-00008

Távora-Vieira, D., Eikelboom, R. H., and Miller, S. (2011). Neuromonics tinnitus treatment for patients with significant level of hearing loss: an adaptation of the protocol. *Int. J. Audiology* 50, 881–886. doi: 10.3109/14992027.2011.606286

Tellegen, A. (1982). *Brief manual for the Multidimensional Personality Questionnaire.* Minneapolis, MN: University of Minnesota.

Tyler, R. S. (2006). *Tinnitus Treatment: Clinical Protocols.* New York, NY: Thieme.

Tyler, R. S., Gogel, S. A., and Gehringer, A. K. (2007). Tinnitus activities treatment. *Prog. Brain Res.* 166, 425–434. doi: 10.1016/S0079-6123(07)66041-5

Tyler, R. S., Noble, W., Coelho, C. B., and Ji, H. (2012). Tinnitus retraining therapy: mixing point and total masking are equally effective. *Ear Hear.* 33, 588–594. doi: 10.1097/AUD.0b013e31824f2a6e

Tyler, R., Coelho, C., Tao, P., Ji, H., Noble, W., and Gehringer, A. (2008). Identifying tinnitus subgroups with cluster analysis. *Am. J. Audiol.* 17, 176–184. doi: 10.1044/1059-0889(2008/07-0044)

Vanneste, S., Song, J. J., and De Ridder, D. (2013). Tinnitus and musical hallucinosis: the same but more. *Neuroimage* 82, 373–383. doi: 10.1016/j.neuroimage.2013.05.107

Vanneste, S., Van de Heyning, P., and De Ridder, D. (2011). The neural network of phantom sound changes over time: a comparison between recent-onset and chronic tinnitus patients. *Eur. J. Neurosci.* 34, 718–731. doi: 10.1111/j.1460-9568.2011.07793.x

Vernon, J. A., and Meikle, M. B. (2000). "Tinnitus masking," in *Tinnitus Handbook*, ed R. S. Tyler (San Diego, CA: Singular Thompson Learning), 313–356.

Watson, D., Clark, L. A., and Tellegan, A. (1988). Development and validation of brief measures of positive and negative affect: the PANAS scales. *J. Pers. Soc. Psychol.* 54, 1063–1070. doi: 10.1037/0022-3514.54.6.1063

Welch, D., and Dawes, P. J. (2008). Personality and perception of tinnitus. *Ear Hear.* 29, 684–692. doi: 10.1097/AUD.0b013e318177d9ac

Wise, K. J. (2012). *Tinnitus and Attention Training, Audiology.* Auckland: University of Auckland.

Wise, K., Kobayashi, K., Magnusson, J., Welch, D., and Searchfield, G. D. (2016). Randomized controlled trial of a perceptual training game for tinnitus therapy. *Games Health J.* 5, 141–149. doi: 10.1089/g4h.2015.0068

Zenner, H. P., Pfister, M., and Birbaumer, N. (2006). Tinnitus sensitization: sensory and psychophysiological aspects of a new pathway of acquired centralization of chronic tinnitus. *Otol. Neurotol.* 27, 1054–1063. doi: 10.1097/01.mao.0000231604.64079.77

Zomeren, A. H., and Brouwer, W. H. (1994). *Clinical Neuropsychology of Attention.* Oxford: Oxford University Press.

2

A Pilot Study of Peripheral Muscle Magnetic Stimulation as Add-on Treatment to Repetitive Transcranial Magnetic Stimulation in Chronic Tinnitus

*Veronika Vielsmeier[1], Martin Schecklmann[2], Winfried Schlee[2], Peter M. Kreuzer[2], Timm B. Poeppl[2], Rainer Rupprecht[2], Berthold Langguth[2] and Astrid Lehner[2]**

[1] Department of Otorhinolaryngology, University of Regensburg, Regensburg, Germany,

[2] Department of Psychiatry and Psychotherapy, University of Regensburg, Regensburg, Germany

Correspondence:
Astrid Lehner
astrid.lehner@medbo.de

While brain stimulation techniques have been examined as treatment options for chronic tinnitus for many years, they have recently been extended to multimodal treatment approaches. As chronic tinnitus is often accompanied by comorbid muscular tension in the neck and back, we performed a one-arm pilot study to explore the feasibility of a new multimodal treatment approach. In detail, repetitive peripheral magnetic stimulation (rPMS) of the back was performed before and after each session of repetitive transcranial magnetic stimulation (rTMS) of the brain. Data of 41 patients were analyzed, all of which were treated with ten sessions of rTMS of the left prefrontal and left temporoparietal cortex followed by rPMS of the neck and back muscles. Tinnitus severity was measured using the tinnitus questionnaire (TQ). Neck pain was assessed using the neck pain and disability scale (NPAD). The new treatment approach was feasible and well accepted by the majority of patients. However, the overall patient group did not improve significantly in either of the questionnaires. If patients were divided in different subgroups depending on whether they were suffering from neck pain or somatosensory tinnitus, explorative *post-hoc* tests suggested differential effects: patients with both neck pain and somatosensory tinnitus had better outcomes than patients without those conditions or with neck pain only. This was true for both the TQ and the NPAD. This effect was of transient nature though: the TQ score went back to its baseline level after a follow-up period of 12 weeks. Based on our results we recommend that in studies that investigate tinnitus treatments targeting somatosensory afferents patients should be stratified according to somatic co-morbidities and somatosensory influence on the tinnitus percept.

Clinical trial registration: www.clinicaltrials.gov, NCT02306447.

Keywords: rPMS, rTMS, tinnitus, brain stimulation, muscle magnetic stimulation, chronic tinnitus

INTRODUCTION

Chronic subjective tinnitus is a very heterogeneous condition with respect to its causes, clinical characteristics and the emotional distress perceived by a patient. Therefore, it has been suggested that there exist various subtypes of tinnitus which might respond to different treatment approaches (Landgrebe et al., 2010). Accordingly, there are also multiple models for tinnitus pathophysiology, all of which might be able to explain different aspects of tinnitus generation or maintenance. While cognitive models highlight the importance of top-down mechanisms such as selective attention, interpretation and emotional evaluation of the phantom sound (McKenna et al., 2014; Elgoyhen et al., 2015; Ghodratitoostani et al., 2016), there are also pathophysiological models of tinnitus which emphasize bottom-up influences by suggesting neuroplastic changes in somatosensory afferents (Shore et al., 2016). The current study seeks to target both bottom-up and top-down mechanisms by using a combined treatment of rPMS (hypothesized bottom-up influence) and rTMS (hypothesized top-down influence via cortical stimulation of DLPFC and temporoparietal cortex).

Tinnitus has been shown to be accompanied by altered activity of and connectivity between different cortical networks including temporal, parietal and frontal cortices (Schlee et al., 2009; Schmidt et al., 2013; Elgoyhen et al., 2015). As rTMS is considered to be able to interfere with alterations of cortical activity, it has been examined as a treatment option for patients suffering from tinnitus (Theodoroff and Folmer, 2013; Lefaucheur et al., 2014). The effect sizes for this treatment remain small (Lefaucheur et al., 2014). Therefore, different strategies have been tried to increase treatment effects such as targeting multiple brain areas with rTMS (Kreuzer et al., 2011; Lehner et al., 2016) or varying the frequency by which the rTMS pulses are applied (Schecklmann et al., 2016). Up to now, the stimulation of temporal and frontal cortical areas has been suggested to exert beneficial effects on tinnitus (Kleinjung et al., 2008; Langguth and De Ridder, 2013).

Besides the importance of auditory and non-auditory cortical structures, there is also strong evidence for the somatosensory bottom-up system to be involved in tinnitus pathophysiology. Even if controversial, one tinnitus subtype might be cervicogenic somatic tinnitus (Bhatt et al., 2015; Michiels et al., 2015). It is known that auditory-somatosensory integration takes place in the cochlear nucleus (Dehmel et al., 2008) and auditory brainstem activity was shown to be modulated by trigeminal and also somatosensory stimulation (Dehmel et al., 2012; Markovitz et al., 2015). Somatosensory inputs are thought to be functionally relevant with respect to suppression of body-generated sounds (Shore and Zhou, 2006). Pathological conditions are supposed to spread into to auditory system via the cochlear nucleus. Actually, plastic changes in this bimodal system have already been observed in animal models of tinnitus (Dehmel et al., 2012). Furthermore, many patients suffering from tinnitus are able to modulate their phantom sound by moving face or neck muscles (Levine et al., 2007; Sanchez and Rocha, 2011). This somatosensory tinnitus component has already been targeted by different treatment approaches. For instance, myofascial trigger point deactivation was shown to bring tinnitus relief for patients with tinnitus and comorbid myofascial pain syndrome (Rocha and Sanchez, 2012). There is also some evidence that the reduction of muscle tension of neck and back muscles can bring relief to some tinnitus patients. For example, it was shown that Qigong—a system of movements, body postures and breathing exercises—leads to an improvement of tinnitus severity especially in patients with somatosensory tinnitus (Biesinger et al., 2010). Additionally, a recent case report describes a patient whose tinnitus disappeared after the application of a cervical collar, underscoring the involvement of cervical muscles in tinnitus generation (Bechter et al., 2016). In a very recent study, Marks et al. (2018) found that bimodal auditory-somatosensory treatment was effective in reducing tinnitus loudness and severity in patients suffering from somatic tinnitus. With respect to rTMS, it has been hypothesized that rTMS effects may also be partly mediated by modulation of somatosensory afferents (Vanneste et al., 2011; Lehner et al., 2012). There is some preliminary evidence that magnetic stimulation can also be used for reducing muscle tension in neck muscles and for inducing analgetic effects (Smania et al., 2003, 2005; Zunhammer et al., 2011; Sollmann et al., 2016).

Only recently, brain stimulation techniques have been extended to multimodal treatment approaches by combining them with e.g., acoustic stimulation (Shekhawat et al., 2015) or relaxation techniques (Kreuzer et al., 2016). Integrating the knowledge about the central nervous dysfunction as well as the importance of the somatosensory system for chronic tinnitus, we investigate a new multimodal treatment approach which targets both systems by combining rTMS with repetitive peripheral magnetic stimulation (rPMS) of the neck muscles. For rTMS, a stimulation protocol was chosen which combines low-frequency stimulation of auditory cortical areas with high-frequency stimulation of the prefrontal cortex and which has already shown promising effects in the past (Kleinjung et al., 2008; Langguth et al., 2014). While low-frequency rTMS of the temporoparietal cortex is a standard procedure (Lefaucheur et al., 2014) high frequency rTMS of the prefrontal cortex is supposed to induce activity changes in the anterior cingulate cortex (Speer et al., 2000) which is thought to be involved in tinnitus distress (Vanneste et al., 2010). rPMS treatment is supposed to bring relief to muscle tension (Smania et al., 2003, 2005) which might alter the somatosensory input to the cochlear nucleus. We investigated the feasibility of this bimodal treatment approach in a one-arm pilot study (Dobie, 1999; Landgrebe et al., 2012).

MATERIALS AND METHODS

Subjects

The study was registered at Clinical Trials (NCT02306447). Inclusion criteria for study participation were age between 18 and 80 years and presence of chronic subjective tinnitus for at least 6 months. Exclusion criteria were objective tinnitus, a treatable cause of tinnitus and the involvement in other treatments for tinnitus at the same time. Furthermore, patients with clinically relevant psychiatric comorbidities, alcohol or drug abuse, acute neck or back pain, neck or back pain with unknown etiology as well as unstable internal or neurological comorbidities were excluded. In addition, general exclusion criteria for rTMS or rPMS stimulation applied (history or evidence of significant brain malformation or neoplasm, head injury, cerebral vascular events, neurodegenerative disorders affecting the brain, prior brain surgery, metal objects in and around the body that cannot be removed, pregnancy). Patients were recruited during routine clinical tinnitus consultations. All data were collected at the Department of Psychiatry and Psychotherapy, University of Regensburg between September 2014 and April 2016 (last follow-up visit). All research participants provided written, informed consent to participate in this research as well as for the data to be used for analysis and publication. Data were gathered and analyzed within the framework of the Tinnitus Research Initiative database (Landgrebe et al., 2010) which was approved by the Ethics Committee of the University Hospital of Regensburg (Germany, reference number 08/046).

Questionnaires and Outcome Measures

Patients completed the below listed questionnaires at four measurement time points: at baseline (treatment day 1), week 2 (treatment day 10, last treatment day), week 4 and week 12 (2 and 10 weeks after the last treatment session, respectively). Tinnitus severity was assessed using the German version of the Tinnitus Questionnaire (TQ, Goebel and Hiller, 1994), the Tinnitus Handicap Inventory (THI, Newman et al., 1996) and five rating scales measuring how loud, uncomfortable, annoying, unpleasant and how easy to ignore the tinnitus was. Those scales ranged from 0 (not at all loud/uncomfortable etc.) to 10 (extremely loud/uncomfortable etc.). In addition, depressive symptoms were assessed by the Major Depression Inventory (MDI) and quality of life was measured by the WHO-QoL BREF (World Health Organization Quality of Life) assessment which is divided into four domains: physical health (domain 1), psychological health (domain 2), social relationships (domain 3), and environment (domain 4). In addition, patients completed the neck pain and disability scale (NPAD, Scherer et al., 2008) at baseline and week 2. The NPAD was only available for a subgroup of 34 patients though. In order to assess demographic and clinical patient characteristics at baseline, patients filled in the Tinnitus Sample Case History Questionnaire (Langguth et al., 2007) and underwent pure-tone audiometry. The mean hearing threshold is reported which represents the average of all thresholds measured bilaterally for frequencies between 125 Hz and 8 kHz.

Primary outcome was defined as the change of tinnitus severity as measured by the TQ from baseline to week 12. Secondary outcomes were changes in TQ, THI, MDI, numeric rating scales, and WHO-QoL over the course of the trial (baseline, week 2, week 4, and week 12). Furthermore the change in the neck pain and disability scale (NPAD) from baseline to week 2 was analyzed.

rTMS and rPMS Treatment

The present clinical trial was designed as a one-arm open-label proof of concept study. Therefore, all patients underwent the same treatment procedures during which they were treated in 10 sessions on 10 consecutive working days with a break over the weekend. Each treatment session consisted of four parts which were applied successively without break in between (apart from the break which was necessary to change coils; see **Figure 1**): (1) rPMS of the neck and back muscles; (2) rTMS stimulation of the left dorso-lateral prefrontal cortex (DLPFC, 2000 stimuli, 20 Hz, which were applied in 20 trains with an intertrain interval of 25 s); (3) rTMS stimulation of the left temporo-parietal cortex (2000 stimuli, 1 Hz). (4) rPMS of the neck and back muscles.

(2) and (3) were done at a stimulation intensity of 110% resting motor threshold using a Medtronic MagPro X100 stimulator (Medtronic, Denmark) and a 70 mm figure-of-eight coil. The temporo-parietal cortex was localized using the 10–20 system: The coil was placed between the temporal (T3) and parietal (P3) EEG electrode sites. The DLFPC was targeted by centring the TMS coil 6 cm anterior from the part of the motor cortex which had been used for defining the motor threshold (Lehner et al., 2013). Combined temporoparietal plus frontal stimulation protocol have been examined before and were shown to be safe (Langguth et al., 2014; Kreuzer et al., 2015; Lehner et al., 2016). The rPMS protocol was based on clinical experience in the use of rPMS in rehabilitative medicine and consisted of four medial-lateral movements starting from the neck (1: left trapezius and deltoid muscle; 2: right trapezius and deltoid muscle; 3: left trapezius and latissimus dorsi muscle; 4: right trapezius and latissimus dorsi muscle) and one cranio-caudal movement over the backbone (see **Figure 2**). The series of those five movements was repeated eight times: the first four repetitions with a stimulation frequency of 5 Hz, the remaining four repetitions with 20 Hz. Each movement consisted of 20 stimulation pulses. As a consequence, the duration of a 20 Hz

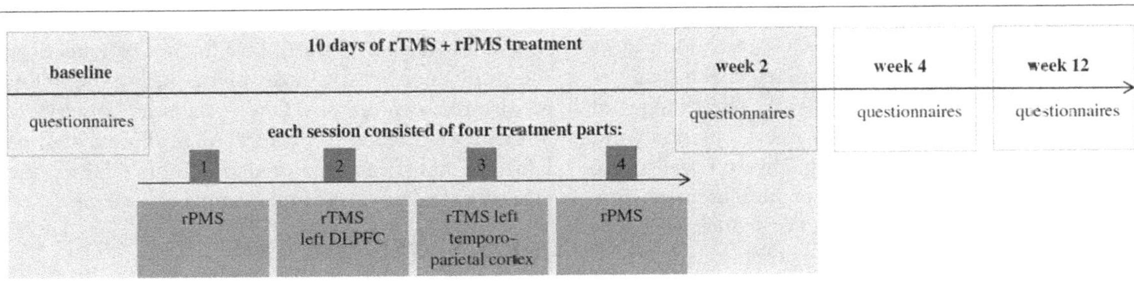

FIGURE 1 | Overall treatment schedule.

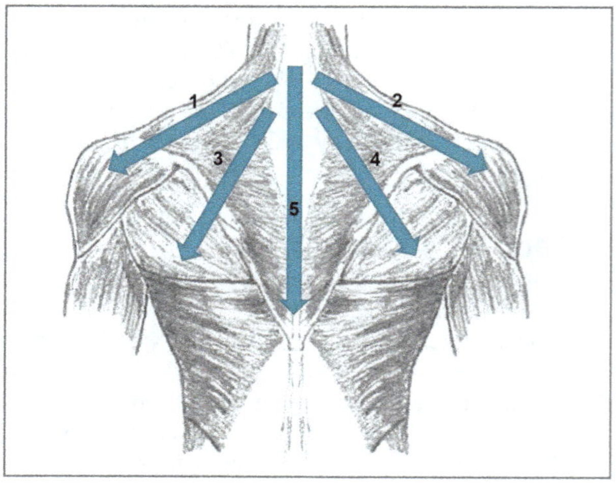

FIGURE 2 | Directions of the movements done during rPMS stimulation. 1, left trapezius and deltoid muscle; 2, right trapezius and deltoid muscle; 3, left trapezius and latissimus dorsi muscle, 4, right trapezius and latissimus dorsi muscle; 5, cranio-caudal movement over the backbone.

movement was 1 s, the duration of a 5 Hz movement was 4 s. Between the movements, there was a 2s interval. In total, one rPMS treatment part had a duration of 100 s. rTMS treatment lasted 2,575 s (2,000 s for the 1 Hz treatment, 575 s for the 20 Hz treatment incl. intertrain intervals). As a consequence, a complete session of two rPMS treatment parts plus rTMS treatment lasted 2,775 s or 46.25 min. rPMS stimulation was done using a round coil with 126 mm outer diameter (MagVenture MMC-140-II) at an intensity that was determined as individually comfortable in a pretest (typically 20–30% of maximal stimulator output). Before the first treatment session, the resting motor threshold was measured. It was defined as the minimal intensity at which at least five of ten motor evoked potentials were 50 μV in amplitude in the right abductor digiti minimi.

Statistical Analysis

For statistical analyses IBM SPSS Statistics for Windows (Version 22.0, Armonk, NY: IBM Corp.) was used. Four missing values were replaced by using a last observation carried forward (LOCF) procedure: The TQ score of one patient was missing for the final visit and the score for the rating scale "annoying" was missing for another patient for week 2. Furthermore, the MDI score for week 2 was missing for one patient and for week 12 for another patient. Recently, we could demonstrate that the LOCF method induces no statistical bias in comparison to linear mixed effects analyses for missing data <10% (Kreuzer et al., 2016). The changes of the TQ score from baseline to week 12 (primary outcome) and of the NPAD score from baseline to week 2 were tested using paired *t*-tests with the within-subjects factor measurement time point. To test for changes in tinnitus severity scores, MDI and WHO-QoL over all four measurement time points an analysis of variance (ANOVA) with the within-subjects factor measurement time point (baseline, week 2, week 4, week 12) was calculated for all questionnaires and rating scales. For the ANOVAs, the sphericity of data was checked with Mauchly Tests (Mauchly, 1940). In case of significant Mauchly-Tests, Greenhouse-Geisser corrections were applied.

In addition to the statistical analyses described above, some exploratory data analyses were conducted in order to understand the results in more detail. To this end, some analyses with a special focus on neck pain and somatosensory tinnitus were done. Patients were divided into different groups depending on whether they were suffering from neck pain ("Do you suffer from neck pain?") and/or from somatosensory tinnitus ("Does any head and neck movement (e.g., moving the jaw forward or clenching the teeth), or having your arms/hands or head touched, affect your tinnitus?"), based on their answers in the Tinnitus Sample Case History Questionnaire (Langguth et al., 2007). A number of 11 patients did not suffer from neck pain or somatosensory tinnitus, 16 patients suffered from neck pain only, and 11 patients reported both neck pain and somatosensory tinnitus. Another 3 patients only reported somatosensory tinnitus. Because of the small sample size, this group was excluded from the following analyses. For the subgroup of 34 patients who filled in the NDPAD, 9 patients did not suffer from neck pain or somatosensory tinnitus, 13 suffered from neck pain only, 9 reported both neck pain and somatosensory tinnitus and 3 reported somatosensory tinnitus only.

Repeated measures ANOVAs were done to compare the resulting three groups with respect to the change of the NPAD score and the TQ from baseline to week 2. The homogeneity of variances between groups was tested with Levene's Tests. In case of significant Levene's Tests, F_{max}-Tests were done. Those tests revealed that an adaptation of the level of significance was not necessary for the ANOVAs with the TQ as dependent variable. For the ANOVA with the NPAD as dependent variable, the significance level had to be adapted to.025.

RESULTS

Dropouts

Forty-nine patients were enrolled in the study. Three patients dropped out of the study during the treatment phase. One of them reported a light subjective cardiac arrhythmia. Although he had had cardiac arrhythmias before and the relation to rPMS seemed to be doubtful, the rPMS treatment was terminated. Another patient dropped out due to an ongoing loudening of the tinnitus percept. The third patient dropped out due to a hypertensive crisis with doubtful relation to rTMS treatment (pre-known hypertension). Five further patients dropped out of the study after the treatment phase during the follow-up phase, all for unknown reasons. One of them had described a transient loudening of the tinnitus before. All in all, data of 41 patients were left to be statistically analyzed (see **Table 1** for demographic and clinical characteristics of this sample at baseline).

Adverse Events

In all treated patients, both the rPMS as well as the rTMS part of the treatment were tolerated without severe side effects. Among the 41 patients who completed the study 5 patients (13%)

TABLE 1 | Demographical data and clinical characteristics at baseline (M ± SD) for the overall patient group and for the three exploratory subgroups.

	Overall patient group ($n = 41$)	Neither neck pain nor somatosensory tinnitus ($n = 11$)	Neck pain ($n = 16$)	Neck pain and somatosensory tinnitus ($n = 11$)
Age (years)	50.70 ± 12.69	48.21 ± 12.67	52.20 ± 11.67	53.62 ± 14.37
Gender	26 m, 15 f	8m, 3f	9m, 7f	6m, 5f
Mean hearing threshold [dB HL]	18.18 ± 11.84 ($n = 40$)	15.01 ± 10.22	21.59 ± 10.89 ($n = 15$)	20.45 ± 13.26
Tinnitus laterality (r/l/l>r/r>l/both/inside head)	6/10/8/6/8/3	0/5/2/0/4/0	2/5/3/1/4/1	3/0/3/4/0/1
Tinnitus duration in years	7.69 ± 7.70 ($n = 38$)	11.07 ± 8.80 ($n = 10$)	4.34 ± 4.93 ($n = 15$)	8.95 ± 9.11 ($n = 10$)
TQ (0–84)	37.83 ± 16.23	25.27 ± 16.62	41.19 ± 16.85	43.27 ± 3.01
THI (0–100)	42.34 ± 21.57	31.73 ± 21.99	44.63 ± 22.71	48.36 ± 16.46
MDI ($N = 40$; 0–50)	7.23 ± 5.43	4.36 ± 4.91	8.44 ± 6.11	8.55 ± 4.59
WHO-QoL Domain 1 (4–20)	15.47 ± 2.57	17.12 ± 2.37	14.52 ± 2.87	15.21 ± 1.77
WHO-QoL Domain 2 (4–20)	14.35 ± 2.66	15.12 ± 3.43	13.98 ± 2.17	14.10 ± 2.90
WHO-QoL Domain 3 (4–20)	15.62 ± 2.85	15.76 ± 3.15	16.10 ± 2.63	15.27 ± 3.00
WHO-QoL Domain 4 (4–20)	16.71 ± 1.62	17.91 ± 1.76	16.16 ± 1.21	16.77 ± 1.49
Rating scales (0–10)				
Strong/loud	6.73 ± 1.88	5.55 ± 2.16	7.13 ± 1.86	7.27 ± 1.49
Uncomfortable	6.76 ± 2.05	5.73 ± 2.01	6.75 ± 2.27	7.55 ± 1.64
Annoying	6.56 ± 2.18	5.27 ± 2.20	7.13 ± 2.28	7.00 ± 1.95
Ignoring	6.20 ± 2.52	4.45 ± 2.30	7.19 ± 2.54	6.55 ± 2.30
Unpleasant	6.68 ± 2.15	5.45 ± 1.92	6.87 ± 2.28	7.45 ± 2.12
Somatosensory tinnitus	14 yes, 27 no			
Suffer from neck pain	27 yes, 14 no			
NPAD score (0–100)	31.47 ± 24.26 ($n = 34$)	4.22 ± 5.97 ($n = 8$)	42.15 ± 19.04 ($n = 13$)	47.33 ± 20.97 ($n = 9$)

Mean hearing threshold (in dB HL): average of all thresholds measured bilaterally ranging from 125 Hz to 8 kHz. Tinnitus laterality is defined in categories: r, right-sided; l, left-sided, l > r, both sides but louder on the left side; r > l, both sides but louder on the right side; both, both sides; inside head, tinnitus is perceived in the middle of/ inside the head. TQ, Tinnitus Questionnaire; THI, Tinnitus Handicap Inventory; MDI, Major Depression Inventory; rating scales ranging from 0 (not at all loud/uncomfortable etc.) to 10 (extremely loud/uncomfortable etc.); WHO-QoL, World Health Organization-Quality of Life; NPAD, neck pain and disability scale.

reported transient headaches and one patient (2.5%) reported headache which was still present at week 12. Furthermore, six patients (14.6%) complained of an increase in tinnitus loudness. In two of them, this increase was still present at week 12. Additionally, one patient reported a transient pain in his fingers.

Statistical Analysis

Concerning the primary outcome (change of the TQ score from baseline to week 12), no significant treatment effect was observed [$t_{(40)} = -0.27$; $p = 0.787$; $d = 0.04$]. The ANOVAs testing for changes in the different questionnaire scores and rating scales over all measurement time points were not significant (see **Figure 3**, **Table 2**). The NPAD score changed marginally from an average total score of 31.47 points at baseline to 28.00 at week 2 [$t_{(33)} = 1.80$; $p = 0.081$; $d = 0.31$).

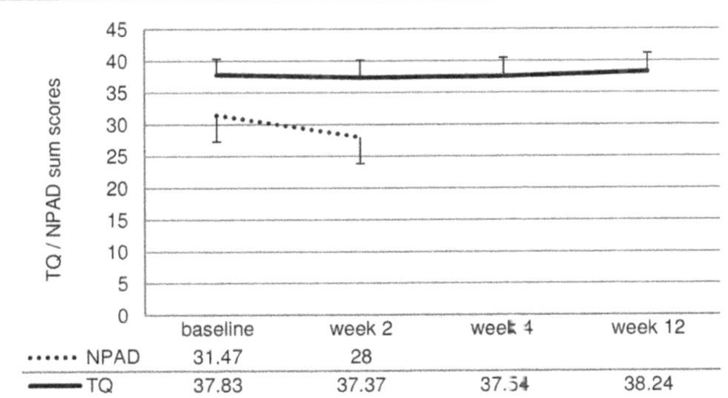

FIGURE 3 | Line chart showing the NPAD and TQ scores over time. Error bars represent standard errors. The change of the NPAD sum score is marginally significant.

Exploratory Data Analysis

If the patients with/without neck pain and/ or somatosensory tinnitus were compared, the interaction effect time*group was significant for the change of the NPAD score from baseline to week 2 [$F_{(2, 28)} = 4.88$; $p = 0.015$; $eta^2 = 0.258$]. For the three *post hoc* t-tests, the Bonferroni-corrected significance level has to be set at 0.016. *Post hoc* t-tests of the mean NPAD differences from baseline to week 2 revealed that patients with both neck pain and somatosensory tinnitus showed more NPAD change ($M = -12.78$; $SD = 10.63$) than patients with neck pain only ($M = 0.85$; $SD = 13.20$). This difference was marginally significant [$t_{(20)} = -2.57$; $p = 0.018$; $d = 1.14$]. Patients with both conditions

TABLE 2 | Results from repeated measures analyses of variance.

	F (df)	*p*	*Eta*^{2}
TQ	$F_{(3, 120)} = 0.18$	0.912	0.004
THI	$F_{(2.28, 91.23)} = 0.27$	0.792	0.007
MDI	$F_{(1.85, 72.09)} = 0.90$	0.404	0.023
Loudness	$F_{(3, 120)} = 0.49$	0.687	0.012
Uncomfortable	$F_{(3, 120)} = 0.11$	0.954	0.003
Annoyance	$F_{(3, 120)} = 0.36$	0.779	0.009
Ignoring	$F_{(3, 120)} = 0.11$	0.952	0.003
Unpleasant	$F_{(3, 120)} = 1.11$	0.348	0.027
WHO-QoL domain 1	$F_{(2.55, 102)} = 1.40$	0.250	0.034
WHO-QoL domain 2	$F_{(2.1, 83.88)} = 0.22$	0.810	0.006
WHO-QoL domain 3	$F_{(2.57, 102.78)} = 1.20$	0.312	0.029
WHO-QoL domain 4	$F_{(2.52, 100.74)} = 1.90$	0.144	0.045

also showed significantly more NPAD change than patients with neither condition [$M = -1.22$; $SD = 2.77$; $t_{(9.09)} = -3.16$; $p = 0.011$; $d = 1.49$]. There was no significant difference between the group with neither condition and the group with neck pain only [$t_{(13.50)} = 0.55$; $p = 0.593$; $d = 0.22$]. See **Figure 4** for an illustration of the NPAD changes in all three groups. Also, the overall group effect was significant [$F_{(2, 28)} = 15.73$, $p < 0.001$; $eta^2 = 0.022$]: patients without neck pain or somatosensory tinnitus scored lower on the NPAD than the other two patient groups. If the change of the TQ score from baseline to week 2 was analyzed, there was also a significant time*group interaction effect [$F_{(2, 35)} = 5.47$; $p = 0.009$; $eta^2 = 0.238$]. Again, *post-hoc t*-tests of the mean TQ differences from baseline to week 2 (Bonferroni-corrected alpha = 0.016) revealed that the group with both conditions ($M = -5.91$; $SD = 6.64$) was significantly different from the group suffering from neither condition [$M = 2.18$; $SD = 5.53$; $t_{(20)} = -3.11$; $p = 0.006$; $d = 1.32$] and different by trend from the group suffering from neck pain only [$M = -0.69$; $SD = 5.46$; $t_{(25)} = -2.24$; $p = 0.034$; $d = 0.86$]. There was no significant difference between the group with neither condition and the group with neck pain only [$t_{(25)} = -1.34$; $p = 0.194$; $d = 0.52$]. Again, the main effect "group" was significant [$F_{(2,35)} = 3.35$; $p = 0.047$; $eta^2 = 0.028$]: patients without neck pain or somatosensory tinnitus scored lower on the TQ than the other two patient groups. If the TQ changes of all three subgroups were compared over all four measurement time points, the ANOVA revealed no significant time*group interaction effect [$F_{(4.46, 78)} = 1.40$; $p = 0.238$; $eta^2 = 0.074$]. There was no significant main effect of time [$F_{(2.23, 78)} = 0.44$; $p = 666$; $eta^2 = 0.012$] but a significant main effect of group [$F_{(2, 35)} = 3.75$; $p = 0.033$; $eta^2 = 0.177$]. See **Figure 5** for an illustration of the TQ changes in all three groups.

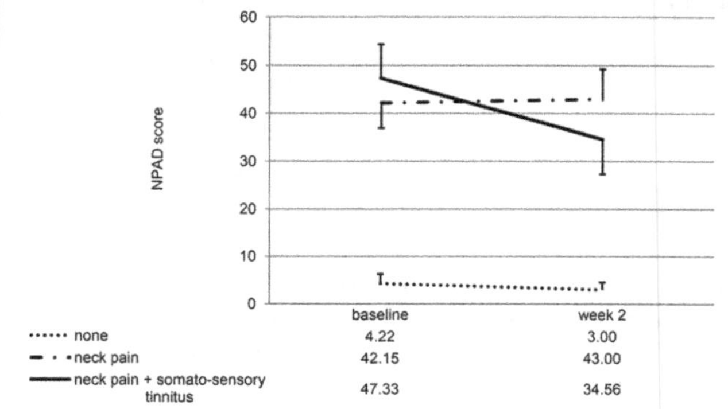

FIGURE 4 | Line chart showing the NPAD score at baseline and week 2 for all three subgroups of patients. Error bars represent standard errors. The NPAD change of patients with both somatosensory tinnitus and neck pain differed significantly from the NPAD change of patients with neither condition. The difference to the change of patients with neck pain only was marginally significant.

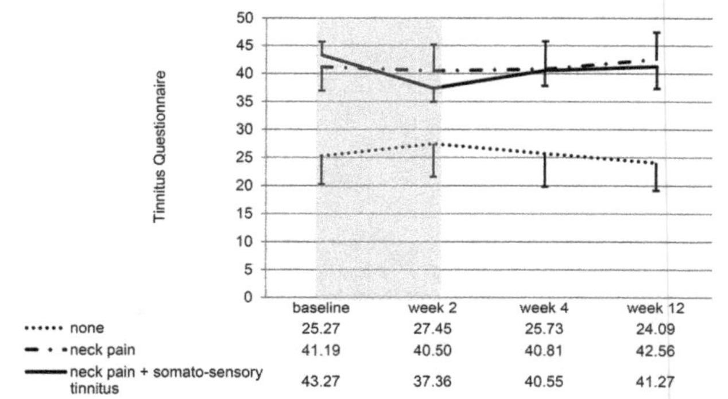

FIGURE 5 | Line chart showing the score at all measurement time points for all three subgroups of patients. Error bars represent standard errors. The 10-day treatment phase is marked in gray color. The TQ change from baseline to week 2 of patients with both somatosensory tinnitus and neck pain differed significantly from the TQ change of patients with neither condition.

DISCUSSION

This is the first study to report combined rTMS and rPMS for the treatment of patients suffering from chronic subjective tinnitus. As it was designed as a pilot study, there are some weaknesses which should be kept in mind when interpreting the results. First, in order to examine the feasibility of the combined treatment, a one-arm trial with no control group was chosen. Second, we chose a well-studied standard rTMS protocol in order to combine it with rPMS treatment. This standard rTMS protocol consisted of left-hemispherical treatment and did not account for tinnitus laterality. The question if and how tinnitus laterality should be considered for the choice of the "right" rTMS treatment protocol has partly been examined for unilateral tinnitus (Khedr et al., 2010) but is still an open question for bilateral tinnitus or tinnitus which is perceived inside the head. A recent study indicates that tinnitus laterality has no association with rTMS response (Lehner et al., 2012). Although important, it was not part of the current study's hypothesis to add to this question. Third, the exploratory analyses were done post-hoc, which means that also the subdivision of patients to the different subgroups was done post-hoc. Therefore, the subgroups were not matched with respect to demographical and clinical characteristics.

It was shown that this treatment approach is feasible in clinical routine. The amount of side effects in the current study is similar to previous results. For example, in Lehner et al. (2016), 12% of the patients treated with triple-site stimulation and 25% of patients treated with standard single-site left temporoparietal stimulation reported transient headaches. In Kreuzer et al. (2015) 16.7% of patients reported headaches after combined left temporoparietal plus left DLPFC stimulation. In the current study, 13% of the patients reported transient, 2.5% ongoing headaches. An increase in tinnitus loudness was reported in 12.5% of the patients treated with single-site stimulation in Lehner et al. (2016), 11.1% in Kreuzer et al. (2015) and in 14.6% of the patients in the current study.

However, there was no significant improvement in tinnitus severity (as measured by the TQ) or neck pain (as measured using the NPAD). This outcome is worse than results of previous studies examining combined frontal plus temporal rTMS stimulation protocols (e.g., Kleinjung et al., 2008; Langguth et al., 2014). One promising approach in increasing treatment effects in chronic tinnitus is the combination of different therapeutic approaches. In tinnitus, several multimodal approaches including rTMS combined with relaxation (Kreuzer et al., 2016), transcranial electric stimulation combined with hearings aids (Shekhawat et al., 2014), tinnitus retraining therapy (Rabau et al., 2015) or tailor-made notched music therapy (Teismann et al., 2014; Lee et al., 2017), vagal nerve stimulation paired with acoustic stimulation (Li et al., 2015) or trigeminal nerve stimulation combined with acoustic stimulation (Hamilton et al., 2016) were introduced. Beside tinnitus other neuropsychiatric disorders were also the focus of combined therapies—for example combined brain stimulation and cognitive training in dementia (Nguyen et al., 2017) or combined brain stimulation and physiotherapy after stroke (Elsner et al., 2017; Salazar et al., 2018). Combination of different neuronal treatments is a challenging task as several open issues have to be resolved. The most important one is the timing or temporal order of both therapies (Padbouj and Padberg, 2014; Martin et al., 2014; Marks et al., 2018). Combining different therapies might not only result in augmentation of effects. Complex interaction effects might also lead to reduced efficacy. The present trial combined rTMS with preceding and succeeding rPMS. This was a pilot study showing the feasibility and efficacy of the combined approach. In this study we found that for the whole group the combined approach had no beneficial effects, neither on neck muscle pain, nor on tinnitus severity. A possible explanation for this result is that the combination of cortical rTMS with rPMS, as it was investigated in this trial, is not synergistic in the overall patient group. Furthermore this combined protocol may act differentially on different subgroups of patients. This is in line with the findings of the exploratory analyses which suggest additive effects, i.e., linear increase of efficacy from the group without additional conditions over the group with neck pain to the group with neck pain and somatosensory tinnitus. Another explanation of course is that TMS is not effective in tinnitus. A recent review article concluded that it is possibly effective (Lefaucheur et al., 2014).

Nonetheless, a reduction of the TQ score of nearly 6 points from baseline to week 2 is rather large as compared to other rTMS studies. For example, Langguth et al. (2014) reported TQ changes of 2 points from baseline to week 2 for left temporal stimulation and of 3.32 points for a combined left temporal plus frontal stimulation. Lehner et al. (2016) reported a difference of 4.59 points in the TQ score from baseline to week 2 for the overall patient group. Up to now, the most effective treatment option for patients suffering from chronic tinnitus is a specialized care treatment protocol as suggested by Cima et al. (2012) where TQ differences of 7.38 points are seen after 3 months and 15.95 points after 12 months. On an individual patient level a reduction of 5 points in the TQ has been identified a minimal clinically important difference (Adamchic et al., 2012). If related to these results, a mean reduction by 6 points seems to be a rather large change which might be worth future research.

Importantly, the subgroups also differed with respect to the treatment outcome concerning neck pain: patients with both neck pain and somatosensory tinnitus improved with respect to the NPAD score while patients with neck pain only did not. All in all, this suggests that tinnitus patients with both conditions might represent a subgroup of patients for which combined rPMS and rTMS might be a promising treatment approach. There are different possible explanations for these findings. There are studies backing the hypothesis that an improvement of muscle tension leads to an improvement of tinnitus severity (Biesinger et al., 2010; Bechter et al., 2016). A recent systematic review has shown that cervical physical therapy is an effective treatment approach for patients with somatosensory tinnitus (Michiels et al., 2016). Furthermore, Marks et al. (2018) reported that a combined auditory-somatosensory treatment was able to reduce tinnitus loudness and severity in patients suffering from somatosensory tinnitus whereas unimodal auditory treatment was not, emphasizing the importance of the somatosensory system in these patients. This bimodal stimulation examined by Marks et al. has been shown to exert its effects via long term depression in the cochlear nucleus. The changes we observed in patients with neck pain and somatosensory tinnitus in our study might be mediated by similar mechanisms. The fact that we observed improvement only in patients with neck pain and somatosensory tinnitus suggests that both altered neuronal input from the neck area and an interaction between the somatosensory system and the tinnitus percept represent a requirement for a beneficial effect of rPMS.

This result emphasizes the relevance of individualized treatment for tinnitus patients. Tinnitus should be understood as a symptom with diverse causes and variable subgroups all of which might benefit from different treatment approaches (Landgrebe et al., 2010). Besides somatic tinnitus (Ward et al., 2015), typewriter tinnitus was defined as a very specific subtype which is responsive to carbamazepine (Levine, 2006). Further subtypes such as trauma-associated tinnitus (Kreuzer et al., 2012) or tinnitus in combination with specific comorbid symptoms such as temporomandibular joint disorders (Vielsmeier et al.,

2011) have been reported. Therefore, bottom-up oriented treatment strategies might be useful for a different group of tinnitus patients than top-down oriented treatment options.

For electromagnetic stimulation, individual differences in the response to different central and peripheral stimulation techniques have already been demonstrated in the past (Vanneste et al., 2011). As brain stimulation effects depend particularly on the excitability state of the stimulated structure (Rossini et al., 2015), individualized treatment might be particularly relevant for treatment with electrical or magnetic stimulation. Moreover the combination of two techniques—such as rPMS plus rTMS—is challenging to explore, as the complexity is increased by additional aspects such as the temporal relationship between peripheral and central stimulation. Consequently, future studies should try to concentrate on subgroup-specific effects of different treatment strategies or, more generally, on individualized treatment programs considering the very specific combination of possible causes and/or tinnitus-related alterations of a particular patient (Kreuzer et al., 2017).

AUTHOR CONTRIBUTIONS

BL and MS conceived the idea of the study. VV, PK, and TP contributed to data acquisition. AL analyzed the data and drafted the manuscript. All authors contributed to the interpretation of the result and revised the manuscript. All authors approved its final version. The authors declare no competing financial interests with respect to the study.

ACKNOWLEDGMENTS

We thank Helene Niebling, Sandra Pfluegl, and Ulrike Stadler for their technical assistance in administering rTMS and rPMS and collecting data.

REFERENCES

Adamchic, I., Tass, P. A., Langguth, B., Hauptmann, C., Koller, M., Schecklmann, M., et al. (2012). Linking the Tinnitus Questionnaire and the subjective Clinical Global Impression: which differences are clinically important? *Health Qual. Life Outcomes* 10:79. doi: 10.1186/1477-7525-10-79

Bajbouj, M., and Padberg, F. (2014). A perfect match: noninvasive brain stimulation and psychotherapy. *Eur. Arch. Psychiatry Clin. Neurosci.* 264(Suppl. 1), S27–S33. doi: 10.1007/s00406-014-0540-6

Bechter, K., Wieland, M., and Hamann, G. F. (2016). Chronic cervicogenic tinnitus rapidly resolved by intermittent use of cervical collar. *Front. Psychiatry* 7:43. doi: 10.3389/fpsyt.2016.00043

Bhatt, J., Ghavami, Y., Lin, H. W., and Djalilian, H. (2015). Cervical spine dysfunctions in patients with chronic subjective tinnitus. *Otol. Neurotol.* 36, 1459–1460. doi: 10.1097/MAO.0000000000000827

Biesinger, E., Kipman, U., Schätz, S., and Langguth, B. (2010). Qigong for the treatment of tinnitus: a prospective randomized controlled study. *J. Psychosom. Res.* 69, 299–304. doi: 10.1016/j.jpsychores.2010.04.013

Cima, R. F., Maes, I. H., Joore, M. A., Scheyen, D. J., El Refaie, A., Baguley, D. M., et al. (2012). Specialised treatment based on cognitive behaviour therapy versus usual care for tinnitus: a randomised controlled trial. *Lancet* 379, 1951–1959. doi: 10.1016/S0140-6736(12)60469-3

Dehmel, S., Cui, Y. L., and Shore, S. E. (2008). Cross-modal interactions of auditory and somatic inputs in the brainstem and midbrain and their imbalance in tinnitus and deafness. *Am. J. Audiol.* 17, S193–209. doi: 10.1044/1059-0889(2008/07-0045)

Dehmel, S., Pradhan, S., Koehler, S., Bledsoe, S., and Shore, S. (2012). Noise overexposure alters long-term somatosensory-auditory processing in the dorsal cochlear nucleus–possible basis for tinnitus-related hyperactivity? *J. Neurosci.* 32, 1660–1671. doi: 10.1523/JNEUROSCI.4608-11.2012

Dobie, R. A. (1999). A review of randomized clinical trials in tinnitus. *Laryngoscope* 109, 1202–1211. doi: 10.1097/00005537-199908000-00004

Elgoyhen, A. B., Langguth, B., De Ridder, D., and Vanneste, S. (2015). Tinnitus: perspectives from human neuroimaging. *Nat. Rev. Neurosci.* 16, 632–642. doi: 10.1038/nrn4003

Elsner, B., Kwakkel, G., Kugler, J., and Mehrholz, J. (2017). Transcranial direct current stimulation (tDCS) for improving capacity in activities and arm function after stroke: a network meta-analysis of randomised controlled trials. *J. Neuroeng. Rehabil.* 14:95. doi: 10.1186/s12984-017-0301-7

Ghodratitoostani, I., Zana, Y., Delbem, A. C., Sani, S. S., Ekhtiari, H., and Sanchez, T. G. (2016). Theoretical tinnitus framework: a neurofunctional model. *Front. Neurosci.* 10:370. doi: 10.3389/fnins.2016.00370

Goebel, G., and Hiller, W. (1994). [The tinnitus questionnaire. A standard instrument for grading the degree of tinnitus. Results of a multicenter study with the tinnitus questionnaire]. *HNO* 42, 166–172.

Hamilton, C., D'Arcy, S., Pearlmutter, B. A., Crispino, G., Lalor, E. C., and Conlon, B. J. (2016). An investigation of feasibility and safety of bi-modal stimulation for the treatment of tinnitus: an open-label pilot study. *Neuromodulation* 19, 832–837. doi: 10.1111/ner.12452

Khedr, E. M., Abo-Elfetoh, N., Rothwell, J. C., El-Atar, A., Sayed, E., and Khalifa, H. (2010). Contralateral versus ipsilateral rTMS of temporoparietal cortex for the treatment of chronic unilateral tinnitus: comparative study. *Eur. J. Neurol.* 17, 976–983. doi: 10.1111/j.1468-1331.2010.02965.x

Kleinjung, T., Eichhammer, P., Landgrebe, M., Sand, P., Hajak, G., Steffens, T., et al. (2008). Combined temporal and prefrontal transcranial magnetic stimulation for tinnitus treatment: a pilot study. *Otolaryngol. Head Neck Surg.* 138, 497–501. doi: 10.1016/j.otohns.2007.12.022

Kreuzer, P. M., Landgrebe, M., Schecklmann, M., Poeppl, T. B., Vielsmeier, V., Hajak, G., et al. (2011). Can temporal repetitive transcranial magnetic stimulation be enhanced by targeting affective components of tinnitus with frontal rTMS? A randomized controlled pilot trial. *Front. Syst. Neurosci.* 5:88. doi: 10.3389/fnsys.2011.00088

Kreuzer, P. M., Landgrebe, M., Schecklmann, M., Staudinger, S., and Langguth, B. (2012). Trauma-associated tinnitus: audiological, demographic and clinical characteristics. *PLoS ONE* 7:e45599. doi: 10.1371/journal.pone.0045599

Kreuzer, P. M., Lehner, A., Schlee, W., Vielsmeier, V., Schecklmann, M., Poeppl, T. B., et al. (2015). Combined rTMS treatment targeting the anterior cingulate and the temporal cortex for the treatment of chronic tinnitus. *Sci. Rep.* 5:18028. doi: 10.1038/srep18028

Kreuzer, P. M., Poeppl, T. B., Bulla, J., Schlee, W., Lehner, A., Langguth, B., et al. (2016). A proof-of-concept study on the combination of repetitive transcranial magnetic stimulation and relaxation techniques in chronic tinnitus. *J. Neural Transm. (Vienna).* 123, 1147–1157. doi: 10.1007/s00702-016-1588-4

Kreuzer, P. M., Poeppl, T. B., Rupprecht, R., Vielsmeier, V., Lehner, A., Langguth, B., et al. (2017). Individualized repetitive transcranial magnetic stimulation treatment in chronic tinnitus? *Front. Neurol.* 8:126. doi: 10.3389/fneur.2017.00126

Landgrebe, M., Azevedo, A., Baguley, D., Bauer, C., Cacace, A., Coelho, C., et al. (2012). Methodological aspects of clinical trials in tinnitus: a proposal for an international standard. *J. Psychosom. Res.* 73, 112–121. doi: 10.1016/j.jpsychores.2012.05.002

Landgrebe, M., Zeman, F., Koller, M., Eberl, Y., Mohr, M., Reiter, J., et al. (2010). The Tinnitus Research Initiative (TRI) database: a new approach for delineation of tinnitus subtypes and generation of predictors for treatment outcome. *BMC Med. Inform. Decis. Mak.* 10:42. doi: 10.1186/1472-6947-10-42

Langguth, B., and De Ridder, D. (2013). Tinnitus: therapeutic use of superficial brain stimulation. *Handb. Clin. Neurol.*, 116, 441–467. doi: 10.1016/B978-0-444-53497-2.00036-X

Langguth, B., Goodey, R., Azevedo, A., Bjorne, A., Cacace, A., Crocetti, A., et al. (2007). Consensus for tinnitus patient assessment and treatment outcome measurement: tinnitus research initiative meeting, Regensburg, July 2006. *Prog. Brain Res.* 166, 525–536. doi: 10.1016/S0079-6123(07)66050-6

Langguth, B., Landgrebe, M., Frank, E., Schecklmann, M., Sand, P. G., Vielsmeier, V., et al. (2014). Efficacy of different protocols of transcranial magnetic stimulation for the treatment of tinnitus: pooled analysis of two randomized controlled studies. *World J. Biol. Psychiatry* 15, 276–285. doi: 10.3109/15622975.2012.708438

Lee, H. Y., Choi, M. S., Chang, D. S., and Cho, C. S. (2017). Combined bifrontal transcranial direct current stimulation and tailor-made notched music training in chronic tinnitus. *J. Audiol. Otol.* 21, 22–27. doi: 10.7874/jao.2017.21.1.22

Lefaucheur, J. P., André-Obadia, N., Antal, A., Ayache, S. S., Baeken, C., Benninger, D. H., et al. (2014). Evidence-based guidelines on the therapeutic use of repetitive transcranial magnetic stimulation (rTMS). *Clin. Neurophysiol.* 125, 2150–2206. doi: 10.1016/j.clinph.2014.05.021

Lehner, A., Schecklmann, M., Greenlee, M. W., Rupprecht, R., and Langguth, B. (2016). Triple-site rTMS for the treatment of chronic tinnitus: a randomized controlled trial. *Sci. Rep.* 6:22302. doi: 10.1038/srep22302

Lehner, A., Schecklmann, M., Kreuzer, P. M., Poeppl, T. B., Rupprecht, R., and Langguth, B. (2013). Comparing single-site with multisite rTMS for the treatment of chronic tinnitus - clinical effects and neuroscientific insights: study protocol for a randomized controlled trial. *Trials* 14:269. doi: 10.1186/1745-6215-14-269

Lehner, A., Schecklmann, M., Landgrebe, M., Kreuzer, P. M., Poeppl, T. B., Frank, E., et al. (2012). Predictors for rTMS response in chronic tinnitus. *Front. Syst. Neurosci.* 6:11. doi: 10.3389/fnsys.2012.00011

Levine, R. A. (2006). Typewriter tinnitus: a carbamazepine-responsive syndrome related to auditory nerve vascular compression. *ORL J. Otorhinolaryngol. Relat. Spec.* 68, 43–46; discussion: 46–47. doi: 10.1159/000090490

Levine, R. A., Nam, E. C., Oron, Y., and Melcher, J. R. (2007). Evidence for a tinnitus subgroup responsive to somatosensory based treatment modalities. *Prog. Brain Res.* 166, 195–207. doi: 10.1016/S0079-6123(07)66017-8

Li, T. T., Wang, Z. J., Yang, S. B., Zhu, J. H., Zhang, S. Z., Cai, S. J., et al. (2015). Transcutaneous electrical stimulation at auricular acupoints innervated by auricular branch of vagus nerve pairing tone for tinnitus: study protocol for a randomized controlled clinical trial. *Trials* 16:101. doi: 10.1186/s13063-015-0630-4

Markovitz, C. D., Smith, B. T., Gloeckner, C. D., and Lim, H. H. (2015). Investigating a new neuromodulation treatment for brain disorders using synchronized activation of multimodal pathways. *Sci. Rep.* 5:9462. doi: 10.1038/srep09462

Marks, K. L., Martel, D. T., Wu, C., Basura, G. J., Roberts, L. E., Schvartz-Leyzac, K. C., et al. (2018). Auditory-somatosensory bimodal stimulation desynchronizes brain circuitry to reduce tinnitus in guinea pigs and humans. *Sci. Transl. Med.* 10:eaal3175. doi: 10.1126/scitranslmed.aal3175

Martin, D. M., Liu, R., Alonzo, A., Green, M., and Loo, C. K. (2014). Use of transcranial direct current stimulation (tDCS) to enhance cognitive training: effect of timing of stimulation. *Exp. Brain Res.* 232, 3345–3351. doi: 10.1007/s00221-014-4022-x

Mauchly, J. W. (1940). Significance test for sphericity of a normal n-variate distribution. *Ann. Math. Statist.* 11, 204–209. doi: 10.1214/aoms/1177731915

McKenna, L., Handscomb, L., Hoare, D. J., and Hall, D. A. (2014). A scientific cognitive-behavioral model of tinnitus: novel conceptualizations of tinnitus distress. *Front. Neurol.* 5:196. doi: 10.3389/fneur.2014.00196

Michiels, S., De Hertogh, W., Truijen, S., and Van de Heyning, P. (2015). Cervical spine dysfunctions in patients with chronic subjective tinnitus. *Otol. Neurotol.* 36, 741–745. doi: 10.1097/MAO.0000000000000670

Michiels, S., Van de Heyning, P., Truijen, S., Hallemans, A., and De Hertogh, W. (2016). Does multi-modal cervical physical therapy improve tinnitus in patients with cervicogenic somatic tinnitus? *Man. Ther.* 26, 125–131. doi: 10.1016/j.math.2016.08.005

Newman, C. W., Jacobson, G. P., and Spitzer, J. B. (1996). Development of the Tinnitus Handicap Inventory. *Arch. Otolaryngol. Head Neck Surg.* 122, 143–148. doi: 10.1001/archotol.1996.01890140029007

Nguyen, J. P., Suarez, A., Kemoun, G., Meignier, M., Le Saout, E., Damier, P., et al. (2017). Repetitive transcranial magnetic stimulation combined with cognitive training for the treatment of Alzheimer's disease. *Neurophysiol. Clin.* 47, 47–53. doi: 10.1016/j.neucli.2017.01.001

Rabau, S., Van Rompaey, V., and Van de Heyning, P. (2015). The effect of Transcranial Direct Current Stimulation in addition to Tinnitus Retraining Therapy for treatment of chronic tinnitus patients: a study protocol for a double-blind controlled randomised trial. *Trials* 16:514. doi: 10.1186/s13063-015-1041-2

Rocha, C. B., and Sanchez, T. G. (2012). Efficacy of myofascial trigger point deactivation for tinnitus control. *Braz. J. Otorhinolaryngol.* 78, 21–26. doi: 10.5935/1808-8694.20120028

Rossini, P. M., Burke, D., Chen, R., Cohen, L. G., Daskalakis, Z., Di Iorio, R., et al. (2015). Non-invasive electrical and magnetic stimulation of the brain, spinal cord, roots and peripheral nerves: Basic principles and procedures for routine clinical and research application. An updated report from an I.F.C.N. Committee. *Clin. Neurophysiol.* 126, 1071–1107. doi: 10.1016/j.clinph.2015.02.001

Salazar, A. P. S., Vaz, P. G., Marchese, R. R., Stein, C., Pinto, C., and Pagnussat, A. S. (2018). Noninvasive brain stimulation improves hemispatial neglect after stroke: a systematic review and meta-analysis. *Arch. Phys. Med. Rehabil.* 99, 355–366. doi: 10.1016/j.apmr.2017.07.009

Sanchez, T. G., and Rocha, C. B. (2011). Diagnosis and management of somatosensory tinnitus: review article. *Clinics (Sao Paulo)* 66, 1089–1094. doi: 10.1590/S1807-59322011000600028

Schecklmann, M., Giani, A., Tupak, S., Langguth, B., Raab, V., Polak, T., et al. (2016). Neuronavigated left temporal continuous theta burst stimulation in chronic tinnitus. *Restor. Neurol. Neurosci.* 34, 165–175. doi: 10.3233/RNN-150518

Scherer, M., Blozik, E., Himmel, W., Laptinskaya, D., Kochen, M. M., and Herrmann-Lingen, C. (2008). Psychometric properties of a German version of the neck pain and disability scale. *Eur. Spine J.* 17, 922–929. doi: 10.1007/s00586-008-0677-y

Schlee, W., Hartmann, T., Langguth, B., and Weisz, N. (2009). Abnormal resting-state cortical coupling in chronic tinnitus. *BMC Neurosci.* 10:11. doi: 10.1186/1471-2202-10-11

Schmidt, S. A., Akrofi, K., Carpenter-Thompson, J. R., and Husain, F. T. (2013). Default mode, dorsal attention and auditory resting state networks exhibit differential functional connectivity in tinnitus and hearing loss. *PLoS ONE* 8:e76488. doi: 10.1371/journal.pone.0076488

Shekhawat, G. S., Kobayashi, K., and Searchfield, G. D. (2015). Methodology for studying the transient effects of transcranial direct current stimulation combined with auditory residual inhibition on tinnitus. *J. Neurosci. Methods* 239, 28–33. doi: 10.1016/j.jneumeth.2014.09.025

Shekhawat, G. S., Searchfield, G. D., and Stinear, C. M. (2014). Randomized trial of transcranial direct current stimulation and hearing aids for tinnitus management. *Neurorehabil. Neural Repair* 28, 410–419. doi: 10.1177/1545968313508655

Shore, S. E., Roberts, L. E., and Langguth, B. (2016). Maladaptive plasticity in tinnitus–triggers, mechanisms and treatment. *Nat. Rev. Neurol.* 12, 150–160. doi: 10.1038/nrneurol.2016.12

Shore, S. E., and Zhou, J. (2006). Somatosensory influence on the cochlear nucleus and beyond. *Hear. Res.* 216-217, 90–99. doi: 10.1016/j.heares.2006.01.006

Smania, N., Corato, E., Fiaschi, A., Pietropoli, P., Aglioti, S. M., and Tinazzi, M. (2003). Therapeutic effects of peripheral repetitive magnetic stimulation on myofascial pain syndrome. *Clin. Neurophysiol.* 114, 350–358. doi: 10.1016/S1388-2457(02)00367-X

Smania, N., Corato, E., Fiaschi, A., Pietropoli, P. Aglioti, S. M., and Tinazzi, M. (2005). Repetitive magnetic stimulation: a novel therapeutic approach for myofascial pain syndrome. *J. Neurol.* 252, 307–314. doi: 10.1007/s00415-005-0642-1

Sollmann, N., Trepte-Freisleder, F., Albers, L., Jung, N. H., Mall, V., Meyer, B., et al. (2016). Magnetic stimulation of the upper trapezius muscles in patients with migraine - A pilot study. *Eur. J. Paediatr. Neurol.* 20, 888–897. doi: 10.1016/j.ejpn.2016.07.022

Speer, A. M., Kimbrell, T. A., Wassermann, E. M., D Repella, J., Willis, M. W., Herscovitch, P., et al. (2000). Opposite effects of high and low frequency rTMS on regional brain activity in depressed patients. *Biol. Psychiatry* 48, 1133–1141. doi: 10.1016/S0006-3223(00)01065-9

Teismann, H., Wollbrink, A., Okamoto, H., Schlaug, G., Rudack, C., and Pantev, C. (2014). Combining transcranial direct current stimulation and tailor-made notched music training to decrease tinnitus-related distress–a pilot study. *PLoS ONE* 9:e89904. doi: 10.1371/journal.pone.0089904

Theodoroff, S. M., and Folmer, R. L. (2013). Repetitive transcranial magnetic stimulation as a treatment for chronic tinnitus: a critical review. *Otol. Neurotol.* 34, 199–208. doi: 10.1097/MAO.0b013e31827b4d46

Vanneste, S., Langguth, B., and De Ridder, D. (2011). Do tDCS and TMS influence tinnitus transiently via a direct cortical and indirect somatosensory modulating effect? A combined TMS-tDCS and TENS study. *Brain Stimul.* 4, 242–252. doi: 10.1016/j.brs.2010.12.001

Vanneste, S., Plazier, M., vander Loo, V., de Heyning, P. V., Congedo, M., and De Ridder, D. (2010). The neural correlates of tinnitus-related distress. *Neuroimage* 52, 470–480. doi: 10.1016/j.neuroimage.2010.04.029

Vielsmeier, V., Kleinjung, T., Strutz, J., Bürgers, R., Kreuzer, P. M., and Langguth, B. (2011). Tinnitus with temporomandibular joint disorders: a specific entity of tinnitus patients? *Otolaryngol. Head Neck Surg.* 145, 748–752. doi: 10.1177/0194599811413376

Ward, J., Vella, C., Hoare, D. J., and Hall, D. A. (2015). Subtyping somatic tinnitus: a cross-sectional UK cohort study of demographic, clinical and audiological characteristics. *PLoS ONE* 10:e0126254. doi: 10.1371/journal.pone.0126254

Zunhammer, M., Busch, V., Griesbach, F., Landgrebe, M., Hajak, G., and Langguth, B. (2011). rTMS over the cerebellum modulates temperature detection and pain thresholds through peripheral mechanisms. *Brain Stimul.* 4, 210–217 e211. doi: 10.1016/j.brs.2010.11.002

3

Tinnitus Treatment with Oxytocin

Andreia Aparecida Azevedo[1], Ricardo Rodrigues Figueiredo[2], Ana Belen Elgoyhen[3,4], Berthold Langguth[5], Norma De Oliveira Penido[1] and Winfried Schlee[5]*

[1] Universidade Federal de São Paulo, São Paulo, Brazil, [2] Faculdade de Medicina de Valença, Valença, Brazil, [3] Instituto de Investigaciones en Ingeniería Genética y Biología Molecular "Dr. Héctor N. Torres", CONICET, Buenos Aires, Argentina, [4] Facultad de Medicina, Instituto de Farmacología, Universidad de Buenos Aires (UBA), Buenos Aires, Argentina, [5] Department of Psychiatry and Psychotherapy, University of Regensburg, Regensburg, Germany

***Correspondence:**
Ricardo Rodrigues Figueiredo
rfigueiredo@otosul.com.br

Introduction: Tinnitus is the perception of sound in the absence of an external stimulus. It is a frequent condition for which there is as yet no pharmacological treatment approved. Auditory and non-auditory pathways are involved in tinnitus' pathophysiology. Oxytocin is a neurohormone and eventual neurotransmitter that plays a complex role in social cognition and behavior.

Objective: To evaluate the potential of oxytocin as a tinnitus treatment.

Study design: Two studies were performed. Study 1 was a long-term open pilot study, while study 2 investigated short-term effects with a double-blinded placebo-controlled cross-over study.

Setting: Ambulatory ENT care.

Subjects and method: In study 1, 15 patients were investigated over a 10-week period in an open pilot study. In study 2, 16 patients were included in a placebo-controlled crossover trial to investigate short-term effects following a single dose.

Results: For the long-term study (study 1), analysis of variance revealed a significant decrease in tinnitus sensation, both for the Tinnitus Handicap Inventory and Clinical Global Impression (CGI). Also, the short-term effects in study 2 revealed a significant reduction of tinnitus because of the oxytocin nasal spray as measured with the Visual Analog Scale and the CGI Scale.

Conclusion: These preliminary studies demonstrated that oxytocin may represent a helpful tool for treating tinnitus and further larger controlled studies are warranted.

Keywords: tinnitus, oxytocin, hearing disorders, pharmacotherapy, nasal sprays

INTRODUCTION

Tinnitus is a phantom auditory sensation that is not generated by an external stimulus. It is a symptom that affects about 25% of American adults, in a frequent basis for around 8% of them (1). According to current trends of thoughts, tinnitus is a central nervous system phenomenon that follows an initial peripheral damage and may be modulated by many concurring neuronal circuits (2). Neuroimaging studies suggest that tinnitus results from the dynamic interaction between auditory and non-auditory pathways, and the result of this interaction, especially when the limbic and autonomous systems are involved, is the trigger of negative emotional associations and appearance of uncomfortable reactions (3). As yet, there is no Food and Drug Administration (FDA)-approved pharmacological treatment for tinnitus. However, various factors structures such as ion channels, neurotransmitters, and receptors have been proposed to be involved in tinnitus pathophysiology (4). Thus, there is no reasonable argument to believe that tinnitus could not be pharmacologically treated (5).

Oxytocin is a neurohormone that may also act as a neurotransmitter, produced by magnocellular neurons in the ventricular nuclei of the hypothalamus (6). Oxytocin's production is stimulated by high estrogen doses and inhibited by high doses of catecholamines (dopamine, epinephrine, and norepinephrine) (7). It is released to the bloodstream by the posterior pituitary. Oxytocin receptors (OTR) are widespread throughout the human body and belong to the family of heterotrimeric G-protein-coupled receptors, which are found in many cell types (8). OTR promote the inhibition of adenilate-cyclase, thus reducing intracellular levels of cyclic-AMP and subsequently opening potassium channels and closing calcium channels, having, thereby, an inhibitory signature (9).

Oxytocin is responsible for important physiological functions, such as uterine contraction, lactation stimulation, sperm transport, and ejaculation (10). In addition, oxytocin plays a complex role in social cognition and behavior. Important aspects of human social interaction such as empathy, trust, and social learning are influenced by oxytocin (11). Among other mechanisms the prosocial effects of oxytocin are mediated by reduction of amygdale activation (12). Recently, it has been shown, that oxytocin also increases the salience of acoustic social stimuli by modulating the inhibitory function in the auditory cortex (13).

Imaging studies have demonstrated that tinnitus loudness and tinnitus distress are reflected by increased activation in networks involving the auditory cortex and the amygdala, respectively (3, 14). Therefore, we hypothesized that oxytocin may influence tinnitus perception and tested in two studies whether its intranasal application reduces tinnitus loudness and distress.

MATERIALS AND METHODS

The trial comprised 2 studies, as follows.

Study 1

Study Design

Study 1 was designed as an open pilot study.

Subjects

Fifteen patients who presented with the primary complaint of tinnitus in a local ENT clinic in São Paulo and Valença were included. Only patients older than 18 years with a continuous perception of tinnitus of at least 6 months duration were included. Patients were excluded if their Tinnitus Handicap Inventory (THI) (15) score in the Brazilian Portuguese validated version (16) was below 16 points. All patients underwent a complete otolaryngological evaluation and were excluded from the study in case of external or media otitis or in the presence of A-s, B, and C tympanogram curves. Also, women in fertile age [up to 49 years old (17)] were excluded from the study, to avoid oxytocin-induced uterine contractions. Informed consent was obtained prior to the study, and the patients were informed about the clinical procedures. Clinical and demographic characteristics of participants (mean age, percentage of females, mean duration of tinnitus in months, laterality and scores on the THI in both studies) are described in **Table 1**.

Experimental Procedure

Oxytocin (Syntocinon) was administered daily for a duration of 10 weeks. Patients were instructed to apply one puff [each puff corresponds to 4 oxytocin IU] of oxytocin in each nostril two times a day, which sums up to a dosage of 16 IU per day. The patients were asked to store the oxytocin in the refrigerator throughout the study period. Subsequent visits were made in weeks 1, 2, 3, 4, 6, 8, and 10 to monitor study progress and screen for side effects. Treatment effects were assessed with the THI (primary outcome measurement) and the Clinical Global Impression (CGI) scale improvement [secondary outcome measurement; CGI-I (18)]. The CGI scale is a well-accepted instrument in clinical research for evaluating the clinical improvement retrospectively. The instruction in the CGI is: "Please rate the total improvement of your tinnitus complaints compared to before beginning of treatment."

Statistical Analysis

For the THI, a mixed model analysis of variance (ANOVA) was calculated with the factor time and a random intercept per patient. A mixed model ANOVA was also calculated for the CGI with the factor time (weeks 1–10) and a random intercept per patient. In case of positive results of the ANOVA further comparisons were calculated.

Study 2

During study 1, five subjects reported an immediate effect (5–10 min after drug administration) on tinnitus sensation (around 50% reduction of tinnitus volume). Considering this unexpected finding, we decided to investigate this tinnitus reduction following one single dose in more detail. Therefore, we performed a second study with a single dose of oxytocin treatment in a double-blind placebo-controlled study using a crossover design. As study 1 turned out with positive results, study 2 was performed with a similar number of patients.

TABLE 1 | Patient groups, clinical and demographic data (mean ± SD).

n	Age	Female (%)	Duration of tinnitus in months	Laterality	THI at baseline
Study 1 (*n* = 15)	60.6 ± 9.6	40	107.8 ± 118.7	5 unilateral 7 bilateral 3 in head	56.8 ± 28.2
Study 2 (*n* = 16)	62.8 ± 10.6	31.3	78.8 ± 147.9	11 unilateral 5 bilateral	52.8 ± 30.5

THI, Tinnitus Handicap Inventory.

Subjects

Study 2 was performed in the same ENT clinic as study 1. Seventeen patients with the primary complaint of tinnitus and who had not participated in study 1 were included.

As in the first study, all patients were older than 18 years and reported chronic tinnitus of more than 6 months duration. Prior to the study, all patients were seen by an experienced ENT doctor. Patients with vascular or muscular origin of their tinnitus, patients with conductive hearing loss and patients with regular intake of other medications during the study period were not included. Patients reporting previous experience with oxytocin nasal spray were not included as well. A further inclusion criterion was a tinnitus loudness rating of at least 4, measured on a scale between 0 and 10.

One patient dropped out of the study because she could not return for the second visit. Clinical and demographic characteristics of the 16 patients, which were included in the analysis, are displayed in **Table 1**. Informed consent was obtained prior to study participation.

Experimental Procedure

In study 2, the effects of nasal oxytocin administration were compared with placebo treatment. The order of drug treatment was counterbalanced. Patients were randomized to receive either a single dosage administration of 16 IU of oxytocin (Syntocinon) or a placebo treatment with a nasal spray containing distilled water, which is indistinguishable to oxytocin nasal spray considering smell and taste. A randomization table was created prior to study start by Winfried Schlee who is not in contact with the study participants. After an interval of 1 week, the patients received a second administration with either placebo (the group who received oxytocin first) or with oxytocin (the group who received placebo first). The patients, as well as the medical doctor who evaluated the results (author 1), were blinded to the treatment assignment. Author 2, who applied oxytocin and placebo, was not blinded. In the oxytocin condition, patients received two puffs of oxytocin in each nostril, which corresponded to 16 IU. Likewise, in the placebo treatment, the patients received two puffs distilled water in each nostril, which is supposed to have no clinical effect.

The primary outcome measurement was a visual analog scale (VAS) asking for the tinnitus loudness (19). The VAS score for tinnitus loudness was assessed directly before administering the nasal spray as well as 30 min and 24 h after the intervention. Additionally, the CGI-I was applied 30 min and 24 h after the intervention as secondary outcome measurement.

Statistical Analysis

For the VAS scores a two-way mixed model ANOVA was calculated with the factors *time* and *treatment*. A random intercept was modeled for each participant. Mixed model ANOVA were also used to analyze the results of the CGI scale. For the CGI scores, again a two-way mixed model ANOVA was calculated with the factors *time* and *treatment*.

The statistical analysis was performed with the statistical software package R, version 3.3.3 [R Core Team (2017). R: a language and environment for statistical computing. R Foundation for Statistical Computing, Vienna, Austria. URL https://www.R-project.org/]. For the mixed models analysis, the "nlme" library (version 3.1-131) was used. A p-value ≤ 0.05 was considered as significant. Correction for multiple comparisons was applied using the stepwise Holm–Bonferroni method (20).

Study Registration

The study was approved by the ethics committee and registered at http://clinicaltrials.gov.

RESULTS

Study 1

Mean scores for the THI and the CGI-I are presented in **Figures 1** and **2**, respectively. Both measures show continuous and significant decreases of tinnitus-related symptoms measured with the THI [$F(7,98) = 7.45$, $p < 0.0001$] as well as global clinical improvement (CGI-I) [$F(6,84) = 5.22$, $p < 0.0001$] over the study period.

For the THI scores, further comparisons using paired t-tests between baseline and all other time points reveal significant differences for the THI measurements at week 1, 2, 3, 4, 6, 8, and 10 (p-values of all comparisons survived the Holm–Bonferroni method for multiple comparisons).

For the CGI-I additional tests were calculated to test if scores were different from the value of 4, which indicates "no change." No significant difference was found for week 1, week 2, and week 3. The comparisons for week 4, 6, 8, and 10; however, survived the Holm–Bonferroni correction for multiple comparisons. For week 4 and 6, the CGI scores indicated a change with high significance ($p < 0.01$), for week 8 and 10, the CGI scores indicated a change with very high significance ($p < 0.001$).

Paired t-tests were calculated to compare the maximum hearing loss of the participants before and after the treatment. The hearing function did not change significantly, neither for the right ear ($p = 0.2$) nor for the left ear ($p = 0.36$).

Study 2

Mean scores of the oxytocin treatment and the placebo intervention are presented in **Figures 3** and **4** for the VAS scores and the CGI-I, respectively.

In the ANOVA for the VAS scores, the main effect of *treatment* was highly significant [$F(1,77) = 9.54$, $p = 0.003$] and the main effect of *time* was significant [$F(2,77) = 4.47$, $p = 0.015$]. The interaction effect *time* × *treatment*, however, failed to reach the level of significance [$F(2,77) = 1.13$, $p = 0.33$]. Cohen's d effect sizes for the VAS ratings were 0.55 (30 min) and 0.56 (24 h) for oxytocin treatment and 0.18 (30 min) and 0.19 (24 h) for placebo treatment, respectively.

Furthermore, the ANOVA using the CGI scores as dependent variable, the main effect *treatment* was highly significant [$F(1,46) = 8.72$, $p = 0.005$], while the main effect *time* did not reach statistical significance [$F(1,46) = 0.60$, $p = 0.44$]. There was no statistically significant interaction effect [$F(1,45) = 0.001$, $p > 0.9$]. Additional t-tests were calculated to confirm the results and showed that there was no statistical significant difference between the two time points (30 m and 24 h after treatment) for the oxytocin ($p > 0.63$) nor for the placebo condition ($p > 0.58$). A t-test testing

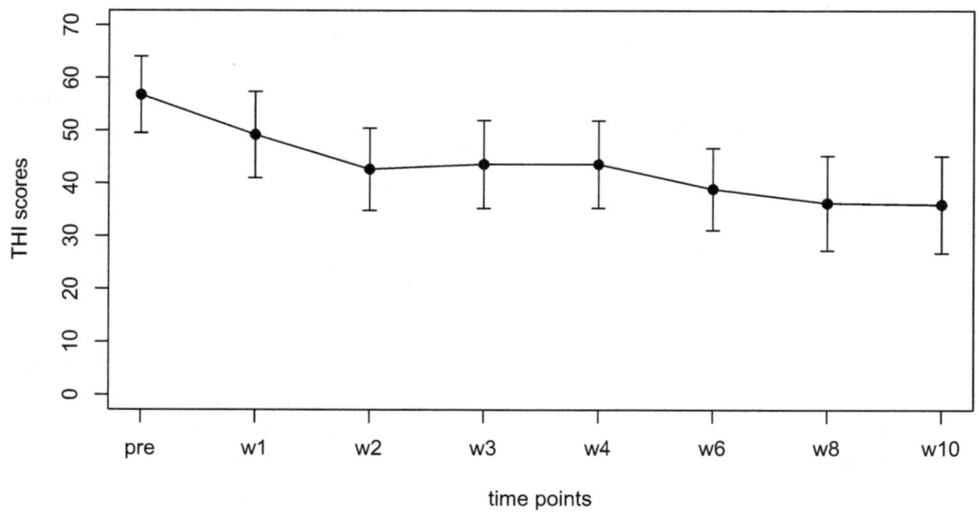

FIGURE 1 | Average scores of the Tinnitus Handicap Inventory (THI) (0–100) before the treatment and at all visits during the study (weeks 1–8). The final assessment was done at the end of treatment in week 10.

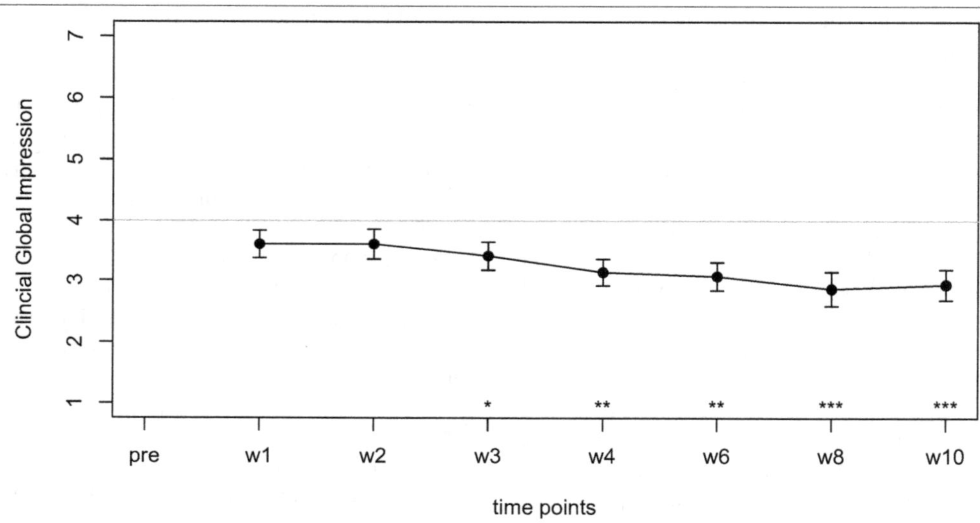

FIGURE 2 | Average scores of the Clinical Global Impression scale (1–7). A rating of 4 on this scale indicates "no change." Smaller numbers indicate an improvement of clinical symptoms (1 = "very much better," 2 = "much better," 3 = "minimally better").

for the difference between the oxytocin and placebo intervention, irrespective of the time point, revealed a statistically significant improvement for the oxytocin treatment ($t = -2.9, p = 0.005$).

DISCUSSION

The present results show that in an exploratory non-controlled study, a 10-week treatment with daily intranasal puffs of oxytocin produced a significant reduction in the THI and CGI in a group of tinnitus patients. Moreover, a double-blind controlled study with a single dose of an intranasal oxytocin, although not significant, exhibited a tendency in a reduction in tinnitus distress, as measured by the CGI.

The presented pilot studies were designed to explore possible effects of oxytocin on tinnitus. The open 10 week treatment study (study 1) suggests that regular intake of oxytocin can reduce tinnitus-related handicap. Open pilot studies have been suggested as a useful screening tool to identify potentially promising pharmacological compounds (21–23). Motivated by the promising results of study 1, we performed also a placebo-controlled crossover trial to investigate the short-term effects of a single dose of oxytocin. Whereas questionnaires represent the gold standard for assessing longer lasting effects of therapeutic interventions (24), short-term effects can be best detected with VAS. While the clinical effects of the short-term oxytocin treatment are much smaller than the long-term effects in study 1, they still suggest

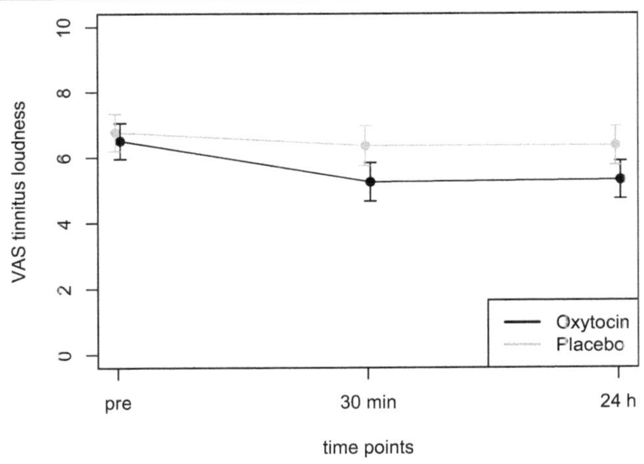

FIGURE 3 | Average scores of the Visual Analogue Scale (0–10) before the treatment and at two time points after the intervention (30 min and 24 h after).

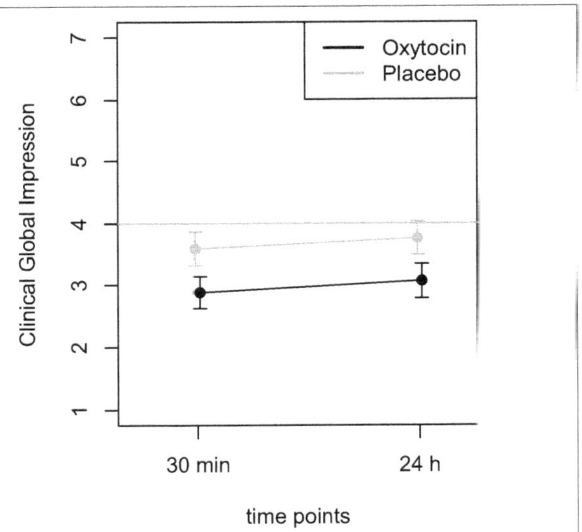

FIGURE 4 | Average scores of the Clinical Global Impression scale (1–7). A rating of 4 on this scale indicates "no change." Smaller numbers indicate an improvement of clinical symptoms (1 = "very much better," 2 = "much better," 3 = "minimally better").

a potential therapeutic role of oxytocin for tinnitus. These preliminary results warrant further controlled studies, which should include more patients and investigate chronic treatments with oxytocin. The results of the presented pilot studies provide an estimation of the effect sizes for both acute and long-term effects of oxytocin to inform the study design of future randomized controlled studies. While the open study with the long-term treatment (study 1) revealed a strong reduction of tinnitus-related distress over time, the short-term treatment (study 2) revealed only small differences between placebo and oxytocin. Further studies on oxytocin treatment for tinnitus should invest in long-term treatment.

A wide variety of compounds are used off-label to treat tinnitus patients (5, 25). However, there is still no US FDA- or European Medicines Agency-approved drug on the market for this clinical unmet use (5). The comprehensive list of compounds includes almost the entire pharmacopeia arsenal, such as anxiolytics, anticonvulsants, antidepressants, *N*-methyl D-aspartate (NMDA) antagonists, cholinergic antagonists, antihistamines, vasodilators, antipsychotics, sodium and calcium channel antagonists, antidiuretics, and herbal medicines, among others (5, 25). In most cases, the pharmacological treatment is used to treat comorbidities which accompany tinnitus, such as frustration, annoyance, anxiety, depression, irritation, concentration difficulties, and sleep disturbances which are most relevant for the perceived tinnitus severity (5, 19). In this context, the exploratory use of oxytocin on tinnitus patients is well justified, since it is a compound with a different mechanism of action from those previously tested.

In particular, Kirsch et al. have shown that when compared with placebo, oxytocin potently reduces activation of the amygdala and coupling of the amygdala to brainstem regions implicated in autonomic and behavioral manifestations of fear (26). In this regard, tinnitus neuroimaging techniques have identified brain networks related to tinnitus associated distress which include the amygdala and the autonomic nervous system (3). Recently, it has been shown that tinnitus distress correlates with enhanced effective connectivity from the amygdala to the auditory cortex (27). An EEG analysis revealed that tinnitus distress is correlated with more synchronized alpha activity in various emotion-related areas, including the subcallosal anterior cingulate cortex, the insula, the parahippocampal area and the amygdale (28). In addition, an MEG functional connectivity analysis has shown long-range coupling between frontal, parietal and cingulate brain areas in alpha and gamma phase synchronization related to tinnitus distress (29). In summary, tinnitus distress has been related to the co-activation of a network which includes amygdala, anterior cingulate cortex, insula, parahippocampal area and which is under direct influence of the posterior cingulate and prefrontal cortex (30, 31). This network partially overlaps with brain areas implicated in distress in patients suffering from pain (32), dyspnea in asthma (33), somatoform disorders (34) and might, therefore, represent a non-specific distress network.

Through source localized resting-state EEG and electrocardiogram recordings, the participation of the autonomic nervous system to tinnitus distress has been investigated, showing that the dorsal and subgenual anterior cingulate, as well as the left and right insula are important in the central control of the autonomic system in tinnitus patients (35, 36). The perceived distress in tinnitus patients seems to be sympathetically mediated. It is of interest that the same areas that are involved in the control of the autonomic system are also involved in salience processing and distress. This suggests that the autonomic nervous system critically influences salience perception and distress associated with tinnitus.

Thus, the observed reduction of tinnitus handicap after long-term oxytocin application could be explained by a modulatory influence of oxytocin on amygdala activity and on a decoupling between amygdala activation and autonomous nervous system regulation. Further studies investigating the effect of oxytocin on perception and simultaneously on brain activity and connectivity could shed further light on the mechanisms by which oxytocin interacts with tinnitus perception and distress.

ETHICS STATEMENT

Comitê de Ética em Pesquisa Médica do Centro Universitário de Volta Redonda—Unifoa/Fundação Parecer No. 42257214.1.0000. 5237/1.017.546 7/4/2015.

AUTHOR CONTRIBUTIONS

Study design: AA, RF, WS, BL, and AE. Data collection: AA and RF. Statistics: WS. Writing: AA, RF, AE, BL, and NP. Manuscript revision: AA, RF, AE, BL, and PS. All contributed for writing and revision: AA, RF, BL, AE, NP, and WS.

FUNDING

This work was supported by a grant from Tinnitus Research Initiative.

REFERENCES

Shargorodsky J, Curhan JC, Farwell WR. Prevalence and characteristics of tinnitus among US adults. *Am J Med* (2010) 123(8):711–8. doi:10.1016/j.amjmed.2010.02.015

Langguth B, Kreuzer PM, Kleinjung T, De Ridder D. Tinnitus: causes and clinical management. *Lancet Neurol* (2013) 12(9):920–30. doi:10.1016/S1474-4422(13)70160-1

Elgoyhen AB, Langguth B, De Ridder D, Vanneste S. Tinnitus: perspectives from human neuroimaging. *Nat Rev Neurosci* (2015) 16(10):632–42. doi:10.1038/nrn4003

Elgoyhen AB, Langguth B, Nowak W, Schecklmann M, De Ridder D, Vanneste S. Identifying tinnitus-related genes based on a side-effect network analysis. *CPT Pharmacometrics Syst Pharmacol* (2014) 3:e97. doi:10.1038/psp.2013.75

LangguthB,SalviR,ElgoyhenAB.Emergingpharmacotherapyoftinnitus.*Expert Opin Emerg Drugs* (2009) 14(4):687–702. doi:10.1517/14728210903206975

Richard P, Moos F, Freund-Mercier MJ. Central effects of oxytocin. *Physiol Rev* (1991) 71(2):331–70.

Wang H, Ward AR, Morris JF. Oestradiol acutely stimulates exocytosis of oxytocin and vasopressin from dendrites and somata of hypothalamic magno- cellular neurons. *Neuroscience* (1995) 68(4):1179–88. doi:10.1016/0306-4522 (95)00186-M

Wettschureck N, Moers A, Hamalainen T, Lemberger T, Schütz G, Offermanns S. Heterotrimeric G proteins of the Gq/11 family are crucial for the induction of maternal behavior in mice. *Mol Cell Biol* (2004) 24(18):8048–54. doi:10.1128/MCB.24.18.8048-8054.2004

Gimpl G, Fahrenholz F. The oxytocin receptor system: structure, function, and regulation. *Physiol Rev* (2001) 81:629–83.

Muin DA, Wolzt M, Marculescu R, Sheikh Rezaei S, Salama M, Fuchs C, et al. Effect of long-term intranasal oxytocin on sexual dysfunction in premenopausal and postmenopausal women: a randomized trial. *Fertil Steril* (2015) 104(3):715–23.e4. doi:10.1016/j.fertnstert.2015.06.010

Meyer-Lindenberg A, Domes G, Kirsch P, Heinrichs M. Oxytocin and vasopressin in the human brain: social neuropeptides for translational medicine. *Nat Rev Neurosci* (2011) 12(9):524–38. doi:10.1038/nrn3044

Kirsch P. Oxytocin in the socioemotional brain: implications for psychiatric disorders. *Dialogues Clin Neurosci* (2015) 17(4):463–76.

Marlin BJ, Mitre M, D'amour JA, Chao MV, Froemke RC. Oxytocin enables maternal behaviour by balancing cortical inhibition. *Nature* (2015) 520(7548):499–504. doi:10.1038/nature14402

De Ridder D, Elgoyhen AB, Romo R, Langguth B. Phantom percepts: tinnitus and pain as persisting aversive memory networks. *Proc Natl Acad Sci U S A* (2011) 108(20):8075–80. doi:10.1073/pnas.1018466108

Newman CW, Jacobson GP, Spitzer JB. Development of the Tinnitus Handicap Inventory. *Arch Otolaryngol Head Neck Surg* (1996) 122(2):143–8. doi:10.1001/ archotol.1996.01890140029007

Paula Erika Alves F, Cunha F, Onishi ET, Branco-Barreiro FC, Ganança FF. TinnitusHandicapInventory:cross-culturaladaptationtoBrazilianPortugue se. *Pro Fono* (2005) 17(3):303–10. doi:10.1590/S0104-56872005000300004

Wallace WHB, Kelsey TW. Human ovarian reserve from conception to the menopause. *PLoS One* (2010) 5(1):e8772. doi:10.1371/journal.ponee.0008772

Guy W, editor. *ECDEU Assessment Manual for Psychopharmacology*. Rockville, MD: US Department of Health, Education and Welfare Public Health Service Alcohol, Drug Abuse, and Mental Health Administration (1976).

Adamchic I, Langguth B, Hauptmann C, Tass PA. Psychometric evaluation of visual analog scale for the assessment of chronic tinnitus. *Am J Audiol* (2012) 21(2):215–25. doi:10.1044/1059-0889(2012/12-0010)

Holm S. A simple sequentially rejective multiple test procedure. *Scand J Stat* (1979) 6:65–70.

Dobie RA. A review of randomized clinical trials in tinnitus. *Laryngoscope* (1999) 109(8):1202–11. doi:10.1097/00005537-199908000-00004

Coelho C, Figueiredo R, Frank E, Burger J, Schecklmann M, Landgrebe M, et al. Reduction of tinnitus severity by the centrally acting muscle relaxant cyclobenzaprine: an open-label pilot study. *Audiol Neurootol* (2012) 17(3): 179–88. doi:10.1159/000335657

Landgrebe M, Azevedo A, Baguley D, Bauer C, Cacace A, Coelho C, et al. Methodological aspects of clinical trials in tinnitus: a proposal for an international standard. *J Psychosom Res* (2012) 73(2):112–21. doi:10.1016/j.jpsychores.2012.05.002

Langguth B, Goodey R, Azevedo A, Bjorne A, Cacace A, Crocetti A, et al. Consensus for tinnitus patient assessment and treatment outcome measurement: Tinnitus Research Initiative meeting, Regensburg, July 2006. *Prog Brain Res* (2007) 166:525–36. doi:10.1016/S0079-6123(07)66050-6

Figueiredo RR, Azevedo AA, Penido NO. Pharmacological treatment of tinnitus. In: Watson J, editor. *Tinnitus*. New York: Nova Science Publishers (2016). p. 25–42.

Kirsch P, Esslinger C, Chen Q, Mier D, Lis S, Siddhanti S, et al. Oxytocin modulates neural circuitry for social cognition and fear in humans. *J Neurosci* (2005) 25(49):11489–93. doi:10.1523/JNEUROSCI.3984-05.2005

Chen YC, Xia W, Chen H, Feng Y, Xu JJ, Gu JP, et al. Tinnitus distress is linked to enhanced resting-state functional connectivity from the limbic system to the auditory cortex. *Hum Brain Mapp* (2017) 38(5):2384–97. doi:10.1002/hbm.23525

Vanneste S, Plazier M, der Loo EV, de Heyning PV, Congedo M, De Ridder D. The neural correlates of tinnitus-related distress. *Neuroimage* (2010) 52(2):470–80. doi:10.1016/j.neuroimage.2010.04.029

Schlee W, Weisz N, Bertrand O, Hartmann T, Elbert T. Using auditory steady state responses to outline the functional connectivity in the tinnitus brain. *PLoS One* (2008) 3(11):e3720. doi:10.1371/journal.pone.0003720

De Ridder D, Vanneste S, Weisz N, Londero A, Schlee W, Elgoyhen AB, et al. An integrative model of auditory phantom perception: tinnitus as a unified percept of interacting separable subnetworks. *Neurosci Biobehav Rev* (2014) 44:16–32. doi:10.1016/j.neubiorev.2013.03.021

Husain FT. Neural networks of tinnitus in humans: elucidating severity and habituation. *Hear Res* (2016) 334:37–48. doi:10.1016/ j.heares.2015.09.010

Price DD. Psychological and neural mechanisms of the affective dimen- sion of pain. *Science* (2000) 288(5472):1769–72. doi:10.1126/science. 288.5472.1769

von Leupoldt A, Sommer T, Kegat S, Baumann HJ, Klose H, Dahme B, et al. Dyspnea and pain share emotion-related brain network. *Neuroimage* (2009) 48(1):200–6. doi:10.1016/j.neuroimage.2009.06.015

Landgrebe M, Barta W, Rosengarth K, Frick U, Hauser S, Langguth B et al. Neuronal correlates of symptom formation in functional somatic syndromes: a fMRI study. *Neuroimage* (2008) 41(4):1336–44. doi:10.1016/j neuroimage.2008.04.171

van der Loo E, Congedo M, Vanneste S, Van De Heyning P, De Ridder D. Insular lateralization in tinnitus distress. *Auton Neurosci* (2011) 165(2):191–4. doi:10.1016/j.autneu.2011.06.007

Vanneste S, De Ridder D. Brain areas controlling heart rate variability in tin- nitus and tinnitus-related distress. *PLoS One* (2013) 8(3):e59728. doi:10.1371/ journal.pone.0059728

4

Unilateral Cochlear Implantation Reduces Tinnitus Loudness in Bimodal Hearing

*Jérôme J. Servais[1], Karl Hörmann[1,2] and Elisabeth Wallhäusser-Franke[2]**

[1] Department of Otorhinolaryngology, Cochlear Implant Centre, University Medicine Mannheim, Mannheim, Germany,
[2] Audiology, Medical Faculty Mannheim, Department of Otorhinolaryngology, Heidelberg University, Mannheim, Germany

Correspondence:
Elisabeth Wallhäusser-Franke
elisabeth.wallhaeusser-franke@medma.uni-heidelberg.de

Perceptive and receptive aspects of subjective tinnitus like loudness and tinnitus-related distress are partly independent. The high percentage of hearing loss in individuals with tinnitus suggests causality of hearing impairment particularly for the tinnitus percept, leading to the hypothesis that restoration of auditory input has a larger effect on tinnitus loudness than on tinnitus-related distress. Furthermore, it is assumed that high levels of depression or anxiety prevent reductions of tinnitus loudness and distress following restoration of activity in the cochlea. This prospective study investigated the influence of unilateral cochlear implant (CI) on tinnitus in 19 postlingually deafened adults during 6 months following implantation. All had bimodal provision with the other ear being continuously supported by a hearing aid. On the day before CI implantation (T1, T2), and at about 3 and 6 months postsurgery (T3, T4), participants were questioned about their current tinnitus. Loudness was rated on a Numeric Rating Scale, distress was assessed by the TQ12 Tinnitus Questionnaire, and depression and anxiety were recorded with the Hospital Anxiety and Depression Scale. At T2, 79% experienced tinnitus, one participant developed tinnitus after implantation. Following implantation, tinnitus loudness was reduced significantly by 42%, while reductions in tinnitus-related distress (−24%), depression (−20%), and anxiety (−20%) did not attain statistical significance. Significant correlations existed between tinnitus measures, and between postimplantation tinnitus-related distress and anxiety and depression scores. Moreover, improvement of hearing in the CI ear was significantly correlated with reduction in tinnitus loudness. A new aspect of this study is the particular influence of CI provision on perceptive aspects of preexisting tinnitus (hypothesis 1), with the effect size regarding postimplant reduction of perceived tinnitus loudness (1.40) being much larger than effect sizes on the reduction of tinnitus-related distress (0.38), depression (0.53), and anxiety (0.53). Contrary to expectation both tinnitus measures reduce even in the majority of CI recipients with increased levels of anxiety or depression. This suggests that reduction of the tinnitus signal by restoring activity in the cochlea cannot be entirely compensated for by central tinnitus mechanisms and results in a reduction of perceptive and less so of reactive aspects of subjective tinnitus.

Keywords: tinnitus, loudness reduction, cochlear implant, bimodal hearing, anxiety, depression, prospective study

INTRODUCTION

This prospective study addresses changes in subjective tinnitus following cochlear implantation. A new aspect is the investigation of bimodal implantees, who hear with the help of a cochlear implant (CI) on one ear and an acoustic hearing aid (HA) on the contralateral ear. This combination of hearing substitution is rather common and provides significant real-world benefit as compared to unilateral CI (1). Moreover, influence on perceived loudness of the tinnitus and tinnitus-related distress are assessed separately and effect sizes are calculated.

Hearing loss is a major risk factor for tinnitus (2), and therefore, it is not surprising that tinnitus is common among CI candidates. On average, as many as 80% of CI candidates experience tinnitus (3, 4). It was realized early that CIs may reduce tinnitus (5) with several authors reporting on tinnitus reduction (6–11). However, the opposite, namely, exacerbation of a preexisting tinnitus, or development of tinnitus with CI use has also been observed (7, 12). The risk of developing tinnitus following CI ranges from 0 to 4%, while worsening of a preexisting tinnitus has been reported in 1–9% of cases (7). As tinnitus may lead to considerable suffering (13–15), the circumstances influencing its suppression, versus its worsening, or even the emergence of new tinnitus with CI use need to be explored.

The tinnitus signal or percept is thought to arise in the central auditory system in response to a hearing deficit, which in most cases can be attributed to impairments in the cochlea (16). The burden experienced by tinnitus extends beyond this percept and was shown to correlate with anxiety and depression (14, 17). Heterogeneity and severity in symptoms associated with tinnitus is reflected in a wide variety of proposed treatments (13) and may be the reason why overall effectiveness of currently available treatments is suboptimal.

Tinnitus is an auditory percept that varies in persistence, can be localized to one or both ears or is heard within the head, and that is perceived with variable loudness. Beyond this, people with tinnitus may suffer from their tinnitus and the amount of suffering cannot solely be determined by the perceptive qualities of the tinnitus, rather appearing to be associated more closely with mental health (14, 17, 18). In agreement, the reactive component, or distress related to the tinnitus percept, was found to be related to alterations in the emotional, attentional, and memory systems of the brain and to altered interactions between these systems and the auditory system: reportably leading to undue salience of the tinnitus signal (19).

We want to address the following hypotheses: first, we propose that because CIs restore input into the central auditory system, CI provision has a stronger effect on perceptive aspects of tinnitus than on reactive aspects. Thus, we expect CIs to primarily reduce tinnitus permanence and perceived loudness, and possibly change its localization if the hearing balance is altered between ears. At the same time, we expect a weaker effect of CI use on tinnitus-related distress, because this aspect of tinnitus is thought to depend mainly on interactions with the non-auditory brain [e.g., Ref. (15, 19)]. Second, we propose that high levels of depression and anxiety counteract CI-induced tinnitus attenuation, resulting in a lesser reduction of tinnitus-related distress and loudness in individuals with high depression and/or anxiety scores.

Moreover, as CIs are constantly improved in terms of type of implant, electrode insertion and positioning, and speech processing strategy, greater tinnitus suppression is expected by newer types of implants (6, 7). Therefore, it is important to explore the tinnitus reducing capacities of currently available CI technology.

The aims of this prospective study are therefore to (i) estimate the change of perceptive and (ii) reactive tinnitus measures separately, and (iii) examine the influence of mental health on the reduction of tinnitus symptoms following unilateral CI implantation in bimodal users.

MATERIALS AND METHODS

Procedure and Inclusion

Between 2014 and 2016, study participants were recruited from the patients at the CI Centre of the University Medical Centre Mannheim. Prospective participants had postlingual onset of profound hearing impairment. Recruitment was independent of reported tinnitus. Inclusion criteria comprised: first-time unilateral CI provision, an Advanced Bionics (HiRes 90K) implant as chosen by the patient, HA use at the other ear, and aged between 18 and 90 years. All patients who fulfilled these criteria were approached for inclusion. Exclusion criteria were assessed during an initial interview (T1) and included: insufficient knowledge of the German language, more than mild cognitive deficit, as assessed by the DemTect Test (20), and use of other implanted devices. Twenty-five patients were included in the study. Two participants discontinued the study following sequential bilateral implantation, one discontinued because of health conditions unrelated to the study or their tinnitus, one decided that study participation after T2 was too much effort, and two discontinued for reasons they did not disclose.

The initial interview, study inclusion (T1), and presurgery examination (T2) took place on the same day, usually the day before surgery (mean [SD]: 3 [7] days). Patients received a CI on their weaker ear while HA use was continued on the other ear. They left hospital on average 3 days postsurgery. Two to three weeks later, they participated in a week-long in-patient program with first fitting of the speech processor, several fitting sessions, and technical instruction on CI use. Until the first formal appointment at the CI Centre of the University Medical Centre Mannheim, 4 weeks following surgery, participants' mean daily processor use was 11 h. Postimplantation assessments T3 and T4 were scheduled for 3 and 6 months postimplantation (T3: 100 [18] days; T4: 221 [70] days).

Before T1, all subjects gave written informed consent in accordance with the Declaration of Helsinki. The protocol was approved by the Medizinische Ethikkommission II of the Medical Faculty Mannheim (approval no. 2014-527N-MA). Study participants were compensated for their participation.

Participant's Characteristics

Etiology of hearing loss varied greatly and was unknown in many cases. The decision which ear was to be implanted was based on various audiological and anatomical criteria and was generally independent of reported tinnitus. Nineteen subjects completed the study. Before implantation, four did not experience tinnitus and three of them did not report tinnitus at any assessment, while one developed tinnitus between T2 and T3.

Study participants focused much more on their hearing problems than their tinnitus. When asked at pre-assessment (T1) what they expected of their CI, none mentioned tinnitus. No expectations were expressed by one participant, whereas the remaining 18 expected their hearing to improve in order to understand spoken language more easily and to participate in social situations again. Further characteristics of study participants are given in **Table 1**.

Measures

Pure tone audiometry (PTA) was conducted in sound field for both ears at 0.5, 1, 2, and 4 kHz both prior to and postsurgery with HA and if applicable CI. Measures across these frequencies were averaged separately for CI and HA ears (PTA-4). If a response could not be obtained because a frequency was not heard by the participant, values were set to 120 dB HL, i.e., 10 dB above the highest sound presentation level used during audiometry. The same questionnaires and audiological tests were used at the assessments preceding implantation (T2), as well as approximately 3 (T3) and 6 (T4) months postsurgery.

In addition to general background and expectations, questions about the presence, persistence, and location of tinnitus, a Numeric Rating Scale (NRS) (21) assessing current subjectively perceived tinnitus loudness (NRS 0–10: tinnitus audible only in silence—tinnitus louder than all other sounds) were used. Additionally, tinnitus-related distress was assessed with the 12-item version of the Tinnitus Questionnaire [TQ12, named MTQ in Ref. (14, 15)]. The TQ12 was developed by Hiller and Goebel (22) according to an optimal combination of high item-total correlations, reliability, and sensitivity for the assessment of changes in tinnitus-related distress. According to Zeman et al. (23), the TQ showed satisfying psychometric results, which were equally good for the long form and for the short TQ12 form. Internal consistency of TQ12 was $\alpha = 0.87$ (23). For a classification of tinnitus-related distress, Hiller and Goebel (22) proposed four grades with: scores 1–7 (grade 1) signifying no clinically relevant distress, a score of 8–12 (grade 2) representing moderate distress, a score of 13–18 (grade 3) representing severe distress, and a score of 19–24 representing the most severe distress due to tinnitus. Grades 3 and 4 are considered to require therapeutic intervention. Depression and anxiety were assessed with the Hospital Anxiety and Depression Scale [HADS (24)] at T2 and T4. For both subscales of the HADS, scores of 8 or above are considered to be indicative of potential problems in these areas (24). For tinnitus patients, internal consistencies of $\alpha = 0.83$ and $\alpha = 0.88$ were determined for the anxiety and depression subscales (25). One question with five options between "very good" (4) and "poor" (0) assessed the subjective impression of a participant regarding his/her general health condition at T2 and T4.

TABLE 1 | Participant's characteristics.

	Tinnitus at T2	No tinnitus at T2
Number	15	4
Gender: male (N)	2	2
Age mean (SD)	55.3 (14.0)	64.3 (19.3)
Cochlear implant (CI) left	9	2
CI ear: years with hearing impairment	25.5 (18.5)	24.0 (13.0)
Hearing aid (HA) ear: years with hearing impairment	21.3 (19.6)	17.0 (11.8)
Pre-OP HA use CI ear (excluding cross)	10	3
Pre-OP HA use other ear	15	4
PTA-4 (dB HL) of CI ear		
Preimplantation	95.9 (17.3)	91.3 (15.0)
Postimplantation	46.6 (12.8)	43.8 (9.7)
PTA-4 (dB HL) of HA ear		
Preimplantation	65.5 (18.6)	70.1 (15.1)
Postimplantation	61.1 (24.0)	72.3 (4.5)
Hospital Anxiety and Depression Scale (HADS) with at least 1 scale ≥8 at T2	6	0
Participants with relevant other health conditions	9	3

Shown are numbers per condition and means with respective SDs. PTA-4 thresholds of the CI ear decrease significantly with implantation indicating much better hearing postimplantation. Although the group without tinnitus is older, duration of hearing impairment at the HA ear is shorter, and hearing on the HA ear is worse, differences between tinnitus and non-tinnitus group are not statistically significant. Another potential difference between those affected by tinnitus and those without may be differences in mental wellbeing. Scores of 8 points or above in the HADS are seen as indicator of potential problems regarding depressiveness and anxiety, respectively, and are present only in the tinnitus group. Other relevant health conditions were, for instance, hypertension, thyroid, cardiologic, depression, and condition following a malignant tumor.

Statistical Analysis

Statistical analysis was performed with IBM SPSS Statistics, version 22 (SPSS/IBM, Chicago, IL, USA). Descriptive statistics included mean and SD. The effect of intracochlear electrical stimulation on tinnitus was assessed by comparing baseline values to the outcomes obtained at the end of the follow-up. Pearson correlation coefficients were calculated, with coefficients <0.5 being considered as weak, coefficients between 0.5 and 0.8 being considered as moderate, and >0.8 being considered as strong. In addition, a general linear model for repeated measurements with Bonferroni correction and in case of non-normality Friedman tests were performed prior to *post hoc* testing with two-sided *t*-tests or Wilcoxon signed-rank tests, respectively. Statistical significance was defined for p values smaller than 0.05, and p-values smaller than 0.01 were considered to be highly significant.

Effect sizes for repeated measures in dependent samples were calculated according to Bortz (26) [see also Ref. (27)] with the following equation:

$$\varepsilon = \frac{\mu_1 - \mu_2}{\hat{\sigma}\sqrt{1-r}}$$

The difference between means (μ_1, μ_2) is divided by the pooled variance ($\hat{\sigma}$). Introduction of the Pearson correlation coefficient (r) serves as a correction for the dependence among means. Effect sizes of >0.2 correspond to weak effects, of >0.5 to moderate, and of >0.8 to strong effects.

RESULTS

Pure Tone Audiometry

Preoperative aided thresholds at 0.5, 1, 2, and 4 kHz (PTA-4) in free sound field could not be determined for 10 of the 24 CI ears and for 1 HA ear due to no response in some or all of these frequencies. For calculation of overall improvement of hearing, values for measurements that did not yield a result were set to 120 dB HL. Pre- and postimplantation PTA-4 averages are shown in **Table 1**. Improvement of hearing thresholds of CI ears with CI use was highly significant ($t = 10.593$; $p < 0.001$), while average thresholds in the HA ear were unchanged ($t = 1.078$; $p = 0.301$). For participants with preexisting tinnitus, the CI ear remained the worse ear for three, became the better hearing ear for seven, and aided hearing levels were similar for both ears in five individuals. For all individuals without tinnitus, the CI ear became the better ear postsurgery.

Tinnitus before CI

Prior to implantation, tinnitus was reported by 79% (15/19) of the study participants. The four participants without tinnitus were older, duration of hearing impairment on the other ear was shorter, preimplantation hearing thresholds were more similar for the two ears, and they were less likely to report high scores in the anxiety and depression scales. Differences to the tinnitus group were not statistically significant, however. In contrast, reported duration of hearing impairment on the ear to be implanted was similar to the average in the tinnitus group (**Table 1**).

Preexisting tinnitus was permanent in 7 cases, and was localized across both ears, or was heard within the head in 10 individuals, while it localized to the future CI ear in 4 and to the HA ear in 1. Perceived loudness was very loud (≥8) for four participants and very low (≤2) for 2, with an average of 4.9 [(2.7), range 1–10] on the 0–10 NRS scale. According to the grading of Hiller and Goebel (22) with TQ12 scores above 12 indicating clinically significant tinnitus-related distress, two participants (13%) expressed clinically significant tinnitus-related distress, while the average score was 7.4 [(6.0), range 1–24], corresponding to low tinnitus-related distress (see **Figure 1**).

Changes in Tinnitus with CI Use

Of the 15 study participants with tinnitus at T2, all but 2 reported a subjective benefit following CI use. In two subjects with tinnitus prior to surgery, an additional tone arose for the CI ear or the HA ear, respectively. One subject developed new tinnitus at the CI ear, which was neither loud or distressing and not permanent by T4. At T2, seven participants reported permanent tinnitus, while this was true for six at T4.

Changes in tinnitus localization after cochlear implantation coincided with improvement of PTA-4 thresholds in the CI ear relative to the HA ear. Whereas tinnitus localization did not change if the CI ear remained the worse ear ($n = 3$), it changed in 50% of the other 12 in whom hearing balance between CI and HA ear was changed by CI use.

For calculations of average scores for the tinnitus and health variables, values obtained from the individual with tinnitus onset after surgery were omitted. On average, tinnitus loudness decreased by 42% between T2 and T4 resulting in an effect size of 1.40, which indicates a strong effect (**Figure 1**). Overall, this reduction was highly significant ($F = 9.161$; $p = 0.012$), and the reduction between T2 and T4 reached significance with *post hoc* testing ($p = 0.035$). Tinnitus loudness was at least halved in 47%. At the end of the study, mean perceived loudness was 2.9 (2.5) and was rated as 5 or below for all except one subject (**Figure 1**). This subject experienced a tinnitus of maximal loudness (10/10) at onset and at the end of the study.

On average, TQ12 scores decreased by 24% between T2 and T4 resulting in an effect size of 0.38 which indicates a weak effect of bimodal provision on tinnitus-related distress (**Figure 1**). The main effect just missed statistical significance ($chi^2 = 5.911$; $p = 0.052$), while *post hoc* tests clearly missed a significance level (T2–T3: $Z = -0.996$; $p = 0.319$; T2–T4: $Z = -1.646$; $p = 0.100$). Between T2 and T4, the TQ12 score decreased by at least 3 points (12.5% on the 0–24 TQ12 scale) for eight participants (53%), was unchanged for 5 (33%), and increased by at least 3 points for two participants. The latter both indicated severe stress independent of their hearing at the end of the study. At T4, all but three participants had tinnitus of the lowest category, grade 1, and one fell into grade 2, indicating mild to moderate tinnitus (**Figure 1**). The remaining two participants did not benefit from CI use in terms of tinnitus-related distress reduction. One of them reported maximal tinnitus-related distress (24/24) both at the beginning and at the end of the study, coinciding with maximal tinnitus loudness (10/10) at both assessments. This participant was diagnosed with an additional attack of sudden sensorineural hearing loss on the non-implanted ear during the study and expressed a high level of anxiety and depression symptoms at all times. The other participant had very low tinnitus loudness and distress prior to CI surgery. With CI use, tinnitus loudness increased from 2 to 3 points on the NRS, whereas the TQ12 score was increased by 17 points at T3 and by 16 points at T4, as compared to pre-CI, reaching a level of severe tinnitus distress (grade 3) at the post-CI assessments. Noteworthy in this participant were the continuously high levels of depression and anxiety. This was despite taking antidepressive medication since T3, prescribed independently of the study.

Anxiety, Depression, and General Health

On average, the levels of anxiety and depression were both reduced by 20% with an effect size of 0.53 indicating moderate effects on both factors (**Figure 1**). Reductions did not reach significance for either factor (anxiety: $t = 1.451$; $p = 0.169$; depression: $Z = -1.307$; $p = 0.191$). At the first assessment prior to implantation, six of the participants with preexisting tinnitus (40%) reported a score of 8 or above, either in one or in both HADS subscales, i.e., indicating potential problems in these areas. At T4, three participants reported a score of ≥8 in one of the HADS scales. During the study, scores dropped below 8 in 4 participants and increased in one, whose initial scores had been inconspicuous. The latter case could be related to events independent of the CI. Despite indications of mental health problems, tinnitus loudness and distress were reduced by more than 50% in four of the six participants who reported increased HADS scores

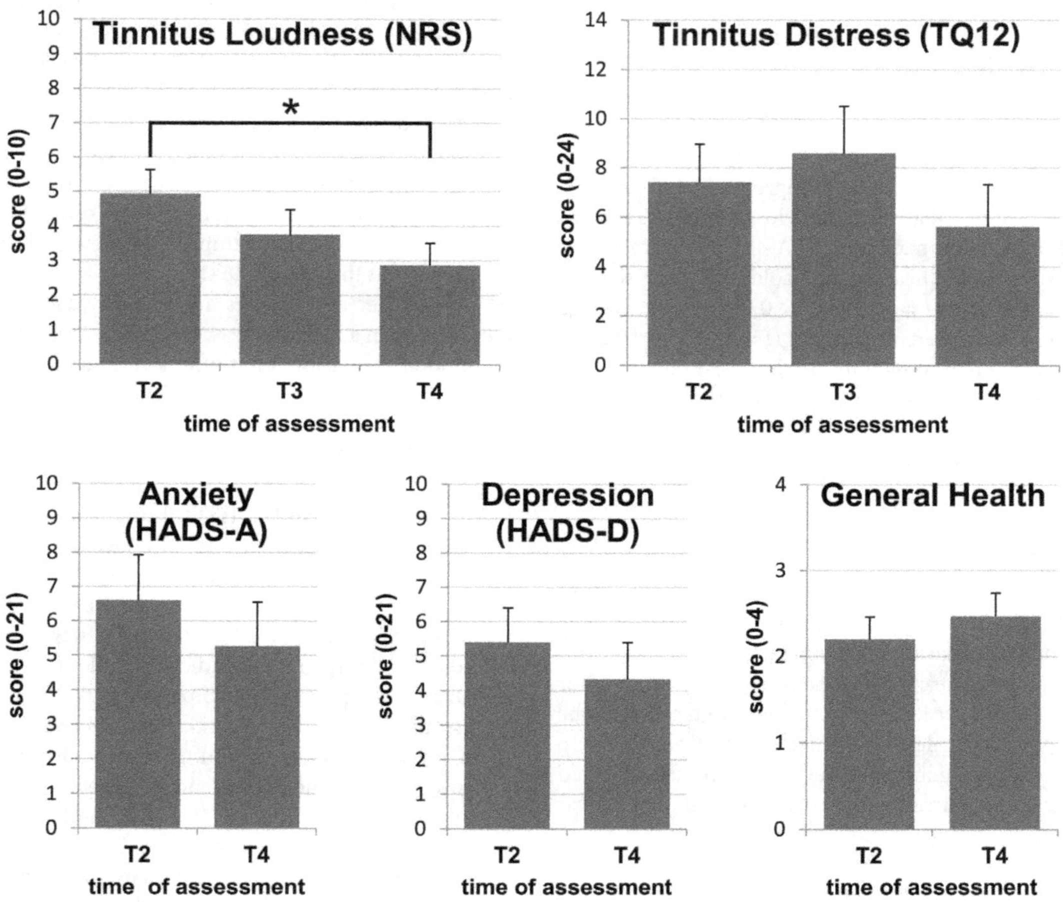

FIGURE 1 | Group means with SEs at assessments T2, T3, and T4: only the reduction of perceived tinnitus loudness reaches statistical significance, while differences between assessments did not attain statistical significance for tinnitus-related distress, anxiety, depression, or general health. Statistically significant differences are indicated by $^{*}p < 0.05$.

at T2, and also in the individual whose HADS scores increased above 8 during the study.

When asked for a judgment of their general health situation, only one individual reported a substantial improvement of 3 points on the 0–4 scale between T2 and T4. On average, general health was considered to be satisfactory at T2, and the majority did not report any improvement, often despite a statement that their hearing ability had improved considerably (**Figure 1**).

Correlation between Measures

In the correlation matrices presented in **Tables 2** and **3**, correlations between subjective tinnitus loudness and tinnitus-related distress peaked between significant to highly significant, but moderate correlations were found at all assessments. In addition, correlations between postimplantation tinnitus-related distress and the level of anxiety at T2 and T4 and also with the level of depression at T2 exhibited significant to highly significant correlations of moderate strength. When correlating changes during the study period, a significant correlation existed between improvement of hearing at the CI ear and the reduction of tinnitus loudness between T2 and T4 ($r = 0.584$; $p = 0.022^{*}$). In addition, time of hearing impairment showed a significant correlation with the improvement in anxiety scores between T2 and T4 (**Table 3**). Age at implantation did not show a significant correlation with any of the above variables, but a significant inverse correlation with general health indicating that older participants had more health problems. According to the reporting of chronic health conditions by the participants, these were mostly unrelated to their hearing (**Table 1**).

DISCUSSION

Tinnitus was common for the hearing-impaired participants of this study. Main findings are a significant reduction in subjective tinnitus loudness between preimplantation and 6 months postimplantation (T2 versus T4), and a significant correlation between improvement of hearing with CI use and the reduction in tinnitus loudness. As predicted by hypothesis 1, restoration of activity in the cochlea had a stronger effect on subjective tinnitus loudness, and less influence on tinnitus-related distress.

TABLE 2 | Correlations between measures.

	T2-TNRS	T3-TNRS	T4-TNRS	T2-TQ12	T3-TQ12	T4-TQ12	T2-HADS-A	T4-HADS-A	T2-HADS-D	T4-HADS-D	T2-Health	T4-Health
Age at implantation	0.044	0.206	0.055	0.253	0.195	0.027	0.068	0.239	0.295	0.083	−0.246	−0.647
	0.875	0.521	0.846	0.363	0.544	0.925	0.810	0.392	0.285	0.768	0.376	0.009**
T2-TNRS	1	0.589	0.697	0.576	0.528	0.274	−0.038	0.146	0.040	−0.121	−0.546	−0.139
		0.044*	0.004**	0.025*	0.078	0.322	0.893	0.603	0.889	0.667	0.035*	0.622
T3-TNRS		1	0.785	0.826	0.767	0.624	0.139	0.383	−0.009	−0.077	−0.043	−0.147
			0.002**	0.001**	0.004**	0.030*	0.666	0.247	0.978	0.813	0.894	0.649
T4-TNRS			1	0.780	0.760	0.756	0.375	0.482	0.237	0.089	−0.472	−0.220
				0.001**	0.004**	0.001**	0.168	0.069	0.395	0.752	0.075	0.432
T2-TQ12				1	0.651	0.495	0.256	0.477	0.059	−0.176	−0.178	−0.244
					0.022*	0.061	0.357	0.072	0.835	0.529	0.526	0.381
T3-TQ12					1	0.851	0.587	0.672	0.510	0.498	−0.421	−0.537
						<0.001**	0.045*	0.017*	0.090	0.100	0.172	0.072
T4-TQ12						1	0.681	0.710	0.558	0.508	−0.411	−0.458
							0.005**	0.003**	0.031*	0.053	0.128	0.086
T2-HADS-A							1	0.725	0.772	0.654	−0.365	−0.524
								0.002**	0.001**	0.008**	0.180	0.045*
T4-HADS-A								1	0.582	0.616	−0.197	−0.643
									0.023*	0.014*	0.482	0.010**
T2-HADS-D									1	0.814	−0.541	−0.648
										<0.001**	0.037*	0.009**
T4-HADS-D										1	−0.258	−0.482
											0.354	0.069
T2-Health											1	0.505
												0.055

Significant correlations exist between subjective tinnitus loudness and tinnitus-related distress. Further significant correlations are observed for postimplantation tinnitus-related distress with anxiety at T2 and T4 and with depression scores at T2. Furthermore, tinnitus loudness and depression at T2 and anxiety scores at T2 and T4 as well as age at implantation show significant inverse correlations with general health.

Pearson correlation coefficients: $^{**}p < 0.01$ (2-tailed); $^{*}p < 0.05$ (2-tailed).

HADS-A, Hospital Anxiety and Depression Scale for anxiety; HADS-D, Hospital Anxiety and Depression Scale for depression.

Moreover, magnitude of influence on tinnitus-related distress was lower than effects on anxiety and depression. Contrary to hypothesis 2 that high levels of anxiety or depression prevent reduction of tinnitus symptoms, these reduced in the majority of participants with high depression and anxiety scores, while failure to reduce or increases could be related to other current sources of distress.

To the best of our knowledge, this is the first longitudinal study on the influence of bimodal provision on tinnitus symptoms. Present findings are in general agreement with findings on unilateral electric amplification of sound by CI as reported in retrospective studies (11, 28–30), reviews (3, 4, 31–33), and a growing body of prospective studies [e.g., Ref. (7, 12, 34–39)]. Although total remission from tinnitus was not observed in the present study, most subjects noticed substantial reduction of their tinnitus, while worsening of a preexisting tinnitus was rare, predominantly pertained tinnitus-related distress, and appeared to be associated with increased levels of anxiety and depression. Emergence of tinnitus only after cochlear implantation was an exception, and as reported before (7, 12), resolved within a few weeks and was experienced as mild at the end of follow-up. In the sample by Pan et al. (12), those who acquired tinnitus had the shortest duration hearing loss and were the oldest implant recipients. This cannot be corroborated by the present results, however.

The effect size for loudness reduction indicates a strong effect comparable to or higher than effect sizes that were reported for generally accepted tinnitus therapies that, however, serve to reduce tinnitus-related distress as opposed to tinnitus loudness (40, 41). Two prospective studies on tinnitus following cochlear implantation addressed tinnitus loudness in a similar way, namely, by a visual analog scale (35, 38). The participants of these studies had severe to profound unilateral or bilateral hearing impairment and were provided unilaterally with a CI while hearing was not amplified at the other ear. Tinnitus loudness was reduced significantly and by a similar amount as in the present study, but effect sizes for the reduction of tinnitus loudness were not reported in these publications.

Bimodal provision was far less effective in reducing tinnitus-related distress. This finding was expected since tinnitus-related distress depends on further influences that cannot directly be influenced by restoration of cochlear activity (19). Furthermore, presurgery tinnitus-related distress was reported as mild to moderate by the majority of the study participants, even if the tinnitus was rather loud. This is in line with earlier studies on CI implantees (36, 39) and may have prevented findings of significant reductions. Taken together, present findings support the assumption that restoration of auditory input primarily reduces the tinnitus signal, whereas it has a weaker influence on tinnitus-related distress, and they support the distinction between perceived tinnitus loudness and distress (14, 15, 42). Furthermore, these findings corroborate the assumption that tinnitus-related distress is influenced by non-auditory factors as suggested previously (15, 17–19, 43).

Acquired hearing impairment represents a risk factor for increased levels of anxiety and depression (44, 45), especially in combination with distressing tinnitus (14, 18). A total of 40% of those with preexisting tinnitus indicated conspicuous levels of anxiety and/or depression before implantation, whereas average

TABLE 3 | Correlations between changes in measures with cochlear implant (CI) use.

	Pre- to postimplantation improvement					
	CI ear: PTA-4	**TNRS**	**TQ12**	**Hospital Anxiety and Depression Scale for anxiety (HADS-A)**	**Hospital Anxiety and Depression Scale for depression (HADS-D)**	**Health**
Age at implantation	−0.239	−0.008	0.211	−0.160	0.389	−0.422
	0.391	0.977	0.451	0.568	0.151	0.117
CI ear: years of hearing impairment	−0.338	−0.315	−0.250	0.580	−0.073	0.220
	0.218	0.253	0.368	0.023*	0.796	0.431
Hearing aid (HA) ear: years of hearing impairment	−0.466	−0.380	−0.319	0.613	−0.129	−0.058
	0.080	0.163	0.246	0.015*	0.647	0.839
CI ear: PTA-4 improvement	1	0.584	0.354	−0.273	−0.191	0.424
		0.022*	0.195	0.325	0.496	0.115
TNRS improvement		1	0.405	−0.312	−0.025	0.231
			0.134	0.258	0.929	0.408
TQ12 improvement			1	−0.364	0.082	−0.002
				0.182	0.772	0.994
HADS-A improvement				1	0.442	0.246
					0.099	0.377
HADS-D improvement					1	0.113
						0.688

Significant correlations are present between improvement of PTA-4 thresholds pre- to postimplantation of the CI ear and improvement, i.e., reduction of subjective tinnitus loudness between T2 and T4, and between years of hearing impairment of the CI and the HA ear and the reduction in anxiety scores between T2 and T4.
*Pearson correlation coefficients: *$p < 0.05$ (2-tailed).*

levels were low which is in accordance with earlier results from CI recipients [e.g., Ref. (28, 29, 35, 36)]. Depression and anxiety scores were reduced by 20% between baseline and the end of follow-up, but these differences did not attain statistical significance. Former reports differ in this aspect with some observing significant reductions whereas others do not, with discrepancies likely being dependent on sample characteristics (28–30, 36). Estimated magnitude of effects for the reduction of anxiety and depression were higher than for the reduction in tinnitus-related distress. This suggests that other aspects of life quality related to anxiety and depression may have been improved by bimodal provision (44, 45). Correlations of postimplant levels of tinnitus-related distress with anxiety and for fewer comparisons also with depression attained significance. An association between these measures has been reported for tinnitus populations with and without cochlear implants (8, 14, 28), and catastrophic interpretations of tinnitus have been associated with fear (46). But increased levels of anxiety or depression did not prevent a reduction in tinnitus loudness and tinnitus-related distress, except in two participants, indicating that a reduction in tinnitus is highly reliant on afferent auditory input. Despite a reduction in tinnitus-related complaints and better hearing in general, individuals with higher scores in the HADS scales were not satisfied with their quality of life. Although low in terms of percentage, CI recipients who do not experience tinnitus relief, or express compromised well-being, need to be taken care of as they might benefit from other types of therapies (13), and this in turn might improve performance with their CI.

The exact mechanism through which CI use suppresses tinnitus symptoms is unknown. Several mechanisms, such as masking, direct electrical nerve stimulation, habituation, and plastic reorganization in the brain have to be considered. Another aspect why CIs appear to be effective in reducing the tinnitus may be the intense auditory training required during rehabilitation. According to current knowledge, tinnitus is the result of maladaptive plasticity in the central auditory pathway in response to auditory deprivation. In the majority of cases, the trigger for tinnitus-related changes in the brain is impairment of the cochlea (16). Experimentally inducing auditory deprivation by exposing healthy subjects to complete silence triggers phantom sounds that are reversible upon restoration of the auditory input (47). In addition, continuous use of earplugs can lead to a reversible perception of tinnitus (48). This suggests that tinnitus can be induced by auditory deprivation and that it can be reversed by restoring input into the central auditory system. Restoration of peripheral input especially at the base of the cochlea which is important for activity in the tinnitus-relevant high-frequency areas of the auditory system can be achieved by CI use or by other types of electrical stimulation (8). Extracochlear (49–51) and intracochlear electrical stimulation (52–54) reduce tinnitus, even when the stimuli are "not audible." A study by Punte et al. (55) suggested that tinnitus suppression does only occur if the full length of the cochlea is electrically stimulated by a CI. On the other hand, continued presence of tinnitus during CI use may be due to the fact that hearing is not completely restored by the implant, or because a memory of the tinnitus has been established in the brain which is partly independent of external input.

Although electrical stimulation of the inner ear effectively suppresses tinnitus for many CI recipients, the reported percentages vary between studies and may depend on characteristics of the samples under study, particularly regarding non-auditory aspects (29). For conscious perception of the tinnitus signal and for the suffering arising from it, involvement of brain areas beyond the auditory system appears to be mandatory (19). Thus, tinnitus is not simply the result of defective auditory input but obviously requires further mechanisms. This may be the reason why some that are hard of hearing, or deaf, do not experience tinnitus: for instance, 21% of the participants of the present study.

Brain regions with alterations related to tinnitus have included the emotional, attentional, and memory systems. These systems are thought to influence processing in the auditory cortex and thus in the auditory system in a top-down manner (19, 56), particularly in those who suffer from their tinnitus (19, 57, 58). Behaviorally, this is evidenced for instance by enhanced levels of depression and anxiety in tinnitus populations especially, among those with distressing tinnitus (14, 15). Remarkably and similar to other studies (28, 35), average depression and anxiety scores are low in the present CI sample. This may be a favorable condition for allowing a reduction of the tinnitus signal in a bottom-up manner and may part explain the extent of tinnitus reduction by CIs. Although tinnitus with a major emphasis on non-auditory mechanisms (19) was thought to respond less to recovery of the auditory input, even individuals with enhanced levels of anxiety and depression responded to bimodal provision with a substantial reduction of tinnitus symptoms, given that there existed no other current sources of severe distress. In the latter, the tinnitus might even worsen despite attenuation of its trace within the auditory system. Noteworthy in this respect are the two individuals whose tinnitus was not positively influenced by bimodal hearing. Whereas in one, the tinnitus retained maximal loudness and distress throughout the study period, in the other negligent tinnitus-related distress before CI provision increased tremendously with CI use. Concomitantly high levels of anxiety and depression at pre- and postsurgical assessment in both individuals and the reporting of severe distress postimplantation are in agreement with the assumption that highly distressing tinnitus may predominantly be a consequence of central top-down processing and that it is therefore, less influenced by attenuation of the tinnitus signal in the ascending auditory pathway.

Taken together, CIs alone as well as in combination with a contralateral HA appear to be effective in reducing the tinnitus signal through influencing neurophysiological processes involved in the generation and maintenance of tinnitus, via compensation of peripheral deafferentation. In addition, enhanced attentiveness to environmental sounds following implantation may lower awareness of the tinnitus. Although psychological factors certainly contribute to the tinnitus relief obtained through implant use, restoring auditory input by electrical stimulation appears to be primary effect. In accordance, loudness is reduced to a larger extent than the tinnitus-related distress. Whether long-term CI use reverses reorganization in the central auditory system associated with peripheral deafferentation and with tinnitus (16) remains to be shown. Tinnitus reduction does not always result in increased well-being, however. In our study sample, individuals with increased levels of anxiety or depression still felt anxious or depressed, despite improvements in their tinnitus and their hearing in general. Such individuals might additionally require psychological help.

Limitations

As in all prospective studies with CI recipients, the sample under investigation is small and therefore, might not be representative. However, our results are in general agreement with the published literature. Study participants were observed in their first 6 months after cochlear implantation. This time may be too short as an endpoint since improvements in auditory comprehension tend to continue thereafter. However, others (35, 38) have shown that reductions of tinnitus loudness occur early after CI provision. Furthermore, as double-blind studies are not feasible in this patient group, this was an open study that is not completely free from bias. It is conceivable, however, that placebo-controlled studies are and will be exceptional in intracochlear electrical stimulation for tinnitus suppression. For our sample, it can be stated that, while amelioration of tinnitus was not the main focus of the participants' concerns or expectations, most experienced relieving tinnitus reduction.

CONCLUSION

Restoration of auditory input by bimodal provision (CI and contralateral HA) appears to be an efficient method of reducing tinnitus: primarily the perceived loudness. At the same time, the risk of worsening or developing tinnitus as a result of implant surgery is low. Therefore, restoration of auditory input in the high-frequency part of the cochlea, as achieved by a CI, can be regarded as an effective means for the reduction of tinnitus, but is only justified in patients with deeply compromised hearing ability. Electrical stimulation of the cochlea independent of CI use might represent a feasible alternative for those with better hearing yet experiencing loud tinnitus.

In addition to an effective stimulation of the tinnitus-relevant high-frequency range of the cochlea, and consequently of central auditory structures, effectiveness of CI use regarding tinnitus reduction might also be related to the low levels of tinnitus-related distress, depression, and anxiety commonly found prior to implantation. Based on our findings, we propose that central mechanisms exacerbating tinnitus have to be expected in individuals who exhibit increased levels of anxiety and depression in particular if they experience severe distress postimplantation. Although those who suffer from their tinnitus and show compromised mental health represent a small percentage of CI recipients with tinnitus, this aspect has to be taken care of. The impact on quality of life, possibly on acceptance of the CI, means that these individuals may require other types of specialized therapeutic interventions, interventions which however are available (13).

AUTHOR CONTRIBUTIONS

JS: data acquisition, interpretation of data, and drafting of the manuscript. KH: critical revision. EW-F: study conception and design, data acquisition, analysis and interpretation of data, and drafting of the manuscript.

ACKNOWLEDGMENTS

We thank our participants for their time and effort. We would like to thank Tanja Sutter for administrative help, and Svetlana Hetjens for her statistical comments.

FUNDING

This work was supported by Advanced Bionics GmbH.

REFERENCES

Fielden CA, Kitterick PT. Contralateral acoustic hearing aid use in adult unilateral cochlear implant recipients: current provision, practice, and clinical experience in the UK. *Cochlear Implants Int* (2016) 17:132–45. doi:10.1080/ 14670100.2016.1162382

Nondahl DM, Cruickshanks KJ, Huang GH, Klein BE, Klein R, Chappell R, et al. Tinnitus and its risk factors in the Beaver Dam offspring study. *Am J Audiol* (2011) 50:313–20. doi:10.3109/14992027.2010.551220

van Zon A, Peters JP, Stegeman I, Smit AL, Grolman W. Cochlear implantation for patients with single-sided deafness or asymmetrical hearing loss: a systematic review of the evidence. *Otol Neurotol* (2015) 36:209–19. doi:10.1097/ MAO.0000000000000681

van Zon A, Smulders YE, Ramakers GG, Stegeman I, Smit AL, Van Zanten GA, et al. Effect of unilateral and simultaneous bilateral cochlear implantation on tinnitus: a prospective study. *Laryngoscope* (2016) 126:956–61. doi:10.1002/ lary.25493

House WF. Cochlear implants. *Ann Otol Rhinol Laryngol* (1976) 85:1–93. doi :10.1177/00034894760850S303

Quaranta N, Wagstaff S, Baguley DM. Tinnitus and cochlear implantation. *Int J Audiol* (2004) 43:245–51. doi:10.1080/14992020400050033

Quaranta N, Fernandez-Vega S, D'elia C, Filipo R, Quaranta A. The effect of unilateral multichannel cochlear implant on bilaterally perceived tinnitus. *Acta Otolaryngol* (2008) 128:159–63. doi:10.1080/00016480701387173

Tyler RS, Rubinstein J, Pan T, Chang SA, Gogel SA, Gehringer A, et al. Electrical stimulation of the cochlea to reduce tinnitus. *Semin Hear* (2008) 29:326–32. doi:10.1055/s-0028-1095892

Punte AK, Vermeire K, Hofkens A, De Bodt M, De Ridder D, Van de Heyning P. Cochlear implantation as a durable tinnitus treatment in single-sided deafness. *Cochlear Implants Int* (2011) 12:S26–9. doi:10.1179/146701011X 13001035752336

Mertens G, Kleine Punte A, De Bodt M, Van de Heyning P. Binaural auditory outcomes in patients with postlingual profound unilateral hearing loss: 3 years after cochlear implantation. *Audiol Neurootol* (2015) 20:67–72. doi:10.1159/000380751

Pierzycki RH, Edmondson-Jones M, Dawes P, Munro KJ, Moore DR, Kitterick PT. Tinnitus and sleep difficulties after cochlear implantation. *Ear Hear* (2016) 37:e402–8. doi:10.1097/AUD.0000000000000341

Pan T, Tyler RS, Ji H, Coelho C, Gehringer AK, Gogel SA. Changes in the tinnitus handicap questionnaire after cochlear implantation. *Am J Audiol* (2009) 18:144–51. doi:10.1044/1059-0889(2009/07-0042)

Langguth B. Treatment of tinnitus. *Curr Opin Otolaryngol Head Neck Surg* (2015) 23:361–8. doi:10.1097/MOO.0000000000000185

Wallhäusser-Franke E, Brade J, Balkenhol T, D'Amelio R, Seegmüller A, Delb W. Tinnitus: distinguishing between subjectively perceived loudness and tinnitus-related distress. *PLoS One* (2012) 7:e34583. doi:10.1371/journal. pone.0034583

Wallhäusser-Franke E, Repik I, Delb W, Glauner A, Hörmann K. Long-term development of acute tinnitus. *Laryngorhinootologie* (2015) 94:759–69. doi:1 0.1055/s-0035-1550039

Eggermont JJ, Roberts LE. The neuroscience of tinnitus: understanding abnormal and normal auditory perception. *Front Syst Neurosci* (2012) 6:53. doi:10.3389/fnsys.2012.00053

Langguth B, Landgrebe M, Kleinjung T, Sand GP, Hajak G. Tinnitus and depression. *World J Biol Psychiatry* (2011) 12:489–500. doi:10.3109/15622975. 2011.575178

Brüggemann P, Szczepek AJ, Rose M, McKenna L, Olze H, Mazurek B. Impact of multiple factors on the degree of tinnitus distress. *Front Hum Neurosci* (2016) 10:341. doi:10.3389/fnhum.2016.00341

De Ridder D, Vanneste S, Weisz N, Londero A, Schlee W, Elgoyhen AB, et al. An integrative model of auditory phantom perception: tinnitus as a unified percept of interacting separable subnetworks. *Neurosci Biobehav Rev* (2014) 44:16–32. doi:10.1016/j.neubiorev.2013.03.021

Kalbe E, Kessler J, Calabrese P, Smith R, Passmore AP, Brand M, et al. DemTect: a new sensitive cognitive screening test to support the diagnosis of mild cognitive impairment and early dementia. *Int J Geriatr Psychiatry* (2004) 19:136–43. doi:10.1002/gps.1042

Meikle MB, Stewart BJ, Griest SE, Henry JA. Tinnitus outcomes assessment. *Trends Amplif* (2008) 12:223–35. doi:10.1177/1084713808319943

Hiller W, Goebel G. Rapid assessment of tinnitus-related psychological distress using the mini-TQ. *Int J Audiol* (2004) 43:600–4. doi:10.1080/ 14992020400050077

Zeman F, Koller M, Schecklmann M, Langguth B, Landgrebe M. Tinnitus assessment by means of standardized self-report questionnaires: psychometric properties of the tinnitus questionnaire (TQ), the tinnitus handicap inventory (THI), and their short versions in an international and multilingual sample. *Health Qual Life Outcomes* (2012) 10:128. doi:10.1186/1477-7525- 10-128

Zigmond AS, Snaith RP. The hospital anxiety and depression scale. *Acta Psychiatr Scand* (1983) 67:361–70. doi:10.1111/j.1600-0447.1983.tb09716.x

Andersson G, Kaldo-Sandström V, Ström L, Strömgren T. Internet administration of the Hospital Anxiety and Depression Scale in a sample of tinnitus patients. *J Psychosom Res* (2003) 55:259–62. doi:10.1016/ S0022-3999(02)00575-5

Bortz J. *Statistik für Sozialwissenschaftler*. Heidelberg: Springer (1993). 137 p.

Cohen J. *Statistical Power Analysis for the Behavioral Sciences*. Hillsdale, NJ: Lawrence Erlbaum (1988).

Andersson G, Freijd A, Baguley DM, Idrizbegovic E. Tinnitus distress, anxiety, depression, and hearing problems among cochlear implant patients with tinnitus. *J Am Acad Audiol* (2009) 20:315–9. doi:10.3766/jaaa.20.5.5

Kloostra FJ, Arnold R, Hofman R, Van Dijk P. Changes in tinnitus after cochlear implantation and its relation with psychological functioning. *Audiol Neurootol* (2015) 20:81–9. doi:10.1159/000365959

Olze H, Szczepek AJ, Haupt H, Förster U, Zirke N, Gräbel S, et al. Cochlear implantation has a positive influence on quality of life, tinnitus, and psychological comorbidity. *Laryngoscope* (2011) 21:2220–7. doi:10.1002/lary. 22145

Blasco MA, Redleaf MI. Cochlear implantation in unilateral sudden deafness improves tinnitus and speech comprehension: meta-analysis and systematic review. *Otol Neurotol* (2014) 35:1426–32. doi:10.1097/ MAO.0000000000000431

Gaylor JM, Raman G, Chung M, Lee J, Rao M, Lau J, et al. Cochlear implantation in adults: a systematic review and meta-analysis. *JAMA Otolaryngol Head Neck Surg* (2013) 139:265–72. doi:10.1001/jamaoto.2013.1744

Vlastarakos PV, Nazos K, Tavoulari EF, Nikolopoulos TP. Cochlear implantation for single-sided deafness: the outcomes. An evidence-based approach. *Eur Arch Otorhinolaryngol* (2014) 271:2119–26. doi:10.1007/s00405-013-2746-z

Bovo R, Ciorba A, Martini A. Tinnitus and cochlear implants. *Auris Nasus Larynx* (2011) 38:14–20. doi:10.1016/j.anl.2010.05.003

Kim DK, Moon IS, Lim HJ, Yoo SY, Heo KW, Bae SC, et al. Prospective, multi- center study on tinnitus changes after cochlear implantation. *Audiol Neurootol* (2016) 21:165–71. doi:10.1159/000445164

Knopke S, Gräbel S, Förster-Ruhrmann U, Mazurek B, Szczepek AJ, Olze H. Impact of cochlear implantation on quality of life and mental comorbidity in patients aged 80 years. *Laryngoscope* (2016) 126:2811–6. doi:10.1002/ lary.25993

Kompis M, Pelizzone M, Dillier N, Allum J, DeMin N, Senn P. Tinnitus before and 6 months after cochlear implantation. *Audiol Neurootol* (2012) 17:161–8. doi:10.1159/000335126

Mertens G, De Bodt M, Van de Heyning P. Cochlear implantation as a long-term treatment for ipsilateral incapacitating tinnitus in subjects with unilateral hearing loss up to 10 years. *Hear Res* (2016) 331:1–16. doi:10.1016/ j.heares.2015.09.016

Vallés-Varela H, Royo-López J, Carmen-Sampériz L, Sebastián-Cortés JM, Alfonso-Collado I. The cochlear implant as a tinnitus treatment. *Acta Otorrinolaringol Esp* (2013) 64:253–7. doi:10.1016/j.otorri.2012. 11.008

Bauer CA, Brozoski TJ. Effect of tinnitus retraining therapy on the loudness and annoyance of tinnitus: a controlled trial. *Ear Hear* (2011) 32:145–55. doi:10.1097/AUD.0b013e3181f5374f

Zenner HP, Delb W, Kröner-Herwig B, Jäger B, Peroz I, Hesse G, et al. A multidisciplinary systematic review of the treatment for chronic idiopathic tinnitus. *Eur Arch Otorhinolaryngol* (2016). doi:10.1007/s00405-016-4401-y

Hiller W, Goebel G. When tinnitus loudness and annoyance are discrepant: audiological characteristics and psychological profile. *Audiol Neurootol* (2007) 12:391–400. doi:10.1159/000106482

Song JJ, Punte AK, De Ridder D, Vanneste S, Van de Heyning P. Neural substrates predicting improvement of tinnitus after cochlear implantation in patients with single-sided deafness. *Hear Res* (2013) 299:1–9. doi:10.1016/j.heares.2013.02.001

Contrera KJ, Wallhagen MI, Mamo SK, Oh ES, Lin FR. Hearing loss health care for older adults. *J Am Board Fam Med* (2016) 29:394–403. doi:10.3122/jabfm.2016.03.150235

Hsu WT, Hsu CC, Wen MH, Lin HC, Tsai HT, Su P, etal. Increasedriskofdepression in patients with acquired sensory hearing loss: a 12-year follow-up study. *Medicine (Baltimore)* (2016) 95:e5312. doi:10.1097/MD.0000000000005312

Cima RF, Crombez G, Vlaeyen JW. Catastrophizing and fear of tinnitus predict quality of life in patients with chronic tinnitus. *Ear Hear* (2011) 32:634–41. doi:10.1097/AUD.0b013e31821106dd

Heller MF, Bergman M. Tinnitus aurium in normally hearing persons. *Ann Otol Rhinol Laryngol* (1953) 62:73–83.

Schaette R, Turtle C, Munro KJ. Reversible induction of phantom auditory sensation through simulated unilateral hearing loss. *PLoS One* (2012) 7:e35238. doi:10.1371/journal.pone.0035238

Kuk FK, Tyler RS, Rustad N, Harker LA, Tye-Murray N. Alternating current at the eardrum for tinnitus reduction. *J Speech Hear Res* (1989) 32:393–400. doi:10.1044/jshr.3202.393

Mielczarek M, Michalska J, Polatyńska K, Olszewski J. An increase in alpha band frequency in resting state eeg after electrical stimulation of the ear in tinnitus patients – a pilot study. *Front Neurosci* (2016) 10:453. doi:10.3389/fnins.2016.00453

Rubinstein JT, Tyler RS, Johnson A, Brown CJ. Electrical suppression of tinnitus with high-rate pulse trains. *Otol Neurotol* (2003) 24:478–85. doi:10.1097/00129492-200305000-00021

Arts RA, George EL, Janssen M, Griessner A, Zierhofer C, Stokroos RJ. Tinnitus suppression by intracochlear electrical stimulation in single sided deafness – a prospective clinical trial: follow-up. *PLoS One* (2016) 11:e0153131. doi:10.1371/journal.pone.0153131

Chang JE, Zeng FG. Tinnitus suppression by electric stimulation of the auditory nerve. *Front Syst Neurosci* (2012) 6:19. doi:10.3389/fnsys.2012.00019

McKerrow WS, Schreiner CE, Snyder RL, Merzenich MM, Toner JG. Tinnitus suppression by cochlear implants. *Ann Otol Rhinol Laryngol* (1991) 100:552–8. doi:10.1177/000348949110000706

Punte AK, De Ridder D, Van de Heyning P. On the necessity of full length electrical cochlear stimulation to suppress severe tinnitus in sin- gle-sided deafness. *Hear Res* (2013) 295:24–9. doi:10.1016/j.heares.2012. 08.003

Leaver AM, Turesky TK, Seydell-Greenwald A, Morgan S, Kim HJ, Rauschecker JP. Intrinsic network activity in tinnitus investigated using functional MRI. *Hum Brain Mapp* (2016) 37:2717–35. doi:10.1002/hbm. 23204

Husain FT. Neural networks of tinnitus in humans: elucidating severity and habituation. *Hear Res* (2016) 334:37–48. doi:10.1016/j.heares.2015. 09.010

Jastreboff PJ. Phantom auditory perception (tinnitus): mechanisms of generation and perception. *Neurosci Res* (1990) 8:221–54. doi:10.1016/j.heares.2015.09.010

5

Heidelberg Neuro-Music Therapy Restores Attention-Related Activity in the Angular Gyrus in Chronic Tinnitus Patients

Christoph M. Krick[1], Heike Argstatter[2], Miriam Grapp[2], Peter K. Plinkert[3] and Wolfgang Reith[1]*

[1] Department for Neuroradiology, Saarland University Hospital, Homburg, Germany, [2] German Research Centre for Music Therapy Research, Heidelberg, Germany, [3] Department of Otorhinolaryngology, Head and Neck Surgery, University Hospital for Ear, Nose, and Throat, University of Heidelberg, Heidelberg, Germany

***Correspondence:**
Christoph M. Krick
christoph.krick@uniklinikum-saarland.de

Background: Tinnitus is the perception of a phantom sound without external acoustic stimulation. Recent tinnitus research suggests a relationship between attention processes and tinnitus-related distress. It has been found that too much focus on tinnitus comes at the expense of the visual domain. The angular gyrus (AG) seems to play a crucial role in switching attention to the most salient stimulus. This study aims to evaluate the involvement of the AG during visual attention tasks in tinnitus sufferers treated with Heidelberg Neuro-Music Therapy (HNMT), an intervention that has been shown to reduce tinnitus-related distress.

Methods: Thirty-three patients with chronic tinnitus, 45 patients with recent-onset tinnitus, and 35 healthy controls were tested. A fraction of these (21/21/22) were treated with the "compact" version of the HNMT lasting 1 week with intense treatments, while non-treated participants were included as passive controls. Visual attention was evaluated during functional Magnet-Resonance Imaging (fMRI) by a visual Continous Performance Task (CPT) using letter-based alarm cues ("O" and "X") appearing in a sequence of neutral letters, "A" through "H." Participants were instructed to respond via button press only if the letter "O" was followed by the letter "X" (GO condition), but not to respond if a neutral letter appeared instead (NOGO condition). All participants underwent two fMRI sessions, before and after a 1-week study period.

Results: The CPT results revealed a relationship between error rates and tinnitus duration at baseline whereby the occurrence of erroneous "GO omissions" and the reaction time increased with tinnitus duration. Patients with chronic tinnitus who were treated with HNMT had decreasing error rates (fewer GO omissions) compared to treated recent-onset patients. fMRI analyses confirmed greater activation of the AG during CPT in chronic patients after HNMT treatment compared to treated recent-onset patients.

Conclusions: Our findings suggest that HNMT treatment helps shift the attention from the auditory phantom percept toward visual cues in chronic tinnitus patients and that this shift in attention may involve the AG.

Keywords: tinnitus, fMRI neuroimaging, Heidelberg model of music therapy, tinnitus distress, tinnitus treatment, attention

INTRODUCTION

Tinnitus is the perception of a phantom sound, such as a pure tone, ringing, buzzing, or other noise, without external acoustic stimulation. However, while the occurrence of tinnitus may be often disturbing, it does not necessarily cause the disease pattern of a mental suffering (Malouff et al., 2011). Conversely, the duration since the tinnitus onset and the gender seem influence the individually reported mental distress (Seydel et al., 2013). Thus, the etiology of tinnitus-related distress depends on a number of poorly understood factors (Møller, 2016) that has led to several models and theories on the pathophysiology of tinnitus (Henry et al., 2014). Findings from Positron Emission Tomography (PET) measurements showed an involvement of auditory and non-auditory networks for maintaining the tinnitus percept (Mirz et al., 1999). The awareness of tinnitus activates those brain centers that are also involved in conscious acoustic perception (Dehaene and Changeux, 2011). Presumably prefrontal and parietal attention networks play a crucial role in conscious perception. The inferior parietal lobe has been found to be a key region for the awareness of an acoustic percept (Sadaghiani et al., 2009). Recent tinnitus research suggested a relationship between these attention processes and maintenance of tinnitus (Roberts et al., 2013). Husain et al. (2015) observed that tinnitus patients' attention networks showed more activation during visual than auditory tasks. These findings suggested a need for rising engagement of the attention system in tinnitus patients while focusing on visual stimuli. It is unclear, however, whether these perceptual changes arose immediately with the tinnitus onset or whether they were gradually provoked by the persisting tinnitus percept. Recent findings on tinnitus distress suggested that the distress-related higher mental effort for attention control may arise primarily from focusing on self-referred emotional signals that were triggered by a network consisting of the amygdala, the anterior cingulate cortex, the insula, and the parahippocampal area (Vanneste et al., 2010). Patients' attention thus shifts from the outside world toward the inner "mental pain" caused by the tinnitus distress (Malouff et al., 2011). Mohamad et al. (2016) summarized attention-related studies in tinnitus sufferers: That review did not tend to generally impaired attention due to tinnitus but some evidence that tinnitus patients performed poorer on selective attention in visual tasks compared to normal hearing controls (Hallam et al., 2004; Stevens et al., 2007), but non-significant findings were mentioned, too (Heeren et al., 2014). Hence, the observations so far remained unclear whether and how the tinnitus percept may claim resources for the visual attention. Selective attention in the visual domain and the respective brain responses can be measured by a Continuous Performance Task (CPT) which requires sustained attention to a sequence of visual stimuli (Hester et al., 2004). In this context, reaction time (RT) and error rates for responses can be measured to assess effects of a musical intervention (Guo et al., 2015).

The inferior parietal lobe plays a key role in conscious awareness of acoustic and visual cues (van Gaal et al., 2011; Igelström et al., 2016). Humphreys and Chechlacz (2015) described a network for attentive visual search which includes the angular gyrus (AG), the middle occipital gyrus, superior and middle temporal gyri, and the insula. The latter is also known as part of the tinnitus network, whereas the temporal regions and the AG are involved in self-awareness and self-perception (De Ridder et al., 2014). Hester et al. (2004) found these regions to be systematically involved in self-monitoring during visual CPT. The AG appears to play a crucial role for binding the attention to the individually most salient sensory stream (Taylor et al., 2011). Visual attention can be disrupted by suppressing AG activity using Transcranial Magnet Stimulation (TMS; Taylor and Thut, 2012). If the AG is involved in driving awareness toward the most salient sensory modality, the attention focus may be strongly driven toward the auditory system in case of tinnitus (De Ridder et al., 2014; Husain et al., 2015). Resting-state functional MRI scans revealed higher amplitude of low-frequency fluctuations in the AG and other attention-related areas (Chen et al., 2015). PET measurements confirmed these findings showing higher AG activity in chronic tinnitus patients (Song et al., 2012). Binding the attention to the auditory sensation in turn may explain the attention deficits in visual tasks as well as the attention conflict in the auditory domain in tinnitus patients (Araneda et al., 2015; Li et al., 2016). Using PET measurements, Plewnia et al. (2007) observed both tinnitus-related hyperactivity in the right AG and TMS-related attenuation of tinnitus after stimulation of this area. This finding indicated that the AG is a key region in understanding the erroneous focus on the phantom noise in clinically decompensated tinnitus patients.

A number of therapy options have been developed for tinnitus treatment, comprising Tinnitus Retraining Therapy, Cognitive Behavioral Therapy, Progressive Tinnitus Management, Biofeedback, Education, and Relaxation Therapies (Herraiz et al., 2007; Hesse and Laubert, 2010; Hesser et al., 2011; Folmer et al., 2014; Grewal et al., 2014; Myers et al., 2014). Most therapies aim to dissuade patients auditory self-monitoring. In those studies, however, there was little consistency in the therapeutic effects and their scientific verifiability. The statistically weak or inconsistent observations may reflect variation in the aberrant mental states of tinnitus patients. With respect to long-lasting neuroplastic changes, starting with the onset of tinnitus (Mühlau et al., 2006; Landgrebe et al., 2009; Schneider et al., 2009; Husain et al., 2011; Leaver et al., 2012; Boyen et al., 2013; Schecklmann et al., 2013), one can assume that the duration of tinnitus is one of several factors for the variable effects in tinnitus relief (Malouff et al., 2011). Relief is not directly related to the loudness of the phantom sound, but to the level of "catastrophizing" its affective experience (Møller, 2016). This in turn corresponds to the strength of an emotionally driven attention shift in tinnitus' pathophysiology causing tinnitus-related distress (Vanneste et al., 2010; Ueyama et al., 2013). The compact approach of the Heidelberg Neuro-Music Therapy (HNMT) has been shown to reduce tinnitus-related distress as assessed by a controlled trial (Argstatter et al., 2015). Its effects have also been shown to be maintained over a long time (Argstatter et al., 2012).

In the current study, we implemented a task that has previously been used in our research unit for examination of adults with attention deficit syndrome, the visual CPT (Schneider et al., 2010). The CPT was implemented as GO/NOGO task, allowing the observation of attention and inhibition control

Attention difficulties can be detected by omitted GO stimuli, whereas decreased inhibition control results in erroneous NOGO reactions. The current paper aims to show the effects of tinnitus duration on the control of visual attention and the effects of HNMT on the visual attention network in tinnitus patients. Thus, we assessed the attention binding to the visual cue that required the participant's decision for action or inhibition. We postulated that HNMT will improve the visual attention in those patients with initial attention impairments.

MATERIALS AND METHODS

Participants

Both recent-onset patients unsuccessfully completing the standard clinical treatment (tinnitus persisting for a maximum of 6 months) and patients with chronic tinnitus (duration of at least 6 months) were invited for participation. Thirty-three patients with chronic tinnitus (12 females), 45 patients with recent-onset tinnitus (19 females), and 35 healthy controls (18 females) participated in the trial (**Table 1**). The group of healthy controls was enrolled after recruitment of the tinnitus groups, according to the patients' gender ratio and age distribution. Mean age was 47.6 ± *SD* 10.4 years in the chronic tinnitus group, 43.1 ± *SD* 10.5 years in the recent-onset tinnitus patients, and 43.4 ± *SD* 14.5 years in healthy controls (**Table 1**). In the group of recent-onset patient there was less variance with respect to the tinnitus duration (mean 8.1 weeks ± *SD* 1.6 weeks), since those participants were systematically included immediately after the standard treatment by otorhinolaryngology. In contrast to this, tinnitus duration in the chronic cases ranged from 1 to 14 years (mean 5.26 years ± *SD* 4.1 years). All participants underwent clinical examination and audiometric testing. The tinnitus patients were additionally examined by a pre-participation evaluation based on the TRI-recommendations (audiological testing, otolaryngological examination, and psychological intake interview). Patients were excluded if the tinnitus was related to anatomic lesions of the ear, retro-cochlear lesions, or to cochlear implants. Further exclusion criteria included clinical diagnosis of a comorbid severe mental disorder, clinical diagnosis of Menière's Disease, severe hyperacusis, or severe hearing impairment (>40 dB) in the tinnitus frequencies region. The latter criterion was defined to allow the participation of HNMT without hearing aids.

The study was conducted in accordance with the Declaration of Helsinki and approved by the local Saarland (Germany) ethics committee (ID-number 111/11). A complete clinical study protocol was compiled according to the ICH guidelines for good clinical practice.

Tinnitus Questionnaire (TQ)

Psychological complaints were assessed using the German version of the "Tinnitus Questionnaire" (TQ) as described by Goebel and Hiller (1998). This well-validated inventory comprises 52 items and records tinnitus related complaints. The items can be aggregated to variables representing the dimensions of mental distress: emotional and cognitive load, tinnitus duration, hearing impairments, sleep disturbance, and somatoform disorders. The global TQ-score ranges between the minimum score of 0 and the maximum score of 84, in which high values indicate high tinnitus related distress. Four levels of severity include: mild (0–30), middle (31–46), severe (47–59), and very severe (60–84) affliction. Cross-correlation between TQ and Tinnitus Handicap Inventory (THI) was reported by Zeman et al. (2012) yielding a Pearson's correlation coefficient of 0.87.

The patients' distress was examined by TQ at the time point of the pre-participation evaluation (T0) as well as before (T1) and after (T2) the study period. In the tinnitus groups, we included adult patients who were diagnosed with disturbing tinnitus (TQ-score > 30), but not completely decompensated tinnitus (TQ-score < 64). At T0, the tinnitus distress as measured by TQ was 43.2 ± 9.6 *SD* in chronic patients and 37.3 ± 15.8 *SD* in recent-onset patients. Since the tinnitus duration is regarded in the TQ score, there was a systematic difference between recent-onset and chronic tinnitus.

Intervention (HNMT)

All participants from the three groups, chronic and recent-onset tinnitus patients as well as healthy controls, were included in the examination of visual attention, but the groups were randomly divided in different treatment cohorts, comprising the participation in the "compact" HNMT in each group. The other option consisted in either no treatment or weekly sessions ("standard" protocol) instead of the compact treatment over 5 days. So, in each group of participants, treatment cohorts with comparable sample sizes were selected for undergoing the compact HNMT application. Thus, 21 chronic tinnitus patients (9 females, tinnitus duration 250 weeks ± 187 *SD*), 21 recent-onset tinnitus patients (9 females, tinnitus duration 8.14 weeks ± 1.85 *SD*), and 22 healthy controls (10 females, no tinnitus) underwent the compact HNMT.

For examination of interaction between tinnitus duration and visual performance, the initial behavioral measurements at T1 from all participants, comprising both treated and non-treated subgroups, were regarded. At this time the conditions were comparable for all participants, since there wasn't yet an influence from the subsequent therapy option. Hence, evaluations from this time point were independent from the therapy option and, hence, used to generally assess influences from the individually pre-existing or not existing tinnitus to the visual attention.

The subgroups treated with the compact HNMT (**Table 1**, marked in bold text) were compared to reveal the duration-specific effect among therapy-related effects on the attention network. The sub-groups of recent-onset tinnitus patients and the "treated" healthy controls have been already included in a previously reported study on structural effects from HNMT, in which we found that HNMT caused a major improvement of 17.7 points on the TQ scale in treated tinnitus patients (**Figure 1**, Krick et al., 2015). In the current study, we analogously evaluated the effects of HNMT in chronic tinnitus patients. As the HNMT has been found to rapidly reduce tinnitus distress (Grapp et al., 2013; Krick et al., 2015), this therapy can be used to assess distress-related effects on brain activation during a short study period.

TABLE 1 | Participants ($n = 113$) and therapy participation.

		Tinnitus			Sum
		Controls	Recent-onset	Chronic	
Music therapy and tinnitus profile	None (*n*)	13 (8f/5m)	24 (10f/14m)		37
	Frequency (*SD*)	None	6,376 (3,176)		
	Duration (*SD*)		0.16 y (0.03)		
	Standard (*n*)			12 (3f/9m)	12
	Frequency (*SD*)			6,200 (3,615)	
	Duration (*SD*)			6.09 y (4.35)	
	Compact (*n*)	**22 (10f/12m)**	**21 (9f/12m)**	**21 (9f/12m)**	**64**
	Frequency (*SD*)	None	5,102 (2,332)	6,785 (2,547)	
	Duration (*SD*)		0.16 y (0.04)	4.80 y (3.56)	
Sum		35	45	33	113

The HNMT was offered weekly (standard) or condensed in 1 week (compact). For fMRI comparison of HNMT effect only participants undergoing the compact treatment were included ($n = 64$; bold). Behavior observations, however, comprised reaction data of all participants at first measurement (before the study period).

The study protocol of the compact version of HNMT consisted of 9 consecutive 50-min sessions of individualized therapy, comprising acoustic training for frequency discrimination, auditory attention control tasks, and guided exercises for mindfulness and distress regulation. Therapy took place on 5 consecutive days (Monday to Friday) with two therapy sessions per day. Music therapy can be divided into two main categories: receptive (music listening based) and active (music making). Each morning and each afternoon session lasted for 50 min, in which there were 25 min of active music therapy and 25 min of receptive music therapy. Two trained music therapists carried out the therapy, in which one therapist performed the active modules and the other performed the receptive modules. The interventions were structured into treatment modules of directive counseling, habituation training, and stress management. A more detailed description can be found in Argstatter et al. (2015) and Grapp et al. (2013).

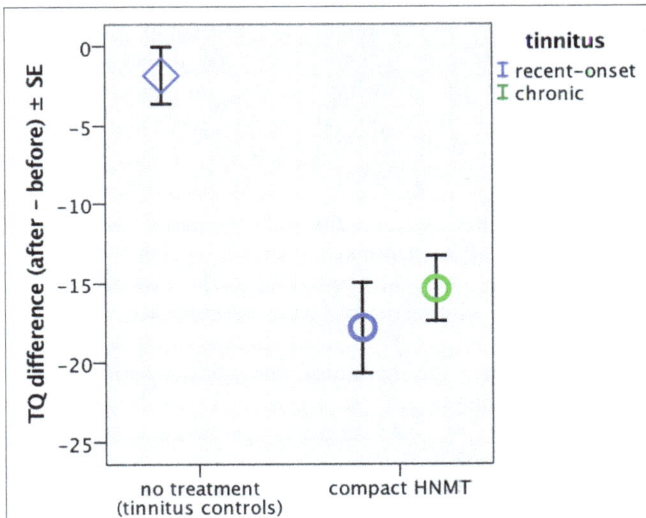

FIGURE 1 | Change in subjective tinnitus distress as measured by TQ. Krick et al. (2015) found that HNMT caused a major improvement in tinnitus distress in recent-onset tinnitus patients (blue circle), as measured by a reduction of near 18 on the TQ scale, an improvement which was not observed in non-treated passive control patients (rhomb). Here we measured the HNMT effect in chronic tinnitus sufferers (green circle), revealing a similar decrease on the TQ score by 15.3 ± *SD* 9.5 ($n = 21$; $Z = -4.3$; $p < 0.0001$). There was no significant difference in the therapy-induced TQ reduction between treated chronic and treated recent-onset patients ($n = 21/21$; $Z = -0.4$; $p > 0.6$).

Experimental Setup

Independently from the assignment to the treatment cohorts, all participants performed a letter-based CPT twice, during two fMRI sessions at T1 and at T2. Capital letters "A" through "H" were used as "neutral" stimuli in a quasi-random order. Letters "O" and "X" were used as alerting events inserted in the letter stream. Each letter was presented for 420 ms on a screen. Participants were instructed to watch the rapid sequence of letters and to look out for the letter "O" as an alarm stimulus. If the next letter following the "O" was an "X," they were asked to press a button (GO condition). In all other cases, the participants were instructed not to press the button. Especially if the letter "O" was followed by a letter different from "X," no reaction (NOGO condition) was required. The response button was counterbalanced for left and right hand in all groups.

Each condition consisted of 30 trials of GO or NOGO events which were randomly inserted among the presentation of 1300 letters over 12.6 min. The letters were projected through a window of the Magnet-Resonance (MR) cabin on a screen placed behind the head-side opening of the scanner. A mirror on the top of the head coil allowed viewing the letters in a light square on black background. The presentation was controlled by a computer synchronized with the imaging pulses.

Data Acquisition and Data Analysis

The 3 tesla MR scanner "Skyra" (Siemens) was used for imaging. Functional scan parameters of the Blood Oxygen Dependent (BOLD) imaging were set to time-to-repeat (TR) of 2.2 s, echo time (TE) to 30 ms, and flip angle of 90°. Thirty slices of 3 mm thickness with a 0.75 mm gap to the next slice covered the whole brain. Each slice was scanned into a 94 × 94 matrix resulting in a voxel volume of 2 × 2 × 3 mm^3. For each run, 348 scans were acquired, including 4 prescans to compensate for magnetization saturation effects. The prescans were later discarded from data processing.

The functional BOLD imaging was conducted at T1 and T2. Two high-resolution anatomical scans over the whole brain were also measured at T1 and at T2, using a Magnetization Prepared Rapid Acquisition of Gradient Echoes (MPRAGE; Mugler and Brookeman, 1990) sequence. This 3D brain image resulted in isometric voxel dimensions of 0.9 × 0.9 × 0.9 mm^3.

Thus, functional and anatomical MRI (fMRI) scans were each conducted in two consecutive MRI sessions before and after the 1-week study period, meaning that all participants underwent the GO/NOGO CPT twice, at T1 and T2. The same hand and the same procedure were used in both consecutive measurements. During the MRI sessions, double ear protection (earmuffs and head phones) was applied to reduce scanner noise. For compensating ametropia, MRI-compatible glasses with adapted diopter for each eye were offered if necessary.

Preprocessing and modeling of MRI measurements were executed using standard procedures of *Statistical Parametric Mapping* (SPM8, Wellcome Trust Centre for Neuroimaging, London). Preparation of the functional scans included:

- slice time and motion correction of functional scans;
- segmentation of the anatomical scan;
- co-registration of the resulting gray matter (GM) compartment to the mean image of corrected functional scans;
- co-registration of the anatomical image to the position of the functional mean image;
- determination of normalization parameters using the anatomical image;
- application of normalization parameters to the functional scans with fitting to the template of the Montreal Neurological Institute (MNI space);
- and Gaussian smoothing using an 8-mm radius in each direction.

For general activation regarding to the alarm stimulus, the visual cue "O" from both GO and NOGO trials of the first run were pooled by a conjunction analysis. The effect of HNMT with respect to the tinnitus duration was estimated using both MRI sessions by a flexible factorial model (2 × 2 ANOVA) with "Time" (T1, T2) as within-subject factors and "Group" (chronic, recent-onset, control) as between-subject factors to explore the effect of treatment in the various participant groups. An assumption of interaction between "Time" and "Group" was predicted due to the effect of HNMT and tinnitus duration on the subjects' brain activity.

The GO and the NOGO conditions were modeled using the canonical hemodynamic response function and its first derivative as evoked by the visual alarm stimulus "O." This first-level "O"-responses of both measurement times (T1 and T2) per participant was included in the flexible factorial model.

Behavioral accuracy and RT from button responses were evaluated separately using SPSS Statistics (IBM). As the error rates from both GO and NOGO conditions did not correspond to a Gaussian distribution, non-parametric tests (Spearman Rho correlation and Wilcoxon test for paired data) were used to investigate the influence from tinnitus duration on the subjects' attention.

RESULTS

Therapy Effect on Subjective Distress Score (TQ)

Participation in HNMT yielded a reduction of 15.3 ± *SD* 9.5 scale points on the TQ score in chronic tinnitus sufferers (n = 21; Mann–Whitney-*U* test: Z = −4.3; $p < 0.0001$) compared to non-treated tinnitus patients (n = 22) which showed only a small test-retest effect of −1.8 score points. In chronic tinnitus patients, the subjective tinnitus distress was similarly reduced after HNMT as previously reported for treated recent-onset patients (Krick et al., 2015; **Figure 1**). When comparing the findings from recent-onset patients with the TQ reduction in treated chronic patients, the effects did not significantly differ between both patient groups (n = 21/21; Z = −0.4; $p >$ 0.6).

Visual Attention Task and Behavioral Accuracy

Regarding the individual tinnitus anamnesis, there was a significant interaction between tinnitus duration and error rates from GO/NOGO task. At T1, error rates for both the GO condition (Spearman-Rho: +0.27; $p < 0.005$) and the NOGO condition (Spearman-Rho: −0.23; $p < 0.05$) depended on the type of tinnitus: chronic or recent-onset. Error rates from GO trials increased with tinnitus duration, whereas error rates from NOGO trials were diminished with chronic tinnitus (**Figure 2A**).

Latencies of the observed reactions also yielded effects of tinnitus duration (**Figure 2B**). Patients with chronic tinnitus exhibited longer RTs compared to healthy controls (Mann–Whitney-U; Z = −5.9; $p < 0.0001$), whereas there was no significant RT difference between controls and patients with recent-onset tinnitus (Mann–Whitney-U; Z = −0.82; $p > 0.4$). A linear regression model showed that the RT latency was delayed by about 42 ms with each year of tinnitus duration ($T = 7.3$; $p <$ 0.0001).

Non-parametric paired Wilcoxon tests were performed to assess differences between HNMT treated and untreated participants. In the non-treated patients, error rates did not differ between start and end of the study period, neither in the GO condition (Wilcoxon Z: −0.01; $p > 0.99$) nor in the NOGO condition (Wilcoxon Z: −1.4; $p > 0.15$). For both groups participating in HNMT, "treated" controls and treated tinnitus patients, there were a measurable effect by the HNMT application in each case, showing each diminishing error rates between T1 and T2. This effect was similar between "treated" controls (GO: Wilcoxon *Z*: −1.68; $p < 0.1$; NOGO: Wilcoxon

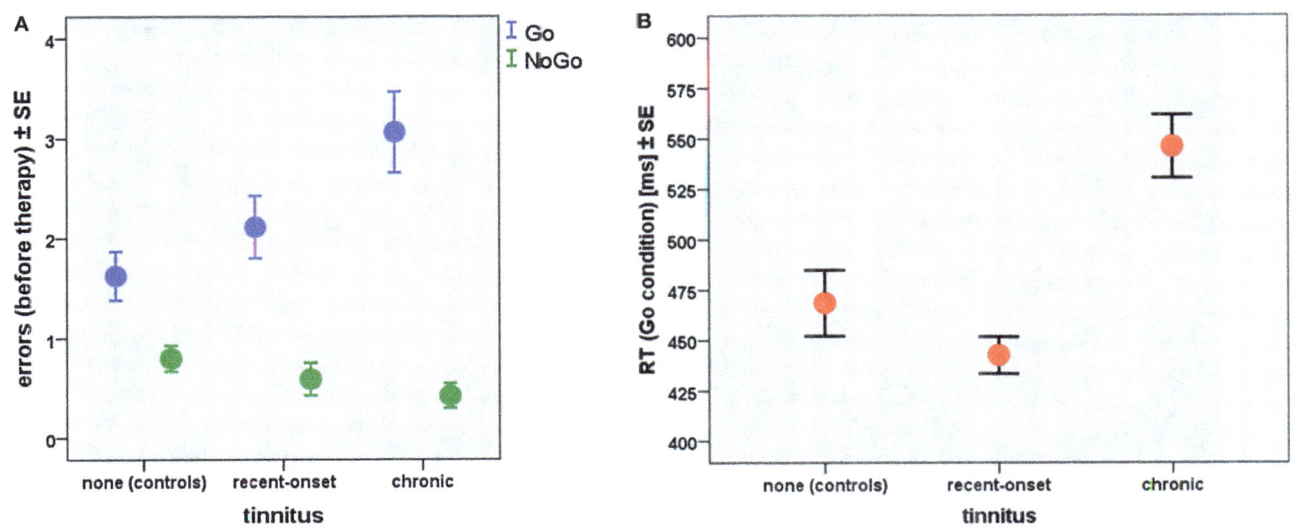

FIGURE 2 | (A) Error rates and **(B)** reaction times (RT) related to tinnitus type at T1 for all participants (35 healthy controls, 45 recent-onset tinnitus patients, and 33 chronic tinnitus patients).

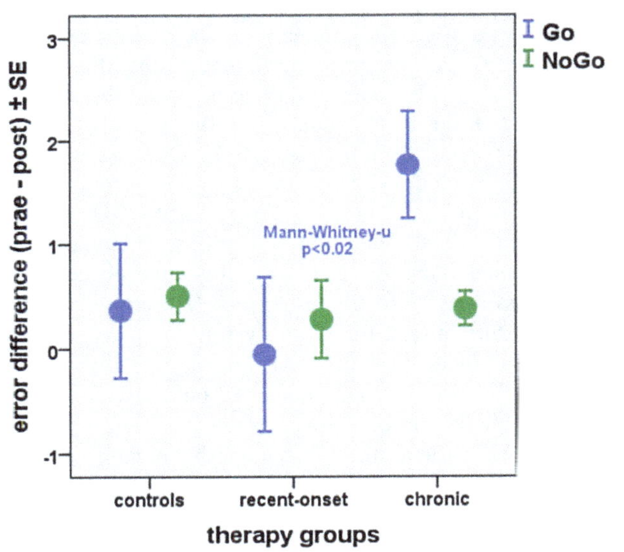

FIGURE 3 | Difference of error rates for GO and NOGO trials before and after HNMT in treated subsamples of healthy controls ($n = 22$), recent-onset tinnitus patients ($n = 21$), and chronic tinnitus sufferers ($n = 21$).

Z: −2.00; $p < 0.05$) and treated patients (GO: Wilcoxon Z: −1.83; $p < 0.1$); NOGO: Wilcoxon Z: −1.74; $p < 0.1$). However, comparing the subgroups of treated tinnitus patients, the reduction of GO errors was significantly more pronounced in chronic compared to recent-onset tinnitus patients (Mann-Whitney Z: −2.3; $p < 0.02$) as shown in **Figure 3**. In contrast to this, there was no effect on the attention-related errors in non-treated participants (GO: Wilcoxon Z: −0.01; $p > 0.9$; NOGO: Wilcoxon Z: −1.41; $p > 0.15$).

Brain Activation

BOLD contrast by the effect of visual attention on the cue "O" was derived from the first MRI session (T1) for all participants ($n = 113$). This analysis was realized by a conjunction (comparable with the statistical intersection by an AND operation) of both GO and NOGO conditions, since both conditions were based on the visual cue "O." We aimed to observe here the brain network for conscious processing and attention binding (Dehaene and Changeux, 2011). Thus, the common activation by the visual cue for both GO and NOGO trials was relevant for observing its interdependency with tinnitus. The brain activations covered dorsolateral inferior frontal areas, the insula, superior and middle temporal regions, the premotor cortex, inferior parietal lobes, and inferior occipital areas in both hemispheres (**Figure 4**). In this network, activation in the right (MNI: +60/−42/+18) and left (MNI: −26/−62/+46) AG scored highest (**Table 2**).

Based on the fact of AG involvement in conscious attention control, a region of interest (ROI) including the left and the right AG was derived from the brain atlas for Automatic Anatomical Labeling (AAL, Tzourio-Mazoyer et al., 2002) using the WFU PickAtlas (Maldjian et al., 2003). The neural base of the observed behavioral differences between long-term tinnitus sufferers and recent-onset tinnitus patients was investigated within this ROI by utilization of the HNMT effects on the distress symptoms. A flexible factorial model for repeated measures with "Time" as within-subject factor and "Group" as between-subject factor was performed in treated patients to reveal effects from the individual tinnitus duration on change in AG activation. Contrasts of the respective activation levels at T1 and T2 exhibited higher activation differences in the right AG (MNI: +50/−64/+28) and left AG (MNI: −50/−68/+24) in chronic patients compared to recent-onset patients (**Figure 5**). The maximum peak regarding this activation difference was located in the right AG, even for a whole-brain analysis (**Table 2**). When reversely contrasting

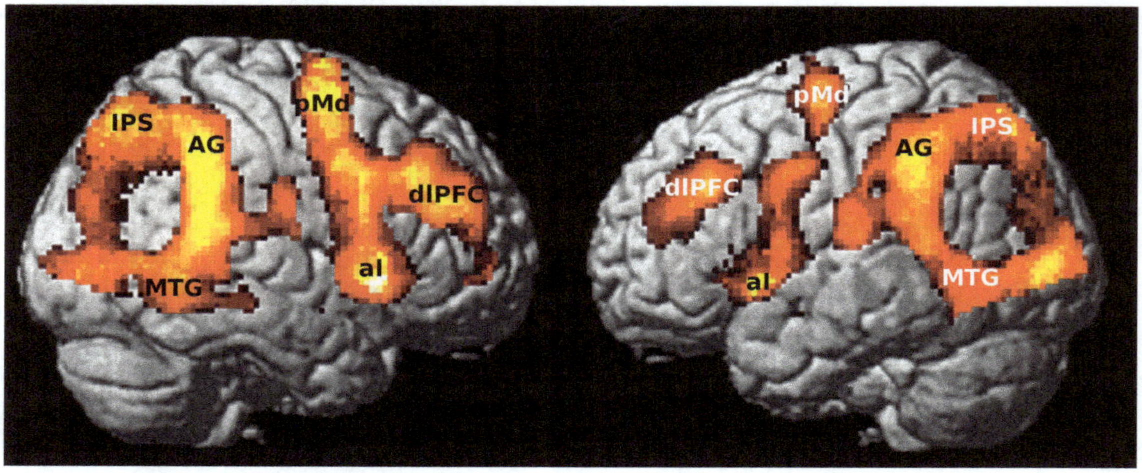

FIGURE 4 | Activated network for to the alarm stimulus ("O") from the first fMRI session (T1) by conjunction of conditions GO & NOGO ($n = 113$). Maximum activation peaked in the right AG ($p < 10^{-10}$ FWE corrected; 20 voxels extent threshold).

the differences in the opposite direction, there were no clusters peaking higher in recent-onset than in chronic patients.

DISCUSSION

The effect of auditory discrimination training and sound-based stimulation have often been discussed in tinnitus therapy (Flor et al., 2004; Herraiz et al., 2010; Hoare et al., 2013) yielding inhomogeneous outcome. While most music-based approaches are passive interventions which are based on listening to computer-modified musical stimuli, the HNMT pursues an active engagement by means of repeated stimulation of the central auditory pathway with sounds in the harmonic spectrum of the individual tinnitus frequency. Thus, the therapeutic sounds are actively performed in aware attention, not as passive listening. Evidence seems to indicate that the amount of attention dedicated to the auditory input is essential (Argstatter et al., 2015). The HNMT combines complementary receptive and active based music interventions to intervene at different levels of the neural tinnitus network. The "Neuroauditive Cortex Training" is a targeted and active auditory training focusing on tone sequences centered around the frequency of the patients' tinnitus frequency. A systematic and targeted training of inaccurately intonated musical sounds enables the patients to exert influence on their auditory processes since they learn to actively filter out irrelevant information and to concentrate on relevant acoustic stimuli. Music-based exercises for mindfulness then promotes desensitization of tinnitus perception. The individual tinnitus sound is embedded in relaxation music and the patients learn to decouple possible negative reactions toward the tinnitus sound or even to completely ignore the acoustic on-top-interference. Being able to disengage from emotional stimuli may reduce the tendency to experience negative affect and redeploying attention has been postulated to lead to a "flexibility of attention" which may free up cognitive resources (Linehan et al., 2007).

Jonker et al. (2013) were able to show that auditory distractors did not provoke a general influence on the visual attention as measured by CPT. This may mean that neither the tinnitus percept nor the MRI noise themselves would be sufficient to induce attention-related effects on the visual perception. However, our results from the visual GO/NOGO attention task yielded rising frequency of omission errors (GO errors) with the duration of tinnitus. In addition, erroneous NOGO responses were reduced with the duration of tinnitus. This observation can be explained in the context of a tinnitus-duration-dependent attention loss relating to the visual task (Husain et al., 2015) due to the shift toward the auditory tinnitus percept (Alpini and Cesarani, 2006). One can then assume that difficulties in monitoring the visual stream concerned both GO and NOGO trials. If the "alarm stimulus" was perceived to a lesser degree in chronic tinnitus patients, the reduced number of false alarms can be interpreted as due to a lack of visual attention rather than from better inhibition control. Following this line of argument, the conjunction of both conditions as a common predictor for visual attention seemed justifiable for the functional analyze regarding the visual cue "O."

Since the attention-related effects as observed by the GO/NOGO task were different with the tinnitus duration, we compared the visual attention and its change due to HNMT in recent-onset and chronic tinnitus patients. HNMT led to a decrease of omission errors in the chronic patients whose attention was most impaired before therapy. The error reduction can be explained in terms of a reinforcement of visual attention. According to this reduction of GO errors response times for the GO condition were also most reduced in chronic tinnitus patients after HNMT (**Figure 6**). The therapy-induced acceleration in cases of chronic tinnitus differed significantly from "treated" controls (Mann–Whitney-U tests; $Z = -2.99$; $p < 0.005$) as well as from treated patients with recent-onset tinnitus ($Z = -2.25$;

TABLE 2 | Activated Clusters for the visual cue "O": (A) general brain activations for the cue "O" and (B) HNMT-induced alterations in relation to tinnitus duration.

Localization	MNI (x y z)			*p* cluster
(A) ACTIVATION DUE TO "O" CUE; CONJUNCTION GO & NOGO, *N* = 113 WHOLE BRAIN ANALYSIS; *P* < 0.00001 FWE CORRECTED				
R angular Gyrus (AG)	60	−42	18	$p < 0.001$ corr
L angular Gyrus (AG)	−26	−62	46	$p < 0.001$ corr
R intraparietal sulcus (IPS)	34	−62	48	$p < 0.001$ corr
L intraparietal sulcus (IPS)	−32	−50	38	$p < 0.001$ corr
R insula	34	20	4	$p < 0.001$ corr
L insula	−32	18	4	$p < 0.001$ corr
R inferior frontal gyrus (IFG)	46	8	22	$p < 0.001$ corr
L inferior frontal gyrus (IFG)	−32	36	10	$p < 0.001$ corr
R premotor cortex (pMd)	46	8	32	$p < 0.001$ corr
L premotor cortex (pMd)	−28	−12	68	$p < 0.001$ corr
R middle frontal gyrus (MFG)	40	34	32	$p < 0.001$ corr
L middle frontal gyrus (MFG)	−44	32	32	$p < 0.001$ corr
posterior medial frontal gyrus	4	8	52	$p < 0.001$ corr
R middle temporal gyrus (MTG)	50	−52	−6	$p < 0.001$ corr
L middle temporal gyrus (MTG)	−50	−66	−2	$p < 0.001$ corr
(B) "O" CUE; T2 > T1; CHRONIC (21) > RECENT-ONSET PATIENTS (21) MASKED WITH ROI COVERING THE AG; SMALL-VOL. CORR.; *P* < 0.001 UNCORR.				
R AG	50	−64	28	$p < 0.05$ corr
L AG	−50	−68	24	n.s.

Localization	MNI (x y z)			Cluster size
(C) "O" CUE; T2 > T1; CHRONIC (21) > RECENT-ONSET PATIENTS (21) WHOLE-BRAIN ANALYSIS; *P* < 0.001 UNCORR.				
R angular gyrus (AG)	50	−64	28	236 voxels
L angular gyrus (AG)	−50	−68	24	41 voxels
L middle temporal gyrus (MTG)	−50	−18	−14	55 voxels
R precuneus	10	−56	20	25 voxels
(D) "O" CUE; T2 > T1; CHRONIC (21) > CONTROLS (22) WHOLE-BRAIN ANALYSIS; *P* < 0.001 UNCORR.				
L frontal eye field (FEF)	−16	−16	64	79 voxels
R frontal eye field (FEF)	−22	−8	68	191 voxels
R premotor cortex (pMC)	10	26	72	81 voxels
(E) "O" CUE; T2 > T1; RECENT-ONSET (21) > CONTROLS (22) WHOLE-BRAIN ANALYSIS; *P* < 0.001 UNCORR.				
no suprathreshold clusters				

The cluster-related significance (p cluster) was calculated after Family-wise Error (FEW) correction for multiple comparisons (abbr. "corr").

$p < 0.05$). Hence, the therapy-induced alteration of attention parameters was dependent on the tinnitus duration. In contrast to this, the therapy-induced TQ change showed no influence from tinnitus duration (**Figure 1**).

The behavioral effect of HNMT coincidentally matched with a higher task-related activation level of the bilateral AG with a right-sided maximum. The role of the AG has previously been established in visual attention control (Taylor et al., 2011; Humphreys and Chechlacz, 2015) and it has been recognized as part of the "tinnitus core" (De Ridder et al., 2014). Dehaene and Changeux (2011) assumed its role as part of a "Global Neural Workspace" for conscious processing. Thus, one can assume that the structural overlap between visual attention network, awareness network, and tinnitus core network mediated between the duration of tinnitus and a diminished awareness in visual attention (Roberts et al., 2013). The evidence of a HNMT-induced reinforcement of AG activation in chronic tinnitus patients underlined the role of this brain area in the context of the central attention control. Therefore, the reduction of omission errors can be explained as a relaxation of the erroneous attention binding to the auditory sensation in chronic tinnitus patients.

In general, the AG is considered to be a cerebral cross-modal hub for multisensory information and for reorienting attention to relevant information (Seghier, 2013). This means that the AG acts as a central gate for reorienting or shifting the attention toward those sensations that gain the highest salience in terms of emotional value or individual meaning (Gottlieb, 2007). The AG seems to include at least two centers: a dorsal and a ventral part (Uddin et al., 2010) which are involved either in multisensory bottom-up tasks, such as reading (Price, 2010; Segal and Petrides, 2013), or in top-down control of self-referential mental concepts (Bahnemann et al., 2010; Kim, 2010). The reactivation of AG found in this study can be anatomically assigned to the ventral part of AG. This region additionally overlaps with parietal areas of the "default-mode network" (Raichle, 2015) and it plays a role in self-relevant memory retrieval (Kim, 2010) as well as in emotional and

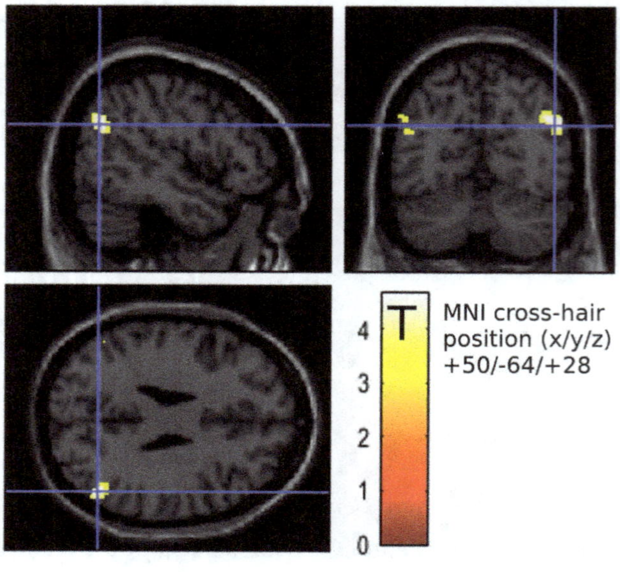

FIGURE 5 | Activation difference (after – before HNMT) yielded stronger effects in chronic ($n = 21$) compared to recent-onset ($n = 21$) patients in the mask covering the left and the right angular gyrus (AG) ($p < 0.001$ uncorrected; 20 voxels extent threshold). The maximum peak was situated in the right AG (crosshairs, neurological view). This cluster peaked in a T score of 4.7 that was significant after FWE correction on cluster level ($p < 0.05$).

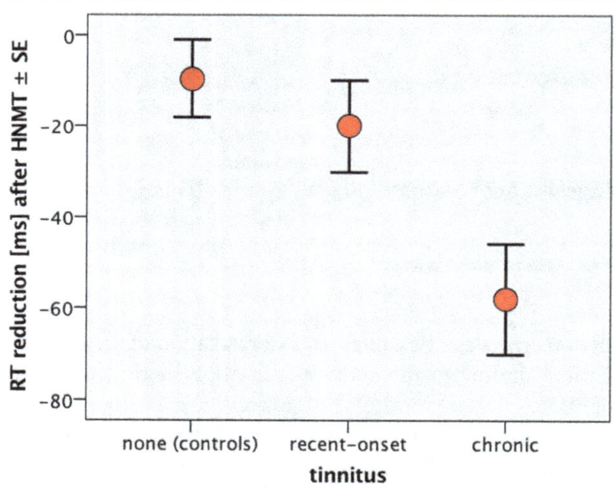

FIGURE 6 | RT difference (after – before) over the 1-week study period in the GO condition. "Treated" healthy participants served as active controls ($n = 22$) to compare the mental acceleration due to the compact HNMT in treated patients with recent-onset ($n = 21$) and chronic tinnitus ($n = 21$). RT was significantly reduced in chronic patients compared to both recent-onset patients (Mann–Whitney-*U* tests; $p < 0.05$) and active controls ($p < 0.005$). There was no significant RT difference between active controls and recent-onset patients ($p > 0.63$).

social perception (Bahnemann et al., 2010; Igelström et al., 2016). Plewnia et al. (2007) located the tinnitus-related activation of right AG (MNI: 52/−66/32) neighboring our findings of task-related reinforcement of the AG activity (MNI: 50/−64/28). This means that the same region is addressed by both monitoring the tinnitus and visual attention control, however, the attention is driven toward different sensory modalities. When suffering from chronic tinnitus, paying attention to a visually presented alarm stimuli seems to be impaired due to a failure to switch the attention toward the visual input. Trevis et al. (2016) recently conformed this finding also using a letter-based behavioral experiment. The long-term effects from the tinnitus duration causing the difficulties in attention switching may be based on structural change among attention-related and self-referencing brain networks (Lanting et al., 2016; Leaver et al., 2016). HNMT has been found to partially redirect these structural brain alterations (Krick et al., 2015). This in turn may explain the sensitivity of HNMT regarding the restored ability to switching attention between auditory and visual perception in chronic tinnitus sufferers.

Since we used temporal jittered ITI, the occurrence of the rare alarm stimuli (60 cues/1,800 letters = 3.33%) was not predictable by the participants. Following the dual-attention model (Corbetta and Shulman, 2002), the participants had to monitor the visual stream by internally guided attention ("top-down control"), whereas the occurrence of an "O" did not match the participant's expectance but happened externally driven ("bottom-up process;" Serences et al., 2005). Hence, regarding more the alarm stimuli rather than the GO/NOGO conditions, this task was similar to an oddball paradigm (Clark et al., 2000). However, activation of the inferior parietal cortex in an oddball task presupposes a relevance to the main task (Downar et al., 2001; Cabeza et al., 2012) that had been defined in turn by the required GO/NOGO decisions. In most studies on perceptual reorienting tasks the naming of the respective inferior parietal areas was traditionally named "tempero-parietal junction" (TPJ) applying a less exact anatomical assignment by subsuming parts of AG, marginal gyrus (MG), and superior temporal areas (STG; Cabeza et al., 2012). In contrast, language-related studies tend to call the same area "angular gyrus" (Cabeza et al., 2012). In this study, the assignment of relevant meaning to the oddball stimulus "O" was realized by letters that in turn may explain the focus on AG but not MG or STG when performing a whole brain analysis (**Table 2**).

The combination of abnormal attention control due to mental focus on an unpleasing percept has been also observed in adults with ADHD symptoms that augmented the predisposition for chronic pain, especially in coincidence with further mental disorders (Stickley et al., 2016). The association between suffering from aversive sensations and attention difficulties may play a fundamental role in chronic tinnitus sufferers as well (Husain et al., 2015). Hence, the interaction between conscious tinnitus experience and deviant attention control may also become relevant in both future tinnitus research and tinnitus treatment.

Limitations

The compared samples of participants, suffering from either chronic or recent-onset tinnitus, differed slightly in age which was 4.5 years higher on average in chronic patients compared to recent-onset participants. However, the age of chronic patients was not correlated with the respective tinnitus duration. The age difference is due to the circumstance that chronic patients suffered from tinnitus over a comparable mean time span. When acting on the assumption of a comparable mean age of onset in both groups, the cohorts seemed representative.

CONCLUSION

Our observations and the hitherto existing knowledge about the AG lead to the conclusion that this region plays a crucial role in both chronic tinnitus and suitable therapies. In particular, chronic tinnitus impaired the patients' attention for a visual task. HNMT has been shown to reinforce visual attention in chronic tinnitus patients by reorienting the activity in the AG to the cognitively demanding task. These effects regarding the role of AG in tinnitus were dependent on the time since the onset of tinnitus. The observed duration-related attention shift indicates a variable of tinnitus diversity that should be considered in therapy concepts.

AUTHOR CONTRIBUTIONS

CK: MRI measurements, analysis of MRI data, data interpretation. HA: Development of Heidelberg Neuro-Music Therapy, therapy management, statistics. MG: therapist, analysis of clinical data, statistics. PK: tinnitus diagnostics, clinical therapy control. WR: neuroradiological screening, coordinator between the facilities, study coordinator.

ACKNOWLEDGMENTS

The study was supported by KTS Klaus Tschira Stiftung gGmbH. Many thanks to Claudia Sarkady and Dr. Carrie Ankerstein for stylistic and linguistic improvements to this paper.

REFERENCES

Alpini, D., and Cesarani, A. (2006). Tinnitus as an alarm bell: stress reaction tinnitus model. *ORL* 68, 31–37. doi: 10.1159/000090488

Araneda, R., De Volder, A. G., Deggouj, N., Philippot, P., Heeren, A., Lacroix, E., et al. (2015). Altered top-down cognitive control and auditory processing in tinnitus: evidences from auditory and visual spatial stroop. *Restor. Neurol. Neurosci.* 33, 67–80. doi: 10.3233/RNN-140433

Argstatter, H., Grapp, M., Hutter, E., Plinkert, P. K., and Bolay, H. V. (2015). The effectiveness of neuro-music therapy according to the Heidelberg model compared to a single session of educational counseling as treatment for tinnitus: a controlled trial. *J. Psychosom. Res* 78, 285–292. doi: 10.1016/j.jpsychores.2014.08.012

Argstatter, H., Grapp, M., Hutter, E., Plinkert, P., and Bolay, H. V. (2012). Long-term effects of the "Heidelberg Model of Music Therapy" in patients with chronic tinnitus. *Int. J. Clin. Exp. Med.* 5, 273–288.

Bahnemann, M., Dziobek, I., Prehn, K., Wolf, I., and Heekeren, H. R. (2010). Sociotopy in the temporoparietal cortex: common versus distinct processes. *Soc. Cogn. Affect. Neurosci.* 5, 48–58. doi: 10.1093/scan/nsp045

Boyen, K., Langers, D. R., de Kleine, E., and van Dijk, P. (2013). Gray matter in the brain: differences associated with tinnitus and hearing loss. *Hear. Res.* 295, 67–78. doi: 10.1016/j.heares.2012.02.010

Cabeza, R., Ciaramelli, E., and Moscovitch, M. (2012). Cognitive contributions of the ventral parietal cortex: an integrative theoretical account. *Trends Cogn. Sci.* 16, 338–352. doi: 10.1016/j.tics.2012.04.008

Chen, Y. C., Xia, W., Luo, B., Muthaiah, V. P., Xiong, Z., Zhang, J., et al. (2015). Frequency-specific alternations in the amplitude of low-frequency fluctuations in chronic tinnitus. *Front. Neural Circuits* 9:67. doi: 10.3389/fncir.2015.00067

Clark, V. P., Fannon, S., Lai, S., Benson, R., and Bauer, L. (2000). Responses to rare visual target and distractor stimuli using event-related fMRI. *J. Neurophysiol.* 83, 3133–3139.

Corbetta, M., and Shulman, G. L. (2002). Control of goal-directed and stimulus-driven attention in the brain. *Nat. Rev. Neurosci.* 3, 201–215. doi: 10.1038/nrn755

De Ridder, D., Vannestea, S., Weisz, N., Londero, A., Schlee, W., Elgoyhen, A. B., et al. (2014). An integrative model of auditory phantom perception: tinnitus as a unified percept of interacting separable subnetworks. *Neurosci. Biobehav. Rev.* 44, 16–32. doi: 10.1016/j.neubiorev.2013.03.021

Dehaene, S., and Changeux, J. P. (2011). Experimental and theoretical approaches to conscious processing. *Neuron* 70, 200–227. doi: 10.1016/j.neuron.2011.03.018

Downar, J., Crawley, A. P., Mikulis, D. J., and Davis, K. D. (2001). The effect of task relevance on the cortical response to changes in visual and auditory stimuli: an event-related fMRI study. *Neuroimage* 14, 1256–1267. doi: 10.1006/nimg.2001.0946

Flor, H., Hoffmann, D., Struve, M., and Diesch, E. (2004). Auditory discrimination training for the treatment of tinnitus. *Appl. Psychophysiol. Biofeedback* 29, 113–120. doi: 10.1023/B:APBI.0000026637.77671.f4

Folmer, R. L., Theodoroff, S. M., Martin, W. H., and Shi, Y. (2014). Experimental, controversial, and futuristic treatments for chronic tinnitus. *J. Am. Acad. Audiol.* 25, 106–125. doi: 10.3766/jaaa.25.1.7

Goebel, G., and Hiller, W. (1998). *Tinnitus-Fragebogen (TF); ein Instrument zur Erfassung von Belastung und Schweregrad bei Tinnitus; Handanweisung.* Göttingen: Hogrefe Verlag für Psychologie.

Gottlieb, J. (2007). From thought to action: the parietal cortex as a bridge between perception, action, and cognition. *Neuron* 53, 9–16. doi: 10.1016/j.neuron.2006.12.009

Grapp, M., Hutter, E., Argstatter, H., Plinkert, P. K., and Bolay, H. V. (2013). Music therapy as an early intervention to prevent chronification of tinnitus. *Int. J. Clin. Exp. Med.* 6, 589–593.

Grewal, R., Spielmann, P. M., Jones, S. E., and Hussain, S. S. (2014). Clinical efficacy of tinnitus retraining therapy and cognitive behavioural therapy in the treatment of subjective tinnitus: a systematic review. *J. Laryngol. Otol.* 128, 1028–1033. doi: 10.1017/S0022215114002849

Guo, W., Ren, J., Wang, B., and Zhu, Q. (2015). Effects of relaxing music on mental fatigue induced by a continuous performance task: behavioral and ERPs evidence. *PLoS ONE* 10:e0136446. doi: 10.1371/journal.pone.0136446

Hallam, R. S., McKenna, L., and Shurlock, L. (2004). Tinnitus impairs cognitive efficiency. *Int. J. Audiol.* 43, 218–226. doi: 10.1080/14992020400050030

Heeren, A., Maurage, P., Perrot, H., De Volder, A., Renier, L., Araneda, R., et al. (2014). Tinnitus specifically alters the top- down executive control sub-component of attention: evidence from the attention network task. *Behav. Brain Res.* 269, 147–154. doi: 10.1016/j.bbr.2014.04.043

Henry, J. A., Roberts, L. E., Caspary, D. M., Theodoroff, S. M., and Salvi, R. J. (2014). Underlying mechanisms of tinnitus: review and clinical implications. *J. Am. Acad. Audiol.* 25, 5–22. doi: 10.3766/jaaa.25.1.2

Herraiz, C., Diges, I., Cobo, P., Aparicio, J. M., and Toledano, A. (2010). Auditory discrimination training for tinnitus treatment: the effect of different paradigms. *Eur. Arch. Otorhinolaryngol.* 267, 1067–1074. doi: 10.1007/s00405-009-1182-6

Herraiz, C., Hernandez, F. J., Toledano, A., and Aparicio, J. M. (2007) Tinnitus retraining therapy: prognosis factors. *Am. J. Otolaryngol.* 28, 225–229 doi: 10.1016/j.amjoto.2006.09.004

Hesse, G., and Laubert, A. (2010). Zur Pharmakotherapie des akuten und chronischen Tinnitus. *HNO* 10, 990–998. doi: 10.1007/s00106-010-2179-6

Hesser, H., Weise, C., Westin, V. Z., and Andersson, G. (2011). A systematic review and meta-analysis of randomized controlled trials of cognitive-behavioral therapy for tinnitus distress. *Clin. Psychol. Rev.* 31, 545–553. doi: 10.1016/j.cpr.2010.12.006

Hester, R., Fassbender, C., and Garavan, H. (2004). Individual differences in error processing: a review and reanalysis of three event-related fMRI studies using the GO/NOGO task. *Cereb. Cortex* 14, 986–994. doi: 10.1093/cercor/bhh059

Hoare, D. J., Adjamian, P., Sereda, M., and Hall, D. A. (2013). Recent technological advances in sound-based approaches to tinnitus treatment: a review of efficacy considered against putative physiological mechanisms. *Noise Health* 15, 107–116. doi: 10.4103/1463-1741.110292

Humphreys, G. W., and Chechlacz, M. (2015). A neural decomposition of visual search using voxel-based morphometry. *J. Cogn. Neurosci.* 27, 1854–1869. doi: 10.1162/jocn_a_00828

Husain, F. T., Akrofi, K., Carpenter-Thompson, J. R., and Schmidt, S. A. (2015). Alterations to the attention system in adults with tinnitus are modality specific. *Brain Res.* 1620, 81–97. doi: 10.1016/j.brainres.2015.05.010

Husain, F. T., Medina, R. E., Davis, C. W., Szymko-Bennett, Y., Simonyan, K., Pajor, N. M., et al. (2011). Neuroanatomical changes due to hearing loss and chronic tinnitus: a combined VBM and DTI study. *Brain Res.* 1369, 74–88. doi: 10.1016/j.brainres.2010.10.095

Igelström, K. M., Webb, T. W., Kelly, Y. T., and Graziano, M. S. (2016). Topographical organization of attentional, social, and memory processes in the human temporoparietal cortex. *eNeuro* 3:ENEURO.0060-16.2016. doi: 10.1523/ENEURO.0060-16.2016

Jonker, T. R., Seli, P., Cheyne, J. A., and Smilek, D. (2013). Performance reactivity in a continuous-performance task: implications for understanding post-error behavior. *Conscious. Cogn.* 22, 1468–1476. doi: 10.1016/j.concog.2013.10.005

Kim, H. (2010). Dissociating the roles of the default-mode, dorsal, and ventral networks in episodic memory retrieval. *Neuroimage* 50, 1648–1657. doi: 10.1016/j.neuroimage.2010.01.051

Krick, C. M., Grapp, M., Daneshvar-Talebi, J., Reith, W., Plinkert, P. K., and Bolay, H. V. (2015). Cortical reorganization in recent-onset tinnitus patients by the Heidelberg Model of Music Therapy. *Front. Neurosci.* 9:49. doi: 10.3389/fnins.2015.00049

Landgrebe, M., Langguth, B., Rosengarth, K., Braun, S., Koch, A., Kleinjung, T., et al. (2009). Structural brain changes in tinnitus: grey matter decrease in auditory and non-auditory brain areas. *Neuroimage* 46, 213–218. doi: 10.1016/j.neuroimage.2009.01.069

Lanting, C., Woźniak, A., van Dijk, P., and Langers, D. R. (2016). Tinnitus- and task-related differences in resting-state networks. *Adv. Exp. Med. Biol.* 894, 175–187. doi: 10.1007/978-3-319-25474-6_19

Leaver, A. M., Seydell-Greenwald, A., Turesky, T. K., Morgan, S., Kim, H. J., and Rauschecker, J. P. (2012). Cortico-limbic morphology separates tinnitus from tinnitus distress. *Front. Syst. Neurosci.* 5:21. doi: 10.3389/fnsys.2012.00021

Leaver, A. M., Turesky, T. K., Seydell-Greenwald, A., Morgan, S., Kim, H. J., and Rauschecker, J. P. (2016). Intrinsic network activity in tinnitus investigated using functional MRI. *Hum. Brain Mapp.* 37, 2717–2735. doi: 10.1002/hbm.23204

Li, Z., Gu, R., Zeng, X., Zhong, W., Qi, M., and Cen, J. (2016). Attentional bias in patients with decompensated tinnitus: prima facie evidence from event-related potentials. *Audiol. Neurootol.* 21, 38–44. doi: 10.1159/000441709

Linehan, M. M., Bohus, M., and Lynch, T. R. (2007). "Dialectical behavior therapy for pervasive emotion dysregulation," in *Handbook of Emotion*, ed J. Gross (New York, NY: Guildford Press), 581–605.

Maldjian, J. A., Laurienti, P. J., Burdette, J. B., and Kraft, R. A. (2003). An automated method for neuroanatomic and cytoarchitectonic atlas-based interrogation of fMRI data sets. *Neuroimage* 19, 1233–1239. doi: 10.1016/S1053-8119(03)00169-1

Malouff, J. M., Schutte, N. S., and Zucker, L. A. (2011). Tinnitus-related distress: a review of recent findings. *Curr. Psychiatry Rep.* 13, 31–36. doi: 10.1007/s11920-010-0163-1

Mirz, F., Pedersen, B., Ishizu, K., Johannsen, P., Ovesen, T., Stødkilde-Jørgensen, H., et al. (1999). Positron emission tomography of cortical centers of tinnitus. *Hear. Res.* 134, 133–144. doi: 10.1016/S0378-5955(99)00075-1

Mohamad, N., Hoare, D. J., and Hall, D. A. (2016). The consequences of tinnitus and tinnitus severity on cognition: a review of the behavioural evidence. *Hear. Res.* 332, 199–209. doi: 10.1016/j.heares.2015.10.001

Møller, A. R. (2016). Sensorineural tinnitus: its pathology and probable therapies. *Int. J. Otolaryngol.* 2016:2830157. doi: 10.1155/2016/2830157

Mugler, J. P. III, and Brookeman, J. R. (1990). Three-dimensional magnetization-prepared rapid gradient-echo imaging (3D MP RAGE). *Magn. Reson. Med.* 15, 152–157. doi: 10.1002/mrm.1910150117

Mühlau, M., Rauschecker, J. P., Oestreicher, E., Gaser, C., Rottinger, M., Wohlschlager, A. M., et al. (2006). Structural brain changes in tinnitus. *Cereb. Cortex* 16, 1283–1288. doi: 10.1093/cercor/bhj070

Myers, P. J., Griest, S., Kaelin, C., Legro, M. W., Schmidt, C. J., Zaugg, T. L., et al. (2014). Development of a progressive audiologic tinnitus management program for Veterans with tinnitus. *J. Rehabil. Res. Dev.* 51, 609–622. doi: 10.1682/JRRD.2013.08.0189

Plewnia, C., Reimold, M., Najib, A., Brehm, B., Reischl, G., Plontke, S. K., et al. (2007). Dose-dependent attenuation of auditory phantom perception (tinnitus) by PET-guided repetitive transcranial magnetic stimulation. *Hum. Brain Mapp.* 28, 238–246. doi: 10.1002/hbm.20270

Price, C. J. (2010). The anatomy of language: a review of 100 fMRI studies published in 2009. *Ann. N. Y. Acad. Sci.* 1191, 62–88. doi: 10.1111/j.1749-6632.2010.05444.x

Raichle, M. E. (2015). The brain's default mode network. *Annu. Rev. Neurosci.* 38, 433–447. doi: 10.1146/annurev-neuro-071013-014030

Roberts, L. E., Husain, F. T., and Eggermont, J. J. (2013). Role of attention in the generation and modulation of tinnitus. *Neurosci. Biobehav. Rev.* 37, 1754–1773. doi: 10.1016/j.neubiorev.2013.07.007

Sadaghiani, S., Hesselmann, G., and Kleinschmidt, A. (2009). Distributed and antagonistic contributions of ongoing activity fluctuations to auditory stimulus detection. *J. Neurosci.* 29, 13410–13417. doi: 10.1523/JNEUROSCI.2592-09.2009

Schecklmann, M., Lehner, A., Poeppl, T. B., Kreuzer, P. M., Rupprecht, R., Rackl, J., et al. (2013). Auditory cortex is implicated in tinnitus distress: a voxel-based morphometry study. *Brain Struct. Funct.* 218, 1061–1070. doi: 10.1007/s00429-013-0520-z

Schneider, M. F., Krick, C. M., Retz, W., Hengesch, G., Retz-Junginger, P., Reith, W., et al. (2010). Impairment of fronto-striatal and parietal cerebral networks correlates with attention deficit hyperactivity disorder (ADHD) psychopathology in adults - a functional magnetic resonance imaging (fMRI) study. *Psychiatry Res.* 183, 75–84. doi: 10.1016/j.pscychresns.2010.04.005

Schneider, P., Andermann, M., Wengenroth, M., Goebel, R., Flor, H., Rupp, A., et al. (2009). Reduced volume of Heschl's gyrus in tinnitus. *Neuroimage* 45, 27–939. doi: 10.1016/j.neuroimage.2008.12.045

Segal, E., and Petrides, M. (2013). Functional activation during reading in relation to the sulci of the angular gyrus region. *Eur. J. Neurosci.* 38, 2793–2801. doi: 10.1111/ejn.12277

Seghier, M. L. (2013). The angular gyrus: multiple functions and multiple subdivisions. *Neuroscientist* 19, 43–61. doi: 10.1177/1073858412440596

Serences, J. T., Shomstein, S., Leber, A. B., Golay, X., Egeth, H. E., and Yantis, S. (2005). Coordination of voluntary and stimulus-driven attentional control in human cortex. *Psychol. Sci.* 16, 114–122. doi: 10.1111/j.0956-7976.2005.00791.x

Seydel, C., Haupt, H., Olze, H., Szczepek, A. J., and Mazurek, B. (2013). Gender and chronic tinnitus: differences in tinnitus-related distress depend on age and duration of tinnitus. *Ear Hear.* 34, 661–672. doi: 10.1097/AUD.0b013e31828149f2

Song, J. J., De Ridder, D., Van de Heyning, P., and Vanneste, S. (2012). Mapping tinnitus-related brain activation: an activation-likelihood estimation metaanalysis of PET studies. *J. Nucl. Med.* 53, 1550–1557. doi: 10.2967/jnumed.112.102939

Stevens, C., Walker, G., Boyer, M., and Gallagher, M. (2007). Severe tinnitus and its effect on selective and divided attention. *Int. J. Audiol.* 46, 208–216. doi: 10.1080/14992020601102329

Stickley, A., Koyanagi, A., Takahashi, H., and Kamio, Y. (2016). ADHD symptoms and pain among adults in England. *Psychiatry Res.* 246, 326–331. doi: 10.1016/j.psychres.2016.10.004

Taylor, P. J. C., and Thut, G. (2012). Brain activity underlying visual perception and attention as inferred from TMSeEEG: a review. *Brain Stimul.* 5, 124–129. doi: 10.1016/j.brs.2012.03.003

Taylor, P. J. C., Muggleton, N. G., Kalla, R., Walsh, V., and Eimer, M. (2011). TMS of the right angular gyrus modulates priming of pop-out in visual search: combined TMS-ERP evidence. *J. Neurophysiol.* 106, 3001–3009. doi: 10.1152/jn.00121.2011

Trevis, K. J., McLachlan, N. M., and Wilson, S. J. (2016). Cognitive mechanisms in chronic tinnitus: psychological markers of a failure to switch attention. *Front. Psychol.* 7:1262. doi: 10.3389/fpsyg.2016.01262

Tzourio-Mazoyer, N., Landeau, B., Papathanassiou, D., Crivello, F., Etard, O., Delcroix, N., et al. (2002). Automated anatomical labeling of activations in SPM using a macroscopic anatomical parcellation of the MNI MRI single-subject brain. *Neuroimage* 15, 273–289. doi: 10.1006/nimg.2001.0978

Uddin, L. Q., Supekar, K., Amin, H., Rykhlevskaia, E., Nguyen, D. A., Greicius, M. D., et al. (2010). Dissociable connectivity within human angular gyrus and intraparietal sulcus: evidence from functional and structural connectivity. *Cereb. Cortex* 20, 2636–2646. doi: 10.1093/cercor/bhq011

Ueyama, T., Donishi, T., Ukai, S., Ikeda, Y., Hotomi, M., Yamanak, N., et al. (2013). Brain regions responsible for tinnitus distress and loudness: a resting-state fMRI study. *PLoS ONE* 8:e67778. doi: 10.1371/journal.pone.0067778

van Gaal, S., Lamme, V. A., Fahrenfort, J. J., and Ridderinkhof, K. R. (2011). Dissociable brain mechanisms underlying the conscious and unconscious control of behavior. *J. Cogn. Neurosci.* 23, 91–105. doi: 10.1162/jocn.2010.21431

Vanneste, S., Plazier, M., der Loo, Ev., de Heyning, P. V., Congedo, M., and De Ridder, D. (2010). The neural correlates of tinnitus-related distress. *Neuroimage* 52, 470–480. doi: 10.1016/j.neuroimage.2010.04.029

Zeman, F., Koller, M., Schecklmann, M., Langguth, B., Landgrebe, M., and TRI Database Study Group (2012). Tinnitus assessment by means of standardized self-report questionnaires: psychometric properties of the Tinnitus Questionnaire (TQ), the Tinnitus Handicap Inventory (THI), and their short versions in an international and multi-lingual sample. *Health Qual. Life Outcomes* 10:128. doi: 10.1186/1477-7525-10-128

6

Positive Association between Tinnitus and Arterial Hypertension

Ricardo Rodrigues Figueiredo[1,2]*, Andréia Aparecida Azevedo[1] and Norma De Oliveira Penido[1]

[1] Otolaryngology, Universidade Federal de São Paulo, São Paulo, Brazil,

[2] Otolaryngology, Faculdade de Medicina de Valença, Valença, Brazil

***Correspondence:**
Ricardo Rodrigues Figueiredo
rfigueiredo@otosul.com.br

Introduction: Tinnitus is the perception of noise in the absence of an external source and is considered by most authors as a multifactorial symptom. A systematic review concerning the association of tinnitus and systemic arterial hypertension retrieved suggestions of a positive association, but the articles included failed to perform a detailed analysis on the theme.

Purpose: To analyze the presence of arterial hypertension in tinnitus and non-tinnitus patients, to analyze differences between tinnitus impact and psychoacoustic measurements in hypertensive and normotensive patients, and to evaluate the association between the presence of tinnitus and the diverse antihypertensive drugs employed.

Materials and methods: This includes cross-sectional transversal study, comparing two groups of subjects (144 in the study group with tinnitus and 140 in the control group without tinnitus). Clinical, demographical, audiometrical, and psychoacoustics characteristics of the subjects were compared.

Results: Hypertension prevalence in tinnitus subjects was 44.4% against 31.4% in subjects without tinnitus ($p = 0.024$). Positive associations with tinnitus were found with hypertension treatment with angiotensin-converting enzyme (ACE) inhibitors ($p = 0.006$), tiazidic diuretics ($p < 0.0001$), potassium-sparing diuretics ($p = 0.016$), and calcium channels blockers ($p = 0.004$).

Conclusion: There is an association between tinnitus and arterial hypertension. This association is particularly strong in older patients. Hypertension treatment with diuretics, ACE inhibitors, and calcium channels blockers were more prevalent in tinnitus patients, suggesting that an eventual ototoxicity of these drugs may be involved in tinnitus pathophysiology, a hypothesis that should be evaluated in further studies.

Keywords: tinnitus, arterial hypertension, hearing loss, cardiovascular diseases, hearing disorders

INTRODUCTION

Tinnitus is the perception of noise, which is not generated by external stimulus (1). It affects approximately 25% of the general population: one third on a frequent basis (2). Tinnitus may be classified as auditory and para-auditory tinnitus with the former representing the majority of cases, and the latter being subdivided into muscular and vascular tinnitus, sometimes referred as somatosounds (3).

According to the most recent trends of thought, tinnitus is considered a symptom which may have multiple causes, sometimes even in a single patient (4, 5). Noise exposure, metabolic and cardiovascular disease, presbycusis, ototoxicity, and cranial and cervical trauma are the most frequently considered causes of tinnitus (5, 6). Caffeine abuse, dietary factors, temporomandibular joint, and cervical disease have also been described as contributing factors (7–9).

Systemic arterial hypertension is a multifactorial clinical condition characterized by raised and sustained arterial pressure levels (10). It is defined as systolic levels equal or greater than 140 mmHg and diastolic levels equal or greater than 90 mmHg (10). The prevalence in Brazil, similar to that in other countries, is estimated to be between 22.3 and 43.9% (32.5% average), raising to 50% between 60 and 69 years old and 75% for 70 years and older (10–12). The presence of comorbidities, such as diabetes mellitus and dyslipidemias, and habits, such as smoking, was demonstrated to increase complications risks (13). Arterial hypertension has been described as a possible cause of tinnitus since 1940s (14). Three principle mechanisms suspected of being involved are: damage to inner ear microcirculation (15), ototoxicity by antihypertension drugs (16), and perception of noise generated by blood vessels (3).

As related to inner ear microcirculation, the *stria vascularis* was demonstrated to be the main cochlear site damaged by arterial hypertension (17). Sodium retention could also lead to an increase of extracellular fluid volume, including the perilymph (18), and the endocochlear potential being reduced in hypertensive rats (19). Moreover, hypertension has been associated with a higher risk of hearing loss in brain ischemia (15) and also with a slower recovery in sudden hearing loss (20).

In considering ototoxicity, an extensive review cited diuretics, beta-blockers, angiotensin-conversing enzyme (ACE) inhibitors, angiotensin II receptors blockers, and calcium channels blockers as possible ototoxic medications (21). Furosemide's ototoxicity is the most studied form, producing a quick and reversible decrease of the endocochlear potential (22).

As for vascular tinnitus, some studies cite hypertension as a causal factor, mainly when vascular abnormalities have been ruled out (3). An anatomopathological study demonstrated a high incidence of bony dehiscence of the carotid canal in the middle ear, which may affect the inner ear microcirculation and also generate vascular noises (23).

According to a systematic review, there is evidence of an association between tinnitus and arterial hypertension, but there is a lack of more comprehensive studies (24). The association is stronger in studies that analyzed the presence of arterial hypertension in patients with tinnitus than in those which analyzed the presence of tinnitus in patients with arterial hypertension.

The main purpose of this study is to analyze the presence of arterial hypertension in tinnitus and non-tinnitus patients. Secondary purposes are to analyze differences between tinnitus impact and psychoacoustic measurements in hypertensive and normotensive patients and to evaluate the association between the presence of tinnitus and the diverse antihypertensive drugs employed.

MATERIALS AND METHODS

This is a transversal case–control study in which individuals of 18 years of age or older with and without tinnitus were selected at the author's ENT clinic from 2011 to 2014. The trial was approved by the Institutional Review Board (number 010/CEP-FMV/2011). This study was carried out in accordance with the recommendations of the aforementioned Institutional Review Board with written informed consent from all subjects. All subjects gave written informed consent in accordance with the Declaration of Helsinki.

Two groups were created: the first included patients with tinnitus of at least 3 months duration and the second included patients without tinnitus (control). The control group was paired with the tinnitus group for gender, age, and race. The time of tinnitus onset as related to arterial hypertension onset was not an exclusion criteria. Patients from both groups were submitted to anamnesis (including demographics, comorbidities, and habits), otorhinolaryngological physical examination, and arterial pressure measurements with a calibrated sphygmomanometer (Erka Perfekt Aneroid, Germany), in order to exclude possible undiagnosed arterial hypertension. The criteria for blood pressure evaluation were those from the VII Joint National Committee on Prevention, Detection, Evaluation, and Treatment of High Blood Pressure, U. S. Department of Health and Human Services, as previously described.

Patients allegedly normotensive with high blood pressure detected at the physical examination were excluded. Patients from both groups also underwent conventional pure tone and speech audiometry.

Tinnitus patients were questioned regarding their tinnitus characteristics (duration, type of sound, laterality, and periodicity) and also classified their tinnitus according to a Visual Analog Scale (VAS), from 1 to 10 (for intensity and distress) and to the Brazilian Portuguese validated version of the Tinnitus Handicap Inventory (THI) (25). They also underwent psychoacoustic measurements of their tinnitus – Pitch Matching (PM) and Minimum Masking Level (MML).

The sample size was determined after the analysis of the arterial hypertension prevalence in a preliminary sample of tinnitus patients ($n = 46$) that was compared to the prevalence of arterial hypertension in the Brazilian general population, obtained from previous studies (10). The minimum number of individuals for each group was determined to be 140.

For whole sample analysis, the comparison of the variables between the tinnitus group and the control group was performed using the Mann–Whitney test for the numerical data and the chi-square or the Fisher test for the categorical data. The Spearman coefficient was performed to analyze the association between the duration of arterial hypertension and the numerical audiometry measurements. The Cochran–Mantel–Haenszel was used to analyze the association between tinnitus and arterial hypertension adjusting for the presence of hearing loss. The significance level was established at 5%, and the statistical analysis was performed with the SAS statistical software, 6.11 version (SAS Institute, Inc., Cary, NC, USA).

RESULTS

The final sample was composed of 144 patients in the tinnitus group and 140 in the control group. The tinnitus group was then divided into two subgroups: one for patients with arterial hypertension and the other without arterial hypertension.

The average age was 57.8 years of age for the tinnitus group and 58.6 for the control group. The averages of tinnitus duration,

VAS for intensity, VAS for distress, and THI scores for the tinnitus group were, respectively, 54.5 months–4.5 years, 5.45, 5.83, and 41.7 points.

Although the duration of arterial hypertension was longer (average of 128.7 months–10.7 years) than the duration of tinnitus (average of 54.5 months), no statistically significant correlation was found, according to the Spearman coefficient. Considering the patients that could ascertain the duration of both arterial hypertension and tinnitus ($n = 56$), for 42 of them (75%) arterial hypertension preceded tinnitus.

Table 1 shows the comparison of numerical variables and **Table 2** shows the categorical variables, the latter confirming the pairing by gender, age, and race. As shown in **Table 2**, arterial hypertension was more prevalent in tinnitus patients ($p = 0.024$), demonstrating an association of tinnitus and arterial hypertension. This association was not found when data were adjusted for the presence of hearing loss ($p = 0.27$, according to the Cochran–Mantel–Haenszel test). Hearing loss was more frequent in the tinnitus group, as shown in **Table 3**, but there was no difference between the two groups as to the type of hearing loss or the shape of the audiogram curve. Sensorineural descendant was the most frequent curve in both groups (75% in the tinnitus patients group and 58% in the control group). Also, there was no difference in the speech recognition index of both groups (100% median in both).

TABLE 1 | Analysis of the numerical variables (age, duration of arterial hypertension, and daily consumption of caffeine) according to the group.

Variable	Tinnitus			No tinnitus			*p*-Value
	n	Median	IQA	*n*	Median	IQA	
Age (years)	144	59	49–69	140	58	50–67	0.97
Arterial hypertension duration (months)	60	**120**	39–216	43	**180**	84–240	**0.019**
Caffeine (ml/day)	144	**100**	50–200	140	**300**	200–400	**0.0001**

Significant values in bold.
IQA, Interquartilic Amplitude: Q1–Q3.

TABLE 2 | Analysis of categorical variables (gender, age, race, and presence of arterial hypertension) according to the groups.

Variable	Category	Tinnitus		No Tinnitus		*p*-Value[a]
		n	%	*n*	%	
Gender	Male	62	43.1	65	46.4	0.57
	Female	82	56.9	75	53.6	
Age (years)	≤40	18	12.5	14	10.0	0.82
	41–59	55	38.2	60	42.9	
	60–69	40	27.8	36	25.7	
	≥70	31	21.5	30	21.4	
Race	White	93	71.5	98	70.0	0.94
	Brown	22	16.9	24	17.1	
	Black	15	11.5	18	12.9	
Arterial Hypertension	Yes	64	**44.4**	44	**31.4**	**0.024**
	No	80	55.6	96	68.6	

Significant values in bold.
[a]*χ^2 or Fisher test.*

The analysis of the antihypertensive drugs used in both groups is shown in **Table 4**.

The analysis of comorbidities and habits demonstrated that dyslipidemia was more frequent in the tinnitus group (*p*-value of 0.003), while the presence of diabetes mellitus, hypothyroidism, noise exposure, caffeine consumption, and smoking was similar in both groups. When considering the coexistence of arterial hypertension and comorbidities and habits, the association of arterial hypertension and caffeine consumption greater than 150 milliliters per day was more frequent in the tinnitus group ($p < 0.0001$).

Table 4 shows data about the antihypertensive drugs used in both groups.

Table 5 shows data from the numerical variables for the tinnitus' patients subgroups, those with and without arterial hypertension.

There was no statistical difference between the two subgroups concerning gender and race. Diabetes mellitus and dyslipidemia were more frequent in the subgroup with tinnitus and arterial hypertension ($p = 0.017$ and 0.02, respectively), while there were no differences concerning hypothyroidism, noise exposure, caffeine consumption, or smoking. Hearing loss was considered to be more prevalent in the subgroup with arterial hypertension (89.1%), although it was also frequent in the normotensive subgroup (75%, $p = 0.032$). No differences concerning the type or curve were found.

TABLE 3 | Prevalence of hearing loss among tinnitus and non-tinnitus patients (χ^2 test).

Variable	Category	Tinnitus		No Tinnitus		*p*-Value
		N (ears)	%	*N* (ears)	%	
Hearing loss	Yes	111	81.3	75	53.6	<0.0001
	No	32	18.7	65	46.4	

TABLE 4 | Analysis of the categorical variable – antihypertensive drugs used according to the groups.

Variable	Category	Tinnitus		No tinnitus		*p*-Value
		n	%	*n*	%	
B-blocker	Yes	19	13.2	21	15.0	0.66
	No	125	86.8	119	85.0	
ACEI	Yes	23	16.0	8	5.7	0.006
	No	121	84.0	132	94.3	
ARB	Yes	34	23.6	24	17.1	0.18
	No	110	76.4	116	82.9	
Loop diuretic	Yes	0	0.0	4	2.9	0.057
	No	144	100.0	136	97.1	
Thiazidic diuretic	Yes	29	20.1	8	5.7	<0.0001
	No	115	79.9	132	94.3	
K sparing diuretic	Yes	6	4.2	0	0.0	0.016
	No	138	95.8	140	100.0	
CCA	Yes	13	9.0	2	1.4	0.004
	No	131	91.0	138	98.6	

χ-squared or Fisher tests.
ACEI, angiotensin-converting enzyme inhibitor; ARB, angiotensin II receptor blocker; CCA, calcium channel antagonist.

TABLE 5 | Analysis of the numerical variables (age, caffeine consumption, tinnitus duration, Visual Analog Scale, Tinnitus Handicap Inventory, Pitch Masking, and Minimum Masking Level) according to the subgroups of tinnitus patients (with and without arterial hypertension).

Variable	Arterial hypertension subgroup			No arterial hypertension subgroup			*p*-Value[a]
	n	Median	IQA	*n*	Median	IQA	
Age (years)	64	**66**	57–72	80	**52.5**	43–65	**0.0001**
Caffeine (ml/day)	58	100	50–200	67	100	100–200	0.78
Tinnitus duration (months)	59	24	9–60	76	18	5.3–60	0.22
VAS volume (points)	63	5	3–7	80	6	4–8	0.37
VAS distress (points)	63	5	3–8	80	6	4–9	0.37
THI score (points)	63	40	18–70	80	38	16.5–61.5	0.75
PM RE (Hz)	40	4000	1000–8000	64	6000	2000–8000	0.58
PM LE (Hz)	45	4000	1500–8000	56	6000	3250–8000	0.27
MML RE (dB SL)	40	15	5–25	63	15	10–30	0.36
MML LE (dB SL)	44	15	5–29	55	15	5–25	0.48

Nineteen patients reported no caffeine consumption, nine patients could not estimate the duration of their tinnitus, and one patient could not report VAS and THI scores.
IQA, interquartilic amplitude: Q1–Q3.
Bold is to highlight the significant data.
[a]Mann–Whitney test.
VAS, Visual Analog Scale; THI, Tinnitus Handicap Inventory; PM, Pitch Masking; MML, Minimum Masking Level; RE, right ear; LE, left ear; dB, decibel; dB SL, decibel Sensation Level.

Table 6 shows the tinnitus characteristics in both subgroups. The most frequently described types of tinnitus were wheezing, whistle, and insect with no differences between the subgroups. The presence of multiple types of sound in the same patient was more frequently found in the hypertensive subgroup ($p = 0.014$). The prevalence of vascular tinnitus was 6.3% in the hypertensive subgroup and 1.3% in the normotensive one ($p = 0.12$) with muscular tinnitus being found in only two cases, both being in normotensive patients.

No significant differences were found between the subgroups concerning the otolaryngologic exam, including evaluation of the temporomandibular joint. Finally, there was no correlation discovered between the duration of arterial hypertension and tinnitus according to the Spearman coefficient ($p = 0.77$).

DISCUSSION

Association studies are key sources of information for the comprehension of how one disorder may affect another. A study on attempt to establish a correlation between arterial hypertension and tinnitus studies will help to elucidate characteristic in common that could be addressed in the diagnosis and therapeutic interventions. However, causal correlate studies would demand a plethora of different cases, including patients without tinnitus or arterial hypertension who were also free from other infirmities or habits which could be linked to tinnitus generation. Oftentimes, this elaborate type of study requires an extensive time period and patients with incredibly varied conditions.

TABLE 6 | Analysis of the categorical variables (tinnitus clinical characteristics) according to the tinnitus' patients' subgroups (with and without arterial hypertension).

Variable	Category	Arterial hypertension subgroup		No arterial hypertension subgroup		*p*-Value[a]
		n	%	*n*	%	
Laterality	RE	13	20.3	22	27.5	0.60
	LE	15	23.4	14	17.5	
	Bilateral	32	50.0	41	51.3	
	Head	4	6.3	3	3.8	
Instalation	Sudden	33	55.0	33	42.9	0.0.16
	Gradual	27	45.0	44	57.1	
Periodicity	Constant	45	70.3	55	69.6	0.93
	Intermittent	19	29.7	24	30.4	

[a]χ^2 or Fisher test.
RE, right ear; LE, left ear.

A systematic review on this subject (24) argued that studies which have evaluated the prevalence of tinnitus among hypertensive patients failed to demonstrate an association (26–29). However, data from this study, along with other studies (2, 30, 31), demonstrated an association between tinnitus and arterial hypertension (hypertension prevalence in tinnitus patients = 44.4% against 31.4% in patients without tinnitus, $p = 0.024$).

The information above may lead one to infer that tinnitus could be a causal factor for hypertension, albeit it seems more reasonable to believe arterial hypertension is more a cofactor than a main cause of tinnitus.

Regarding hearing loss, the results are in conformity with prior studies, which found a high prevalence among tinnitus patients, as well as the higher prevalence of sensorineural pattern with descending configuration curves (2, 5).

Once hearing loss was added to (adjusted for) the statistical analysis, the association between tinnitus and arterial hypertension was no longer positive, suggesting that arterial hypertension may be a cause of hearing loss, which is related to most cases of tinnitus, as previously reported (1, 6). Having said so, if we think about tinnitus prevention, arterial hypertension may still be regarded as a possible important causal factor.

Arterial hypertension may affect the inner ear microcirculation, and it is known that comorbidities, such as diabetes mellitus and dyslipidemia, may enhance vascular impairment due to hypertension (10). Although dyslipidemia was more prevalent in the tinnitus group, there was no difference concerning the concomitancy of arterial hypertension and dyslipidemia. Diabetes mellitus also affects the inner ear microcirculation, but it may also have direct metabolic effects on cochlea (4, 5, 20). There was a statistical tendency in favor of a higher prevalence of the concomitancy of diabetes and hypertension in the tinnitus group. As for hypothyroidism, another metabolic disease frequently cited as related to tinnitus (6), no differences between the two groups were found, either as an isolated factor or in association with arterial hypertension. The comparison between the tinnitus subgroups (with and without hypertension) demonstrated that diabetes mellitus and dyslipidemia were more prevalent in hypertensive tinnitus patients, suggesting that these diseases may act synergically upon the generation, maintenance and/or aggravation of tinnitus.

The excessive consumption of caffeine is believed to have a negative impact on hypertension control (32), but its association with tinnitus has been doubted by recent studies (9, 33, 34). Data from this study failed to demonstrate any association between tinnitus and caffeine consumption. In fact, the concomitancy of hypertension and caffeine intake greater than 150 ml per day was more prevalent in the control group, which may reflect the widespread patients' concept that caffeine worsens tinnitus. Smoking, which is believed to worsen both tinnitus and hypertension, probably by impairing macro and microcirculation (10, 35), was more prevalent in the tinnitus group, either as an isolated factor or concomitant to hypertension.

Considering these findings, one might speculate that vascular changes, which may affect cochlear microcirculation, leading to hair cells damage and, consequently, tinnitus is probably a common pathophysiological scenario for many conditions, such as arterial hypertension, dyslipidemia, diabetes mellitus, smoking, and caffeine abuse. These conditions are not infrequently found in a single patient and may act sinergically, multiplying the damage to the auditory system.

Although noise exposure is considered as one of the main causes of tinnitus (4, 6), data from this study failed to establish an association between noise exposure and tinnitus, either isolated or concomitant to hypertension. This finding should be considered with caution, being that the study was performed in an industrial city where many workers are exposed to industrial or recreational noise.

The average age of patients with tinnitus and arterial hypertension was significantly higher than the age of those in the group with tinnitus and no arterial hypertension. In the hypertension tinnitus subgroup most of the patients were 60 years or older, while the opposite was verified in the subgroup without hypertension. Both tinnitus and arterial hypertension are more prevalent in the elderly (2, 10), but these findings may also be due to some synergistic action of presbycusis and arterial hypertension contributing to tinnitus generation and, eventually, aggravation.

The difference concerning arterial hypertension duration, which was significantly lower in the tinnitus group, may be due to a lack of proper control of blood pressure in the first years, which may lead to perfusion and reperfusion vascular events in the cochlea. More studies are needed to clarify these findings.

The median of the pitch masking was higher (6 kHz) in the subgroup without hypertension than when compared to the hypertension subgroup (4 kHz), although this difference was not statistically significant. Both measures are in agreement with most of the references, tinnitus ranging from 3 to 8 kHz, which corresponds to the usually most affected frequencies in hearing loss (36, 37). As for the MML, the averages of both subgroups were the same (15 dB SL), which is somewhat higher than the usually reported sensation level of 5–10 dB SL (37). No differences were demonstrated concerning the degree of intensity and distress due to tinnitus in both subgroups, considering the VAS and the THI.

The tinnitus' characteristics were similar in both groups, including the type of sound perceived by the patients. The fact that multiple sounds' tinnitus was more prevalent in the hypertensive patients may reflect the multicausality of tinnitus, hypertension being one of the possible factors involved.

Although the average duration of arterial hypertension was longer than the duration of tinnitus and for most of the patients the onset of hypertension preceded the onset of tinnitus, the methodology of this case–control does not allow the conclusion that hypertension is a causal factor for tinnitus.

The ototoxicity of many antihypertension medications has been well established, especially with diuretics (21, 22). Data from this study demonstrated that the use of ACE inhibitors, thiazidic diuretics, potassium-sparing diuretics, and calcium channels blockers was more prevalent in the tinnitus hypertensive patients than in the control group. These findings have a partial correspondence with prior studies (16) and, although they are not strong enough to justify a correlation between an eventual ototoxicity of these drugs and the presence of tinnitus (for example, multidrug therapy for hypertension is very frequent), it appears that further, more detailed studies on this subject should be performed.

CONCLUSION

There is an association between tinnitus and arterial hypertension. This association is particularly strong in older patients and cannot be dissociated from the hearing loss, which was also more prevalent among tinnitus patients. The use of thiazidic and potassium-sparing diuretics, ACE inhibitors, and calcium channels blockers was more prevalent in tinnitus patients.

The clinical and psychoacoustic characteristics of tinnitus in hypertensive and normotensive patients were similar, as well as tinnitus-related distress.

AUTHOR CONTRIBUTIONS

RF – study design, data collection, and writing. AA – data collection. NP – study design and writing.

ACKNOWLEDGMENTS

Rosângela Martins, for the statistics. Lisa Morrison Thuler, for the manuscript English revision.

FUNDING

This work was supported by a grant from CAPES – Coordenação de Aperfeiçoamento de Pessoal de Nível Superior – Governo Federal do Brasil.

REFERENCES

Heller AJ. Classification and epidemiology of tinnitus. *Otolaryngol Clin North Am* (2003) 36(2):239–48. doi:10.1016/S0030-6665(02)00160-3

Shargorodsky J, Curhan GC, Farwell WR. Prevalence and characteristics of tinnitus among US adults. *Am J Med* (2010) 123(8):711–8. doi:10.1016/j amjmed.2010.02.015

Herraiz C, Aparicio JM. Diagnostic clues in pulsatile tinnitus (somato- sounds). *Acta Otorrinolaringol Esp* (2007) 58(9):426–33. doi:10.1016/ S0001-6519(07)74960-9

Langguth B, Kreuzer PM, Kleinjung T, De Ridder D. Tinnitus: causes and clinical management. *Lancet Neurol* (2013) 12(9):920–30. doi:10.1016/ S1474-4422(13)70160-1

Tunkel DE, Bauer CA, Sun GH, Rosenfeld RM, Chandrasekhar SS, Cunningham ER Jr, et al. Clinical practice guideline: tinnitus. *Otolaryngol Head Neck Surg* (2014) 151(2 Suppl):S1–40. doi:10.1177/0194599814545325

Henry JA, Dennis KC, Schechter MA. General review of tinnitus: preva- lence, mechanisms, effects and management. *J Speech Lang Hear Res* (2005) 48(5):49–70. doi:10.1044/1092-4388(2005/084)

Rocha CB, Sanchez TG. Efficacy of myofascial trigger point deactiva- tion for tinnitus control. *Braz J Otorhinolaringol* (2012) 78(6):21–6. doi:10.5935/1808-8694.20120028

Ferendiuk E, Zajdel K, Pihut M. Incidence of otolaryngological symptoms in patients with temporomandibular joint dysfunctions. *Biomed Res Int* (2014) 2014:824684. doi:10.1155/2014/824684

Figueiredo RR, Rates MJ, Azevedo AA, Moreira RK, Penido NO. Effects of the reduction of caffeine consumption on tinnitus perception. *Braz J Otorhinolaryngol* (2014) 80(5):416–21. doi:10.1016/j.bjorl.2014.05.033

Nobre F, Amodeo C, Consolim-Colombo FA. VI Diretrizes Brasileiras de Hipertensão. *Rev Bras Hipert* (2010) 17(1):7–60.

Barreto SM, Passos VMA, Firmo JOA, Guerra HL, Vidigal PG, Lima-Costa MFF. Hypertension and clustering of cardiovascular risk factors in a com- munity in Southest Brazil – The Bambuí Health and Ageing Study. *Arq Bras Cardiol* (2001) 77(6):576–81. doi:10.1590/S0066-782X20010001200008

Cesarino CB, Cipullo JP, Martin JFV, Ciorlia LA, de Godoy MRP, Cordeiro JA, et al. Prevalência e fatores sociodemográficos em hipertensos de São José do Rio Preto – SP. *Arq Bras Cardiol* (2008) 91(1):31–5. doi:10.1590/ S0066-782X2008001300005

Zanchetti A, Hanson L, Dahlöf B, Elmfeldt D, Kjeldsen S, Kolloch R, et al. Effects of individual risk factors on the incidence of cardiovascular events in the treated hypertensive patients of the Hypertension Optimal Treatment Study. HOT Study Group. *J Hypertens* (2001) 19(6):1149–59. doi:10.1097/00004872-200106000-00021

Johnson LF, Zonderman B. The hearing acuity, tinnitus and ver- tigo in essential hypertension. *Laryngoscope* (1948) 58(5):374–9. doi:10.1288/00005537-194805000-00002

Przewoźny T, Gasecki D, Narozny W, Nyka W. Risk factors of sensorineural hearing loss in patients with ischemic stroke. *Otol Neurotol* (2008) 29(6):745– 50. doi:10.1097/MAO.0b013e318181336c

Borghi C, Brandolini C, Prandin MG, Dormi A, Modugno GC, Pirodda Prevalence of tinnitus in patients with hypertension and the impact of different antihypertensive drugs on the incidence of tinnitus: a prospective, single-blind, observational study. *Curr Ther Res Clin Exp* (2005) 66(5):420–32. doi:10.1016/j.curtheres.2005.10.001

Tachibana M, Yamamichi I, Nakae S. The site of involvement in hyper- tension within the cochlea. *Acta Otolaryngol* (1984) 97(3):257–65. doi:10.3109/00016488409130987

Marková M. The cochleovestibular syndrome in hypertension. *Cesk Otolaryngol* (1990) 39(2):89–97.

Mosnier I, Teixeira M, Loiseau A, Fernandes I, Sterkes O, Amiel C, et al. Effects of acute and chronic hypertension on the labyrinthine barriers in rat *Hear Res* (2001) 151(1–2):227–36. doi:10.1016/S0378-5955(00) 00229-X

Nagaoka J, Anjos MF, Takata TT, Chaim RM, Barros F, Penido NO. Idiopathic sudden sensorineural hearing loss: evolution in the presence of hyperten- sion, diabetes mellitus and dyslipidemias. *Braz J Otorhinolaryngol* (2010) 76(3):363–9. doi:10.1590/S1808-86942010000300015

Cianfrone G, Pentangelo D, Cianfrone F, Mazzei F, Turchetta R, Orlando MP, et al. Pharmacological drugs inducing ototoxicity, vestibular symptoms and tinnitus: a reasoned and updated guide. *Eur Rev Med Pharmacol Sci* (2011) 15(6):601–36.

Rybak LP. Furosemide ototoxicity: clinical and experimental aspects. *Laryngoscope* (1985) 95(9 Pt 2 Suppl 38):1–14. doi:10.1288/00005537-198509010-00001

Penido NO, Borin A, Fukuda Y, Lion CN. Microscopic anatomy of the carotid canal and its relation with cochlea and middle ear. *Braz J Otorhinolaryngol* (2005) 71(4):410–4. doi:10.1016/S1808-8694(15)31191-5

Figueiredo RR, Azevedo AA, Penido NO. Tinnitus and arterial hypertension: a systematic review. *Eur Arch Otorhinolaryngol* (2015) 272(11):3089–94. doi:10.1007/s00405-014-3277-y

Ferreira PEA, Cunha F, Onichi ET, Branco-Barreiro FCA, Ganança FF. Tinnitus Handicap Inventory: adaptação cultural para o português brasileiro. *Pro Fono* (2005) 17(3):303–10. doi:10.1590/S0104-56872005000300004

Fasce E, Flores M, Fasce F. Prevalence of symptoms associated with blood pressure in normal and hypertensive population. *Rev Med Chil* (2002) 130(2):160–6. doi:10.1016/j.curtheres.2005.10.001

Baraldi GS, Almeida LC, Borges ACLC. Hearing loss and hypertension findings in an older by group. *Braz J Otorhinolaryngol* (2004) 70(5):640–4. doi:10.1590/S0034-72992006000400016

Marchiori LLM. Zumbido e hipertensão no processo de envelhecimento. *Rev Bras Hipert* (2009) 16(1):5–8.

Mondelli MFCG, Lopes AC. Relação entre a hipertensão arterial e a deficiên- cia auditiva. *Arq Int Otorrinolaringol* (2009) 13(1):63–8.

Lasisi AO, Abiona T, Gureje O. Tinnitus in the elderly: profile, correlates and impact on the Nigerian Study of Ageing. *Otolaryngol Head Neck Surg* (2010) 143(4):510–5. doi:10.1016/j.otohns.2010.06.817

Negrila-Mezei A, Enache R, Sarafoleanu C. Tinnitus in elderly population: clinic correlations and impact upon QoL. *J Med Life* (2011) 4(4):412–6.

Kalyoncu ZB, Pars H, Bora-Günes N, Karabulut E, Aslan D. A systematic review of nutrition-based practices in prevention of hypertension among healthy young. *Turk J Pediatr* (2014) 56(4):335–46.

Claire LS, Stothart G, McKenna L, Rogers PJ. Caffeine abstinence: an ineffec- tive and potentially distressing tinnitus therapy. *Int J Audiol* (2010) 49(1):24–9. doi:10.3109/14992020903160884

Glicksman JT, Curhan SG, Curhan GC. A prospective study of caffeine intake and risk of incident tinnitus. *Am J Med* (2014) 127(8):739–43. doi:10.1016/j. amjmed.2014.02.033

Martines F, Sireci F, Cannizzaro E, Constanzo R, Martines E, Mucia M, et al. Clinical observations and risk factors for tinnitus in a Sicilian cohort. *Eur Arch Otorhinolaryngol* (2014) 272(10):2719–29. doi:10.1007/s00405-014-3275-0

Penner MJ. Two-tone forward masking patterns for tinnitus. *J Speech Hear Res* (1980) 23(4):779–86. doi:10.1044/jshr.2304.779

Meikle MB. The interaction of central and peripheral mechanisms in tinnitus. In: Vernon JA, Møller A, editors. *Mechanisms of Tinnitus*. Needham Heights, MA: Allyn & Bacon (1995). p. 181–206.

7

Individualized Repetitive Transcranial Magnetic Stimulation Treatment in Chronic Tinnitus?

Peter M. Kreuzer[1,2], Timm B. Poeppl[1,2], Rainer Rupprecht[1], Veronika Vielsmeier[2,3], Astrid Lehner[1,2], Berthold Langguth[1,2] and Martin Schecklmann[1,2]*

[1] Department of Psychiatry and Psychotherapy, University of Regensburg, Regensburg, Germany, [2] Interdisciplinary Tinnitus Center of the University of Regensburg, Regensburg, Germany, [3] Department of Otorhinolaryngology, University of Regensburg, Regensburg, Germany

***Correspondence:**
Peter M. Kreuzer
peter.kreuzer@medbo.de

Background: Prefrontal and temporo-parietal repetitive transcranial magnetic stimulation (rTMS) in patients suffering from chronic tinnitus have shown significant but only moderate effectiveness with high interindividual variability in treatment response. This open-label pilot study was designed to examine the general feasibility of an individualized fronto-temporal rTMS protocol and to explore what criteria are needed for a more detailed evaluation in randomized clinical studies.

Methods: During the first session of a 2-week rTMS protocol, we applied different rTMS protocols to the left and right temporo-parietal and dorsolateral prefrontal cortex (DLPFC) in 25 tinnitus patients. Short trains of 1, 5, 10, and 20 Hz and continuous theta burst stimulation were applied, and patients were asked for immediate tinnitus reductions after each train. If a patient reported such improvements, rTMS treatment was applied over nine sessions with a combined protocol consisting of the most effective frontal and the most effective temporo-parietal stimulation protocol. Those patients who did not improve after the test session were treated with a standard prefrontal plus temporo-parietal protocol (20 Hz over left DLPFC + 1 Hz over temporo-parietal cortex).

Results: Almost half of the patients (12 of 25) reported immediate tinnitus reductions during the test session. In this group, the mean pre- to post-treatment amelioration in the tinnitus questionnaire was higher (medium to high effect sizes) in contrast to the patients who did not respond to the test session. Treatment outcome remained stable over a follow-up period of 10 weeks.

Discussion: Individualized rTMS was shown to be feasible and effective in chronic tinnitus. The results obtained from this study provide tentative evidence in support of an individualized rTMS treatment approach and might provide a basis for a "tailored" application of rTMS in tinnitus and other neuropsychiatric disorders.

Keywords: chronic tinnitus, repetitive transcranial magnetic stimulation, individualized repetitive transcranial magnetic stimulation, neuromodulation, neurostimulation

INTRODUCTION

Chronic Tinnitus

Subjective tinnitus is characterized by the perception of sound in the absence of a corresponding sound source (1). Approximately 1% of the general population report severe tinnitus-related impairment of daily living (2) and seek medical help (3). In contrast to auditory hallucinations that occur in mental disorders and mainly refer to the perception of voices, tinnitus sensations are usually of an unformed acoustic nature such as buzzing, hissing, or ringing (4). Severe tinnitus is frequently associated with depressive symptoms (5), anxiety (6, 7), and insomnia (8), and its socioeconomic relevance is illustrated by the dramatically increased risk for disability pension among tinnitus patients (9). The available evidence-based treatments for tinnitus have only small effect sizes (4, 10, 11), indicating the urgent need for the development and optimization of innovative therapeutic attempts.

Neurobiological Underpinnings of Chronic Tinnitus

Formerly considered as an otological disorder, tinnitus treatment approaches exclusively targeting the cochlea have led to discouraging results in most cases (12). However, during the last years, advances in neuroimaging and the development of animal models have shifted the perspective toward the neuronal pathologies underlying the different forms of tinnitus (13). There is convincing evidence emerging from functional imaging (14) and neurophysiological studies (15, 16) that tinnitus is not only related to abnormal functioning of the central auditory system (1) but also related to abnormal activity of non-auditory brain regions (17, 18) and abnormal functional connectivity between these regions (19–22). Imaging studies have shown that coactivation of prefrontal areas might especially be related to the affective components of tinnitus (5, 22, 23). It has been further proposed that limbic and paralimbic structures may form a fronto-thalamic gating system for tinnitus perception (24). According to this model, increased neuronal activity arises in the auditory pathways as a consequence of deafferentation due to hearing loss. If altered activity in auditory networks is connected to activation of motivational and emotional brain networks, the inhibitory influence from this fronto-thalamic gating system is downregulated, thus allowing the tinnitus signal to propagate to the auditory cortices, which finally leads to conscious perception. This is in line with electrophysiological studies that demonstrated the relevance of dysfunctional top–down inhibitory mechanisms originating in the prefrontal lobe for tinnitus generation (22, 25, 26). Therefore, two potential targets for brain stimulation can be identified: first, the frontal cortex with the aim to enhance the activity of the fronto-striato-thalamic gating mechanism, and second, the temporal cortex with the aim to reduce cortical activity in the auditory cortex. In line with this notion, tinnitus reduction has been demonstrated after repetitive transcranial magnetic stimulation (rTMS), tDCS, and direct cortical stimulation of both frontal and temporal cortices (27, 28).

rTMS in Chronic Tinnitus

On the basis of initial findings of abnormal functioning of central auditory structures (1), rTMS of the temporal and temporo-parietal cortex has been proposed as a potential treatment for chronic tinnitus (29). Several clinical studies showed a sham-controlled reduction of tinnitus severity after repeated 1 Hz rTMS applied to the left temporal cortex (30–34), but some studies were also negative (35, 36). In a meta-analysis, treatment effects were shown to be significant, but effect sizes were moderate at best and interindividual variability in treatment response is high (37).

The *Status Quo*

As mentioned above, rTMS treatment results in chronic tinnitus are currently burdened by only moderate improvement (38) and high interindividual variability indicating the need for optimization strategies. No demographic or clinical criteria could be identified as a predictor for rTMS treatment response in large samples of patients with chronic tinnitus (39). Several studies reported transient tinnitus suppression after a single session of rTMS (40). When the effects of different rTMS protocols over the temporal cortex were compared, it has been shown that the protocol with the best tinnitus suppressing effect differed from patient to patient (41). However, the individually best protocols induced similar changes of oscillatory brain activity (42). Although single rTMS sessions reduced tinnitus only transiently for seconds to minutes, repeated daily rTMS stimulation resulted in longer lasting tinnitus reduction up to several months (30, 43, 44) in some patients. Most studies investigating repeated sessions of rTMS used low-frequency rTMS with 1 Hz, even though two studies comparing the effects of 1 Hz rTMS with those of 10 and 25 Hz revealed similar treatment effects for high-frequency rTMS (45, 46).

In light of these data, the question arises whether a test session, in which the immediate effects of different TMS protocols are evaluated, may be a feasible and useful approach for selecting the rTMS protocol for repeated rTMS sessions. To our knowledge, this question has not yet been addressed by any study, even if the sham-controlled response to single rTMS sessions has been used as a selection criterion for surgical implantation with epidural electrodes (47).

Both auditory and non-auditory brain regions are involved in tinnitus (48, 49), and combined frontal and temporal stimulation protocols exerted best effects in previous studies (22, 50, 51). Thus, the aim of the present study was to investigate the feasibility of an rTMS treatment approach that is (i) individualized based on the effects of single test sessions and that (ii) comprises both prefrontal and temporo-parietal cortices.

MATERIALS AND METHODS

Study Design and Conduct

The study was conducted following a two-armed pilot study design. As a first step, an initial rTMS testing session was conducted in which 1, 5, 10, and 20 Hz; continuous theta burst rTMS; and sham were applied to (i) the left dorsolateral prefrontal cortex (DLPFC), (ii) the right DLPFC, (iii) the left temporo-parietal junction area, and (iv) the right temporo-parietal junction area. The number of applied stimuli during the rTMS testing session on day 1 was 200 stimuli for each stimulation frequency and location (exception: 50 stimuli at 1 Hz frequency), resulting in a total of up to 4,200 stimuli. After the application of each protocol, patients were asked whether they had experienced a change in their tinnitus and were asked to rate the changes on a percentage level regarding to loudness. Patients wore insert earplugs during the testing session and were instructed to report immediate tinnitus changes in form of percentage values. The most effective protocol of each of the four stimulation locations was (i) repeated to assure retest validity and (ii) controlled by sham stimulation (applying the same paradigm with a tilted coil angle of 90° with one wing of the figure-of-eight coil on the head and magnetic field main direction, thus paralleling the scalp surface). Thus, sham conditions were different for each stimulation site and patient during the testing phase. For patients reporting the same tinnitus reduction for different stimulation protocols for the left and right frontal or for the left and right temporo-parietal stimulation sites, equally effective protocols were repeated and contrasted directly. Patients reporting immediate tinnitus modulation during the testing session on day 1 (Monday) were consecutively treated by application of 9 further daily (only working days) combined stimulation sessions consisting of the most effective prefrontal stimulation protocol (2,000 stimuli) at the left or right hemisphere followed by the most effective temporo-parietal stimulation protocol (left or right, 2,000 stimuli/session). Patients who did not experience immediate tinnitus modulation during the testing session on day 1 were treated by a "standard" combined treatment consisting of 2,000 stimuli of 20 Hz rTMS delivered to the left DLPFC followed by 2,000 stimuli of 1 Hz rTMS of the left temporo-parietal junction area ($n = 3$) or a "triple" paradigm consisting of 2,000 stimuli of 20 Hz rTMS of the left DLPFC followed by rTMS (1,000 stimuli left, 1,000 stimuli right) of the bilateral temporo-parietal junction area ($n = 9$) (52). Due to ethical reasons, we switched treatment for the standard group as it turned out during the course of the present study that the triple stimulation is more effective than the former standard treatment (53). The treatment sessions following the testing session consisted of a total of 4,000 stimuli/day for both the individualized and the standard group and were conducted on nine subsequent working days. Follow-up-visits were conducted 2 and 10 weeks after the end of the stimulation period (=week 4 and week 12 visit, respectively).

Stimulation was performed with a 70-mm figure-of-8 (=butterfly) coil (Cool-B65, Magventure A/S, Denmark) in 40 trains with 50 stimuli and an intertrain interval of 25 s (exception: 1 Hz stimulation was administered in one train). The coil was powered by a MagPro ×100 stimulator (Magventure A/S, Denmark). Stimulation was performed at 110% resting motor threshold (RMT) but not higher than 60% maximum stimulator output. RMT was defined as the lowest intensity sufficient to produce left abductor digiti minimi muscle activation (magnetic evoked potentials >50 μV) with a single pulse delivered to the motor cortex in at least 5 of 10 trials and was determined before the testing session on day 1. For treatment of the left DLPFC, the conventional butterfly coil was positioned 6 cm anterior of the left motor hotspot in a sagittal direction with the handle pointing backward in a 45° angle toward the midline (28). Temporo-parietal cortex localization was conducted following a protocol suggested by Khedr et al. (46) positioning the coil between the temporal (T3/T4-electrode location) and parietal (P3/P4-location) (54) according the 10–20 EEG-positioning system (55). Coil positioning was tangential to the scalp with the handle pointing upward.

All participants gave written informed consent after a comprehensive explanation of the study procedures that data were gathered and analyzed for the Tinnitus Research Initiative database (56), which was approved by the Ethics Committee of the University Hospital of Regensburg (Germany, reference number 08/046). All study procedures were carried out in accordance with the approved guidelines.

Patient Enrollment

Inclusion criterion was subjective tinnitus with duration of more than 6 months. Exclusion criteria comprised objective tinnitus (with a treatable cause), ongoing other tinnitus treatments during or 3 months before study enrollment, the presence of clinically relevant psychiatric comorbidities or unstable medical conditions, history or evidence of significant brain malformation or neoplasm, history of head injuries, cerebral vascular events, the presence of irremovable metal objects in and around the body, pregnancy, alcohol abuse or intake of illicit substances, and history of prior TMS treatment. Patients were recruited for participation in the study after presentation in the outpatient clinic of the Interdisciplinary Tinnitus Centre at the University of Regensburg, Regensburg, Germany. The study was conducted between November 2011 and June 2012.

Outcome Measures and Data Presentation

The outcome parameters were change in tinnitus distress and loudness measured with the tinnitus questionnaire (TQ; range 0–84) (57) and a numeric rating scale (range 0–10), respectively. We present change from baseline to the week 2 visit to measure immediate treatment effects and also from pretreatment to post-treatment defined as a mean value of the screening and baseline visits (pretreatment) and of the week 2, 4, and 12 visits (post-treatment). In addition, we demonstrate the number of treatment responders defined as a minimal reduction of 5 points in the TQ (58). Further objectives were the assessment of adverse events and safety information at all visits. Data were assessed according to international standards (59) and registered in a tinnitus database following ICH-GCP regulations (60, 61). We contrasted the group of patients who reported changes in tinnitus after a single session with the group of patients with no response.

All data are displayed as mean ± SD if not otherwise labeled. In case of missing data, the last observation was carried forward, and participants who did not complete rTMS treatment (dropouts) were excluded from analysis ($n = 1$). Due to the pilot character of the study, we focus on the feasibility and identification of modifications for future studies (62, 63). For this purpose, we report raw data and basic statistical tests for rough estimation of the efficacy of the tested treatments. All statistical tests were conducted two tailed, unadjusted for multiple comparisons, and a value of $p < 0.05$ was assumed as statistically significant. For group comparisons, we calculated Student's t-tests for independent measures. Effect sizes are reported according to G*Power 3.1.2 (64). Statistical data analysis was performed using IBM SPSS Statistics for Windows, version 22.0 (released 2013; IBM Corp., Armonk, NY, USA).

RESULTS

Feasibility

Twenty-five patients were recruited for participation in the study. One participant aborted the treatment after the first day due to headache after finishing the testing session on day 1 (without reporting immediate effects). Exactly 50% of the 24 remaining patients ($n = 12$) reported immediate modulation of their tinnitus percept during day 1 testing procedures and were therefore allocated to the individualized treatment arm receiving combined rTMS of prefrontal and temporo-parietal cortical areas for another 9 consecutive working days. Nine of the 12 patients who perceived a tinnitus change after TMS were able to indicate the change in a percentage value (ranging between 3 and 70%). The other three patients provided only vague estimations like "better" (see **Table 1**). Two patients experiencing the most pronounced improvement after active rTMS reported similar improvement after sham TMS during the testing session. No other patient reported tinnitus improvement after sham TMS. Also, these patients were assigned to the individualized arm (subject number 1 and 7 in **Table 1**). Three patients in each of the study groups were under a psychotropic medication (individualized group: 1× citalopram 40 mg/day, 1× venlafaxine 225 mg/day, 1× opipramol 100 mg/day; control group: 1× citalopram 40 mg/day + trimipramine 40 mg/day, 1× agomelatine 25 mg/day, 1× opipramol 100 mg/day).

Concerning the other 12 patients without immediate tinnitus changes during the testing rTMS session, 3 were treated with the "standard double protocol" consisting of 2,000 stimuli to the left DLPFC at 20 Hz frequency followed by 2,000 stimuli to the left temporo-parietal cortex at 1 Hz and 9 were treated with the "standard triple protocol" consisting of high-frequency rTMS of the left prefrontal cortex (2,000 stimuli, 20 Hz) followed by low-frequency rTMS of the bilateral temporo-parietal junction areas (total of 2,000 stimuli, 1 Hz). For graphical illustration of the study conduct, see **Figure 1**.

The comparison of participants of both treatment groups revealed no differences in the clinical and demographic baseline characteristics. Detailed information is provided in **Table 2**. In three patients (all from the individualized group), screening and baseline visits were performed at the same visit resulting in only one pretreatment assessment. One patient did not provide data for visit week 4 (standard treatment). These missing values were added by LOCF using data from the screening visit. For the other patients, interval between screening and baseline was between

TABLE 1 | Individual data for treatment with individualized repetitive transcranial magnetic stimulation (rTMS) and average group data for individualized and standard rTMS (each subject was stimulated with 4,000 pulses per day).

	Subject order	Kind of prefrontal stimulation	Single-session tinnitus reduction[a]	Kind of temporo-parietal stimulation	Single-session tinnitus reduction[a]	Resting motor threshold (RMT); stimulation intensity (stimulator output)[b]	Change in tinnitus questionnaire (TQ) total score from baseline to week 2 visit[d]	Change in TQ total score from pretreatment to posttreatment[c,d]
Individualized treatment (single subject data)	1	Right continuous theta burst stimulation (cTBS)	70%	Right 5 Hz	50%	42%; 46%	24 (–)	20.33 (–)
	3	Right 10 Hz	"Better"	Left cTBS	"Better"	34%; 37%	7 (–)	2.50 (+)
	5	Left cTBS	40%	Left 10 Hz	40%	43%; 47%	0 (+)	1.17 (+)
	7	Left 20 Hz	50%	Left 5 Hz	40%	46%; 51%	11 (–)	15.17 (–)
	9	Left 5 Hz	20%	Right cTBS	10%	37%; 41%	11 (–)	3.17 (+)
	10	Left 20 Hz	2%	Right 10 Hz	2%	33%; 36%	–3 (+)	–8.33 (+)
	13	Left 20 Hz	"Not sure"	Left 20 Hz	"Good"	50%; 55%	9 (–)	9.33 (–)
	16	Right 20 Hz	30%	Left 5 Hz	100%	57%; 60%	–9 (+)	20.83 (–)
	17	Left 5 Hz	"Shortly better"	Right cTBS	"Shortly off"	30%; 33%	20 (–)	5.67 (–)
	18	Left cTBS	10%	Left cTBS	10%	38%; 42%	3 (+)	9.83 (–)
	23	Left 20 Hz	10%	Right 20 Hz	10%	52%; 57%	10 (–)	8.33 (–)
	24	Left 20 Hz	3%	Left 10 Hz	4%	42%; 46%	3 (+)	5.33 (–)
Individualized treatment (mean ± SD)	n.a.	9/12 left; 5 Hz ($n = 2$), 10 Hz ($n = 1$), 20 Hz ($n = 6$), cTBS ($n = 3$)	n.a.	7/12 left; 5 Hz ($n = 3$), 10 Hz ($n = 3$), 20 Hz ($n = 2$), cTBS ($n = 4$)	n.a.	42 ± 8; 46 ± 9	7.17 ± 9.24 (58% responder)	8.57 ± 8.92 (67% responder)
Standard protocol (mean ± SD)	n.a.	Left 20 Hz	n.a.	Left and/or right 1 Hz	n.a.	43 ± 17; 43 ± 9	3.42 ± 7.04 (42% responder)	1.46 ± 8.48 (42% responder)

[a]*Numbers indicate the percent of tinnitus reduction after a single-session stimulation; verbal statements are indicated by quotation marks.*

[b]*Stimulation intensity was 110% of RMT; for safety reasons, 60% was the upper limit for stimulation intensity; RMT and stimulation intensity were comparable in the standard protocol group as two subjects had thresholds highly above 60%.*

[c]*Visits after treatment (week 2 + week 4 + final visit) minus visits before treatment (screening + baseline).*

[d]*Responder information in brackets (+ = yes, – = no).*

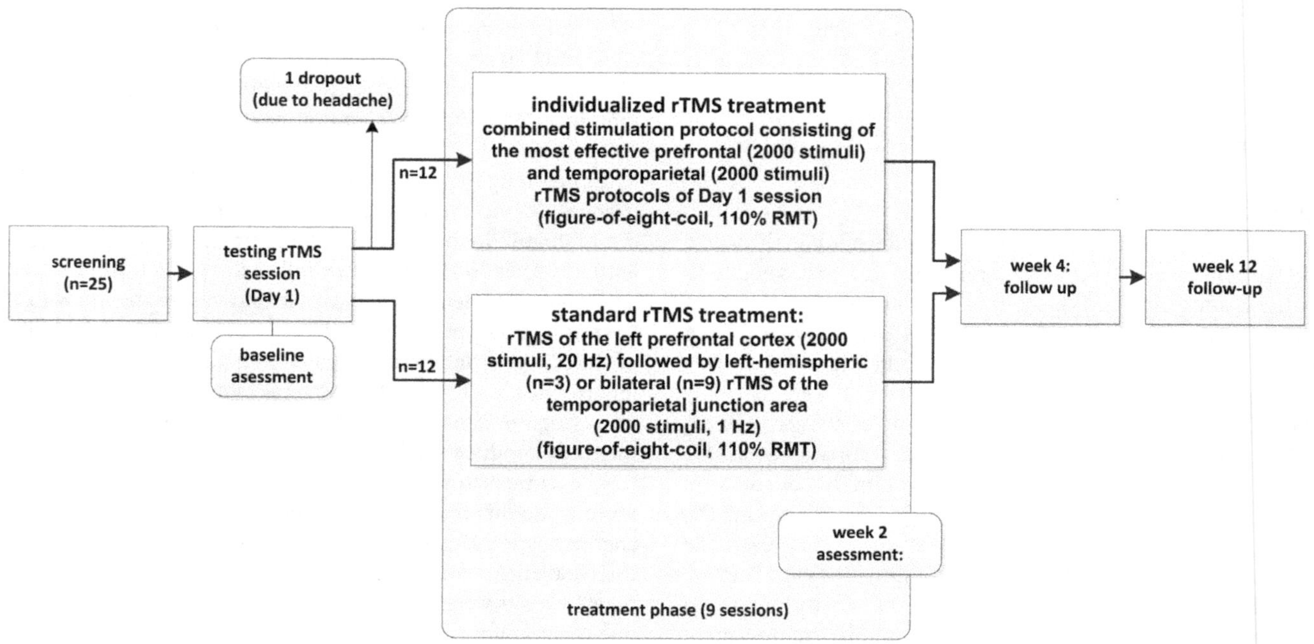

FIGURE 1 | **Study structure and patient flow (for detailed information, see Materials and Methods).**

TABLE 2 | **Group comparisons of the two treatment arms.**

	Individualized rTMS (n = 12)	Standard rTMS (n = 12)	Statistics: individualized vs. standard rTMS
Gender (female/male)	2/10	2/10	n.a.
Age (years)	57.1 ± 7.4	50.6 ± 12.1	$t(22) = 1.582$; $p = 0.128$
Mean hearing level (dB HL)	25.7 ± 15.9	22.9 ± 13.4	$t(22) = 0.476$; $p = 0.639$
Tinnitus duration (months)	108.2 ± 98.9	154.3 ± 106.8	$t(21) = 1.072$; $p = 0.296$
Tinnitus laterality (right/left/both)	0/2/10	0/2/10	n.a.
TQ (baseline minus week 2)	7.2 ± 9.2	3.4 ± 7.0	$t(22) = 1.118$; $p = 0.276$; $d = 0.465$
TQ (screening/ baseline minus week 2/4/12)	8.6 ± 8.9	1.5 ± 8.5	$t(22) = 2.002$; $p = 0.058$; $d = 0.816$
NRS loudness (baseline minus week 2)	0.8 ± 1.9	1.4 ± 2.5	$t(22) = 0.649$; $p = 0.289$; $d = 0.270$
NRS loudness (screening/baseline minus week 2/4/12)	0.9 ± 1.9	1.0 ± 1.5	$t(22) = 0.181$; $p = 0.858$; $d = 0.058$

TQ, tinnitus questionnaire (scale: 0–84); NRS, numeric rating scale (scale: 0–10); rTMS, repetitive transcranial magnetic stimulation.

13 and 349 days (or screening and baseline was the same visit) with a mean of 81.4 and a SD of 86.03 (median = 53). In the individualized treatment group, we had 10 right-handed patients and 2 ambidextrous patients; in the standard group, we had 8 right-handed patients, 2 left-handed patients, and 2 ambidextrous patients. A statistical comparison with the Fisher's exact test shows no difference between groups with respect to handedness ($p = 0.329$). In the individualized group, three patients chose right frontal and nine left frontal stimulation as a best stimulation site ($\chi^2 = 2.222$; df = 2; $p = 0.045$) and five right temporal and seven left temporal stimulation as a best stimulation site ($p = 0.470$), indicating an association of right-handedness with left frontal stimulation. However, this association of left frontal stimulation with right-handedness is from correlational nature, but highlights the need for accounting handedness in rTMS trials.

Safety

No severe adverse events occurred during the course of the study. One participant withdrew his consent to participate due to the experience of headache during the testing session on day 1. This patient did not report changes in tinnitus loudness after single rTMS sessions and was determined as dropout for the standard treatment arm (see **Figure 1**). A deterioration of tinnitus was reported by two patients in the testing session, but did not lead to an interruption of the treatment. These patients were treated with the standard protocol. Further adverse events included headache in two patients (one on 1 day of treatment and one in 2 days of treatment) of the standard treatment and in one patient in the individualized group on 1 treatment day. One patient of the standard treatment missed two treatment days due to a common cold.

Results of the Test Session

For the majority of patients, the testing session revealed best results for left-sided stimulation for both frontal and temporal stimulation resulting in predominant left-hemispheric treatment location in the individualized treatment group (**Table 1**).

With respect to tinnitus localization, two patients of both treatment groups had purely left-sided tinnitus, and the other patients had tinnitus either in both ears or within the head. No patient had reported purely right-sided tinnitus (**Table 2**). In the majority of the patients, high-frequency stimulation protocols or TBS revealed best results in the testing session (**Table 1**).

Efficacy

The mean reduction of tinnitus severity measured by the TQ (57) was numerically higher for the individualized treatment group in contrast to the standard group (**Table 2**). Number of responders was also higher in the individualized group (**Table 1**). Graphical information on the TQ score at the different assessment time points is depicted in **Figure 2**. Decrease in tinnitus loudness was in the same range for the individualized and the standard group (**Table 2**). On a statistical level, individualized treatment (vs. standard treatment) showed numerically superior efficacy with medium or high effect size on a non-significant level contrasting week 2 and baseline or postvisits and previsits, respectively (screening and baseline vs. week 2, 4, and 12) as elicited by the TQ. Changes in tinnitus loudness were not significantly different between groups with small or negligible effects sizes.

DISCUSSION

From this pilot study examining the feasibility of an individualized treatment approach in patients suffering from chronic tinnitus, three main conclusions can be drawn:

(i) The application of a testing rTMS session with different frequencies and stimulation sites has proven to be feasible with almost 50% of the patients reporting immediate effects in our study sample.

(ii) An individualized treatment approach following this testing session was well tolerated by the majority of patients. Adverse events and dropout rates were comparable among both study arms and matched prior observations (28).

(iii) The clinical efficacy of an individualized treatment approach exceeded the results of a standard treatment approach on a descriptive level. Effects for TQ were not significant, but showed medium to high effect sizes. Improvement was stable for several weeks after the treatment.

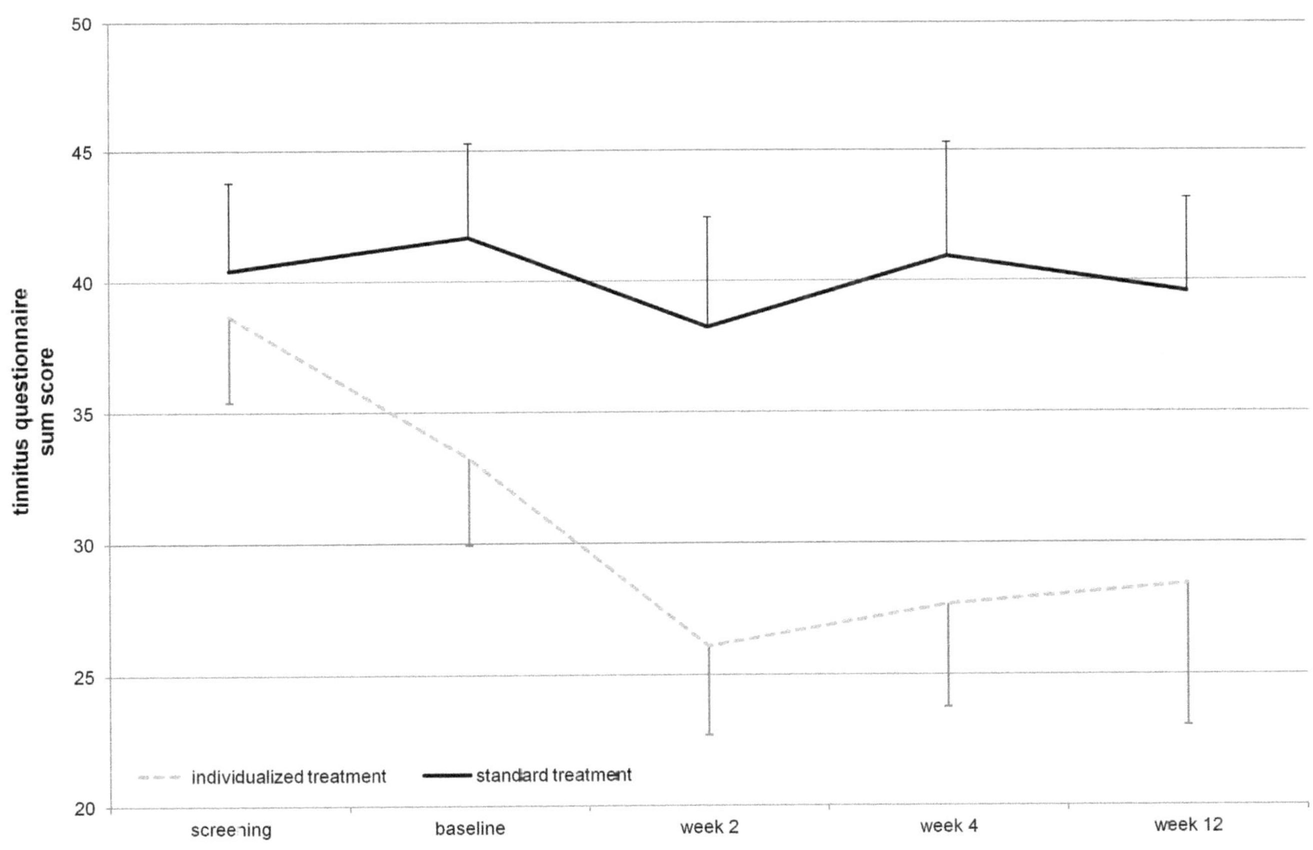

FIGURE 2 | Tinnitus questionnaire total score over the time course of the study (displayed mean ± SEM). Repetitive transcranial magnetic stimulation treatment took place from baseline until week 2 visit. Week 4 and week 12 assessments represent follow-up.

This pilot study addressed the question to what extent clinical effects of a single session may serve as predictors for treatment response of repeated sessions of rTMS. On a descriptive level, the individualized treatment group reported a higher reduction of tinnitus severity than the control group treated with a standard combined rTMS paradigm.

Our finding that response to a single session may predict treatment outcome of prolonged stimulation has similarly been detected in the approach to use a single session of rTMS as a selection criterion for the implantation of epidural electrodes for intractable tinnitus (48, 49). Among patients who responded to a single session of TMS, two-third had also long-term benefit from epidural stimulation (48). Notably, epidural stimulation in chronic tinnitus has been only conducted in few cases of intractable tinnitus, and the results should not carelessly be transferred to our sample and settings. However, this ratio corresponds nicely to our finding that most patients who responded to the testing sessions also responded to repeated rTMS application.

Our finding that the effect of testing sessions predicts the effect of daily treatment is of high clinical relevance as rTMS treatment results are characterized by high interindividual variability and no demographic or clinical tinnitus baseline characteristics could be identified as predictors of rTMS treatment response yet (65). The high interindividual variability in rTMS treatment response in previous studies has been mainly interpreted as an expression of the variability of tinnitus pathophysiology (40). If this was correct, it would be plausible that different patients might respond to different stimulation paradigms, thus profiting from individualized "trial-and-error" treatment attempts (65). Even, if the individualized treatment showed higher efficacy in contrast to standard treatment, the SD of TQ change in the two groups was similar for both treatment arms. This indicates a similar variability in treatment response and suggests that individualized treatment does not increase efficacy by reducing interindividual variability.

One discussable issue is the identification of the most efficient protocol in the testing session. In each patient, 20 different protocols were tested (5 different frequencies at 4 different sites). For practical reasons, the intervals between the different protocols were rather short. Investigators were instructed to wait until the tinnitus returned to baseline level before applying the next protocol. Thus, the interval between different protocols was typically in the range between 1 and 5 min. A testing session, therefore, took approximately 1 h per individual, in some cases even longer. However, we are aware that it cannot be excluded that the effects of the different protocols were influenced by after-effects of the preceding protocols. Thus, the increased responsiveness to high frequency and TBS stimulation may have been partly due to the accumulation of stimulation effects as the order of the different protocols was not randomized during the testing session. It could also be the case that it took some time for the individuals to acclimate to the testing scenario. However, it is unlikely that the effects were only driven by accumulation of stimuli or habituation to the testing situation as TBS was always applied as the last protocol, but not every patient reported best improvement with TBS. Nevertheless, future studies investigating individualized TMS should take a potential order effect into account and follow a randomized protocol regarding the sequence of stimulation frequencies and stimulated hemispheres.

A certain dissociation of the effects of a single session and repeated sessions was observed. Although patients reported loudness reductions of their tinnitus during the testing session, daily treatment had only an effect on tinnitus distress but not on tinnitus loudness. Possible reasons might be related to differences in the applied scales for tinnitus loudness (percentage change after a single session vs. 11 graded numeric rating for tinnitus loudness). Furthermore, ratings during a single session were conducted with inserted earplugs, whereas clinical evaluation over the course of the treatment was done without hearing protection obscuring possible changes in tinnitus loudness.

We are well aware that the comparison between the individualized treatment group and the standard treatment group does not enable us to disentangle whether the response in the testing session serves as a general predictor for response to repeated rTMS sessions or whether the individualized protocol was relevant for the good outcome in the individualized treatment group. In other words, the test session might have only served for the identification of responders at the starting point of the rTMS treatment period. To further address this issue, future studies should be conducted in which patients, who respond to TMS testing sessions, are randomized into standard treatment vs. individualized treatment.

Notably, the present study was designed as a proof-of-concept pilot study, which should primarily evaluate the feasibility and tolerability of an individualized rTMS treatment regime in chronic tinnitus. Thus, we are well aware about the limiting factor of the lack of a sham-controlled study group. It cannot be excluded that the improved outcome in the individualized group was driven by non-specific effects. Patients who experienced tinnitus improvement in the testing session might have developed higher expectations with respect to the daily treatment, which could have contributed to the better outcome. However, active control conditions have especially been recommended in rTMS studies due to the inherent limitations of sham conditions (36, 66, 67). For future studies using this individualized approach, we would suggest the splitting of the patients reporting changes in tinnitus perception into two arms—one arm treated with the individualized protocol and one arm treated with a standard protocol. An optimal design would also include a third sham arm (68).

In summary, our pilot data confirm the potential of individualized rTMS treatment as a non-invasive, safe, and well-tolerated method of brain stimulation in the treatment of chronic tinnitus. Descriptive analyses indicate a remarkable superior effect of the individualized treatment in contrast to standard treatment even if the standard treatment with two or three stimulation sites was shown to be more effective than single-site stimulations (36, 66, 67, 69). Individualized rTMS in chronic tinnitus might provide a basis for an individualized, "tailored" rTMS-based therapeutic approach also in other neuropsychiatric disorders. Combining a single session with electroencephalography during the first treatment day (70) might help to identify neuronal markers, which might enable reliable predictions regarding treatment response after daily rTMS. This approach could eventually be useful in identifying successful TMS protocols based on EEG markers also in those patients, who were not able to detect perceptual improvements in the test session.

AUTHOR CONTRIBUTIONS

PK, BL, RR, and MS: conception of the study, data interpretation, and manuscript edition. AL and MS: statistics and data management. PK, VV, and TP: patient recruitment and conduction of clinical visits.

ACKNOWLEDGMENTS

The authors thank Sandra Pfluegl, Ulrike Stadler, Helene Niebling, Susanne Staudinger, Jarmila Gerxhaliu-Holan, and Jan Brauner for their assistance in administering rTMS and data management. Most of all, they want to thank their patients for participating in their studies and allowing them to use their data for analyses.

FUNDING

The study was supported by the Tinnitus Research Initiative.

REFERENCES

Moller AR. Pathophysiology of tinnitus. *Otolaryngol Clin North Am* (2003) 36:249–266, v–vi. doi:10.1016/S0030-6665(02)00170-6

Harter M, Maurischat C, Weske G, Laszig R, Berger M. [Psychological stress and impaired quality of life in patients with tinnitus]. *HNO* (2004) 52(2):125–31. doi:10.1007/s00106-003-0889-8

Coles RR. Epidemiology of tinnitus: (1) prevalence. *J Laryngol Otol Suppl* (1984) 9:7–15. doi:10.1017/S1755146300090041

Langguth B, Kreuzer PM, Kleinjung T, De Ridder D. Tinnitus: causes and clinical management. *Lancet Neurol* (2013) 12:920–30. doi:10.1016/ S1474-4422(13)70160-1

Langguth B, Landgrebe M, Kleinjung T, Sand GP, Hajak G. Tinnitus and depression. *World J Biol Psychiatry* (2011) 12(7):489–500. doi:10.3109/1562 2975.2011.575178

Krog NH, Engdahl B, Tambs K. The association between tinnitus and mental health in a general population sample: results from the HUNT Study. *J Psychosom Res* (2010) 69:289–98. doi:10.1016/j.jpsychores.2010.03.008

Langguth B. A review of tinnitus symptoms beyond 'ringing in the ears': a call to action. *Curr Med Res Opin* (2011) 27:1635–43. doi:10.1185/03007995. 2011.595781

Cronlein T, Langguth B, Geisler P, Hajak G. Tinnitus and insomnia. *Prog Brain Res* (2007) 166:227–33. doi:10.1016/S0079-6123(07)66021-X

Friberg E, Jansson C, Mittendorfer-Rutz E, Rosenhall U, Alexanderson K. Sickness absence due to otoaudiological diagnoses and risk of disability pension: a nationwide Swedish prospective cohort study. *PLoS One* (2012) 7:e29966. doi:10.1371/journal.pone.0029966

Hoare DJ, Kowalkowski VL, Kang S, Hall DA. Systematic review and meta-analyses of randomized controlled trials examining tinnitus manage- ment. *Laryngoscope* (2011) 121:1555–64. doi:10.1002/lary.21825

Kreuzer PM, Vielsmeier V, Langguth B. Chronic tinnitus: an interdisciplinary challenge. *Dtsch Arztebl Int* (2013) 110:278–84. doi:10.3238/arztebl. 2013.0278

Dobie RA. A review of randomized clinical trials in tinnitus. *Laryngoscope* (1999) 109:1202–11. doi:10.1097/00005537-199908000-00004

Shore SE, Roberts LE, Langguth B. Maladaptive plasticity in tinnitus – triggers, mechanisms and treatment. *Nat Rev Neurol* (2016) 12:150–60. doi:10.1038/ nrneurol.2016.12

Elgoyhen AB, Langguth B, De Ridder D, Vanneste S. Tinnitus: perspectives from human neuroimaging. *Nat Rev Neurosci* (2015) 16:632–42. doi:10.1038/ nrn4003

Weisz N, Dohrmann K, Elbert T. The relevance of spontaneous activity for the coding of the tinnitus sensation. *Prog Brain Res* (2007) 166:61–70. doi:10.1016/ S0079-6123(07)66006-3

Weisz N, Muller S, Schlee W, Dohrmann K, Hartmann T, Elbert T. The neural code of auditory phantom perception. *J Neurosci* (2007) 27:1479–84. doi:10.1523/JNEUROSCI.3711-06.2007

Lanting CP, De Kleine E, Van Dijk P. Neural activity underlying tinnitus generation: results from PET and fMRI. *Hear Res* (2009) 255:1–13. doi:10.1016/ j.heares.2009.06.009

Leaver AM, Renier L, Chevillet MA, Morgan S, Kim HJ, Rauschecker JP. Dysregulation of limbic and auditory networks in tinnitus. *Neuron* (2011) 69:33–43. doi:10.1016/j.neuron.2010.12.002

Schlee W, Weisz N, Bertrand O, Hartmann T, Elbert T. Using auditory steady state responses to outline the functional connectivity in the tinnitus brain. *PLoS One* (2008) 3:e3720. doi:10.1371/journal.pone.0003720

Schlee W, Hartmann T, Langguth B, Weisz N. Abnormal resting-state cortical coupling in chronic tinnitus. *BMC Neurosci* (2009) 10:11. doi:10.1186/1471-2202-10-11

Schlee W, Mueller N, Hartmann T, Keil J, Lorenz I, Weisz N. Mapping cortical hubs in tinnitus. *BMC Biol* (2009) 7:80. doi:10.1186/1741-7007-7-80

De Ridder D, Elgoyhen AB, Romo R, Langguth B. Phantom percepts: tinnitus and pain as persisting aversive memory networks. *Proc Natl Acad Sci U S A* (2011) 108:8075–80. doi:10.1073/pnas.1018466108

Vanneste S, Plazier M, Der Loo E, De Heyning PV, Congedo M, De Ridder D. The neural correlates of tinnitus-related distress. *Neuroimage* (2010) 52:470–80. doi:10.1016/j.neuroimage.2010.04.029

Rauschecker JP, Leaver AM, Muhlau M. Tuning out the noise: limbic-auditory interactions in tinnitus. *Neuron* (2010) 66:819–26. doi:10.1016/ j.neuron.2010.04.032

Norena A, Cransac H, Chery-Croze S. Towards an objectification by classification of tinnitus. *Clin Neurophysiol* (1999) 110:666–75. doi:10.1016/ S1388-2457(98)00034-0

Schecklmann M, Landgrebe M, Poeppl TB, Kreuzer P, Manner P, Marienhagen J, et al. Neural correlates of tinnitus duration and distress: a positron emission tomography study. *Hum Brain Mapp* (2013) 34:233–40. doi:10.1002/ hbm.21426

Vanneste S, Plazier M, Ost J, Van Der Loo E, Van De Heyning P, De Ridder D. Bilateral dorsolateral prefrontal cortex modulation for tinnitus by transcranial direct current stimulation: a preliminary clinical study. *Exp Brain Res* (2010) 202:779–85. doi:10.1007/s00221-010-2183-9

Frank E, Schecklmann M, Landgrebe M, Burger J, Kreuzer P, Poeppl TB, et al. Treatment of chronic tinnitus with repeated sessions of prefrontal transcranial direct current stimulation: outcomes from an open-label pilot study. *J Neurol* (2011) 259(2):327–33. doi:10.1007/s00415-011-6189-4

Eichhammer P, Langguth B, Marienhagen J, Kleinjung T, Hajak G. Neuronavigated repetitive transcranial magnetic stimulation in patients with tinnitus: a short case series. *Biol Psychiatry* (2003) 54:862–5. doi:10.1016/ S0006-3223(02)01896-6

Kleinjung T, Eichhammer P, Langguth B, Jacob P, Marienhagen J, Hajak G, et al. Long-term effects of repetitive transcranial magnetic stimulation (rTMS) in patients with chronic tinnitus. *Otolaryngol Head Neck Surg* (2005) 132 566–9. doi:10.1016/j.otohns.2004.09.134

Plewnia C, Reimold M, Najib A, Reischl G, Plontke SK, Gerloff C. Moderate therapeutic efficacy of positron emission tomography-navigated repetitive transcranial magnetic stimulation for chronic tinnitus: a randomised, con- trolled pilot study. *J Neurol Neurosurg Psychiatry* (2007) 78:152–6. doi:10.1136/ jnnp.2006.095612

Rossi S, De Capua A, Ulivelli M, Bartalini S, Falzarano V, Filippone G, et al Effects of repetitive transcranial magnetic stimulation on chronic tinnitus:

a randomised, crossover, double blind, placebo controlled study. *J Neurol Neurosurg Psychiatry* (2007) 78:857–63. doi:10.1136/jnnp.2006.105007

Smith JA, Mennemeier M, Bartel T, Chelette KC, Kimbrell T, Triggs W, et al. Repetitive transcranial magnetic stimulation for tinnitus: a pilot study. *Laryngoscope* (2007) 117:529–34. doi:10.1097/MLG.0b013e31802f4154

Folmer RL, Theodoroff SM, Casiana L, Shi Y, Griest S, Vachhani J. Repetitive transcranial magnetic stimulation treatment for chronic tinnitus: a randomized clinical trial. *JAMA Otolaryngol Head Neck Surg* (2015) 141:716–22. doi:10.1001/jamaoto.2015.1219

Piccirillo JF, Kallogjeri D, Nicklaus J, Wineland A, Spitznagel EL Jr, Vlassenko AG, et al. Low-frequency repetitive transcranial magnetic stimulation to the temporoparietal junction for tinnitus: four-week stimulation trial. *JAMA Otolaryngol Head Neck Surg* (2013) 139:388–95. doi:10.1001/jamaoto.2013.233

Langguth B, Landgrebe M, Frank E, Schecklmann M, Sand PG, Vielsmeier V, et al. Efficacy of different protocols of transcranial magnetic stimulation for the treatment of tinnitus: pooled analysis of two randomized controlled studies. *World J Biol Psychiatry* (2014) 15:276–85. doi:10.3109/15622975.2012.708438

Soleimani R, Jalali MM, Hasandokht T. Therapeutic impact of repetitive transcranial magnetic stimulation (rTMS) on tinnitus: a systematic review and meta-analysis. *Eur Arch Otorhinolaryngol* (2016) 237:1663–75. doi:10.1007/ s00405-015-3642-5

Frank E, Eichhammer P, Burger J, Zowe M, Landgrebe M, Hajak G, et al. Transcranial magnetic stimulation for the treatment of depression: feasibility and results under naturalistic conditions: a retrospective analysis. *Eur Arch Psychiatry Clin Neurosci* (2011) 261(4):261–6. doi:10.1007/s00406-010-0137-7

Peng Z, Chen XQ, Gong SS. Effectiveness of repetitive transcranial magnetic stimulation for chronic tinnitus: a systematic review. *Otolaryngol Head Neck Surg* (2012) 147(5):817–25. doi:10.1177/0194599812458771

Lefaucheur JP, Andre-Obadia N, Antal A, Ayache SS, Baeken C, Benninger DH, et al. Evidence-based guidelines on the therapeutic use of repetitive transcranial magnetic stimulation (rTMS). *Clin Neurophysiol* (2014) 125:2150–206. doi:10.1016/j.clinph.2014.05.021

De Ridder D, Verstraeten E, Van Der Kelen K, De Mulder G, Sunaert S, Verlooy J, et al. Transcranial magnetic stimulation for tinnitus: influence of tinnitus duration on stimulation parameter choice and maximal tinnitus suppression. *Otol Neurotol* (2005) 26:616–9. doi:10.1097/01.mao.0000178146. 91139.3c

Muller N, Keil J, Obleser J, Schulz H, Grunwald T, Bernays RL, et al. You can't stop the music: reduced auditory alpha power and coupling between auditory and memory regions facilitate the illusory perception of music during noise. *Neuroimage* (2013) 79:383–93. doi:10.1016/j.neuroimage.2013. 05.001

Khedr EM, Rothwell JC, El-Atar A. One-year follow up of patients with chronic tinnitus treated with left temporoparietal rTMS. *Eur J Neurol* (2009) 16:404–8. doi:10.1111/j.1468-1331.2008.02522.x

Burger J, Frank E, Kreuzer P, Kleinjung T, Vielsmeier V, Landgrebe M, et al. Transcranial magnetic stimulation for the treatment of tinnitus: 4-year fol- low-up in treatment responders – a retrospective analysis. *Brain Stimul* (2011) 4:222–7. doi:10.1016/j.brs.2010.11.003

Khedr EM, Rothwell JC, Ahmed MA, El-Atar A. Effect of daily repetitive transcranial magnetic stimulation for treatment of tinnitus: comparison of different stimulus frequencies. *J Neurol Neurosurg Psychiatry* (2008) 79:212–5. doi:10.1136/jnnp.2007.127712

Khedr EM, Abo-Elfetoh N, Rothwell JC, El-Atar A, Sayed E, Khalifa H. Contralateral versus ipsilateral rTMS of temporoparietal cortex for the treatment of chronic unilateral tinnitus: comparative study. *Eur J Neurol* (2010) 17:976–83. doi:10.1111/j.1468-1331.2010.02965.x

Vanneste S, De Ridder D. Differences between a single session and repeated sessions of 1 Hz TMS by double-cone coil prefrontal stimulation for the improvement of tinnitus. *Brain Stimul* (2013) 6:155–9. doi:10.1016/j.brs.2012.03.019

De Ridder D, Vanneste S, Kovacs S, Sunaert S, Menovsky T, Van De Heyning P, et al. Transcranial magnetic stimulation and extradural electrodes implanted on secondary auditory cortex for tinnitus suppression. *J Neurosurg* (2011) 114:903–11. doi:10.3171/2010.11.JNS10197

De Ridder D, Vanneste S, Plazier M, Menovsky T, Van De Heyning P, Kovacs S, et al. Dorsolateral prefrontal cortex transcranial magnetic stimulation and electrode implant for intractable tinnitus. *World Neurosurg* (2012) 77:778–84. doi:10.1016/j.wneu.2011.09.009

Langguth B, Eichhammer P, Wiegand R, Marienhegen J, Maenner P, Jacob P, et al. Neuronavigated rTMS in a patient with chronic tin- nitus. Effects of 4 weeks treatment. *Neuroreport* (2003) 14:977–80. doi:10.1097/00001756-200305230-00014

Plewnia C, Bartels M, Gerloff C. Transient suppression of tinnitus by transcranial magnetic stimulation. *Ann Neurol* (2003) 53:263–6. doi:10.1002/ana.10468

Lehner A, Schecklmann M, Poeppl TB, Kreuzer PM, Vielsmeier V, Rupprecht R, et al. Multisite rTMS for the treatment of chronic tinnitus: stimulation of the cortical tinnitus network – a pilot study. *Brain Topogr* (2013) 26:501–10. doi:10.1007/s10548-012-0268-4

Lehner A, Schecklmann M, Greenlee MW, Rupprecht R, Langguth B. Triple-site rTMS for the treatment of chronic tinnitus: a randomized controlled trial. *Sci Rep* (2016) 6:22302. doi:10.1038/srep22302

Hoffman RE, Boutros NN, Berman RM, Roessler E, Belger A, Krystal JH, et al. Transcranial magnetic stimulation of left temporoparietal cortex in three patients reporting hallucinated "voices". *Biol Psychiatry* (1999) 46:130–2. doi:10.1016/S0006-3223(98)00358-8

Jasper HH. The ten-twenty electrode system of the international federation. *Electroencephalogr Clin Neurophysiol* (1958) 10:371–5.

Landgrebe M, Zeman F, Koller M, Eberl Y, Mohr M, Reiter J, et al. The Tinnitus Research Initiative (TRI) database: a new approach for delineation of tinnitus subtypes and generation of predictors for treatment outcome. *BMC Med Inform Decis Mak* (2010) 10:42. doi:10.1186/1472-6947-10-42

Goebel G, Hiller W. The tinnitus questionnaire. A standard instrument for grading the degree of tinnitus. Results of a multicenter study with the tinnitus questionnaire. *HNO* (1994) 42:166–72.

Adamchic I, Tass PA, Langguth B, Hauptmann C, Koller M, Schecklmann M, et al. Linking the Tinnitus Questionnaire and the subjective clinical global impression: which differences are clinically important? *Health Qual Life Outcomes* (2012) 10:79. doi:10.1186/1477-7525-10-79

World's Health Organization. *WHOQOL-BREF: Introduction, Administration, Scoring*. Geneva, Switzerland: WHO (1996).

Langguth B, Goodey R, Azevedo A, Bjorne A, Cacace A, Crocetti A, et al. Consensus for tinnitus patient assessment and treatment outcome measurement: Tinnitus Research Initiative meeting, Regensburg, July 2006. *Prog Brain Res* (2007) 166:525–36. doi:10.1016/S0079-6123(07)66050-6

Landgrebe M, Azevedo A, Baguley D, Bauer C, Cacace A, Coelho C, et al. Methodological aspects of clinical trials in tinnitus: a proposal for an international standard. *J Psychosom Res* (2012) 73:112–21. doi:10.1016/j.jpsychores.2012.05.002

Leon AC. Implications of clinical trial design on sample size requirements. *Schizophr Bull* (2008) 34:664–9. doi:10.1093/schbul/sbn035

Leon AC, Davis LL, Kraemer HC. The role and interpretation of pilot studies in clinical research. *J Psychiatr Res* (2011) 45:626–9. doi:10.1016/j.jpsychires.2010.10.008

Faul F, Erdfelder E, Lang AG, Buchner A. G*Power 3: a flexible statistical power analysis program for the social, behavioral, and biomedical sciences. *Behav Res Methods* (2007) 39:175–91. doi:10.3758/BF03193146

Lehner A, Schecklmann M, Landgrebe M, Kreuzer PM, Poeppl TB, Frank E, et al. Predictors for rTMS response in chronic tinnitus. *Front Syst Neurosci* (2012) 6:11. doi:10.3389/fnsys.2012.00011

Kleinjung T, Eichhammer P, Landgrebe M, Sand P, Hajak G, Steffens T, et al. Combined temporal and prefrontal transcranial magnetic stimulation for tinnitus treatment: a pilot study. *Otolaryngol Head Neck Surg* (2008) 138:497–501. doi:10.1016/j.otohns.2007.12.022

Lehner A, Schecklmann M, Kreuzer PM, Poeppl TB, Rupprecht R, Langguth Comparing single-site with multisite rTMS for the treatment of chronic tinnitus – clinical effects and neuroscientific insights: study protocol for a ran- domized controlled trial. *Trials* (2013) 14:269. doi:10.1186/1745-6215-14-269

Duecker F, Sack AT. Rethinking the role of sham TMS. *Front Psychol* (2015) 6:210. doi:10.3389/fpsyg.2015.00210

Kreuzer PM, Landgrebe M, Schecklmann M, Poeppl TB, Vielsmeier V, Hajak G, et al. Can temporal repetitive transcranial magnetic stimulation be enhanced by targeting affective components of tinnitus with frontal rTMS? A randomized controlled pilot trial. *Front Syst Neurosci* (2011) 5:88. doi:10.3389/ fnsys.2011.00088

Schecklmann M, Lehner A, Gollmitzer J, Schmidt E, Schlee W, Langguth Repetitive transcranial magnetic stimulation induces oscillatory power changes in chronic tinnitus. *Front Cell Neurosci* (2015) 9:421. doi:10.3389/fncel.2015.00421

10 Hz Amplitude Modulated Sounds Induce Short-Term Tinnitus Suppression

Patrick Neff[1, 2], Jakob Michels[3], Martin Meyer[1, 2, 4], Martin Schecklmann[5], Berthold Langguth[5] and Winfried Schlee[5]*

[1] Neuroplasticity and Learning in the Healthy Aging Brain (HAB LAB), Department of Psychology, University of Zurich, Zurich, Switzerland, [2] University Research Priority Program "Dynamics of Healthy Aging", University of Zurich, Zurich, Switzerland, [3] Department of Medicine, University of Regensburg, Regensburg, Germany, [4] Cognitive Psychology Unit, University of Klagenfurt, Klagenfurt, Austria, [5] Department of Psychiatry and Psychotherapy, University of Regensburg, Regensburg, Germany

***Correspondence:**
Winfried Schlee
winfried.schlee@gmail.com

Objectives: Acoustic stimulation or sound therapy is proposed as a main treatment option for chronic subjective tinnitus. To further probe the field of acoustic stimulations for tinnitus therapy, this exploratory study compared 10 Hz amplitude modulated (AM) sounds (two pure tones, noise, music, and frequency modulated (FM) sounds) and unmodulated sounds (pure tone, noise) regarding their temporary suppression of tinnitus loudness. First, it was hypothesized that modulated sounds elicit larger temporary loudness suppression (residual inhibition) than unmodulated sounds. Second, with manipulation of stimulus loudness and duration of the modulated sounds weaker or stronger effects of loudness suppression were expected, respectively.

Methods: We recruited 29 participants with chronic tonal tinnitus from the multidisciplinary Tinnitus Clinic of the University of Regensburg. Participants underwent audiometric, psychometric and tinnitus pitch matching assessments followed by an acoustic stimulation experiment with a tinnitus loudness growth paradigm. In a first block participants were stimulated with all of the sounds for 3 min each and rated their subjective tinnitus loudness to the pre-stimulus loudness every 30 s after stimulus offset. The same procedure was deployed in the second block with the pure tone AM stimuli matched to the tinnitus frequency, manipulated in length (6 min), and loudness (reduced by 30 dB and linear fade out). Repeated measures mixed model analyses of variance (ANOVA) were calculated to assess differences in loudness growth between the stimuli for each block separately.

Results: First, we found that all sounds elicit a short-term suppression of tinnitus loudness (seconds to minutes) with strongest suppression right after stimulus offset [$F_{(6,\ 1331)} = 3.74$, $p < 0.01$]. Second, similar to previous findings we found that AM sounds near the tinnitus frequency produce significantly stronger tinnitus loudness suppression than noise [vs. Pink noise: $t_{(27)} = -4.22$, $p < 0.0001$]. Finally, variants of the AM sound matched to the tinnitus frequency reduced in sound level resulted in less suppression while there was no significant difference observed for a longer stimulation duration. Moreover, feasibility of the overall procedure could be confirmed as scores of both tinnitus loudness and questionnaires were lower after the experiment [tinnitus loudness: $t_{(27)} = 2.77$, $p < 0.01$; Tinnitus Questionnaire: $t_{(27)} = 2.06$, $p < 0.05$; Tinnitus Handicap Inventory: $t_{(27)} = 1.92$, $p = 0.065$].

Conclusion: Taken together, these results imply that AM sounds, especially in or around the tinnitus frequency, may induce larger suppression than unmodulated sounds. Future studies should thus evaluate this approach in longitudinal studies and real life settings. Furthermore, the putative neural relation of these sound stimuli with a modulation rate in the EEG α band to the observed tinnitus suppression should be probed with respective neurophysiological methods.

Keywords: tinnitus, acoustic stimulation, sound therapy, amplitude modulation, frequency modulation, residual inhibition, entrainment, alpha

1. INTRODUCTION

Subjective tinnitus is defined as "the perception of sound(s) in the absence of an external sound source" (Eggermont and Roberts, 2004; Erlandsson and Dauman, 2013) and is deemed chronic after 12 months since first occurrence (Mazurek et al., 2010). No less than 35% of the general (US) population are haunted by this phantom auditory perception at some point during their lifetime (Jastreboff, 1990). 10–15% report their tinnitus percept as being frequent or continuous and ~1–2% suffer heavily under the condition (Langguth et al., 2013). With a steadily aging demographic, tinnitus is becoming increasingly prevalent and relevant (Hoffman and Reed, 2004; Nondahl et al., 2012). Besides the tantalizing phantom sound or comorbidities like depression, stress and anxiety (Langguth et al., 2013), tinnitus also impacts daily life functions in healthy aging as impaired hearing, sound localization and speech perception can lower the quality of life in tinnitus sufferers (Moon et al., 2015; Gilles et al., 2016; Hyvärinen et al., 2016).

In the majority of cases tinnitus manifests as a single tone, ringing or noise with a definable pitch and loudness, which is perceived bilaterally or with a slight preference to one side, or alternatively lateralized to one ear (Lockwood et al., 2002). Tinnitus pitch, laterality and loudness can be therefore considered as the main (subjective) perceptual parameters of interest in addition to maskability and residual inhibition by external sounds (Henry and Meikle, 2000). Usually, tinnitus is considered to be caused by either objective (Eggermont and Roberts, 2004; Schaette and Kempter, 2006; Mazurek et al., 2010) or hidden hearing loss (Weisz et al., 2006; Schaette and McAlpine, 2011; Adjamian et al., 2012; Xiong et al., 2013), where loss of cochlear hair cells in objective hearing loss has been shown to lead to maladaptive plasticity throughout the auditory pathway and brain. Tinnitus pitch seems to average near the frequency of maximal hearing loss, especially in sufferers with pure-tone tinnitus (Schecklmann et al., 2012). Related to this maladaptive plasticity, a similarity of tinnitus to phantom limb or general phantom (pain) perception following sensory deafferentation has also been proposed (De Ridder et al., 2011). Although models of pathogenesis and physiology are still being debated and are limited by an underlying inherent heterogeneity of the disorder, it can be stated with confidence that both the inner ear and the brain are involved (Jastreboff, 1990; Eggermont and Roberts, 2004; Adjamian et al., 2009; De Ridder et al., 2011, 2014; Vanneste and De Ridder, 2012; Elgoyhen et al., 2015).

Acoustic stimulations have been used in various forms to counteract or alleviate the malicious phantom percept (Jastreboff, 2007). From a clinical routine perspective, acoustic stimulation or sound therapies are proposed as symptom-oriented treatment options besides cognitive behavioral therapy and neuromodulation or -stimulation if chronic subjective tinnitus persists after standard clinical assessment and intervention (Langguth et al., 2013). Traditionally, masking approaches using broadband or narrow-band noise, or pure tones, were established first (Feldmann, 1971; Vernon, 1977; Watanabe et al., 1997; Henry et al., 2004; Hazell and Wood, 2009). These maskers have also been administered in hearing aids (Vernon and Meikle, 2003) with slightly better effects than hearing aids without maskers as shown in a study by Henry et al. (2015). In recent times, two major acoustic stimulation techniques for long-term, daily intervention have been developed building on the model of lateral inhibition (Pantev et al., 2012; Adamchic et al., 2014). Following peripheral hearing loss, central tonotopic map reorganization and hyperactivity in regions of the reorganization responsible for the tinnitus sensation (Eggermont and Komiya, 2000; Eggermont and Roberts, 2004), lateral inhibition is theorized to counteract or reverse this maladaptive hyperactivity. Pantev and colleagues therefore proposed to apply a notch filter in a single octave band around the tinnitus frequency to music. The energy of the sound signal at the edges of the notch filter is theorized to inhibit the frequencies around the tinnitus pitch therefore reversing the maladaptive plasticity, which has been shown to be effective in long-term intervention (Okamoto et al., 2010). The width of the notch filter did not significantly influence treatment effects in a further study (Wunderlich et al., 2015b) while the spectral contrast (i.e., increased sound pressure at frequencies neighboring the filter edges) seems to improve the treatment effects as shown in a further follow up study (Stein et al., 2015). Building on similar reasoning about frequencies neighboring the tinnitus pitch and lateral inhibition, Tass and colleagues (Tass et al., 2012) established a method where sine tones are presented in a randomized fashion around the tinnitus frequency for several hours a day with similar longitudinal therapeutic effects.

While the established approaches focus on the retraining of auditory and related cortical structures in longitudinal therapeutic interventions (Pantev et al., 2012; Adamchic et al., 2014), only few studies looked at the effect of sounds on the temporary suppression of tinnitus (Roberts et al., 2006, 2008; Reavis et al., 2012) to identify possible candidates for future tinnitus sound therapies. Acoustic stimulation with amplitude modulation (AM) and frequency modulation (FM) (Reavis et al., 2012; Tyler et al., 2014) has just recently entered this line of research building on results of electrical stimulation of the cochlea (Zeng et al., 2011). The results of these studies indicate that especially AM sounds in the higher, tinnitus-relevant frequencies of 3,000–9,000 Hz produce a more pronounced tinnitus suppression during and after the stimulation compared to their unmodulated pendants or white noise. In any case, longitudinal data on efficacy and long-term as well as momentary neuroplastic alterations of continuous modulated or patterned, sounds is missing. Therefore, approaches showing efficacy and feasibility in single session experiments with short stimulation duration measuring tinnitus suppression (i.e., residual inhibition) should be tested in longitudinal, prospective placebo-controlled studies to assess long-term efficacy. While recent studies with AM and/or FM sounds, used 40 Hz for the modulation rate (Reavis et al., 2012; Tyler et al., 2014), which is known to produce the largest neural responses in auditory cortex through entrainment as shown in auditory steady-state response (ASSR) paradigms (Picton et al., 2003), no former study tested the influence of lower modulation rates in different carrier sounds, including the tinnitus pitch, for tinnitus suppression. Of special interest here, several reviewed studies in Picton et al. (2003) could also show entrainment effects for different bands including the alpha frequency band. Cortical auditory α activity has been shown to be decreased in tinnitus patients in MEG (Weisz et al., 2005; Schlee et al., 2014), EEG (Moazami-Goudarzi et al., 2010) and possibly also reduced in variability (Schlee et al., 2014). Looking at modulation depth of the stimuli and strength of (entrainment) effect as measured by EEG or MEG, several studies have reliably shown entrainment effects of monaural AM stimuli (100% modulation depth) superior to binaural AM stimuli (Picton et al., 2003; Schwarz and Taylor, 2005; Draganova et al., 2008; Becher et al., 2015). A modulation rate in the α frequency band as well as monaural stimuli with a maximized entrainment effect may therefore enable a normalization of reduced auditory α and thereby concomitantly reduce the tinnitus percept. Based on this preliminary reasoning we here investigated the effects of AM sounds in the α band for tinnitus sound therapy. Yet, the focus of this study was set on the behavioral level to proof the concept and feasibility in the absence of neurophysiological methods.

In the exploratory study at hand, we therefore tested the influence of 10 Hz AM sounds (two pure tones, noise, music and FM sounds) and unmodulated sounds (pure tone, noise) on the temporary suppression of subjective tinnitus loudness in participants with tonal tinnitus in block 1 of the experiment. We hypothesize that all sounds may elicit a short-term suppression of tinnitus loudness (seconds to minutes) with strongest suppression right after stimulus offset (Roberts et al., 2006, 2008; Reavis et al., 2012; Tyler et al., 2014). Given the different types of modulated and unmodulated sounds with frequencies in or around the actual tinnitus pitch, we expect to find differential suppression patterns between the stimuli with AM sounds possibly eliciting enhanced suppression (Reavis et al., 2012). Additionally, with the manipulation of stimulation length and loudness in block 2 of the experiment, we anticipate more pronounced or weaker effects of tinnitus loudness suppression, respectively.

2. METHODS

2.1. Participants

Patients with chronic tonal tinnitus (>12 months tinnitus duration), who had consulted the multidisciplinary Tinnitus Clinic of the University of Regensburg, were included in the study if their age was between 18 and 75 years. Patients with history or presence of severe and relevant somatic, neurological, or mental disorders were excluded. Intake of psychotropic medication or ongoing participation in tinnitus therapies were further exclusion criteria. The study was approved by the Ethics Committee of the University of Regensburg (16-101-0061). All participants gave written informed consent after a comprehensive explanation of the procedures.

After signing the consent, form all participants completed the tinnitus questionnaire (TQ) (Hallam et al., 1988; Goebel and Hiller, 1994), the Tinnitus Handicap Inventory (THI) (Newman et al., 1996), and a visual analog scale (VAS) (Adamchic et al., 2012) with respect to tinnitus loudness (spanning from inaudibility to maximal imaginable loudness). The Tinnitus Sample Case History Questionnaire (TSCHQ) was used to gather clinical and demographic data of all patients (Langguth et al., 2007). Furthermore, hearing level was measured with a standard audiogram using frequencies ranging from 125 Hz to 8 kHz in octave steps with semi-octave steps between 2 and 4 (i.e., 3 kHz), and 4 and 8 kHz (i.e., 6 kHz), respectively (Madsen Midimate 622D; GN Otometrics, Denmark). Headphones used for audiometry, tinnitus matching, as well as for the stimulation procedure were quasi-linear in their frequency response over the whole audible spectrum (Sennheiser HDA 2000; Sennheiser, Germany).

Questionnaire scores and participants characteristics are listed in **Table 1**. The distribution of sexes in the sample was slightly skewed with 11 female and 18 male participants. 3 participants reported a purely left-sided, 2 participants a purely right-sided tinnitus. The majority of participants indicated some form of bilateral or diffuse tinnitus location, with 8 participants indicating tinnitus in both ears, 4 inside the head, 7 both ears with a tendency to the left side, and 4 with a tendency to the right side. A specific tinnitus laterality was not considered as an inclusion criterion due to the diotic presentation of the stimuli. Hearing thresholds slightly differed between ears [right side: mean $= 40.63$, $SD = 13.24$; left side: mean $= 39.46$, $SD = 12.17$; $t_{(28)} = 2.10$, $p = 0.044$].

2.2. Tinnitus Matching

After filling in the questionnaires and audiometry, participants were seated in front of a screen with a computer mouse and

TABLE 1 | Participants characteristics ($n = 29$).

	Mean	SD[a]	Median	Minimum	Maximum
Age (years)	52.34	12.78	54	24	75
Tinnitus duration (months)	123.66	117.74	71	12	431
Hearing Loss (both ears, dB)	38.29	11.78	37.27	15.91	62.73
TQ[b] total score (0–84)	39.41	14.06	40	10	69
THI[c] total score (0–100)	43.97	18.48	44	10	92
Tinnitus loudness (%)	67.59	14.74	70	30	100
VAS[d] loudness (0–100)	54.93	17.26	55	22	86
Tinnitus awareness (%)	66.55	26.73	60	0	100
Tinnitus frequency (matching, Hz)	5,334.77	2,904.96	6,000	911	10,500
Tinnitus loudness (matching, dBA)	45.46	14.92	43.90	23.50	81.60

[a]*SD, Standard Deviation;* [b]*TQ, Tinnitus Questionnaire (Goebel and Hiller, 1994);* [c]*THI, Tinnitus Handicap Inventory (Newman et al., 1996);* [d]*VAS, visual analog scale.*

instructed for the tinnitus matching via software. The matching procedure was designed around a sine tone generator (Meyer et al., 2014) where pitch (in single Hz resolution), amplitude and laterality (panning) could be defined and controlled using MAX software (MAX 7; Cycling'74, USA). First, the loudness and lateralization of the tinnitus was roughly defined followed by the actual pitch by the study personnel (Penner and Bilger, 1992; Henry and Meikle, 2000). Participants were then made familiar with the handling of the pitch dial on the graphical user interface and informed about the possibility to adjust the tinnitus pitch in 1 Hz steps while holding down the shift key on the keyboard. Following that, participants proceeded with the actual pitch matching self-reliantly. To ensure reliability and validity of the procedure, the final pitch indicated by the participant was shifted an octave down and up and checked with the participant, respectively, to control for possible octave confusion. Finally, the matched tone was evaluated in a short discussion with the study personnel and rated on a 5 point likert scale (1 = not at all matching the tinnitus percept, 5 = perfect fit). Frequency and loudness results of the matching procedure are listed in **Table 1**.

2.3. Sound Stimuli

A set of 3 amplitude modulated, 2 notch filter amplitude modulated as well as 2 unmodulated sounds were prepared in MATLAB (Matlab R2015a; Mathworks, USA). Besides sine tones in 4 and noise in 2 conditions, a variety of popular music songs was provided to the participants out of which they could choose their favorite song for notch filter modulated presentation in one condition. A sum total of 7 acoustic stimuli or conditions with 3 min of duration was therefore produced for each participant for block 1. In the remainder of this manuscript, including tables and figures, we termed the different stimuli as follows: "AMTinnitus" for AM sounds centered at the tinnitus frequency (**Figure 1A**), "Tinnitus pure tone" for unmodulated sounds centered at the tinnitus frequency (**Figure 1B**), "AMFM" for the AM FM sound (**Figure 1C**), "AMLow" for AM of the 108 Hz sound (**Figure 1D**), "AMMusic" for the AM of musical songs (**Figure 1E**), "AMPinknotch" for the filter AM of pink noise (**Figure 1F**), and "Pink noise" for the pink noise sound (**Figure 1G**). For block 2, participants could choose their favorite stimulus, besides AM in the tinnitus frequency (AMTinnitus), after completing block 1. The AMTinnitus and the chosen stimulus were then manipulated in length, or loudness, or faded (linear fade out in the last minute of the stimulus) resulting in 3 conditions for two stimuli in block 2.

For AMTinnitus, a carrier sine tone was generated and amplitude modulated (100% modulation depth) with a sinusoidal function according to the following principle, where the first part of the equation represents the carrier sound and the second part the modulator. Note that the information in brackets in the legend of the equation is indicative of study-specific settings:

$$s = ca * \sin(2 * \pi * cf * t) * mia * \cos(2 * \pi * mf * t + \phi) \quad (1)$$

where:

s	sinusoidally amplitude modulated sound
ca	carrier amplitude
cf	carrier frequency (=tinnitus frequency)
t	time
mia	modulator index/amplitude (=1)
mf	modulator frequency (=10 Hz)
ϕ	phase

For the AMPinknotch and AMMusic sounds the target of the 10 Hz modulator was the notch filter amplitude. The notch filter used (Butterworth, filter order = 4) was centered around the matched tinnitus frequency with a filter bandwidth of 1 octave (Okamoto et al., 2010; Wunderlich et al., 2015a). With the filter amplitude modulation applied, the resulting sounds where rhythmically suppressed in the octave around the tinnitus frequency, giving the acoustic impression of a slight flutter in the stimulus.

For the AMFM sound, a FM sweep from 0 Hz up to the tinnitus frequency with a modulation rate of 10 Hz served as the carrier sound, which was then amplitude modulated like AMTinnitus (i.e., 100% modulation depth). AMLow with a low frequency carrier sound (108 Hz instead of tinnitus frequency) was generated analogously to AMTinnitus. Finally, the unmodulated stimuli, namely Tinnitus pure tone and Pink noise, were generated. Possible transient artifacts were avoided in the beginning and the end of the stimuli through ramping (linear

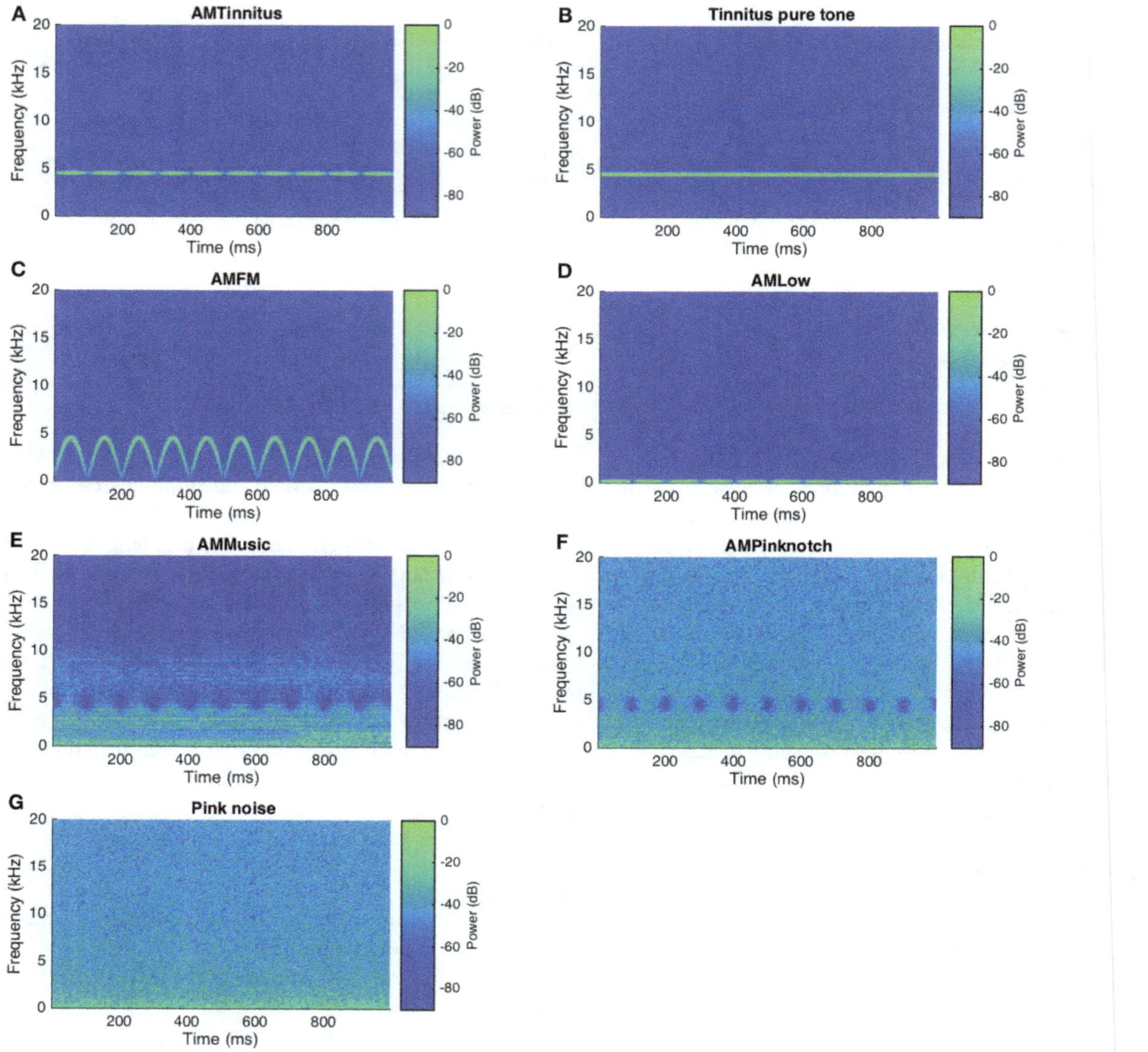

FIGURE 1 | Spectrograms of all sound stimuli (1 s snippets). For all of the plotted representative stimuli an arbitrary tinnitus frequency of 4,500 Hz was chosen and stimuli normalized to full digital displacement. The modulation rate was constant at 10 Hz in modulated sounds **(A,C–F)** whereas **(B,G)** represent the unmodulated stimuli. Stimulus presentation was set to 3 min for all stimuli and block 1. In block 2 AMTinnitus **(A)** underwent loudness (loudness reduction by 30 dB and linear fade out) and temporal (duration of 6 min) manipulations resulting in 4 stimuli including the standard AMTinnitus stimulus from block 1.

fade with 100 ms window). Stimuli were then normalized in sound level and finally exported for the experimental procedure.

2.4. Acoustic Stimulation Procedure

All stimuli were presented at sound levels of 60 dB SL in block 1 (i.e., in broadband stimuli noise and music to the average hearing threshold, whereas in frequency specific stimuli the nearest frequency of the audiogram was chosen as reference for the level adjustment). For block 2, the AMTinnitus and the stimulus of choice were (1) presented for 6 min, (2) reduced in sound level (30 instead of 60 dB SL) and (3) processed with a linear sound level fade out in the last minute of the stimulus. By varying these core parameters of stimulation length and sound level in block 2, we tested differential tinnitus suppression patterns within single stimuli classes with a focus on AMTinnitus. To ensure comfort and safety of the participants, 80 dBA was the upper limit for the sound level of all stimuli. Sound level was carefully checked with an SPL meter (NTi Audio XL2; NTi Audio, Lichtenstein) before actual stimulation. Participants were reminded of the option to interrupt the procedure whenever a sound was deemed uncomfortable at any point of the experiment.

For the acoustic stimulation procedure participants were seated comfortably facing a window with a view on trees to avoid distraction and ensure calmness. No particular instruction was given to focus their attention on either the sound or tinnitus. The presentation sequence of the stimuli was randomized in the two blocks for each participant. Participants were instructed to relax during the acoustic stimulation and to rate the loudness of their tinnitus in percent, compared to the pre-stimulation loudness, after each stimulation at time points 0, 30, 60, 90, 120, 150, and 180 s. A similar approach of tinnitus loudness growth was used in the study by Reavis and colleagues (Reavis et al., 2012). However, we diverged from the former study by not measuring suppression during acoustic stimulation, having no reference tones in and after the stimulation and deploying a loudness regime tied to hearing loss with 60 dB SL (Reavis et al. (2012) presented stimuli slightly below matched tinnitus loudness). There was a short break between the blocks to maintain vigilance and comfort of the participants. At the end of the study after block 2, the VAS for tinnitus loudness and tinnitus questionnaires were again filled in by the participants. Participants were then thanked for their participation and finally dismissed.

2.5. Data Analysis

A repeated measures mixed model analysis of variance (ANOVA) was calculated with the factors time and condition as well as a random intercept per participant to assess the effect of temporary tinnitus suppression in the loudness growth paradigm. *Post hoc* tests of the ANOVA controlled for multiple comparisons contrasting the suppression profiles between the stimuli were performed using the Tukey method. Finally, paired two-tailed *t*-tests were used to compare tinnitus questionnaire scores and tinnitus loudness VAS before and after acoustic stimulation procedure. As the 3 variables subjected to the paired comparisons were considered within an independent analysis and not part of any primary outcome statistical model or search space, we refrained from a correction for multiple comparisons (e.g., bonferroni) for this secondary analysis. R statistic toolbox with the supplementary libraries "nlme" and "lsmeans" was used for all statistical calculations (R version 3.3.2; R Foundation for Statistical Computing, Austria).

TABLE 2 | Results of ANOVA block 1 ($n = 28$).

	numDF[a]	denDF[b]	*F*-value	*p*-value
(Intercept)	1	1,331	2,845.28	<0.0001
Condition	6	1,331	5.40	<0.0001
Time	1	1,331	185.81	<0.0001
Condition:Time	6	1,331	3.74	0.0011

[a] *numDF, degrees of freedom of numerator;* [b] *denDF, degrees of freedom of denominator.*

TABLE 3 | *Post-hoc* contrasts block 1 ($n = 28$, Tukey-adjusted).

Contrast	Estimate	*t*-value	*p*-value
AMFM - AMMusic	**−5.204**	**−3.31**	**0.016**
AMFM - AMPinknotch	−2.245	−1.43	0.786
AMFM - AMLow	−4.082	−2.60	0.127
AMFM - Pink noise	**−4.898**	**−3.12**	**0.031**
AMFM - AMTinnitus	1.735	1.11	0.927
AMFM - Tinnitus pure tone	−2.041	−1.30	0.852
AMMusic - AMPinknotch	2.959	1.88	0.491
AMMusic - AMLow	1.122	0.72	0.992
AMMusic - Pink noise	0.306	0.20	>0.999
AMMusic - AMTinnitus	**6.939**	**4.42**	**<0.0001**
AMMusic - Tinnitus pure tone	3.163	2.01	0.406
AMPinknotch - AMLow	−1.837	−1.17	0.906
AMPinknotch - Pink noise	−2.653	−1.69	0.623
AMPinknotch - AMTinnitus	3.98	2.53	0.148
AMPinknotch - Tinnitus pure tone	0.204	0.13	>0.999
AMLow - PinkNoise	−0.816	−0.52	0.999
AMLow - AMTinnitus	**5.816**	**3.70**	**0.004**
AMLow - Tinnitus pure tone	2.041	1.30	0.852
Pink noise - AMTinnitus	**6.633**	**4.22**	**0.001**
Pink noise - Tinnitus pure tone	2.857	1.82	0.535
AMTinnitus - Tinnitus pure tone	−3.776	−2.40	0.193

Degrees of freedom = 1,331; Standard error = 1.517; Significant differences are highlighted in bold.

3. RESULTS

3.1. Tinnitus Loudness Growth after Acoustic Stimulation

The results of the ANOVA for the tinnitus loudness growth curves of all stimuli in block 1 are shown in **Table 2** and respective corrected *post-hoc* contrasts in **Table 3**. Notably, there was a significant effect of condition, time, and interaction condition*time on the tinnitus loudness. Mean tinnitus loudness suppression curves are plotted in **Figure 2**.

Post hoc contrasts between each of the 7 stimuli elicited significant differences ($p < 0.05$) for AMMusic vs. AMTinnitus [$t_{(27)} = 4.42$, $p < 0.0001$], Pink noise vs. AMTinnitus [$t_{(27)} = 4.22$, $p = 0.001$], AMLow vs. AMTinnitus [$t_{(27)} = 3.70$, $p = 0.004$], AMFM vs. AMMusic [$t_{(27)} = -3.31$, $p = 0.016$], and AMFM vs. Pink Noise [$t_{(27)} = -3.12$, $p = 0.031$], respectively. These results are indicative of a pattern of enhanced tinnitus suppression of AMTinnitus and AMFM compared to Pink Noise, AMMusic, and AMLow [except AMFM vs. AMLow with $t_{(27)} = -2.60$, $p = 0.127$].

To counteract possible effects of the stimulation sequence in block 1, we furthermore tested the data for order effects with no significant results for position [$F_{(1, 1317)} = 0.05$, $p = 0.832$], condition*position [$F_{(6, 1317)} = 0.94$, $p = 0.468$], time*position [$F_{(1, 1317)} = 3.05$, $p = 0.081$], and interaction condition*time*position [$F_{(6, 1317)} = 0.70$, $p = 0.646$].

For block 2, we report the results for tinnitus loudness growth of the manipulated variations of AMTinnitus (long (6 min of duration), fade, and reduced sound level) with the addition of the data of AMTinnitus of block 1 (standard) in **Table 4**. *Post-hoc* contrasts are indicated in **Table 5** and mean tinnitus loudness suppression curves are plotted in **Figure 3**. Of special interest and according to our expectations, longer stimulation (long, 6 min) resulted in a larger suppression compared to stimulations reduced in sound level [fade vs. long: $t_{(27)} = 3.88$, $p = 0.00065$; reduced sound level vs. long: $t_{(27)} = 4.00$, $p = 0.00041$] but no significant differences with the AMTinnitus stimulation for

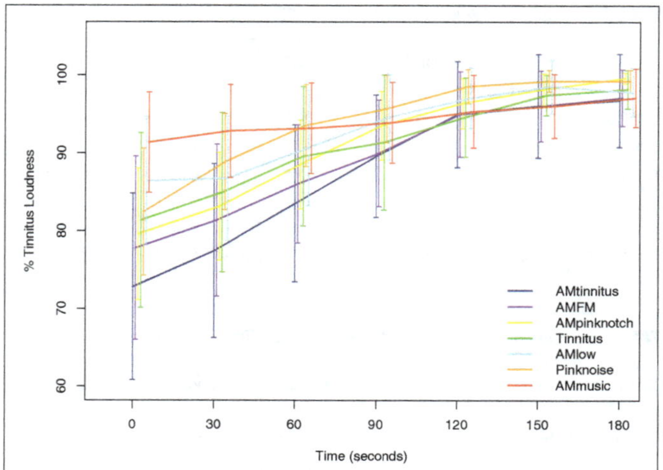

FIGURE 2 | Mean tinnitus loudness suppression after stimulus offset of all sound stimuli in block 1. Confidence intervals at 95% are plotted for each condition and time point. Notably, after 90–120 s tinnitus loudness suppression generally diminishes and curves of the different stimuli converge. Significant differences between stimuli (conditions) are listed in **Table 3**.

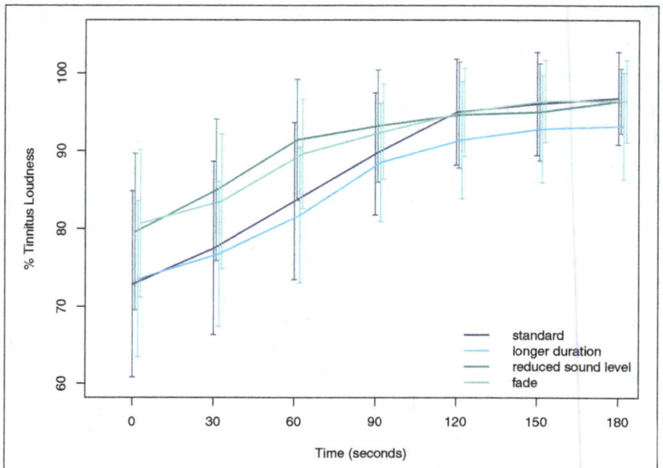

FIGURE 3 | Mean tinnitus loudness suppression after stimulus offset of AMTinnitus and its variations in block 2. Confidence intervals at 95% are plotted for each condition and time point. Standard and longer duration of the stimulus are colored in blue whereas stimuli with reduced sound level or fade out are colored in green. Significant differences between stimuli (conditions) are listed in **Table 5**.

TABLE 4 | Results of ANOVA for AMTinnitus in block 2 ($n = 28$).

	numDF[a]	denDF[b]	*F*-value	*p*-value
(Intercept)	1	749	746.20	<0.0001
Condition	3	749	7.62	0.0001
Time	1	749	201.14	<0.0001
Condition:Time	3	749	2.70	0.0443

[a]numDF, degrees of freedom of numerator; [b]denDF, degrees of freedom of denominator.

TABLE 5 | *Post-hoc* contrasts block 2 ($n = 28$, Tukey-adjusted).

Contrast	Estimate	*t*-value	*p*-value
Fade - Reduced sound level	−0.153	−0.12	0.999
Fade - Long	**5.153**	**3.88**	**0.00065**
Fade - Standard	3.265	2.46	0.067
Reduced sound level - Long	**5.306**	**4.00**	**0.00041**
Reduced sound level - Standard	**3.418**	**2.57**	**0.050**
Long - Standard	−1.887	−1.42	0.486

Degrees of freedom = 749; Standard error = 1.328; Significant differences are highlighted in bold.

3 min from block 1 [long vs. standard: $t_{(27)} = -1.42$, $p = 0.486$]. Furthermore, AMTinnitus elicited marginally increased suppression compared to the faded stimulus [fade vs. standard: $t_{(27)} = 2.46$, $p = 0.067$, trend] and the stimulus with reduced sound level [reduced sound level vs. standard: $t_{(27)} = 2.57$, $p = 0.050$]. The comparison of the two stimuli with manipulated sound level resulted in no significant difference [fade vs. reduced sound level: $t_{(27)} = -0.12, p = 0.999$].

3.2. Responder Patterns and Overall Feasibility

The evaluation of the matched tinnitus pitch resulted in a mean of 4.0 ($SD = 0.55$, with 5 indicating perfect fit) highlighting the reasonable quality of the matching procedure. The response criterion for temporary tinnitus suppression was set to any suppression per stimuli (here at t0, right after the offset of the auditory stimulation) as similarly done before (Reavis et al., 2012). Applying this criterion, the following descriptive responder pattern emerges: In the AMTinnitus condition 19 out of 28 participants indicated a suppression at t0, in AMPinknotch 19/28, in AMFM 16/28, in Pink noise 16/28, in AMLow 13/28, in Tinnitus pure tone 13/28, and in AMMusic 8/20.

Differences in tinnitus loudness (VAS) and total scores of standardized questionnaires (TQ and THI) comparing assessments before and after experimental procedures are listed in **Table 6** and summarized in the following: Tinnitus loudness (VAS) was significantly reduced after experimental procedures compared to the baseline assessment [$t_{(27)} = 2.774$, $p = 0.01$]. Furthermore, TQ and THI scores measuring tinnitus-related distress were also both lower after the experiment. While TQ scores are below the p-value threshold of $p = 0.05$, we can only report a trend for the THI [TQ: $t_{(27)} = 2.062$, $p = 0.049$; THI: $t_{(27)} = 1.922, p = 0.065$]. It has to be noted though, that the effects reported here are based on the possible influence of all amplitude modulated sounds as well as unmodulated "control" sounds and this secondary analysis serves safety and feasibility purposes.

4. DISCUSSION

Acoustic stimulation or sound therapy is proposed as a main treatment option for chronic subjective tinnitus (Langguth et al.,

TABLE 6 | Differences in tinnitus loudness and questionnaire scores before (pre) and after (post) experimental procedures.

Measure	Mean score pre	SD[a] pre	Mean score post	SD post	df	*t*-value	*p*-value
VAS loudness (mm)	54.46	17.39	48.25	17.48	27	2.774	0.01
TQ total score (0–84)	38.36	13.09	35.07	14.78	27	2.062	0.049
THI total score (0–100)	42.25	16.3	38.29	16.95	27	1.922	0.065

[a]*SD, Standard Deviation.*

2013). Numerous approaches for acoustic stimulation exist, be it in experimental studies (e.g., Roberts et al., 2006; Reavis et al., 2012; Hoare et al., 2014), longitudinal clinical trials (e.g., Okamoto et al., 2010; Adamchic et al., 2014), fitted hearing aids or sound players (e.g., Vernon and Meikle, 2003), mobile apps or webpages, and various user-driven self-administered forms. As of yet, there is neither an established general-purpose acoustic stimulation to abolish or reduce tinnitus nor a working strategy for subtypization of responder profiles. To further probe the field of acoustic stimulations for tinnitus therapy, the purpose of this exploratory study was to compare 10 Hz AM sounds (pure tones, noise, music and FM sounds) and unmodulated sounds (pure tone, noise) regarding their temporary suppression of tinnitus loudness in participants with tonal tinnitus.

First we found that all sounds elicit a short-term suppression of tinnitus loudness (seconds to minutes) with strongest suppression right after stimulus offset . Adding to this, feasibility of the overall procedure could be confirmed as scores of both tinnitus questionnaires as well as the VAS for tinnitus loudness were lower after the experiment . Furthermore, no adverse events or persisting increase in tinnitus loudness or distress during and after the experimental procedure were noted. Second, akin to the findings of Reavis et al. (2012), while not directly comparable (due to higher presentation loudness in our study, frequency ranges instead of matched tinnitus pitch and white noise instead of pink noise in the former study), we found that AMTinnitus and AMFM produced a significantly stronger tinnitus loudness suppression than noise.

Furthermore, both AMTinnitus and AMFM produced superior suppression than AMMusic condition with the amplitude modulated notch filter.

Finally, AMTinnitus resulted in a clearly more pronounced suppression than AMLow.

Taken together, these results imply that AM sounds, especially in or around the tinnitus frequency (i.e., AMTinnitus and AMFM, Schaette et al., 2010), may produce larger suppression than unmodulated sounds. Yet, the direct contrast between AMTinnitus and Tinnitus pure tone did not result in a significant difference, but the direction and the size of the statistical values may point to a significant contrast in future studies (see **Figure 2** and **Table 3**). Possible cumulative effects of tinnitus suppression over the entire acoustic stimulation procedure in block 1 can be largely ruled out as there were no order effects . Third, with the manipulations of the AMTinnitus stimulus in block 2 either increasing the stimulus duration to 6 min, or reducing either overall sound level (30 dB), or fading of the stimulus in the last minute, we could partly show that these manipulations led to an altered tinnitus suppression: Standard AMTinnitus produced significantly more tinnitus suppression than both of the sound level-manipulated variations according to our expectations (i.e., reduced sound level, see **Figure 3** and **Table 5**), yet the longer version of the very same stimulus failed to show increased overall tinnitus suppression . However, comparing the loudness growth curves of the standard AMTinnitus with the version longer in duration, there may be a difference in suppression depth from 90 s onwards after stimulation offset. While the initial suppression at 0 s seems to be in similar range in both stimuli, the longer version may sustain the suppression for a longer time as reflected in the flatter curve. This effect could be topic of possible future studies where stimulation duration undergoes respective manipulation.

Looking at the AMFM stimulus we noticed both a good suppression potential second to AMTinnitus and a promising tolerance as participants clearly preferred AMFM over all other stimuli for block 2 (10/28 chose AMFM out of the 7 alternative options). On the other hand, it is challenging to interpret these results given the lack of a direct control sound (i.e., 10 Hz FM without AM). Finally, the sounds with amplitude modulated notch filter (AMPinknotch and AMMusic) were designed to test possible short-term suppression effects of the established long-term sound therapy with notch-filtered music (Pantev et al., 2012). AMMusic clearly exhibited the least overall suppression probably due to missing energy of the sounds in and around the filtered frequency range inherent to the presented songs, as music is both spectrally and temporally highly variable in amplitude (see **Figure 1E**). To a lesser degree, this is also true of (pink) noise so that both of the notch-filtered AM sounds are not straight-forwardly comparable in acoustic morphology and putative suppression effects to the pure tone sounds. Furthermore, given the tonal nature of the tinnitus in participants, this result certainly was expectable. All in all, the weaker suppression effect of these filter gain modulated sounds may be due to missing energy in the critical frequency bands of the notch filter, which is not surprising given the long-term application and its putatively induced reversal of maladaptive map plasticity through residual inhibition (Pantev et al., 2012; Tass et al., 2012).

Generally, between 90 and 120 s after stimulus offset, or even earlier in some stimuli (i.e., AMMusic, Pink noise, AMPinknotch, AMLow), tinnitus loudness reaches 90% of the baseline loudness and tends to reach 100% after 180 s, which equals the stimulation duration. A similar pattern was observed by Reavis et al. (2012) in representative, individual suppression profiles, while group statistics are not performed in a comparable manner to our study. First, we did not focus on responders for statistical analyses like the previous study as all subjects, conditions and time points were included in our study. Second, no transformation on the variables or other adjustments to the raw data were performed. Yet, given the various differences in the study design of Reavis et al. (2012), namely measuring suppression during acoustic stimulation, having reference tones in and after the stimulation and applying a loudness regime slightly below matched tinnitus, results are still deemed comparable and we may substantiate the former findings that AM (and partly FM) sounds elicit better tinnitus suppression than traditional maskers (i.e., unmodulated white noise and pure tones).

4.1. Limitations

In the following we would like to consider some issues, which may be regarded as shortcomings of our study, while not being detrimental given the exploratory scope of this study. First, looking at the sound stimuli, unlike Reavis et al. (2012) we did not use white noise as (control) masking sounds, which may limit the interpretation of especially the contrast to AMTinnitus, as in white noise there is more sound energy in the high frequency bands where tinnitus usually manifests. Besides, there also was no direct, unmodulated control sound to AMLow and noise was not amplitude modulated over the entire audible frequency range. Future studies should therefore define respective a priori contrasts with only a single or few parameters manipulated in the stimuli to ensure optimal comparability. Second, sound presentation may be updated with consideration of tinnitus laterality (contra- vs. ipsi- vs. bilateral presentation) (Feldmann, 1971) and with related adjustments for asymmetrical hearing loss (Roberts et al., 2008), loudness weighting reconsidered (i.e., application of more detailed loudness contour curves (ISO 226) to the stimuli instead of dbA weighting), and finally matching sounds alongside the active stimuli to evaluate loudness growth independent from tinnitus (Reavis et al., 2012). Third, to both identify and analyze tinnitus subgroups as well as responder profiles, it would be advantageous to include further questionnaires to probe comorbidities and (general) quality of life (Langguth et al., 2007) and, more importantly, questionnaires elucidating personal profiles, like the NEO-PI-R (Costa and McCrae, 2008), possibly related to tolerance and acceptance of sound therapy in tinnitus. Fourth, given the behavioral nature of the current study, both neurophysiological models for cortical and subcortical responses to these stimuli and possible beneficial effects for tinnitus have to be specifically tested in fitting paradigms in future studies. Finally, in block 2, we could not test for order effects because the conditions with the stimuli chosen by the participants were deliberately left out in the analysis of the data. Given the inexistence of such order effects in block 1 and identical randomization strategies used in both blocks, we do not expect an order effect in the trimmed analysis of block 2.

4.2. Conclusion and Outlook

Given the results of the present study in the context of previous findings, we conclude (and partly replicate) that amplitude modulated sounds with various carrier sounds in and around tinnitus frequency are feasible for short-term tinnitus suppression. With a modulation rate of 10 Hz in the EEG α band, we expect indirect neuromodulation and normalization of the endogeneous (also: individual) α rhythm which has been shown to be reduced in patients with tinnitus. Exact mechanisms of this auditory entrainment should therefore be investigated by means of respective neurophysiological methods (MEG/EEG) to test if and how auditory entrainment and possibly related tinnitus suppression is reflected by neural oscillations. Beyond that, longitudinal studies in real life should be performed to evaluate the envisioned long-term goal of this approach, namely to develop individually-customized mobile tinnitus sound therapies with aesthetically appealing sounds.

AUTHOR CONTRIBUTIONS

PN and WS: substantial contribution to the design of the study, data analysis, drafted and revised the manuscript. JM: substantial contribution to the design of the study and data acquisition. MM: substantial contribution to the discussion of the approach and paradigm. MS and BL: drafted and revised the manuscript.

FUNDING

This research was supported by by the University Research Priority Program "Dynamics of Healthy Aging" of the University of Zurich, the "Fonds zur Förderung des akademischen Nachwuchses" (FAN) des "Zürcher Universitätsvereins" (ZUNIV) and by TINNET-COST Action BM1306 "Better Understanding the Heterogeneity of Tinnitus to Improve and Develop New Treatments."

REFERENCES

Adamchic, I., Langguth, B., Hauptmann, C., and Tass, P. A. (2012). Psychometric evaluation of visual analog scale for the assessment of chronic tinnitus. *Am. J. Audiol.* 21, 215–225. doi: 10.1044/1059-0889(2012/12-0010)

Adamchic, I., Toth, T., Hauptmann, C., and Tass, P. A. (2014). Reversing pathologically increased EEG power by acoustic coordinated reset neuromodulation. *Hum. Brain Mapp.* 35, 2099–2118. doi: 10.1002/hbm.22314

Adjamian, P., Sereda, M., and Hall, D. A. (2009). The mechanisms of tinnitus: perspectives from human functional neuroimaging. *Hear. Res.* 253, 15–31. doi: 10.1016/j.heares.2009.04.001

Adjamian, P., Sereda, M., Zobay, O., Hall, D. A., and Palmer, A. R. (2012). Neuromagnetic indicators of tinnitus and tinnitus masking in patients with and without hearing loss. *J. Assoc. Res. Otolaryngol.* 13, 715–731. doi: 10.1007/s10162-012-0340-5

Becher, A. K., Höhne, M., Axmacher, N., Chaieb, L., Elger, C. E., and Fell, J. (2015). Intracranial electroencephalography power and phase synchronization changes during monaural and binaural beat stimulation. *Eur. J. Neurosci.* 41, 254–263. doi: 10.1111/ejn.12760

Costa, P. T., and McCrae, R. R. (2008). The revised neo personality inventory (neo-pi-r). *SAGE Handb. Pers. Theory Assess.* 2, 179–198. doi: 10.4135/9781849200479.n9

De Ridder, D., Elgoyhen, A. B., Romo, R., and Langguth, B. (2011). Phantom percepts: tinnitus and pain as persisting aversive memory networks *Proc. Natl. Acad. Sci. U.S.A.* 108, 8075–8080. doi: 10.1073/pnas.1018466108

De Ridder, D., Vanneste, S., Weisz, N., Londero, A., Schlee, W., Elgoyhen, A. B., et al. (2014). An integrative model of auditory phantom perception: tinnitus as a unified percept of interacting separable subnetworks. *Neurosci. Biobehav. Rev.* 44, 16–32. doi: 10.1016/j.neubiorev.2013.03.021

Draganova, R., Ross, B., Wollbrink, A., and Pantev, C. (2008). Cortical steady-state responses to central and peripheral auditory beats. *Cereb. Cortex* 18, 1193–1200. doi: 10.1093/cercor/bhm153

Eggermont, J. J., and Komiya, H. (2000). Moderate noise trauma in juvenile cats results in profound cortical topographic map changes in adulthood. *Hum. Audit. Neuroimaging* 142, 89–101. doi: 10.1016/S0378-5955(00)00024-1

Eggermont, J. J., and Roberts, L. E. (2004). The neuroscience of tinnitus. *Trends Neurosci.* 27, 676–682. doi: 10.1016/j.tins.2004.08.010

Elgoyhen, A. B., Langguth, B., De Ridder, D., and Vanneste, S. (2015). Tinnitus: perspectives from human neuroimaging. *Nat. Rev. Neurosci.* 16, 632–642. doi: 10.1038/nrn4039

Erlandsson, S., and Dauman, N. (2013). Categorization of tinnitus in view of history and medical discourse. *Int. J. Qual. Stud. Health Well Being* 8:55. doi: 10.3402/qhw.v8i0.23530

Feldmann, H. (1971). Homolateral and contralateral masking of tinnitus by noise-bands and by pure tones. *Audiology* 10, 138–144. doi: 10.3109/00206097109072551

Gilles, A., Schlee, W., Rabau, S., Wouters, K., Fransen, E., and Van de Heyning, P. (2016). Decreased speech-in-noise understanding in young adults with tinnitus. *Front. Neurosci.* 10:288. doi: 10.3389/fnins.2016.00288

Goebel, G., and Hiller, W. (1994). The tinnitus questionnaire A standard instrument for grading the degree of tinnitus. results of a multicenter study with the tinnitus questionnaire. *HNO* 42, 166–172.

Hallam, R., Jakes, S., and Hinchcliffe, R. (1988). Cognitive variables in tinnitus annoyance. *Br. J. Clin. Psychol.* 27, 213–222. doi: 10.1111/j.2044-8260.1988.tb00778.x

Hazell, J. W. P., and Wood, S. (2009). Tinnitus masking-a significant contribution to tinnitus management. *Br. J. Audiol.* 15, 223–230. doi: 10.3109/03005368109081442

Henry, J. A., Frederick, M., Sell, S., Griest, S., and Abrams, H. (2015). Validation of a novel combination hearing aid and tinnitus therapy device. *Ear Hear.* 36, 42–52. doi: 10.1097/AUD.0000000000000093

Henry, J. A., and Meikle, M. B. (2000). Psychoacoustic measures of tinnitus. *J. Am. Acad. Audiol.* 11, 138–155.

Henry, J. A., Rheinsburg, B., and Zaugg, T. (2004). Comparison of custom sounds for achieving tinnitus relief. *J. Am. Acad. Audiol.* 15, 585–598. doi: 10.3766/jaaa.15.8.6

Hoare, D. J., Searchfield, G. D., El Refaie, A., and Henry, J. A. (2014). Sound therapy for tinnitus management: practicable options. *J. Am. Acad. Audiol.* 25, 62–75. doi: 10.3766/jaaa.25.1.5

Hoffman, H. J., and Reed, G. W. (2004). "Epidemiology of tinnitus," in *Tinnitus: Theory and Management*, ed J. B. Snow (Hamilton, BC: Decker), 16–41.

Hyvärinen, P., Mendonça, C., Santala, O., Pulkki, V., and Aarnisalo, A. A. (2016). Auditory localization by subjects with unilateral tinnitus. *J. Acoust. Soc. Am.* 139, 2280–2289. doi: 10.1121/1.4946897

Jastreboff, M. M. (2007). Sound therapies for tinnitus management. *Prog. Brain Res.* 166, 435–440. doi: 10.1016/S0079-6123(07)66042-7

Jastreboff, P. J. (1990). Phantom auditory perception (tinnitus): mechanisms of generation and perception. *Neurosci. Res.* 8, 221–254. doi: 10.1016/0168-0102(90)90031-9

Langguth, B., Goodey, R., Azevedo, A., Bjorne, A., Cacace, A., Crocetti, A., et al. (2007). Consensus for tinnitus patient assessment and treatment outcome measurement: tinnitus research initiative meeting, regensburg, july 2006. *Prog. Brain Res.* 166, 525–536. doi: 10.1016/S0079-6123(07)66050-6

Langguth, B., Kreuzer, P. M., Kleinjung, T., and De Ridder, D. (2013). Tinnitus: causes and clinical management. *Lancet Neurol.* 12, 920–930. doi: 10.1016/S1474-4422(13)70160-1

Lockwood, A. H., Salvi, R. J., and Burkard, R. F. (2002). Tinnitus. *N. Engl. J. Med.* 347, 904–910. doi: 10.1056/NEJMra013395

Mazurek, B., Olze, H., Haupt, H., and Szczepek, A. J. (2010). The more the worse: the grade of noise-induced hearing loss associates with the severity of tinnitus. *Int. J. Environ. Res. Public Health* 7, 3071–3079. doi: 10.3390/ijerph7083071

Meyer, M., Luethi, M. S., Neff, P., Langer, N., and Büchi, S. (2014). Disentangling tinnitus distress and tinnitus presence by means of EEG power analysis. *Neural Plast.* 2014:468546. doi: 10.1155/2014/468546

Moazami-Goudarzi, M., Michels, L., Weisz, N., and Jeanmonod, D. (2010). Temporo-insular enhancement of EEG low and high frequencies in patients with chronic tinnitus. *BMC Neurosci.* 11:40. doi: 10.1186/1471-2202-11-40

Moon, I. J., Won, J. H., Kang, H. W., Kim, D. H., An, Y. H., and Shim, H. J. (2015). Influence of tinnitus on auditory spectral and temporal resolution and speech perception in tinnitus patients. *J. Neurosci.* 35, 14260–14269. doi: 10.1523/JNEUROSCI.5091-14.2015

Newman, C. W., Jacobson, G. P., and Spitzer, J. B. (1996) Development of the tinnitus handicap inventory. *Arch. Otolaryngol. Head Neck Surg.* 122, 143–148. doi: 10.1001/archotol.1996.01890140029007

Nondahl, D. M., Cruickshanks, K. J., Huang, G.-H., Klein, B. E. K., Klein, R., Tweed, T. S., et al. (2012). Generational differences in the reporting of tinnitus. *Ear Hear.* 33, 640–644. doi: 10.1097/AUD.0b013e31325069e8

Okamoto, H., Stracke, H., Stoll, W., and Pantev, C. (2010). Listening to tailor-made notched music reduces tinnitus loudness and tinnitus-related auditory cortex activity. *Proc. Natl. Acad. Sci. U.S.A.* 107, 1207–1210. doi: 10.1073/pnas.0911268107

Pantev, C., Okamoto, H., and Teismann, H. (2012). Music-induced cortical plasticity and lateral inhibition in the human auditory cortex as foundations for tonal tinnitus treatment. *Front. Syst. Neurosci.* 6:50. doi: 10.3389/fnsys.2012.00050

Penner, M. J., and Bilger, R. C. (1992). Consistent within-session measures of tinnitus. *J. Speech Hear. Res.* 35, 694–700. doi: 10.1044/jshr.3503.694

Picton, T. W., John, M. S., Dimitrijevic, A., and Purcell, D. (2003). Human auditory steady-state responses: respuestas auditivas de estado estable en humanos. *Int. J. Audiol.* 42, 177–219. doi: 10.3109/14992020309101316

Reavis, K. M., Rothholtz, V. S., Tang, Q., Carroll, J. A., Djalilian, H., and Zeng F.-G. (2012). Temporary suppression of tinnitus by modulated sounds. *J. Assoc. Res. Otolaryngol.* 13, 561–571. doi: 10.1007/s10162-012-0331-6

Roberts, L. E., Moffat, G., Baumann, M., Ward, L. M., and Bosnyak, D. J. (2008). Residual inhibition functions overlap tinnitus spectra and the region of auditory threshold shift. *J. Assoc. Res. Otolaryngol.* 9, 417–435. doi: 10.1007/s10162-008-0136-9

Roberts, L. E., Moffat, G., and Bosnyak, D. J. (2006). Residual inhibition functions in relation to tinnitus spectra and auditory threshold shift. *Acta oto-laryngologica Suppl.* 126, 27–33. doi: 10.1080/03655230600895358

Schaette, R., and Kempter, R. (2006). Development of tinnitus-related neuronal hyperactivity through homeostatic plasticity after hearing loss: a computational model. *Eur. J. Neurosci.* 23, 3124–3138. doi: 10.1111/j.1460-9568.2006.04774.x

Schaette, R., König, O., Hornig, D., Gross, M., and Kempter, R. (2010). Acoustic stimulation treatments against tinnitus could be most effective when tinnitus pitch is within the stimulated frequency range. *Hear. Res.* 269, 95–101. doi: 10.1016/j.heares.2010.06.022

Schaette, R., and McAlpine, D. (2011). Tinnitus with a normal audiogram: physiological evidence for hidden hearing loss and computational model. *J. Neurosci.* 31, 13452–13457. doi: 10.1523/JNEUROSCI.2156-11.2011

Schecklmann, M., Vielsmeier, V., Steffens, T., Landgrebe, M., Langguth, B., Kleinjung, T., et al. (2012). Relationship between audiometric slope and tinnitus pitch in tinnitus patients: insights into the mechanisms of tinnitus generation *PLoS ONE* 7:e34878. doi: 10.1371/journal.pone.0034878

Schlee, W., Schecklmann, M., Lehner, A., Kreuzer, P. M., Vielsmeier, V., Poeppl T. B., et al. (2014). Reduced variability of auditory alpha activity in chronic tinnitus. *Neural Plast.* 2014:436146. doi: 10.1155/2014/436146

Schwarz, D. W. F., and Taylor, P. (2005). Human auditory steady state responses to binaural and monaural beats. *Clin. Neurophysiol.* 116, 658–668. doi: 10.1016/j.clinph.2004.09.014

Stein, A., Engell, A., Lau, P., Wunderlich, R., Junghoefer, M., Wollbrink, A., et al. (2015). Enhancing inhibition-induced plasticity in tinnitus-spectral energy contrasts in tailor-made notched music matter. *PLoS ONE* 10:e0126494. doi: 10.1371/journal.pone.0126494

Tass, P. A., Adamchic, I., Freund, H.-J., Stackelberg, T. V., and Hauptmann, C. (2012). Counteracting tinnitus by acoustic coordinated reset neuromodulation. *Restorat. Neurol. Neurosci.* 30, 137–159. doi: 10.3233/RNN-2012-110218

Tyler, R., Stocking, C., Secor, C., and Slattery, W. H. (2014). Amplitude modulated S-tones can be superior to noise for tinnitus reduction. *Am. J. Audiol.* 23, 303–308. doi: 10.1044/2014_AJA-14-0009

Vanneste, S., and De Ridder, D. (2012). The auditory and non-auditory brain areas involved in tinnitus. An emergent property of multiple parallel overlapping subnetworks. *Front. Syst. Neurosci.* 6:31. doi: 10.3389/fnsys.2012.00031

Vernon, J. (1977). Attempts to relief tinnitus. *Ear Hear.* 2:124.

Vernon, J. A., and Meikle, M. B. (2003). Masking devices and alprazolam treatment for tinnitus. *Otolaryngol. Clin. North Am.* 36, 307–320.

Watanabe, K., Kamio, T., Ohkawara, D., Aoki, H., Baba, S., and Yagi, T. (1997). [Suppression of tinnitus by band noise masker–a study of 600 cases]. *Nihon Jibiinkoka Gakkai kaiho* 100, 920–926. doi: 10.3950/jibiinkoka.100.920

Weisz, N., Hartmann, T., Dohrmann, K., Schlee, W., and Norena, A. (2006). High-frequency tinnitus without hearing loss does not mean absence of deafferentation. *Hear. Res.* 222, 108–114. doi: 10.1016/j.heares.2006.09.003

Weisz, N., Moratti, S., Meinzer, M., Dohrmann, K., and Elbert, T. (2005). Tinnitus perception and distress is related to abnormal spontaneous brain activity as measured by magnetoencephalography. *PLoS Med.* 2:e153. doi: 10.1371/journal.pmed.0020153

Wunderlich, R., Lau, P., Stein, A., Engell, A., Wollbrink, A., Rudack, C., et al. (2015a). Impact of spectral notch width on neurophysiological plasticity and clinical effectiveness of the tailor-made notched music training. *PLoS ONE* 10:e0138595. doi: 10.1371/journal.pone.0138595

Wunderlich, R., Stein, A., Engell, A., Lau, P., Waasem, L., Shaykevich, A., et al. (2015b). Evaluation of iPod-based automated tinnitus pitch matching. *J. Am. Acad. Audiol.* 26, 205–212. doi: 10.3766/jaaa.26.2.9

Xiong, H., Chen, L., Yang, H., Li, X., Qiu, Z., Huang, X., et al. (2013). Hidden hearing loss in tinnitus patients with normal audiograms: implications for the origin of tinnitus. *J. Clin. Otorhinolaryngol. Head Neck Surg.* 27, 362–365.

Zeng, F.-G., Tang, Q., Dimitrijevic, A., Starr, A., Larky, J., and Blevins, N. H. (2011). Tinnitus suppression by low-rate electric stimulation and its electrophysiological mechanisms. *Hum. Audit. Neuroimaging* 277, 61–66. doi: 10.1016/j.heares.2011.03.010

9

Outpatient Tinnitus Clinic, Self-Help Web Platform, or Mobile Application to Recruit Tinnitus Study Samples?

Thomas Probst[1,2], Rüdiger C. Pryss[2], Berthold Langguth[3], Myra Spiliopoulou[4], Michael Landgrebe[3,5], Markku Vesala[6], Stephen Harrison[6], Johannes Schobel[2], Manfred Reichert[2], Michael Stach[2] and Winfried Schlee[3]*

[1]Georg-Elias-Müller Institute for Psychology, Georg-August University Göttingen, Göttingen, Germany, [2]Institute of Databases and Information Systems, Ulm University, Ulm, Germany, [3]Department of Psychiatry and Psychotherapy of the University of Regensburg at Bezirksklinikum Regensburg, University of Regensburg, Regensburg, Germany, [4]Department of Technical and Business Information Systems, Otto-von-Guericke-University Magdeburg, Magdeburg, Germany, [5]Clinic Lech-Mangfall, Agatharied, Germany, [6]Tinnitus Hub Ltd, Hemsworth, UK

***Correspondence:**
Thomas Probst
thomas.probst@ur.de

For understanding the heterogeneity of tinnitus, large samples are required. However, investigations on how samples recruited by different methods differ from each other are lacking. In the present study, three large samples each recruited by different means were compared: *N* = 5017 individuals registered at a self-help web platform for tinnitus (crowdsourcing platform Tinnitus Talk), *N* = 867 users of a smart mobile application for tinnitus (crowdsensing platform TrackYourTinnitus), and *N* = 3786 patients contacting an outpatient tinnitus clinic (Tinnitus Center of the University Hospital Regensburg). The three samples were compared regarding age, gender, and duration of tinnitus (month or years perceiving tinnitus; subjective report) using chi-squared tests. The three samples significantly differed from each other in age, gender and tinnitus duration ($p < 0.05$). Users of the TrackYourTinnitus crowdsensing platform were younger, users of the Tinnitus Talk crowdsourcing platform had more often female gender, and users of both newer technologies (crowdsourcing and crowdsensing) had more frequently acute/subacute tinnitus (<3 months and 4–6 months) as well as a very long tinnitus duration (>20 years). The implications of these findings for clinical research are that newer technologies such as crowdsourcing and crowdsensing platforms offer the possibility to reach individuals hard to get in contact with at an outpatient tinnitus clinic. Depending on the aims and the inclusion/exclusion criteria of a given study, different recruiting strategies (clinic and/or newer technologies) offer different advantages and disadvantages. In general, the representativeness of study results might be increased when tinnitus study samples are recruited in the clinic as well as via crowdsourcing and crowdsensing.

Keywords: tinnitus, recruitment, crowdsourcing, crowdsensing, clinical data

INTRODUCTION

Tinnitus is characterized by the perception of a sound without a corresponding external sound source (Baguley et al., 2013; Langguth et al., 2013). A recent review on prevalence rates of tinnitus in 16 countries found that between 5.1% and 42.7% of the population report tinnitus (McCormack et al., 2016). The prevalence rates typically vary depending on the age, the birth cohort

(Nondahl et al., 2012; Martinez et al., 2015), and the definition of tinnitus used in the epidemiological study (McCormack et al., 2016). A recent US study found that 9.6% of Americans experienced tinnitus in the last year and that only 49.4% discussed the tinnitus with a physician (Bhatt et al., 2016). In case tinnitus patients seen by physicians are not representative for the whole sample of individuals perceiving tinnitus, the representativeness of studies recruiting patients only in medical practices or hospitals might be limited. In the area of anxiety and depression, for example, researchers found differences between patients contacting an outpatient clinic, patients being treated in an Internet-based clinic, and individuals with anxiety or depressive disorders from a national epidemiological survey (Titov et al., 2010). Another study on Internet-based psychotherapy for depression found that patients recruited by online advertisements differed from patients recruited by newspaper advertisements in demographics and depression severity (Lindner et al., 2015).

In the case of tinnitus, several patient databases have been established with the aim to better understand the heterogeneity of tinnitus (Meikle, 1997; Landgrebe et al., 2010; Witsell et al., 2011). However, all these databases collect data from patients who present themselves at a tinnitus clinic. For investigating tinnitus heterogeneity, it is of high importance to know how samples recruited by different methods vary and which recruitment methods are most efficient for the recruitment of specific tinnitus subgroups.

Although the recruitment of individuals not contacting physicians is traditionally difficult, online-recruitment has been shown to be promising in clinical and health science to overcome this obstacle (e.g., Morgan et al., 2013; Bevelander et al., 2014; Gioia et al., 2016; Kayrouz et al., 2016; Thornton et al., 2016; Topolovec-Vranic and Natarajan, 2016). In a recent review on online-recruitment in health studies, Lane et al. (2015) stated, though, that "more empirical evidence is needed to make specific recommendations" (p. 1). The claim for more empirical research might be especially relevant for the relatively new participant-led research paradigm (Vayena and Tasioulas, 2013) including crowdsourcing (e.g., Swan, 2012; Ranard et al., 2014; Chandler and Shapiro, 2016) and crowdsensing (e.g., Ganti et al., 2011; Guo et al., 2014, 2015). "Crowdsourcing is a type of participative online activity in which an individual, an institution, a non-profit organization, or company proposes to a group of individuals of varying knowledge, heterogeneity, and number, via a flexible open call, the voluntary undertaking of a task. The undertaking of the task, of variable complexity and modularity, and in which the crowd should participate bringing their work, money, knowledge and/or experience, always entails mutual benefit. The user will receive the satisfaction of a given type of need, be it economic, social recognition, self-esteem, or the development of individual skills, while the crowdsourcer will obtain and utilize to their advantage what the user has brought to the venture, whose form will depend on the type of activity undertaken" (Estellés-Arolas and González-Ladrón-de-Guevara, 2012, p. 197). Guo et al. (2015) defined mobile crowdsensing and computing (MCSC) as follows: "MCSC extends the vision of participatory sensing by leveraging both participatory sensory data from mobile devices (offline) and user-contributed data from mobile social networking services (online). Further, it explores the complementary roles and presents the fusion/collaboration of machine and human intelligence in the crowdsensing and computing processes" (Guo et al., 2015, p. 1). In contrast to crowdsourcing, crowdsensing relies solely on mobile technology and integrates sensors to collect data, for example, behavioral (e.g., physical activity level, gait pattern), physiological (e.g., heart rate, electrodermal activity), and environmental (e.g., environmental sound level, GPS location) variables.

As it remains unclear whether online-recruitment by crowdsourcing and crowdsensing offers the potential to reach individuals with tinnitus that are different from the ones directly consulting a physician, the study at hand compared tinnitus patients visiting an outpatient tinnitus clinic, users of a tinnitus crowdsourcing platform (moderated self-help web platform) and users of a tinnitus crowdsensing platform (mobile application).

MATERIALS AND METHODS

Samples

The following three samples were investigated:

1. Tinnitus crowdsourcing sample "Tinnitus Talk": Tinnitus Hub[1] operates the moderated self-help platform Tinnitus Talk[2]. The platform was established in March 2011 by Markku Vesala. With 16,500 registered participants (as of December 2016) and over 210,000 unique readers every month, Tinnitus Talk is one of the most active tinnitus-dedicated platforms for information delivery, experience exchange, and self-help among individuals with tinnitus. The data of the present study relies on a survey ran from February 8th till March 13th 2016.
2. Tinnitus crowdsensing sample "TrackYourTinnitus": TrackYourTinnitus (TYT; Pryss et al., 2015a,b)[3] is an application for mobile-devices (iOS and Android) that allows the tracking of tinnitus in daily life by ecological momentary assessments. Although monitoring tinnitus repeatedly directs the attention towards the tinnitus, Schlee et al. (2016) showed that using TYT does not deteriorate the tinnitus. Other studies on TYT investigated the role of emotional states (Probst et al., 2016a) as well as emotion dynamics (Probst et al., 2016b) in tinnitus. The data presented here was collected from April 2014 to June 2016.
3. Outpatient tinnitus clinic sample "Tinnitus Center Regensburg": The University Hospital Regensburg hosts a tinnitus center[4], established 2007, and having about 300 tinnitus patients per annum. To date (December 2016), the Tinnitus database encompasses medical records for about 3000 patients.

[1] www.tinnitushub.com
[2] www.tinnitustalk.com
[3] www.trackyourtinnitus.org
[4] www.tinnituszentrum-regensburg.de

At the Tinnitus Center Regensburg, patients gave written informed consent that data were gathered and analyzed for the Tinnitus Research Initiative Database, which was approved by the Ethics Committee of the University Hospital of Regensburg. The material and the methods of TrackYourTinnitus were approved by the Ethics Committee of the University Hospital Regensburg and were carried out in accordance with the approved guidelines; written consent, however, was not possible to obtain for the users of TrackYourTinnitus. Information that the data will be used for scientific analyses is included in the mobile applications as well as on the website and, therefore, the TrackYourTinnitus users were informed that the data will be used for scientific purposes. Written informed consent was also not possible to obtain for the users of Tinnitus Hub/Tinnitus Talk, but the "Terms and Rules" of the website informed the users that the collected data will be analyzed for scientific purposes. All the data were saved anonymously.

Measures

Three variables were assessed in the three samples by self-reports: age, gender, and duration of tinnitus (month or years perceiving tinnitus; subjective report). In the Tinnitus Talk survey, the variables age (<18 years, 18–24 years, ...; see **Table 1**) and tinnitus duration (<3 months, 4–6 months, ...; see **Table 1**) were assessed in categories. Therefore, the metric scores of age and tinnitus duration as assessed in the Tinnitus Center Regensburg and TrackYourTinnitus were categorized accordingly to be able to perform statistical analyses.

Statistical Analysis

Chi-squared tests were performed with R and the significance value was set to $p < 0.05$.

TABLE 1 | Description of the three samples and comparisons between the samples.

	Tinnitus Talk	TrackYour Tinnitus	Tinnitus Center Regensburg	Between-group statistics
Total number	5017	867	3786	
Age in years				$X^2 = 366.7$;
% <18	1.0	1.6	0.5	$p < 0.001$
% 18–24	5.4	4.4	2.4	
% 25–34	11.4	20.7	6.6	
% 35–44	13.6	22.5	15.7	
% 45–55	20.9	26.5	29.6	
% 55–64	30.2	18.9	26.7	
% 65–74	15.1	5.2	15.5	
% >75	2.4	0.3	3.1	
Gender				$X^2 = 103.5$;
% female	42.8	27.1	35.1	$p < 0.001$
% male	57.2	72.9	64.9	
Tinnitus duration				$X^2 = 393.7$;
% <3 months	6.4	14.2	2.1	$p < 0.001$
% 4–6 months	5.7	6.8	3.4	
% 6–12 months	10.1	7.0	9.3	
% 1–2 years	14.7	7.6	16.2	
% 3–5 years	13.1	15.4	20.6	
% 5–10 years	18.3	16.0	17.1	
% 10–20 years	15.3	16.9	20.7	
% >20 years	16.4	16.1	10.6	

RESULTS

The three samples comprised $N = 9670$ individuals. Information on age was available for $n = 8766$ individuals, information on gender for $n = 9607$, and information on tinnitus duration for $n = 8409$. Full descriptions of the samples are presented in **Table 1**.

Age

A chi-squared test was calculated to test whether the distribution of age (see **Table 1**; **Figure 1**) is different between the samples. With an $X^2 = 366.7$, the hypothesis that the samples had an equal age distribution was rejected ($p < 0.001$). The most obvious differences emerged in the percentage of individuals with an age between 25 and 44 years as well as in the percentage of individuals with an age between 55 and 74 years. The 25–44 years aged individuals were more often among the TrackYourTinnitus users (25–34 years: 20.7%; 35–44 years: 22.5%) than among the Tinnitus Talk users (25–34 years: 11.4%; 35–44 years: 13.6%) and among the patients of the Tinnitus Center Regensburg (25–34 years: 6.6%; 35–44 years: 15.7%). Yet, the 55–74 years aged adults were more frequently among the Tinnitus Talk users (55–64 years: 30.2%; 65–74 years: 15.1%) and among the patients at the Tinnitus Center Regensburg (55–64 years: 26.7%; 65–74 years: 15.5%) than among the TrackYourTinnitus users (55–64 years: 18.9%; 65–74 years: 5.2%).

Gender

A chi-squared test was also calculated to investigate whether the gender distribution of the three sample groups is equal or different (see **Table 1**; **Figure 2**). Based on an $X^2 = 103.5$, the hypothesis of an equal gender distribution was rejected ($p < 0.001$). Although the participants were more frequently men than women in all three samples, TrackYourTinnitus

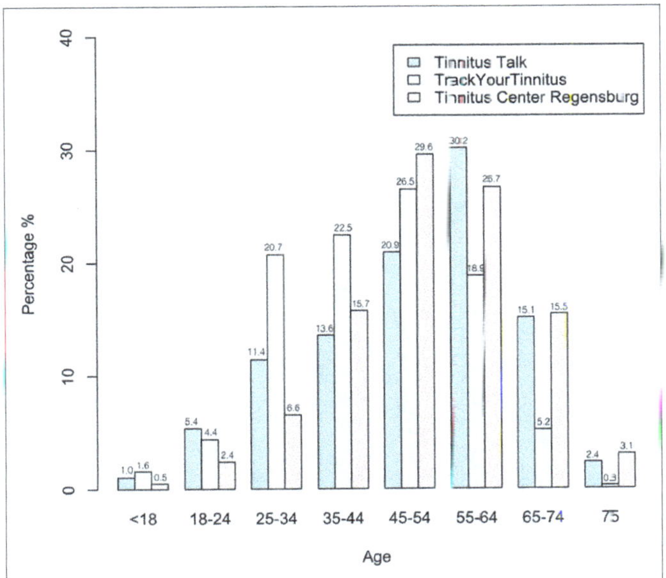

FIGURE 1 | Distribution of age in the three samples.

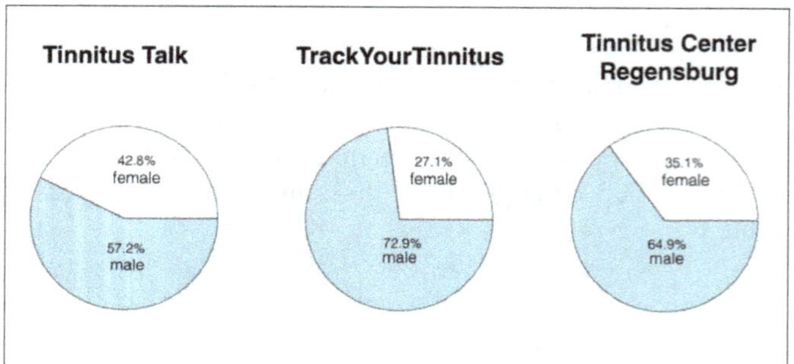

FIGURE 2 | Distribution of gender in the three samples.

had the lowest rate of females (27.1%) and Tinnitus Talk the highest (42.8%).

Tinnitus Duration

Again a chi-squared test was calculated to test whether the distribution of tinnitus duration is equal or different between the three samples (see **Table 1**; **Figure 3**). With an X^2 of 393.7, the hypothesis of an equal tinnitus duration distribution was rejected ($p < 0.001$). Differences were apparent for individuals with a tinnitus duration <3 months: 14.2% of the TrackYourTinnitus users were in this category, but only 6.4% of the Tinnitus Talk users and only 2.1% of the Tinnitus Center Regensburg patients. However, TrackYourTinnitus users reported less often 1–2 years of tinnitus duration (7.6%) than Tinnitus Talk users (14.7%) and patients at the Tinnitus Center Regensburg (16.2%). The Tinnitus Center Regensburg patients reported more often 3–5 years and 10–20 years of tinnitus duration (3–5 years: 20.6%; 10–20 years: 20.7%) than Tinnitus Talk users (3–5 years: 13.1%; 10–20 years: 15.3%) and TrackYourTinnitus users (3–5 years: 15.4%; 10–20 years: 16.9%). The individuals with tinnitus duration >20 years, however, were more frequently among the Tinnitus Talk users (16.4%) and the TrackYourTinnitus users (16.1%) than among the patients at the Tinnitus Center Regensburg (10.6%).

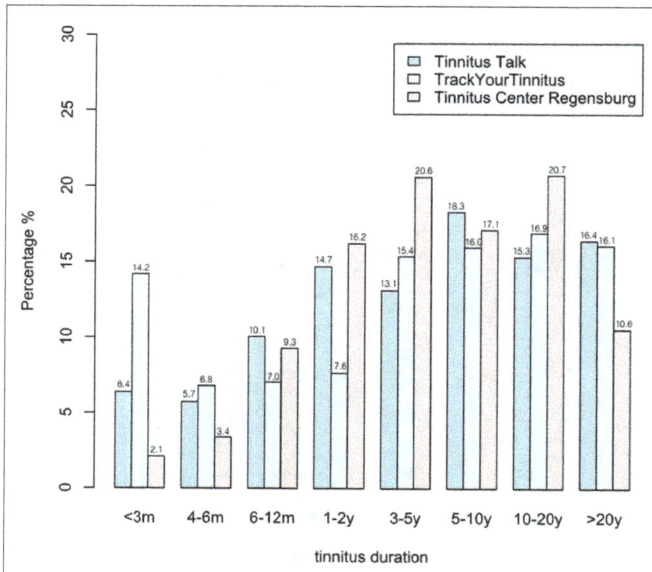

FIGURE 3 | Distribution of tinnitus duration in the three samples.

DISCUSSION

The study at hand compared individuals contacting an outpatient tinnitus clinic (Tinnitus Center Regensburg), individuals registered at a self-help web platform (crowdsourcing platform Tinnitus Talk) and users of an application for mobile devices (crowdsensing platform TrackYourTinnitus). The aim of the study was to investigate whether newer technologies (crowdsourcing and/or crowdsensing) offer possibilities for future studies to reach individuals with tinnitus that are different from the ones directly contacting an outpatient clinic. In summary, we found that the samples differed in the investigated variables. The result that patients of an outpatient clinic differed from users of newer technologies is in line with a study on anxiety and depression comparing patients of an outpatient clinic with those attending an Internet clinic (Titov et al., 2010). Moreover the results of the current study correspond with a recent review (Topolovec-Vranic and Natarajan, 2016), which reported that populations recruited by traditional methods were not comparable to samples recruited by newer technologies (the review focused on social media) in most of the studies (12 vs. 2).

One of the variables investigated in the present study was age. The results revealed that younger individuals (≤44 years) used more frequently the crowdsensing platform for tinnitus, whereas older individuals (≥55 years) were more often among the users of the crowdsourcing platform for tinnitus as well as among the patients of an outpatient tinnitus clinic. Thus, crowdsensing might be potent to recruit younger individuals but not as suited for the recruitment of older individuals. Nevertheless, crowdsensing might be appropriate to recruit older individuals in the future as the younger generation (which now uses crowdsensing) becomes older.

Another evaluated variable in the current study was gender. Gender was predominately male in all three samples and this result is in line with previous research on tinnitus: "In fact, most previous studies, but not all … showed higher tinnitus prevalence in men than in women" (Gallus et al., 2015; p. 16). The crowdsourcing platform Tinnitus Talk had the highest percentage of female individuals, whereas the crowdsensing platform TrackYourTinnitus had the lowest. Therefore, crowdsourcing might be more appropriate than crowdsensing when aiming to recruit women by newer technologies.

The third investigated variable in the study at hand was tinnitus duration (month or years perceiving tinnitus; subjective report). Duration of tinnitus is clinically and scientifically relevant to define acute, subacute and chronic tinnitus. The results of the current study revealed that acute and subacute tinnitus are more frequent among the users of crowdsourcing and crowdsensing platforms than among the patients of an outpatient clinic. Long waiting times for appointments in specialized tinnitus clinic might contribute to this effect.

Regardless the reasons for the delay in seeing a specialist, our data indicate that individuals with tinnitus search for information or help in the Internet already early after symptom onset. As interventions are already helpful in the acute and subacute stages of tinnitus (Nyenhuis et al., 2013b) and might prevent a chronic course, offering helpful interventions for individuals with acute and subacute tinnitus is crucial. As more of these individuals can be reached by crowdsourcing or crowdsensing platforms than by an outpatient clinic, the implementation of appropriate self-help interventions in crowdsourcing or crowdsensing platforms might be promising (e.g., Heron and Smyth, 2010; Donker et al., 2013). The finding that Internet-based self-help is as effective as face-to-face interventions for tinnitus patients (e.g., Nyenhuis et al., 2013a; Jasper et al., 2014; Andersson, 2015) supports this line of argumentation. Another interesting result in the context of tinnitus duration was that individuals who perceived their tinnitus for a very long time (>20 years), were more frequent among the crowdsourcing and crowdsensing samples than among the sample of the outpatient clinic. It could be speculated that these individuals experienced past treatments as ineffective and consequently gave up seeking medical or psychological help (learned helplessness; Abramson et al., 1978) or have already established effective coping strategies. These individuals will not contact a physician or a clinic, although interventions, which these individuals have not tried yet, might be helpful. These findings at least suggest that it might be useful to provide information about interventions and current innovative treatment approaches in crowdsourcing or crowdsensing platforms.

One limitation of the study at hand is that we analyzed only one crowdsourcing platform for tinnitus, only one crowdsensing platform for tinnitus, and only one outpatient tinnitus clinic. Although our samples are relatively large, even more representative results might be obtained by multicenter studies including several clinics and several crowdsourcing (two crowdsourcing platforms were investigated, for example, by Briones and Benham, 2017) as well as several crowdsensing platforms. Another shortcoming of the crowdsourced and crowdsensed data is that the robustness and accuracy of the online-collected data is difficult to verify. Previous studies could, however, provide support for the trustworthiness of web-based research (e.g., Meyerson and Tryon, 2003; Gosling et al., 2004). Moreover comparisons with data from population-based epidemiological studies (see Titov et al., 2010) would be desirable to identify how representative the three samples of the current study are for the total tinnitus population. We abstained from such a comparison, since data from available epidemiological studies are highly variable (McCormack et al., 2016). Finally, since clinical variables were not assessed in all three samples, we could not compare the three samples regarding clinical characteristics of tinnitus (e.g., tinnitus severity). Tinnitus severity is usually important in the recruitment process of clinical studies and usually is measured by psychometrically sound instruments such as the "Tinnitus Handicap Inventory" (THI; Newman et al., 1996). Those who use an app or online site may have less bothersome tinnitus and may have no intention of seeking medical attention. At least some may be just curious but not need any treatment or intervention. Comparing the severity of these groups is an important task for future research to clarify whether recruiting individuals with tinnitus using a tinnitus app or website will aid our understanding of bothersome tinnitus. Such further studies will aid to find the best recruitment strategy for a given study.

Despite these limitations, the current study is the first one comparing tinnitus patients of an outpatient clinic with users of crowdsourcing and crowdsensing platforms for tinnitus. We showed that these newer technologies offer promising perspectives to reach individuals hard to get in contact with at an outpatient tinnitus clinic (e.g., individuals with acute/subacute tinnitus, younger individuals, as well as individuals perceiving tinnitus for a very long time).

AUTHOR CONTRIBUTIONS

TP substantially contributed to the design of the study and data preparation, drafted and revised the manuscript. RCP substantially contributed to the design of the study, data preparation, the TrackYourTinnitus platform and revised the manuscript. BL substantially contributed to the design of the study, data collection at the Tinnitus Center Regensburg, the TrackYourTinnitus platform and revised the manuscript. MS substantially contributed to the design of the study and revised the manuscript. ML substantially contributed to the data collection at the Tinnitus Center Regensburg and revised the manuscript. MV and SH substantially contributed to the Tinnitus Talk platform, and revised the manuscript. JS, MR and MS substantially contributed to the TrackYourTinnitus platform, and revised the manuscript. WS substantially contributed to the design of the study, the TrackYourTinnitus platform, drafted and revised the manuscript, and performed the statistical analyses.

ACKNOWLEDGMENTS

This work was supported by the German Research Foundation (DFG) within the funding programme Open Access Publishing. The authors would like to thank Ankur Bahre (Otto-von-Guericke-University Magdeburg) for providing helpful references and Vishnu Unnikrishnan (Otto-von-Guericke-University Magdeburg) for the statistical work with the three samples.

REFERENCES

Abramson, L. Y., Seligman, M. E., and Teasdale, J. D. (1978). Learned helplessness in humans: critique and reformulation. *J. Abnorm. Psychol.* 87, 49–74. doi: 10.1037/0021-843x.87.1.49

Andersson, G. (2015). Clinician-supported internet-delivered psychological treatment of tinnitus. *Am. J. Audiol.* 24, 299–301. doi: 10.1044/2015_AJA-14-0080

Baguley, D., McFerran, D., and Hall, D. (2013). Tinnitus. *Lancet* 382, 1600–1607 doi: 10.1016/S0140-6736(13)60142-7

Bevelander, K. E., Kaipainen, K., Swain, R., Dohle, S., Bongard, J. C., Hines, P. D., et al. (2014). Crowdsourcing novel childhood predictors of adult obesity. *PLoS One* 9:e87756. doi: 10.1371/journal.pone.0087756

Bhatt, J. M., Lin, H. W., and Bhattacharyya, N. (2016). Prevalence, severity, exposures and treatment patterns of tinnitus in the United States. *JAMA Otolaryngol. Head. Neck. Surg.* 142, 959–965. doi: 10.1001/jamaoto.2016.1700

Briones, E. M., and Benham, G. (2017). An examination of the equivalency of self-report measures obtained from crowdsourced versus undergraduate student samples. *Behav. Res. Methods* 49, 320–334. doi: 10.3758/s13428-016-0710-8

Chandler, J., and Shapiro, D. (2016). Conducting clinical research using crowdsourced convenience samples. *Annu. Rev. Clin. Psychol.* 12, 53–81. doi: 10.1146/annurev-clinpsy-021815-093623

Donker, T., Petrie, K., Proudfoot, J., Clarke, J., Birch, M. R., and Christensen, H. (2013). Smartphones for smarter delivery of mental health programs: a systematic review. *J. Med. Internet Res.* 15:e247. doi: 10.2196/jmir.2791

Estellés-Arolas, E., and González-Ladrón-de-Guevara, F. (2012). Towards an integrated crowdsourcing definition. *J. Inf. Sci.* 38, 189–200. doi: 10.1177/0165551512437638

Gallus, S., Lugo, A., Garavello, W., Bosetti, C., Santoro, E., Colombo, P., et al. (2015). Prevalence and determinants of tinnitus in the Italian adult population. *Neuroepidemiology* 45, 12–19. doi: 10.1159/000431376

Ganti, R. K., Ye, F., and Lei, H. (2011). Mobile crowdsensing: current state and future challenges. *IEEE Commun. Mag.* 49, 32–39. doi: 10.1109/mcom.2011.6069707

Gioia, C. J., Sobell, L. C., Sobell, M. B., and Agrawal, S. (2016). Craigslist versus print newspaper advertising for recruiting research participants for alcohol studies: cost and participant characteristics. *Addict. Behav.* 54, 24–32. doi: 10.1016/j.addbeh.2015.11.008

Gosling, S. D., Vazire, S., Srivastava, S., and John, O. P. (2004). Should we trust web-based studies? A comparative analysis of six preconceptions about internet questionnaires. *Am. Psychol.* 59, 93–104. doi: 10.1037/0003-066x.59.2.93

Guo, B., Wang, Z., Yu, Z., Wang, Y., Yen, N. Y., Huang, R., et al. (2015). Mobile crowd sensing and computing: the review of an emerging human-powered sensing paradigm. *ACM Comput. Surv.* 48:7. doi: 10.1145/2794400

Guo, B., Yu, Z., Zhou, X., and Zhang, D. (2014). "From participatory sensing to mobile crowd sensing," in *2014 IEEE International Conference on Pervasive Computing and Communications Workshops (PERCOM Workshops)* (Budapest), 593–598.

Heron, K. E., and Smyth, J. M. (2010). Ecological momentary interventions: incorporating mobile technology into psychosocial and health behaviour treatments. *Br. J. Health Psychol.* 15, 1–39. doi: 10.1348/135910709X466063

Jasper, K., Weise, C., Conrad, I., Hiller, W., Andersson, G., and Kleinstäuber, M. (2014). Internet-based guided self-help versus cognitive behavioral group therapy for chronic tinnitus: a randomized controlled trial. *Psychother. Psychosom.* 83, 234–246. doi: 10.1159/000360705

Kayrouz, R., Dear, B. F., Karin, E., and Titov, N. (2016). Facebook as an effective recruitment strategy for mental health research of hard to reach populations. *Internet Interv.* 4, 1–10. doi: 10.1016/j.invent.2016.01.001

Landgrebe, M., Zeman, F., Koller, M., Eberl, Y., Mohr, M., Reiter, J., et al. (2010). The Tinnitus Research Initiative (TRI) database: a new approach for delineation of tinnitus subtypes and generation of predictors for treatment outcome. *BMC Med. Inform. Decis. Mak.* 10:42. doi: 10.1186/1472-6947-10-42

Lane, T. S., Armin, J., and Gordon, J. S. (2015). Online recruitment methods for web-based and mobile health studies: a review of the literature. *J. Med. Internet Res.* 17:e183. doi: 10.2196/jmir.4359

Langguth, B., Kreuzer, P. M., Kleinjung, T., and De Ridder, D. (2013). Tinnitus: causes and clinical management. *Lancet Neurol.* 12, 920–930. doi: 10.1016/S1474-4422(13)70160-1

Lindner, P., Nyström, M. B. T., Hassmén, P., Andersson, G., and Carlbring, P. (2015). Who seeks ICBT for depression and how do they get there? Effects of recruitment source on patient demographics and clinical characteristics. *Internet Interv.* 2, 221–225. doi: 10.1016/j.invent.2015.04.002

Martinez, C., Wallenhorst, C., McFerran, D., and Hall, D. A. (2015). Incidence rates of clinically significant tinnitus: 10-year trend from a cohort study in England. *Ear Hear.* 36, e69–e75. doi: 10.1097/AUD.0000000000000121

McCormack, A., Edmondson-Jones, M., Somerset, S., and Hall, D. (2016). A systematic review of the reporting of tinnitus prevalence and severity. *Hear. Res.* 337, 70–79. doi: 10.1016/j.heares.2016.05.009

Meikle, M. B. (1997). Electronic access to tinnitus data: the Oregon Tinnitus Data Archive. *Otolaryngol. Head Neck Surg.* 117, 698–700. doi: 10.1016/s0194-5998(97)70055-x

Meyerson, P., and Tryon, W. W. (2003). Validating internet research: a test of the psychometric equivalence of internet and in-person samples. *Behav. Res. Methods Instrum. Comput.* 35, 614–620. doi: 10.3758/bf03195541

Morgan, A. J., Jorm, A. F., and Mackinnon, A. J. (2013). Internet-based recruitment to a depression prevention intervention: lessons from the Mood Memos study. *J. Med. Internet Res.* 15:e31. doi: 10.2196/jmir.2262

Newman, C. W., Jacobson, G. P., and Spitzer, J. B. (1996). Development of the tinnitus handicap inventory. *Arch. Otolaryngol. Head Neck Surg.* 122, 143–148. doi: 10.1001/archotol.1996.01890140029007

Nondahl, D. M., Cruickshanks, K. J., Huang, G. H., Klein, B. E., Klein, R., Tweed, T. S., et al. (2012). Generational differences in the reporting of tinnitus. *Ear Hear.* 33, 640–644. doi: 10.1097/AUD.0b013e31825069e8

Nyenhuis, N., Golm, D., and Kröner-Herwig, B. (2013a). A systematic review and meta-analysis on the efficacy of self-help interventions in tinnitus. *Cogn. Behav. Ther.* 42, 159–169. doi: 10.1080/16506073.2013.803496

Nyenhuis, N., Zastrutzki, S., Weise, C., Jäger, B., and Kröner-Herwig, B. (2013b). The efficacy of minimal contact interventions for acute tinnitus: a randomised controlled study. *Cogn. Behav. Ther.* 42, 127–138. doi: 10.1080/16506073.2012.655305

Probst, T., Pryss, R., Langguth, B., and Schlee, W. (2016a). Emotional states as mediators between tinnitus loudness and tinnitus distress in daily life: results from the "TrackYourTinnitus" application. *Sci. Rep.* 6:20382. doi: 10.1038/srep20382

Probst, T., Pryss, R., Langguth, B., and Schlee, W. (2016b). Emotion dynamics and tinnitus: daily life data from the "TrackYourTinnitus" application. *Sci. Rep.* 6:31166. doi: 10.1038/srep31166

Pryss, R., Reichert, M., Herrmann, J., Langguth, B., and Schlee, W. (2015a). "Mobile crowd sensing in clinical and psychological trials—a case study," in *28th IEEE Int'l Symposium on Computer-Based Medical Systems* (São Carlos), 23–24.

Pryss, R., Reichert, M., Langguth, B., and Schlee, W. (2015b). "Mobile crowd sensing services for tinnitus assessment, therapy and research," in *2015 IEEE 4th International Conference on Mobile Services* (New York, NY), 352–359.

Ranard, B. L., Ha, Y. P., Meisel, Z. F., Asch, D. A., Hill, S. S., Becker, L. B., et al. (2014). Crowdsourcing—harnessing the masses to advance health and medicine, a systematic review. *J. Gen. Intern. Med.* 29, 187–203. doi: 10.1007/s11606-013-2536-8

Schlee, W., Pryss, R., Probst, T., Schobel, J., Bachmeier, A., Reichert, M., et al. (2016). Measuring the moment-to-moment variability of tinnitus: the TrackYourTinnitus smart phone app. *Front. Aging Neurosci.* 8:294. doi: 10.3389/fnagi.2016.00294

Swan, M. (2012). Crowdsourced health research studies: an important emerging complement to clinical trials in the public health research ecosystem. *J. Med. Internet Res.* 14:e46. doi: 10.2196/jmir.1988

Thornton, L., Batterham, P. J., Fassnacht, D. B., Kay-Lambkin, F., Calear, A. L., and Hunt, S. (2016). Recruiting for health, medical or psychosocial research using Facebook: systematic review. *Internet Interv.* 4, 72–81. doi: 10.1016/j.invent.2016.02.001

Titov, N., Andrews, G., Kemp, A., and Robinson, E. (2010). Characteristics of adults with anxiety or depression treated at an internet clinic: comparison with a national survey and an outpatient clinic. *PLoS One* 5:e10885. doi: 10.1371/journal.pone.0010885

Topolovec-Vranic, J., and Natarajan, K. (2016). The use of social media in recruitment for medical research studies: a scoping review. *J. Med. Internet Res.* 18:e286. doi: 10.2196/jmir.5698

Vayena, E., and Tasioulas, J. (2013). Adapting standards: ethical oversight of participant-led health research. *PLoS Med.* 10:e1001402. doi: 10.1371/journal.pmed.1001402

Witsell, D. L., Schulz, K. A., Moore, K., Tucci, D. L., and CHEER Investigators. (2011). Implementation and testing of research infrastructure for practice-based research in hearing and communication disorders. *Otolaryngol. Head Neck Surg.* 145, 565–571. doi: 10.1177/0194599811406369

10

Results of an Interdisciplinary Day Care Approach for Chronic Tinnitus Treatment: A Prospective Study Introducing the Jena Interdisciplinary Treatment for Tinnitus

Daniela Ivansic[1], Christian Dobel[1], Gerd F. Volk[1], Daniel Reinhardt[1], Boris Müller[1], Ulrich C. Smolenski[2] and Orlando Guntinas-Lichius[1]*

[1] Tinnitus-Centre, Department of Otorhinolaryngology, Jena University Hospital, Jena, Germany,

[2] Institut of Physiotherapy, Jena University Hospital, Jena, Germany

Correspondence:
Daniela Ivansic
daniela.ivansic@med.uni-jena.de

Objective: Considering the heterogeneity of the symptoms shown by patients suffering from chronic tinnitus, there are surprisingly few interdisciplinary treatments available, and mostly available only for inpatients. In order to provide an interdisciplinary treatment, we developed a day care concept in which each patient was treated by an ENT doctor, a cognitive behavioral therapist, a specialist for medical rehabilitation and an audiologist (Jena Interdisciplinary Treatment for Tinnitus, JITT). The aim of this study was to observe the changes of tinnitus related distress due to interdisciplinary day care treatment and to determine which factors mediate this change.

Subjects and Methods: Tinnitus annoyance was measured using the Tinnitus Questionnaire on 308 patients with chronic tinnitus. They were treated in the day care unit over five consecutive days between July 2013 and December 2014. Data were collected before treatment when screened (T0), at the beginning (T1) and at the end of the 5 day treatment (T2), as well as 20 days (T3) and 6 months after treatment (T4).

Results: Overall, tinnitus annoyance improved significantly from the screening day to the beginning of treatment, and to a much larger degree from the beginning to the end of treatment. The treatment outcome remained stable 6 months after treatment. Patients with the following symptoms displayed higher tinnitus annoyance at T0: dizziness at tinnitus onset, tinnitus sound could not be masked with background noise, tinnitus worsening during physical stress, comorbid psychiatric diagnosis, higher age and higher hearing loss. Loudness of tinnitus perceived in the right ear correlated with tinnitus annoyance significantly. Demographic, tinnitus and strain variables could only explain 12.8% of the variance of the change in tinnitus annoyance from T0 to T4. Out of 39 predictors, the only significant ones were "sick leave 6 months before treatment" and "tinnitus annoyance at T0."

Conclusion: The newly developed JITT represents a valuable treatment for chronic tinnitus patients with improvement remaining stable for at least 6 months after treatment. Using a large number of variables did not allow predicting treatment outcome which underlines the heterogeneity of tinnitus.

Keywords: chronic tinnitus, treatment, interdisciplinary, day care, prediction, tinnitus questionnaire

INTRODUCTION

Tinnitus is widely prevalent and is characterized by experiencing ringing, hissing or similar noises in one or both ears without an external acoustic source. This symptom is in its mild form most often transient, but persists in about 5–10% of the population, leading patients to seek treatment (Henry et al., 2005). As tinnitus is a sensory phenomenon, patients usually consult a physician. Moreover, since tinnitus is a symptom that can arise as a consequence of several disorders, it makes the diagnosis and the resulting treatment rather complex. Some of the possible tinnitus causes are exposure to loud noise, presbyacusis, cardiovascular and cerebrovascular diseases, drugs or medication, ear infections/inflammation, head or neck trauma, hyper- and hypo-thyroidism, Menière's disease, otosclerosis, sudden deafness, or vestibular schwannoma (Hoffman and Reed, 2004). The goal within the first 3 months (acute tinnitus) is to find the cause for the symptomatology and to treat it accordingly. However, in almost 50% of cases no physical origin of the tinnitus can be found (Feldmann, 1992; Lenarz, 1992), leaving the medical practitioner without causal treatment options. To make matters worse, the assumed cause of tinnitus is often successfully treated, but without any influence on the tinnitus itself. This argues in favor of a multifactorial cause, which is supported by the high heterogeneity seen in tinnitus patients.

When lasting more than 3 months and no response to medical treatment can be observed, tinnitus is generally considered as a chronic condition. While most people with chronic tinnitus are able to ignore the sound and do not feel impaired by it, approximately 3–5% of the general adult population perceive tinnitus as extremely bothersome, often to such an extent that it is difficult for them to carry out everyday activities (Davis and El Rafaie, 2000). The most prevalent complaints are concentration problems, mood changes as well as problems with sleep and hearing (Tyler and Baker, 1983; Henry et al., 2005). Additionally, high rates of comorbid psychiatric disorders such as depression, anxiety or somatoform disorders are observed in the group of tinnitus patients with bothersome tinnitus (Sullivan et al., 1988; Zöger et al., 2001). Thus, overall the patients are characterized by a rather large heterogeneity of associated symptoms.

One driving question for the development of therapeutic approaches is why some patients suffer from chronic tinnitus and others do not. Auditory aspects such as pitch, loudness and maskability have been found to be insufficient to explain tinnitus distress (Biesinger and Heiden, 1999; Bleich et al., 2001; Hausotter, 2004; Konzag et al., 2006; Hesse and Schaaf, 2007). One theory that tries to explain the co-occurrence of tinnitus and distress is the neurophysiological model of tinnitus (Jastreboff et al., 1996). According to this model, damage to the auditory pathways plays a crucial role in the development of tinnitus, while other parts of the nervous system (e.g. the limbic system) are responsible for developing tinnitus annoyance. Thus, the dysfunctional interplay between the two systems is responsible for the impact of the impairment on everyday life.

Currently, there is no scientifically proven therapy available that can be considered as a cure for chronic tinnitus. According to the American and German tinnitus guidelines (e.g., American Academy of Otolaryngology-Head Neck Surgery, 2014; German Society of Otorhinolaryngology Head, and Neck Surgery, 2015), the only realistic therapeutic goal is the determination of the tinnitus sensitizing antecedents and their therapeutic manageability, as well as the long term habituation to the phantom noise. Taken together, due to the high heterogeneity of tinnitus and the associated symptoms, an interdisciplinary approach for treatment recommends itself. A recent multidisciplinary systematic review emphasizes the combination of tinnitus specific counseling and cognitive behavior therapy. In the case of hearing loss, additional auditory therapeutic measures (e.g. hearing aids or cochlear implants) should be considered. Comorbidities such as depression should be treated additionally and, if necessary, with drugs (Zenner et al., 2016).

Despite the high prevalence of the impairment, there are only few specialized treatment centers in Germany, and the few existing recommendations for treatment are only rarely fulfilled in clinical practice (Hoare et al., 2012). Very often only inpatients receive interdisciplinary treatments, which is a financially expensive approach. To avoid high expenses, we implemented an interdisciplinary tinnitus treatment in our day care unit. The goal of the treatment was to reduce tinnitus annoyance by addressing the most frequent symptoms that patients with chronic tinnitus complain about: fear of tinnitus, problems with sleep and hearing, inability to relax and concentration problems. The individual treatment was tailored to the specific needs of a patient to account for the individual occurrence and combination of symptoms. Accordingly, we call this approach Jena Interdisciplinary Treatment for Tinnitus (JITT).

The aim of this study was (a) to observe the changes of tinnitus-related distress due to JITT, (b) to investigate in which patients tinnitus annoyance was most strongly expressed at the beginning of the treatment and (c) to explore if treatment success can be predicted.

MATERIALS AND METHODS

Assessment of Patients

The study was conducted in the Tinnitus-Center at the ENT department of Jena University Hospital, including one screening day, 5 days of day care treatment as well as two follow-up examinations (20 days and 6 months after treatment).

On the screening day all tinnitus patients underwent an examination by an ENT doctor, including ear microscopy, tinnitus case history and history of other ENT symptoms (particularly dizziness). All patients received routine audiometric evaluation including discrete-tone threshold testing and speech audiometry. Audiometry and tinnitus matching were done with calibrated audiometer (MAICO KS5) over Telephonics (TDH 39) headphones. Hearing level (HL in dB) was determined at following frequencies: 125, 250, 500, 750, 1,000, 1,500, 2,000, 3,000, 4,000, 6,000, and 8,000 Hz for the right and left ear for each individual. Pure tone average thresholds (4 PTA) were calculated over the frequencies of 500, 1,000, 2,000, and 4,000 Hz according to the WHO-standard (International Bureau for Audiophonology, 2017). In a second step, the frequency/pitch of the tinnitus was determined. When the patient reported binaural tinnitus, pitch was matched for each ear individually. In case of multiple tinnitus it was suggested that one should concentrate on the most troublesome tinnitus. The patients were asked whether the tinnitus sounds like a pure tone as just perceived during the audiometry, or if it sounds like a broad band or a narrow band noise. Under this directive pure tones or narrow bands of noise or broad band noise were presented to the tinnitus ear. If the pure tone threshold was too high to perceive a test signal at the side of the tinnitus, the contralateral better ear was used to present the sound. When tinnitus pitch was determined, subject's threshold was determined at that frequency. The procedure started at the frequency determined during pitch matching and at a level just below threshold. Then the intensity was increased in 1-dB steps until the patient signaled a match.

In cases of dizziness, vestibular testing was conducted. If indicated (e.g., asymmetric hearing loss, vertigo, headache), other diagnostic procedures (e.g., magnetic resonance imaging) or drug treatment were performed prior to treatment.

Tinnitus-related distress was assessed with the Tinnitus Questionnaire (TQ; Goebel and Hiller, 1998), a standard measure to differentiate patients with mild and severe tinnitus distress based on Hallam's Tinnitus-Questionnaire (Hallam, 1996). Specific fields of distress were assessed by subscales labeled as emotional and cognitive distress, intrusiveness, hearing problems, sleep disturbances, and somatic complaints evoked by the tinnitus. A total sum score ranging 0–30 implies mild tinnitus annoyance (grade 1), 31–46 moderate tinnitus annoyance (grade 2), 47–59 severe tinnitus annoyance (grade 3) and 60–84 very severe tinnitus annoyance (grade 4). The TQ is a standard questionnaire in tinnitus research showing good reliability in terms of retest-reliability ($r = 0.94$) and internal consistency (Cronbachs $\alpha = 0.94$). Validity coefficients are moderate to high for psychological distress ($r = 0.5$ up to >0.7) and high for tinnitus annoyance ($r = 0.69$–0.74). There is no agreement regarding which treatment-related change in the TQ-score is needed in order for a tinnitus condition to be considered as "improved" (Hall, 2016). The given relevant improvement of the score ranges from an absolute reduction of 5 points to a relative 20% reduction in TQ (Hiller and Haerkötter, 2005; Langguth et al., 2014).

Tinnitus is considered to be at a decompensated level (permanent annoyance and psychological strain) with a TQ score of 47 points or higher (grade 3 and 4) and to be at a compensated level (low secondary symptoms) at 46 points or lower (grade 1 and 2) (Lenarz, 1992; Goebel and Hiller, 1998; Stobik et al., 2005; Mazurek et al., 2009). Therefore, we defined a clinically relevant change as a change from a decompensated to a compensated level, i.e., below 47 points.

Screening of psychological symptoms included a semi-structured interview with a clinical psychologist as well as the full German version of the Patient Health Questionnaire (PHQ; Spitzer et al., 1999), consisting of somatic symptom, depressive mood, anxiety and stress scales. Patients with acute suicidal tendencies or severe psychiatric diagnoses, which prevented a benefit from the day care program, were referred to other specialists.

For the treatment to be covered by health insurance, two main inclusion criteria were mandatory: moderate to very severe tinnitus-related distress (measured by TQ) and tinnitus duration of more than 3 months (chronic tinnitus). Tinnitus patients who fulfilled these inclusion criteria and who accepted the treatment goal of tinnitus habituation were included. On average, one out of three tinnitus patients with an appointment in the ENT outpatient department fulfilled the inclusion criteria for the day care treatment. From those not included in the treatment, only 115 patients provided informed consent that the gathered data can be analyzed for scientific purposes. These data are presented in **Table 1**. The most frequent reasons for exclusion in this group were unwillingness to accept habituation as treatment goal (35%), low tinnitus-related distress measured by TQ (23%) or acute tinnitus (10%). If symptoms of anxiety or depression appeared too severe for treatment participation, patients were transferred to the psychiatric or psychotherapeutic department. Patient flow is shown in **Figure 1**.

Patient Sample and Treatment

Participants were 308 patients with chronic tinnitus, who fulfilled the above inclusion criteria and were treated in the day care unit of the ENT department of Jena University Hospital between July 2013 and December 2014 (the Tinnitus Center was founded in July 2013 and December 2014 served as the deadline for patient inclusion in the current study). Fifty-two Percent were male participants. The mean age of the sample was 57.08 years (±12.05, ranging from 22 to 81 years). Tinnitus onset was approximately 7 years (85.22 ± 94.88 months, ranging from 3 to 602 months) before treatment. At the first appointment, the tinnitus annoyance indexed by the TQ was 52.39 ± 11.92 points, which is considered as severe. Baseline characteristics of the patient population can be found in **Table 1**.

The interdisciplinary day care treatment lasted for 5 days (Monday to Friday) with an average of 7 h of therapy per day. Group therapy has been shown to be as effective as individual therapy (universality of the symptom, interpersonal learning, imparting of information, direct advice, imitative behavior, and instillation of hope for more see Yalom, 1995; Andersson and Lyttkens, 1999; Olderog, 1999). For this reason, about 80% (23 h/Week) of our day care treatment was conducted in closed

TABLE 1 | Baseline characteristics of tinnitus sample ($N = 308$) and excluded tinnitus-patients ($N = 115$).

Parameter		**Experimental Group ($N = 308$)**		**Excluded ($N = 115$)**		
Gender: male		52%		50%		
Age (M ± sd)		57.08 ± 12.05		58.53 ± 16.55		
Tinnitus duration (M ± sd)		85.22 ± 94.88		104. 95 ± 120.77		
Tinnitus-annoyance (TQ)		52.39 ± 11.92		48.68 ± 14.17		
Tinnitus grade	2 (mild)	32.8%		46.4%		
	3 (severe)	39.9%		28.2%		
	4 (very severe)	27.3%		22.7%		
Tinnitus duration	<1 year	16.6%		20.0%		
	1–5 years	37.3%		27.3%		
	>5 years	46.1%		52.7%		
Number of tinnitus sounds	1	74.7%		–		
	2	21.4%		–		
	3	1.9%		–		
Hyperacusis		57.1%		–		
Comorbid psychiatric disorder		20.5%		10%		
Parameter		**Ear: Left**	**Right**	**Ear: Left**	**Right**	
Hearing loss in dB (4 PTA: M ± sd)		28.58 ± 18.79	29.63 ± 21.22	33.27 ± 19.29	31.28 ± 16.57	
Parameter	**Left**	**Right**	**Both**	**Left**	**Right**	**Both**
Tinnitus localization	20.5%	15.9%	63.6%	15.2%	14.3%	70.5%
Hearing aid at baseline	5.3%	3.9%	41.9%			
Sound generator at baseline	0.3%	0.3%	0.3%			
Cochlear implant at baseline	0	0.3%	0			

4 PTA, pure tone average for 500 Hz, 1, 2, and 4 kHz; dB, decibel; M, arithmetic mean; sd, standard deviation.

groups of four to six tinnitus patients. Apart from the group therapy, every patient received several individual therapy sessions (6–7 h/Week) and was treated by an ENT doctor, a cognitive behavioral therapist, a specialist for medical rehabilitation and an audiologist. Therefore, the treatment was conducted within 4 modules, which will be described below. The selection of the modules is based on the "Algorithm for the Diagnostic & Therapeutic Management of Tinnitus" (Tinnitus Research Initiative: Biesinger et al., 2008) and the German S3 guideline for chronic tinnitus, in accordance with the recommendations from Zenner et al. (2015).

Module 1: ENT Counseling

Tinnitus-specific counseling has been repeatedly proven to be an effective way of diminishing tinnitus-related distress (Coles, 1995; Henry and Wilson, 1996; Hall and Ruth, 1999; Mazurek et al., 2006). For this reason, ENT doctors conducted tinnitus-specific counseling in a group setting according to the neurophysiological model of tinnitus (Jastreboff et al., 1996). The anatomy of the ear and auditory system, hearing processes as well as hearing impairment and possible mechanisms of tinnitus generation were explained. The benefit of sound therapy with sound enrichment, masker and hearing aids were discussed and patients' questions were answered. ENT counseling was performed in 3 h in group settings. In the individual sessions with ENT doctors, the tinnitus case history was taken into account and all diagnostic outcomes were explained in detail, setting a basis for an individual tinnitus model from a somatic point of view. Individual treatment options for the time after tinnitus day care treatment were discussed and planed.

Module 2: Cognitive Behavioral Therapy (CBT)

Considering the problems reported as tinnitus related (concentration loss, sleeping disorder, inability to relax, anxiety, depression, fear of aggravation, etc.), it is no surprise that CBT is one of the most validated treatments that reduces tinnitus-related distress (Frenzel, 1998; Andersson and Lyttkens, 1999; Olderog et al., 2004; Martines-Devesa et al., 2010; Cima et al., 2012; for a systematic review see Hesser et al., 2011b). There is a series of studies evidencing the effectiveness of CBT as an internet-based version (Andersson et al., 2002; Kaldo et al., 2008, 2013; Abbott et al., 2009; Hesser et al., 2011b, 2012; Jasper et al., 2014; Weise et al., 2016).

CBT was based on Delb et al. (2002) and Ivansic-Blau (2012) and was administered in 8 group sessions in closed group over 4 days. At first, the roles of attention and emotion in hearing process were explored. The vicious circle of tinnitus distress was explained and factors increasing/decreasing tinnitus awareness were explored. The habitation model of

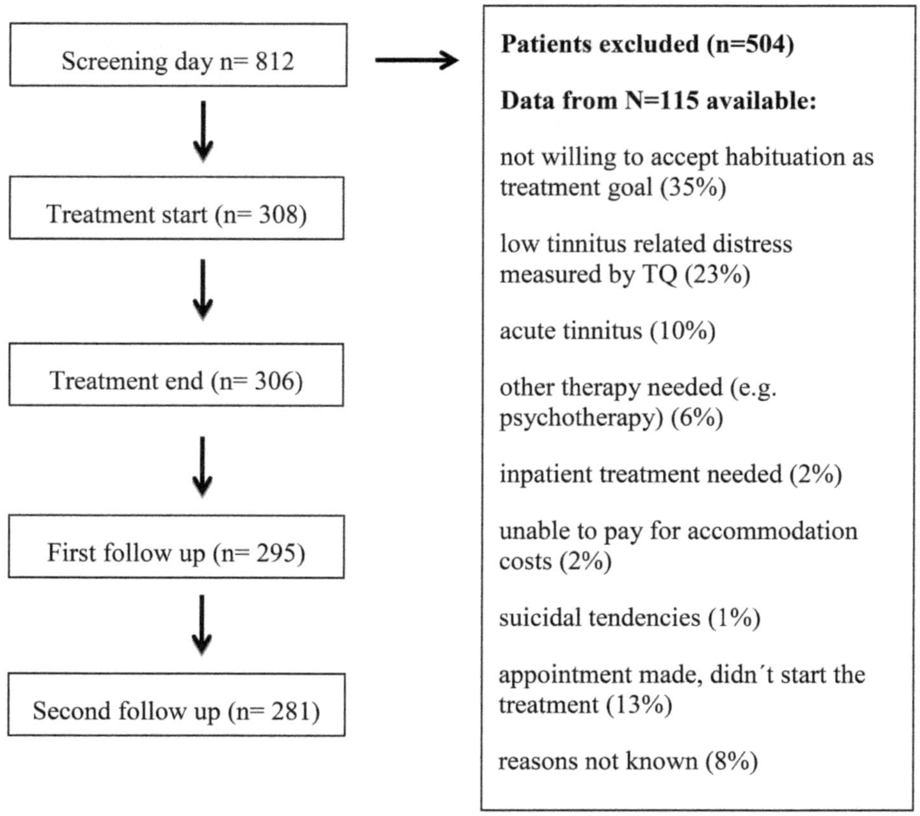

FIGURE 1 | Patient flow chart.

tinnitus (Hallam et al., 1984) was presented, which states that every unknown sound induces an orientation reaction of our body and increases attention to it. If the signal does not change, appears repeatedly and is not considered important, the amount of attention to the signal will reduce as a consequence of habituation. Most tinnitus patients habituate well to their tinnitus sound. Beliefs and emotions hindering habituation were analyzed. The ABC model from Rational-emotive therapy (RET; Ellis, 1993) was introduced and adapted to tinnitus. According to this model, people's beliefs (B) about one activating event (A) strongly affect their emotional and behavioral functioning (C), and not the event itself. Attention switching techniques were learned. Patients were educated about acute/chronic stress responses and about stress reduction techniques. Many tinnitus patients suffering from sleep problems consume alcohol or some medication to improve sleep. We taught our patients about normal sleep patterns and discussed how tinnitus influences sleep. Sleep hygiene recommendations were given and a beneficial sleeping environment (e.g., sound enriched) for tinnitus patients was explored.

In the individual therapy sessions with the CBT therapist an individual tinnitus model was developed, taking into account the following questions: Which individual factors accounted for the tinnitus onset? Which factors helped in dealing with tinnitus? What prevented the implementation of positive management strategies in everyday life? If necessary, patients were encouraged to apply for outpatient psychotherapy subsequent to the treatment in the Tinnitus-Center.

Module 3: Physiotherapy

One subtype of tinnitus is related to a dysfunction of the cervical spine, called cervicogenic somatic tinnitus. Previous research has shown that cervicogenic somatic tinnitus is present in 36–43% of the overall tinnitus population (Abel and Levine, 2004; Fabijanska et al., 2014; Ostermann et al., 2014; Michiels et al., 2015). For that reason, all tinnitus patients underwent physical examination by specialists for medical rehabilitation. In addition to a routine checkup, the influence of head movement, chewing or posture on tinnitus was examined. Individual therapy options for the time after the treatment were discussed and trained. Group physiotherapy was administrated on three consecutive days in 9 sessions, in duration of 50 min each. A physiotherapist conducted one session progressive muscle relaxation (Jacobson, 2006), one session back therapy training and one session physical therapy every day. The goal of the physiotherapy module was to teach patients stress reduction techniques on the one hand, and to expose the patients to ameliorating movement patterns on the other hand. As dysfunctional movements are a common cause for tinnitus aggravation, many tinnitus patients avoid exercise, losing in turn methods for stress reduction.

Module 4: Hearing Therapy

Hearing problems are one of most prevalent complaints of tinnitus patients. Significant hearing loss is found in 70–80% of tinnitus patients (Henry et al., 2005; Hesse and Schaaf, 2015) and the tinnitus frequency is usually within the range of the greatest hearing loss (Noreña et al., 2002). Hearing levels are displayed in **Figure 2**. However, inner ear damage is not necessarily obvious in the pure tone audiogram (Weisz et al., 2006; Schaette and McAlpine, 2011; Epp et al., 2012; Tan et al., 2013). Tinnitus patients with normal hearing thresholds have also more difficulties to understand speech in situations with background noise than persons without tinnitus (Hennig et al., 2011). Increased excitation, plasticity, and connectivity along the entire central auditory path can be compensatory responses to the reduced sensory input (De Ridder et al., 2011; Galazyuk et al., 2012; Stein et al., 2013).

To increase the sensory input, at the beginning of day care treatment, every patient was binaurally fitted with hearing aids and received Terzo® hearing therapy (Funk et al., 2008). Terzo® hearing therapy was originally developed for patients with profound hearing loss and combines hearing aid fitting with auditory speech-in-noise training (Terzo® auditory training). In this 1 h per day training, different stimuli and tasks (e.g., a sentence) were administered from a CD player and the responses (e.g., so-called "key words") were written down in a workbook. Similar to everyday life listening situations, tasks were presented with competing background noise. The Terzo® auditory training was available in three different difficulty levels defined by the initial signal-to-noise ratio (SNR). Depending on listening and comprehension abilities without hearing aids, the suitable training was individually selected. Signal-to-noise-ratio was adaptive and reduced every 2 days in 2 dB SNR. A key section of the workbook contained answers to all exercises, giving the tinnitus patients an important feedback of what was said in the particular sentences. This should increase the awareness for personal hearing (dis)ability. The hearing therapy lasted for 25 days starting at the first day of day care treatment and was continued at home. Terzo® hearing therapy is currently under evaluation; the results will be presented elsewhere.

Follow-up

The first follow-up measurement took part 20 days after the end of the day care treatment. All patients completed the TQ and gave anonymous feedback about the treatment, involving ratings of each treatment module as "very helpful," "helpful," "somewhat helpful," and "not helpful." Hearing aid log data were uploaded and Terzo® hearing therapy workbooks were evaluated. In an individual session with an ENT doctor, it was considered whether patients wanted to continue wearing hearing aids in the future or not. If so, hearing aids were subscribed.

The second follow-up was conducted 6 months after the end of day care treatment. In the individual session with an ENT doctor the treatment was evaluated once more, and patients had a possibility to ask questions or inquire about further help. In a group session with a CBT therapist the personally most useful strategies for reduction of tinnitus-related distress were summarized and problems with implementation of the new, favorable behaviors in everyday life were discussed. All patients completed the TQ once more.

Data were collected before the treatment when each patient was screened (T0), at the beginning (T1) and at the end of the 5 day treatment (T2), as well as 20 days (T3) and 6 months after treatment (T4). In case of missing data (**Figure 1**), we used the last observation carried forward method (Bortz and Döring, 2006). The dependent variable was tinnitus annoyance measured with TQ and its subscales (emotional and cognitive distress, intrusiveness, hearing problems, sleep disturbance, and somatic complains). To identify differences over time, repeated measures analysis of variance (ANOVA) was performed. When significant, *post hoc* testing with Bonferroni correction was performed. To determine the magnitude of change between two points of assessment, effect sizes (ES) using the *d* statistic of Cohen (1992) were calculated; ES between 0.2 and 0.5 are considered as small, from 0.5 to 0.8 as medium and higher than 0.8 as large. The possible impact of patient characteristics on tinnitus annoyance at T0 was tested with Wilcoxon rank sum tests for dichotomized values or with correlations for variables with an interval scale. Regression analysis was used to investigate factors associated with a change in tinnitus annoyance due to treatment. The dependent variable in the regression analysis was change in TQ scores between T0 and T4. The following variables were included in the first regression analysis as independent variables:

- Demographics: age, gender
- Tinnitus-related: duration, localization, frequency, type of onset, subjective loudness, maskability, type of sound, number of sounds, presence during the day, change due to somatic factors like head or jaw movements, change to psychological factors like stress
- Strain variables: baseline TQ score, hearing loss, sound intolerance, sick leave 6 months before treatment, somatic symptoms, depressive mood, anxiety, stress, comorbid psychological disorder
- Otological comorbidity: Menière's disease, dizziness, ear barotrauma, sudden hearing loss, otosclerosis, chronic otitis media, vestibular schwannoma, acoustic trauma

In a second regression analysis, we additionally included "early change" as a predictor. This variable was defined as the TQ change from T0 to T1, i.e., before the actual day care treatment began.

This study was carried out in accordance with the recommendations of ICH harmonized tripartite guideline for Good Clinical Practice, as well as the Declaration of Helsinki. All 308 study participants gave their written informed consent that they were willing to take part in the treatment and that the gathered data can be analyzed for scientific purposes. The protocol was approved by the ethics committee of the Jena University Hospital (4366-03/15).

RESULTS

Treatment Compliance

Overall, treatment compliance was excellent with very low dropout rates (0.6%, $N = 2$) and with 95.2% of patients taking

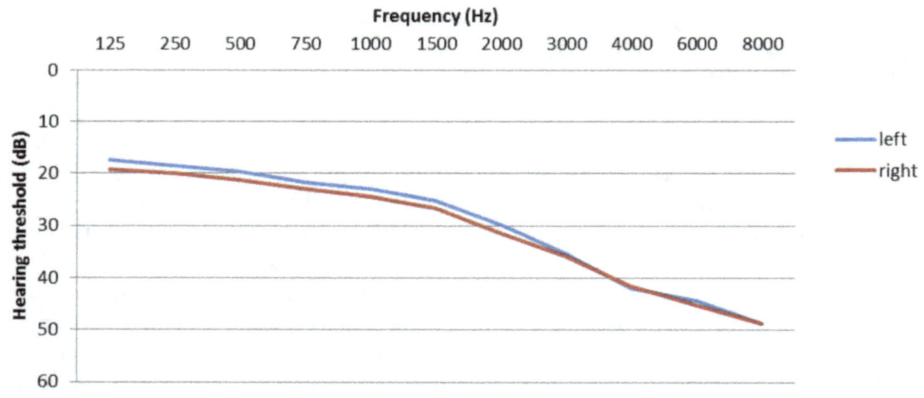

FIGURE 2 | Hearing thresholds.

part in all sessions. According to data logs from the hearing aids at the first follow-up, hearing aids were used for 7.80 ± 4.13 h/day for 21.64 ± 7.79 days (87% of intended 25 days). Almost 90% (89.86%) of the patients completed all tasks of the hearing training.

The anonymous questioner ratings of treatment modules at the end of the treatment showed that all modules were mostly rated as "very helpful" or "helpful": ENT counseling 99%, CBT 99%, physiotherapy 92%, and hearing therapy 92%. As an example, 99% of patients indicated that they would recommend the treatment to family members if they would suffer from chronic tinnitus.

General Treatment Effects

Our treatment goal was to reduce the tinnitus-related annoyance. The repeated measures ANOVA showed that there was a statistical significant difference in tinnitus annoyance measured with TQ over time ($F_{(4,\,304)} = 202.201, p < 0.001$).

The *post hoc* analysis for tinnitus distress showed a significant reduction from T0 to T1 ($t_{(307)} = 6.737, p < 0.001$; from 52.36 ± 11.95 to 48.79 ± 13.74; Cohen's $d = 0.29$, i.e., a small effect), and an even larger reduction from T1 to T2 ($t_{(307)} = 22.710, p < 0.001$; from 48.79 ± 13.74 to 34.29 ± 14.98; Cohen's $d = 1.51$, i.e., a large effect). In comparison to T2, significant changes in tinnitus distress were observed neither at T3 ($t_{(307)} = 0.021, p = 0.983$), nor at T4 ($t_{(307)} = 0.378, p = 0.706$), implying that the outcome remained stable for at least 6 months.

To investigate in more detail which specific tinnitus-related problems did undergo changes over time, we performed repeated measures ANOVA for each TQ subscale. The results are summarized in **Table 2**. The overall changes over time in all TQ subscales were significant ($p < 0.001$). The *post hoc* analyses showed that the results in 4 subscales (emotional and cognitive distress, intrusiveness and sleep disturbance) were significantly reduced from T0 to T1 and from T2 to T3, but remained stable from T2 to both T3 and T4. In two subscales, namely in subscales "hearing problems" and "somatic complains," no change appeared from T0 to T1, but there was a significant reduction from treatment begin (T1) to treatment end (T2), remaining stable at T3 and T4.

Predictors of Tinnitus Annoyance at Baseline

To identify which patient subgroups suffer more from tinnitus, we dichotomized the tinnitus patients in subgroups according to baseline characteristics (e.g., tinnitus onset involving/not involving pressure in ears), and compared differences in tinnitus annoyance between these subgroups at T0. If variables were continuous (e.g., tinnitus duration), we correlated them with TQ sum scores at T0. The results are presented in **Tables 3, 4**.

Patients with the following symptoms displayed higher tinnitus annoyance at T0: dizziness at tinnitus onset, tinnitus sound could not be masked with background noise, tinnitus worsening during physical stress (e.g., exercise), subjective hearing loss, comorbid psychiatric diagnosis (ICD-10) as well as acute multiple somatic complaints, depressive mood, anxiety and high stress level according to PHQ (Spitzer et al., 1999). Higher tinnitus annoyance at the first appointment was correlated with higher age and higher hearing loss. While tinnitus loudness (tinnitus matching, dB) in the right ear correlated with tinnitus annoyance at T0 significantly, there was no correlation for the left ear.

Predictors of Treatment Success

To learn if all tinnitus annoyance subgroups benefit from treatment, patients were classified into 3 groups (moderate, severe, and very severe tinnitus annoyance) depending on their TQ scores at T0, and repeated measures ANOVAs were performed for each subgroup. As can be seen in **Table 5** as well as in **Figure 3**, all three subgroups had a significant overall change in tinnitus annoyance over time (see Data Sheet 1 in the Supplementary Material for individual change in each subgroup). *Post hoc* t-tests with Bonferroni correction showed the following:

In the subgroup with *moderate tinnitus annoyance* there was no change in tinnitus annoyance from T0 to T1, but from T1 to T2 tinnitus annoyance reduced significantly by 11 points at TQ, changing the grading of tinnitus annoyance from "moderate" to

TABLE 2 | Tinnitus Questionnaire subscale scores over time and results of repeated measures analysis of variance (ANOVA).

TQ subscales (Min-Max)	T0 Baseline M (sd)	T1 Therapy begin M (sd)	T2 Therapy end M (sd)	T3 1st follow up (2.5 weeks) M (sd)	T4 2nd follow up (6 months) M (sd)	F	df	p*
Hearing problems (0–14)	7.21 (3.59)	7.36 (3.37)	5.57^{a,b} (3.22)	5.49^{a,b} (3.37)	5.40^{a,b} (3.42)	53.18	4/304	**<0.001**
Emotional distress (0–24)	14.77 (4.31)	13.23^{a} (4.82)	8.84^{a,b} (4.88)	8.74^{a,b} (5.26)	8.57^{a,b} (5.55)	189.37	4/304	**<0.001**
Cognitive distress (0–16)	10.15 (3.28)	8.94^{a} (3.71)	5.41^{a,b} (3.82)	5.67^{a,b} (4.02)	5.84^{a,b} (4.18)	184.20	4/304	**<0.001**
Intrusiveness (0–16)	12.62 (2.22)	12.05^{a} (2.61)	9.07^{a,b} (3.22)	9.08^{a,b} (3.60)	9.18^{a,b} (3.79)	133.97	4/304	**<0.001**
Sleep disturbance (0–8)	4.67 (2.36)	4.41^{a} (2.42)	3.30^{a,b} (2.54)	3.21^{a,b} (2.59)	3.11^{a,b} (2.56)	68.16	4/304	**<0.001**
Somatic complains (0–6)	2.91 (1.85)	2.81 (1.91)	2.10^{a,b} (1.76)	2.09^{a,b} (1.88)	1.93^{a,b} (1.80)	39.02	4/304	**<0.001**

*TQ, Tinnitus Questionnaire (Goebel and Hiller, 1998); M, arithmetic mean; sd, standard deviation; Min–Max, Range of subscale; [a]Significant change ($p < 0.05$ corrected) to baseline according to paired t-test with Bonferroni correction; [b]Significant change ($p < 0.05$ corrected) to T1 according to paired t-test with Bonferroni correction; *Significant values ($p < 0.05$) in bold.*

TABLE 3 | Baseline difference in tinnitus annoyance measured with Tinnitus Questionnaire between patient-subgroups.

Variable	Tinnitus annoyance M ± sd (N)				p (Mann-Whitney U-Test)
Gender	**Male**		**Female**		
	52.49 ± 12.12	(156)	52.22 ± 11.81	(152)	0.824
Tinnitus onset	**Subtle**		**Sudden**		
	52.48 ± 11.58	(114)	52.91 ± 12.39	(130)	0.727
Symptom reported by patient	**Yes**		**No**		
Tinnitus onset involving pressure in ears	54.39 ± 11.73	(61)	52.02 ± 11.98	(184)	0.129
Tinnitus onset involving hearing loss	53.43 ± 11.10	(67)	52.52 ± 12.20	(178)	0.433
Tinnitus onset involving dizziness	**56.59 ± 12.53**	**(51)**	**51.70 ± 11.49**	**(196)**	**0.007**
Tinnitus masked trough background noise	**51.59 ± 11.80**	**(208)**	**54.67 ± 12.06**	**(78)**	**0.050**
Tinnitus gets louder in noise	53.83 ± 12.83	(88)	52.01 ± 11.62	(146)	0.233
Noise sensitivity	53.76 ± 12.42	(176)	53.45 ± 11.11	(107)	0.111
Physical stress leads to tinnitus change	**54.54 ± 12.37**	**(109)**	**51.32 ± 11.40**	**(179)**	**0.029**
Emotional stress leads to tinnitus change	52.70 ± 11.97	(211)	52.05 ± 11.93	(77)	0.576
Jaw movement leads to tinnitus change	51.14 ± 12.73	(42)	52.74 ± 11.66	(234)	0.273
Head movement leads to tinnitus change	52.33 ± 11.31	(39)	52.41 ± 11.99	(241)	0.971
Sudden hearing loss in the past	52.57 ± 11.36	(49)	52.32 ± 12.07	(259)	0.739
Current subjective hearing loss	**53.66 ± 11.57**	**(196)**	**49.27 ± 12.52**	**(66)**	**0.015**
Comorbid psychiatric disorder (ICD-10 Checklist)	**Yes**		**No**		
	57.65 ± 12.86	**(63)**	**50.91 ± 11.28**	**(244)**	**<0.001**
Psychological symptoms (PHQ)	**High**		**Low**		
Depressive mood	**49.31 ± 11.28**	**(112)**	**57.96 ± 11.65**	**(173)**	**<0.001**
Anxiety	**50.36 ± 11.50**	**(78)**	**57.62 ± 12.60**	**(207)**	**<0.001**
Somatic complains	**49.64 ± 11.68**	**(138)**	**55.97 ± 11.86**	**(147)**	**<0.001**
Stress	**51.92 ± 12.19**	**(49)**	**56.18 ± 11.64**	**(237)**	**0.029**

PHQ, Patient Health Questionnaire (Spitzer et al., 1999); M, arithmetic mean; sd, standard deviation; N, number of patients in each category. Significant values ($p < 0.05$) in bold.

"mild" and remaining constant at T3 and T4. Cohen's effect size of this change from T0 to T4 is $d = 1.66$.

In the subgroup with *severe tinnitus annoyance* a significant reduction of tinnitus annoyance from T0 to T1 by 4 points in TQ was observed, but grading of the tinnitus annoyance did not change. During treatment the significant change of tinnitus annoyance in TQ (17 points) was observed, shifting tinnitus grading from "severe" to "moderate," achieving a clinical change and remaining stable at T3 and T4. Cohen's effect size of this change from T0 to T4 is $d = 1.91$.

TABLE 4 | Correlation with tinnitus annoyance measured with Tinnitus Questionnaire at baseline.

Variable	Pearson's *r*	*p*
Age	**0.131**	**0.022**
Tinnitus duration	0.109	0.057
Number of tinnitus sounds	**0.152**	**0.008**
Hearing loss in left ear (4 PTA)	**0.247**	**<0.001**
Hearing loss in right ear (4 PTA)	**0.263**	**<0.001**
Tinnitus frequency right	−0.130	0.633
Tinnitus frequency left	−0.101	0.562
Tinnitus loudness dB right	**0.631**	**0.021**
Tinnitus loudness dB left	0.125	0.494

4 PTA, pure tone average for 500 Hz, 1, 2 and 4 kHz. Significant values ($p < 0.05$) in bold.

In the subgroup with *very severe tinnitus annoyance* there was a significant reduction in tinnitus annoyance from T0 to T1 by 7 points in TQ, without the change in grading of the tinnitus annoyance. During treatment a further change of tinnitus annoyance in TQ (14 points) was observed leading to a change in tinnitus grading from "very severe" to "severe" with no further reduction at T3 and T4. Cohen's effect size of this change from T0 to T4 is $d = 1.47$.

To analyze, which factors predict the change of tinnitus annoyance during treatment, we used the difference between T0 and T4 in TQ sum score as dependent variable (Bonate, 2000). After including various personal, tinnitus and strain variables as independent variables in a multiple regression analysis, the model could explain only 12.8% of the variance (R Square = 0.128) if all predictors were used. Because this model explained only so little of the variance despite the large number of predictors used, we refrained from using stepwise procedures. The only significant predictors were "sick leave 6 months before treatment onset" (B = 7.190, SE B = 3.268, ß = 0.148, $p = 0.016$) and "tinnitus annoyance at T0" (B = 0.204, SE B = 0.081, ß = 0.171, $p = 0.012$). Including "early change" as a predictor in second regression analysis allowed to explain 27.4% (R Square = 0.274) of the variance with "early change" being the strongest predictor (B = −0.661, SE B = 0.90, ß = −0.429, $p < 0.001$).

DISCUSSION AND CONCLUSION

For most patients with tinnitus annoyance, the only available therapy option at the moment is a basic ENT examination, because all other guideline recommended therapies are hardly available (at least in Germany). Even though German public health insurance covers the cost for CBT for decompensated chronic tinnitus, the barrier to seek help at a psychotherapist (e.g., public, perceived and self-stigmatizing attitudes to mental illness or difficulty identifying the symptoms of mental illness; for more see Gulliver et al., 2010) is high. This significantly reduces the number of those taking part in CBT. Only patients with very severe tinnitus annoyance and comorbid psychiatric diagnosis receive interdisciplinary stationary treatment covered by the German public health insurance.

A fixed duration for a given intervention and the subsequent decrease in the resources needed for accommodation (overnight rooms, beds, meals, night-shift employees, etc.) would reduce the overall costs and makes them predictable. For this reason we developed a 5-day day care treatment program (JITT), in order to fill the need for a broadly available interdisciplinary treatment for tinnitus. We measured the changes in tinnitus annoyance from an initial consultation (T0) up to 6 months after the end of treatment (T4). To summarize the results briefly, the developed treatment is highly promising in reducing tinnitus annoyance and treatment effects remained stable until at least 6 months after the end of the day care program. This was indexed by the generally high compliance and the overall measure for tinnitus annoyance from the TQ. While inspecting this questionnaire in more detail, it turned out that complaints about emotional and cognitive distress, intrusiveness and disturbed sleep, already improved to some degree after initial consultation (T0), but improved even more in response to the day care treatment (T1–T4). In contrast, complaints about hearing and somatic problems improved only upon treatment. High annoyance was characterized at T0 by several somatic and psychiatric symptoms, but predicting the outcome of treatment proved unsatisfactory. We will discuss each of these aspects below.

General Treatment Effects and Compliance

The general index for tinnitus annoyance demonstrated a considerable reduction from the first consultation (T0) to the final measurement (T4). There was not only a reduction upon the treatment itself, but already earlier, i.e., between the first appointment (T0) and the start of the daycare treatment (T1) corresponding to 4 points in TQ. We assume that this reduction is the outcome of the extensive diagnostic procedures paired with a first, very brief counseling, reassuring the patient that no severe physical abnormality was detected. This information by itself obviously provided some relief. Support for this assumption is provided by a change in the subscales on emotional and cognitive distress as well as intrusiveness and sleep disturbance, but not in the scales addressing hearing and somatic problems. Similarly, waiting for the treatment and certainty of "getting help soon" could have induced this reduction (T0–T1). A meta-analysis of 11 studies included 314 individuals with tinnitus distress that were randomly allocated to a waiting phase lasting 6–12 weeks (Hesser et al., 2011a). The patients revealed a mean decrease in symptom severity between 3 and 8% (Hedges' $g = 0.17$). Thus, already in response to a waiting period tinnitus patients improve slightly on psychometrically robust tinnitus-specific measures.

In our study, the effect size of the overall change before the start of the day care treatment is considered as small. Consequently, at the beginning of treatment the mean tinnitus annoyance was on average still severe. This means that broad and interdisciplinary (ENT doctor, psychologist and audiologist) diagnostics and counseling leads to a significant reduction of tinnitus annoyance, but it does not lead to patients reaching the non-severe range. Perhaps this is why many patients reported during treatment that they were already somewhat relieved after the primary consultation in our clinic or elsewhere, but that they did not know how to cope better with tinnitus in the future.

TABLE 5 | TQ sum scores over time and results of repeated measures analysis of variance (ANOVA) as well as *post hoc* *t*-tests.

Tinnitus annoyance	T0 Baseline	T1 Therapy begin	T2 Therapy end	T3 1st follow up (2.5 weeks)	T4 2nd follow up (6 months)	*F*	*df*	*p**
	M (sd)	*M* (sd)	*M* (sd)	(M sd)	*M* (sd)			
Moderate ($N = 101$)	38.77 (4.46)	37.24 (9.14)	25.38^{a,b} (10.06)	25.98^{a,b} (11.84)	24.13^{a,b} (11.64)	56.21	4/97	**<0.001**
Severe ($N = 123$)	53.24 (3.83)	49.46^{a} (10.09)	32.07^{a,b} (12.00)	31.77^{a,b} (13.37)	32.49^{a,b} (14.91)	118.96	4/119	**<0.001**
Very severe ($N = 84$)	67.39 (5.29)	61.71^{a} (10.77)	47.52^{a,b} (15.10)	48.32^{a,b} (17.05)	48.17^{a,b} (17.59)	49.45	4/80	**<0.001**

[a]*Significant change (p < 0.05 corrected) to baseline according to paired t-test with Bonferroni correction;* [b]*Significant change (p < 0.05 corrected) to T1 according to paired t-test with Bonferroni correction; *significant values (p < 0.05) in bold.*

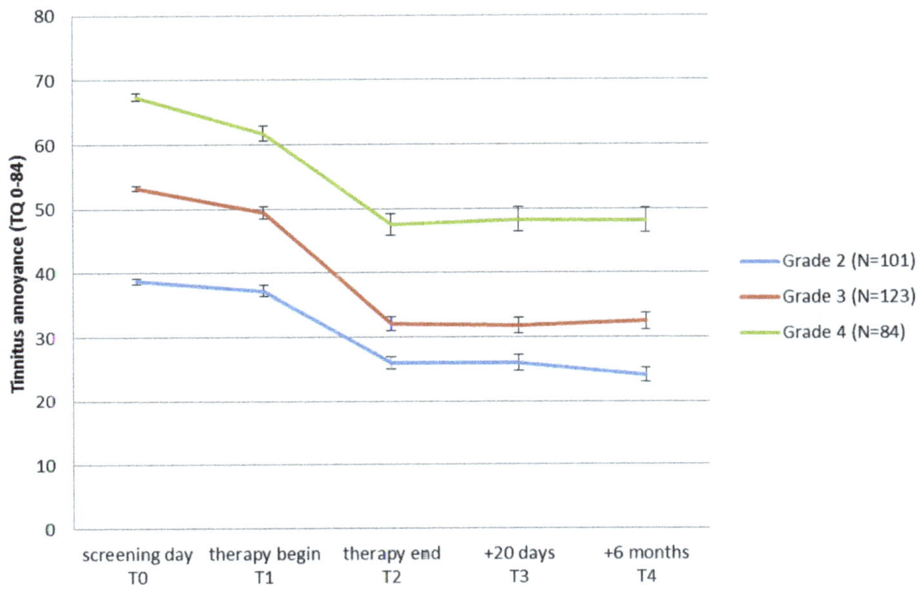

FIGURE 3 | Change of tinnitus annoyance measured with Tinnitus Questionnaire (TQ: Goebel and Hiller, 1998) over time. A higher score represents a higher annoyance. Mean values for patient-groups which started the JITT with moderate (grade 2), severe (grade 3), and very severe (grade 4) tinnitus annoyance are shown. Standard errors of mean are plotted for each point in time and group.

The change in tinnitus annoyance from the beginning (T1) to the end of treatment (T2) is in comparison to the earlier effect considerable, reaching a large effect size with a change in the TQ sum score of further 15 points (in total 18 points); i.e., the mean tinnitus annoyance at treatment end is in the moderate range. This clinically relevant improvement from a decompensated, clinically severe state to a compensated, moderate state remained stable at follow-ups 20 days as well as 6 months later. In contrast to the different responsiveness of subscales for the early change, all TQ subscales reduced significantly upon treatment. Currently, we have no evidence on which of the modules proved more or less successful, but patients considered all modules important.

In general, reported TQ changes in response to different therapeutic approaches differ widely: between 5.2 points (Rief et al., 2005), 7.8 points (Goebel, 1995), 13 points (Haerkötter, 2001), 18.6 points (Weise, 2008), and up to 23.2 points (Weise et al., 2007). Most often the changes at follow-up are smaller compared to the end of treatment, but still significantly larger compared to the onset of treatment (Jakes et al., 1992). As such, JITT seems highly promising, but we also would like to point out several difficulties in directly comparing the different approaches.

The efficacy of most tinnitus management interventions recommended for clinical practice remains to be demonstrated. Currently, only few studies allow making informed conclusions. The efficacy of therapist-delivered CBT appears to be reasonably established (e.g., Hoare et al., 2011). A multidisciplinary CBT-based approach, in which professionals in audiology and psychology share treatment goals aimed at coping with tinnitus through education and counseling, is likely to optimize the benefit for patients (Cima et al., 2012). Thus, multidisciplinary approach was recommended for some time (Henry and Wilson, 1996; El Refaie et al., 2004; Andersson et al., 2005; Henry et al., 2005; Cima et al., 2009; Hoare et al., 2011).

Nevertheless, there are only few researchers reporting the effects of multidisciplinary treatment, often with the limitation that only inpatients of a specialized hospital were examined (Goebel, 1998, 2008; Hiller and Goebel, 1999; Goebel et al., 2006;

Schaaf et al., 2017). These patients are known to be generally more severely impaired and suffer from more psychological complaints than the average patients of ENT practitioners or audiological outpatient departments (Hiller and Goebel, 1999). Therefore, results obtained from inpatient treatment do not seem representative of an outpatient population.

Mazurek et al. (2005) described a 7-day day care interdisciplinary tinnitus-treatment and evaluated it on 46 outpatients. Tinnitus annoyance was reduced significantly from 33.8 points to 27.8 points after 7 days and continued to attenuate to 25.2 points 6 months after treatment. A significant reduction in TQ was observed up to 3 years after treatment (Seydel et al., 2015).

In a large randomized clinical trial, a multidisciplinary stepped care approach involving counseling and elements of CBT and tinnitus retraining therapy (TRT) demonstrated a significant reduction in tinnitus severity (from 49.39 points in TQ to 36.47 points in TQ after 8 months) and tinnitus impairment, as well as improvement of health-related quality of life as compared to usual care (Cima et al., 2012).

Even though the optimal exposure-response relation between number of hours in treatment and outcome remains unknown (Andersson, 2002), the burden for patients and clinicians, as well as the cost-benefit ratio are important (Hoare et al., 2011). JITT lasted 5 days with 2 follow-ups, while other authors report up to 2 years of contact with patients (e.g., Von Wedel and von Wedel, 2000). The very low dropout rate in our study (<1%) suggests that tinnitus patients were generally satisfied with the treatment and that 5 days of treatment seemed to be a reasonable amount of time patients were willing to invest. Such a low dropout rate is remarkable given the much higher rates reported in a review of CBT for tinnitus patients with dropouts ranging between 5 and 22% (Martines-Devesa et al., 2010). These rates were even higher when CBT was delivered via internet (51% in Andersson et al., 2002; 75% in Abbott et al., 2009), even though there was no difference in the reduction of tinnitus annoyance between internet-delivered or therapist-delivered CBT (Kaldo et al., 2008).

Predictors of Tinnitus Annoyance

To describe the heterogeneity of tinnitus patients and in the search for factors related to tinnitus annoyance at T0, we found that patients with the following symptoms displayed higher tinnitus annoyance at the beginning of treatment: dizziness at tinnitus onset, tinnitus sound could not be masked with background noise, tinnitus worsening during physical stress (e.g., exercise), subjective hearing loss, comorbid psychiatric diagnosis (ICD-10) as well as acute multiple somatic complaints, depressive mood, anxiety and high stress level according to PHQ (Spitzer et al., 1999). Additionally, higher tinnitus annoyance at the first appointment was correlated with higher age and greater hearing loss and tinnitus loudness (only for the right ear). This relation is supported by a series of studies that we will briefly review below.

The association between hearing loss and tinnitus corroborates earlier research and is a long standing finding. Prevalence of hearing loss increases with age (Davis, 1995), hearing loss increases the risk for developing tinnitus (Hoffman and Reed, 2004), and on a population level there is a linear increase in tinnitus annoyance with increasing age (Davis and El Rafaie, 2000; Andersson et al., 2005). Studies indicate that 70–80% of tinnitus patients have significant hearing difficulties (Henry et al., 2005; Hesse and Schaaf, 2015). Other studies also reported the positive link between higher hearing loss and higher tinnitus distress (e.g., Goebel and Hiller, 1999; Davis and El Rafaie, 2000; Stobik et al., 2003). For example, Savastano (2008) investigated 520 persons suffering from tinnitus and compared tinnitus patients with and without hearing loss. The author found that subjective discomfort is higher in the presence of hearing loss than in the case of normal hearing (according to Bureau International D'Audiophonologie pure tone average for 500 Hz, 1, 2, and 4 kHz < 20 dB). Among subjects with normal hearing, the level of disturbance was mostly in the moderate range, whereas among subjects with hearing loss, the level of disturbance was mostly elevated. Savastano concluded that the presence of hearing loss increases the complaint of tinnitus considerably, even if the hearing deficit is not severe.

Similarly, the correlation of tinnitus annoyance with otological symptoms reported here corroborates earlier research. Goebel and Hiller (2007) found a strong association between otological conditions and the development of high annoyance: subjects with additional hearing loss and dizziness/vertigo reported both higher loudness and higher annoyance. When subjects with high versus low annoyance were compared, the following odds ratios (OR) were found: hearing loss OR = 5.64 and dizziness/vertigo OR = 3.76. Hallam and Stephens (1985) found that tinnitus patients who complained of dizziness also suffered from higher emotional distress. Both Erlandsson et al. (1992) and Langenbach et al. (2005) observed a worsening of mood and tinnitus symptoms when tinnitus was accompanied by vertigo. The latter study also confirms our finding that loudness of the tinnitus perceived in the right ear correlated with higher tinnitus annoyance at the first appointment. Thus, the sound perceived in the right ear has a stronger impact on the associated emotional processes. This mechanism is not well understood and should be investigated in future studies.

The association between high tinnitus annoyance and poor maskability was also reported in several studies. Goebel and Hiller (1999) reported higher tinnitus annoyance when maskability was poor. Maskability of tinnitus at admission to CBT was a predictor of tinnitus-related distress at a 5-year follow-up (Andersson et al., 2001). Stobik et al. (2005) compared patients with low/moderate and severe/very severe tinnitus distress and also found that patients with severe/very severe tinnitus reported greater difficulty to mask their tinnitus with background sounds.

The relationship between tinnitus and emotional distress or psychiatric problems has long been recognized and is well documented, at least in the help-seeking group (Harrop-Griffiths et al., 1987; Dobie et al., 1992; Andersson, 2002). Sixty-three to seventy-seven percent of tinnitus inpatients have at least one psychiatric diagnosis (mostly mood or anxiety disorder; Kaldo, 2008). The prevalence of concurrent depression or mood disorders ranges between 39 and 60%, whereas the lifetime prevalence amounts to 62–78% (Andersson, 2002). Other psychological causes of distress associated with tinnitus include anxiety, depression, irritability, anger, and insomnia (Wilson et al., 1991). Approximately half of the patients with tinnitus without severe hearing impairment also suffer from psychiatric disorders, the most frequent being anxiety disorders and mood disorders (Zöger et al., 2001). Belli et al. (2008) applied the Structured Clinical Interview for DSM-III-R at 90 acute tinnitus patients and found that 24.4% had at least one axis-I psychiatric diagnosis. The most prevalent disorders were anxiety, somatoform and mood disorders. Only 6% of controls without tinnitus had at least one axis-I psychiatric diagnosis. Depression, sleep disorders and difficulties in concentration were significant predictors of tinnitus annoyance (Scott et al., 1990). Erlandsson and Hallberg (2000) investigated in 122 tinnitus inpatients which factors predict quality of life, and found that impaired concentration, feeling depressed and perceived negative attitudes were the most significant predictors and explained most of the variance in quality of life. In the study from Langenbach et al. (2005) on acute tinnitus, insomnia attributed to tinnitus was the best predictor and accounted for 34% of the variance of tinnitus distress 6 months after tinnitus onset. Anxiety in the acute phase accounted for 30% of variance of tinnitus distress, while life satisfaction and somatic complaints accounted together for 41% of the variance.

We conclude that our results of predicting tinnitus annoyance corroborate previous results. Taking Jastreboff's neurophysiological model of tinnitus into account, the negative impact of these symptoms on developing tinnitus annoyance is quite obvious. As the frequency of the individually perceived tinnitus is very likely to be in the range with the highest hearing loss (Henry et al., 1999; Noreña et al., 2002), the masking of tinnitus with background sounds is, in the case of hearing loss, not possible any more. Habituation inhibits tolerance to a stimulus because of its unpredictability. This is possibly why the variability of tinnitus during physical stress attracts attention to the phantom sound, making it difficult to habituate, which in turn leads to higher annoyance. If a person experiences tinnitus onset simultaneously with dizziness, the fear evoked by dizziness will be associated with the noise according to the principles of classical conditioning. Whenever tinnitus is perceived as a danger, no habituation can be achieved. This risk certainly gets higher, due to the belief that hearing loss or dizziness is caused by tinnitus, which is something that many of our patients reported. In the same direction, emotional distress or psychiatric problems are generally regarded as factors hindering habituation.

Predictors of Treatment Outcome

Inspecting changes in tinnitus annoyance in response to treatment, data from patients with moderate, severe and very severe tinnitus annoyance reached high effect sizes. But if we consider only a clinically significant change, JITT displays the strongest effects in patients with severe tinnitus (grade 3). Although tinnitus annoyance is significantly reduced in patients with very severe tinnitus (grade 4), the 5-day treatment is not sufficient to lead to a clinically significant change in this group. Perhaps this group of patients needs an extended duration of JITT or some other outpatient therapeutic approaches. Another possibility would be intensive inpatient care, which however removes patients from their daily routine. Also other researchers found that patients with high tinnitus annoyance at baseline were more often non-responders (Rübler, 1997; Frenzel, 1998) in outpatient setting.

Demographic, tinnitus and strain variables explained only 12.8% of the variance of the change in tinnitus annoyance from T0 to T4. The only predictors for reduction of tinnitus-related distress were "sick leave 6 months before the treatment onset" and "tinnitus annoyance at T0." Patients who were on sick leave before the treatment or with high tinnitus annoyance at T0 showed less improvement in tinnitus annoyance from treatment begin to the final follow-up. We did not inquire further why the patients were on sick leave, but they most likely experienced somatic/psychological symptoms to such an extent that they were unable to continue with their daily activities. The 5-day treatment was perhaps too short for this subgroup. It is yet unclear if they would benefit from a longer treatment duration or a combination of treatments as suggested below. Including "early change" as a predictor allowed to explain 27.4% of the variance, i.e., considerably more. Early change has generally proven to be a strong predictor in psychotherapy and CBT in particular (Schibbye et al., 2014). We did not include this variable in the first regression analysis, because it already requires knowledge about the responsiveness of a patient which was not given at T0. Nevertheless, it constitutes an early and easy calculable indicator who will respond to treatment and who is more resilient. Providing knowledge about early change to therapists could result in more effective treatment (Lambert and Ogles, 2003). Measuring early change seems well constituted for psychiatric disorders (Schibbye et al., 2014; Koffmann, 2017 for recent references), but it is less known in tinnitus research. We propose to integrate such measures in clinical settings for tinnitus treatment. As examples, the Clinical Outcomes in Routine Evaluation questionnaire (CORE, Evans et al., 2000) and the Outcome Questionnaire-45 (OQ-45; Lambert et al., 2004) in combination with the TQ as a disorder specific measure provide validated tools.

Even though the low predictability for treatment success is unsatisfactory, previous studies similarly failed to predict therapy outcome. Rief et al. (2005) found that age and illness duration had only marginal associations with treatment success. Baseline scores of tinnitus annoyance (TQ), gender of the patient or comorbidity with mental disorders were not significant predictors of outpatient psychological treatment. Neither duration of tinnitus nor the level of sleep disturbance, comorbid psychopathology, hearing problems, or experienced stress level affected the outcome of outpatient treatment (Kröner-Herwig et al., 2006). On the other hand, patients with high tinnitus annoyance and comorbid psychopathology at baseline were more often non-responders (Rübler, 1997; Frenzel, 1998). Goebel (2008) conducted a 15-year follow-up after inpatient tinnitus therapy on 271 tinnitus patients. Noise-induced tinnitus, gender and comorbid psychopathology explained 7.6% of the variance in tinnitus annoyance. Male tinnitus sufferers as well as patients with noise-induced tinnitus and high psychopathology reported higher tinnitus annoyance 15 years after the treatment.

Consequently, it appears that there is only little agreement on what can predict treatment outcome, but in no study was predictability good. The complexity of these processes was again stressed by Caffier et al. (2006). In their study, severely affected tinnitus sufferers showed clear improvements in TQ scores without any age-specific differences. In comparison, the groups of younger and older patients with mild tinnitus severity showed higher reductions in TQ scores in comparison to middle-aged patients between 46 and 56 years. Regarding preexisting tinnitus duration, patients with mild tinnitus annoyance demonstrated a particularly strong reduction of annoyance when the tinnitus lasted for less than 1 year. In contrast, in severely affected tinnitus sufferers, preexisting tinnitus duration did not seem to play a role for treatment success.

These results indicate that in order to predict treatment success by patient characteristics, we have to make subgroups and investigate which combinations of subgroup characteristics lead to better/poorer treatment success. Therefore, the next milestone in tinnitus research should be to update large data registries, into which standardized variables can be entered by independent tinnitus researchers. A tinnitus database has already been established by the Tinnitus Research Initiative (http://www.tinnitusresearch.org/index.php/for-researchers/tinnitus-database) and will be improved and enlarged by the TINNET European research network funded by the COST program (http://tinnet.tinnitusresearch.net/). Such a central database will enable the specification of subgroups of tinnitus patients worldwide, making it more possible to develop individually tailored treatments for tinnitus patients.

LIMITATIONS

Due to the lack of a control group receiving a different treatment, we cannot indicate how effective the present approach is compared to other possible treatments or, in the worst case, if it is due to a placebo effect or the mere passing of time. The interdisciplinary treatment comprised several modules, but whether one of them or a specific combination contributed to the reported effects remains to be tested. Future studies might adopt a dismantling approach, leaving out potentially redundant treatment components. Furthermore, cost-effectiveness studies and equivalence trials should be performed.

Even though the results of this study speak in favor of JITT, it must be noted that 35% of the tinnitus patients seen at the ENT department did not accept "habituation to tinnitus" as an objective of the intervention. Therefore, specific treatment approaches adapted to such patients should also be developed. We propose a combination of two therapeutic methods, one addressing tinnitus distress and the other the symptom itself. As an example for the latter, some evidence was presented that tailor-made notched music training reduces tinnitus loudness (Stein et al., 2016). Neurophysiological models (Jastreboff et al., 1996) suggest the proposed combination as a valuable approach that would also satisfy the needs of patients. As an alternative, there are also non-invasive stimulation methods that seem to ameliorate tinnitus symptoms (for a recent case study see Richter et al., 2017).

CONCLUSION

Our interdisciplinary day care tinnitus treatment represents a treatment for patients with chronic tinnitus that reduces tinnitus annoyance. After initial interdisciplinary diagnostic procedures and a first brief tinnitus-specific counseling, a small reduction in tinnitus annoyance was found. A clinically relevant change in tinnitus annoyance was observed between the beginning and the end of treatment and remained stable at least for 6 months.

The best treatment outcome was reached by patients with moderate and severe tinnitus. The improvement in tinnitus annoyance in patients with sick leave within 6 months before treatment onset or with very severe tinnitus annoyance was smaller than for the rest of the investigated population.

Given the high heterogeneity of tinnitus, we predict that the development of adapted JITT to individual needs will be challenging. Additional measurements of neurophysiological correlates might help in understanding which aspects of the symptomatology and the underlying neural network undergo changes in response to treatment and which do not.

AUTHOR CONTRIBUTIONS

DI: Substantial contributions to the conception and design of the work; the acquisition, analysis and interpretation of data for the work; drafting the work and revising it critically for important intellectual content. Wrote the manuscript. CD: Contribution to the analysis and interpretation of data; drafting the work and revising it critically for important intellectual content. Wrote the manuscript. GV, BM and DR: Substantial contributions to the acquisition and interpretation of data for the work; revising the work critically for important intellectual content. US: Substantial contributions to the conception of the work; revising the work critically for important intellectual content. OG: Substantial contributions to the conception and design of the work; the acquisition, analysis and interpretation of data for the work; revising the work critically for important intellectual content. All authors gave their final approval of the version to be published and agree to be accountable for all aspects of the work in ensuring that questions related to the accuracy or integrity of any part of the work are appropriately investigated and resolved.

ACKNOWLEDGMENTS

The authors would like to thank Marlen Hagemann for the support in acquisition of data and Holger Pickel for organizing the database.

REFERENCES

Abbott, J. A. M., Kaldo, V., Klein, B., Austin, D., Hamilton, C., Piterman, L., et al. (2009). A cluster randomized trial of an Internet-based intervention program for tinnitus distress in an industrial setting. *Cogn. Behav. Ther.* 38, 162–173. doi: 10.1080/16506070902763174

Abel, M. D., and Levine, R. A. (2004). Muscle contractions and auditory perception in tinnitus patients and nonclinical subjects. *Cranio* 22, 181–191. doi: 10.1179/crn.2004.024

American Academy of Otolaryngology-Head and Neck Surgery (2014). *Clinical Practice Guideline: Tinnitus.* Available online at: https://www.guideline.gov/summaries/summary/48751 (Accessed November 23, 2016).

Andersson, G. (2002). Psychological aspects of tinnitus and the application of cognitive–behavioral therapy. *Clin. Psychol. Rev.* 22, 977–990 doi: 10.1016/S0272-7358(01)00124-6

Andersson, G., Baguley, D. M., McKenna, L., and McFerran, D. J. (2005). *Tinnitus: A Multidisciplinary Approach.* London: Whurr.

Andersson, G., and Lyttkens, L. (1999). A meta-analytic review of psychological treatments for tinnitus. *Br. J. Audiol.* 33, 201–210. doi: 10.3109/03005369909090101

Andersson, G., Strömgren, T., Ström, L., and Lyttkens, L. (2002). Randomized controlled trial of Internet-based cognitive behavior therapy for distress associated with tinnitus. *Psychosom. Med.* 64, 810–816. doi: 10.1097/00006842-200209000-00014

Andersson, G., Vretblad, P., Larsen, H. C., and Lyttkens, L. (2001). Longitudinal follow-up of tinnitus complaints. *Arch. Otolaryngol. Head Neck Surg.* 127, 175–179. doi: 10.1001/archotol.127.2.175

Belli, S., Belli, H., Bahcebasi, T., Ozcetin, A., Alpay, E., and Ertem, U. (2008). Assessment of psychopathological aspects and psychiatric comorbidities in patients affected by tinnitus. *Eur. Arch. Otorhinolaryngol.* 265,279–285. doi: 10.1007/s00405-007-0440-8

Biesinger, E., Del Bo, L., De Ridder, D., Goodey, R., Herraiz, C., Kleinjung, T., et al. (2008). *Algorythm for the Diagnostic & Therapeutic Management of Tinnitus.* TRI Tinnitus Clinic Network. Available online at: http://tinnitusresearch.org/index.php/for-clinicians/diagnostic-flowchart (Accessed March 10, 2017).

Biesinger, E., and Heiden, C. (1999). Die Bedeutung der Retrainingtherapie bei Tinnitus. *Deutsches Ärzteblatt.* 96, 2817–2825.

Bleich, T., Lamprecht, F., Lamm, H., and Jäger, B. (2001). Der Langzeitverlauf des chronischen Tinnitus aurium. *Zeitschrift für Medizinische Psychologie* 2, 79–36.

Bonate, P. L. (2000). *Analysis of Pretest-Posttest Designs.* London: *Taylor & Francis.*

Bortz, J., and Döring, N. (2006). *Forschungsmethoden und evaluation für Human- und Sozialwissenschaftler.* Heidelberg: Springer Medizin Verlag.

Caffier, P. P., Haupt, H., Scherer, H., and Mazurek, B. (2006). Outcomes of long-term outpatient tinnitus-coping therapy: psychometric changes and value of tinnitus-control instruments. *Ear Hear.* 27, 619–627. doi: 10.1097/01.aud.0000240504.77861.1a

Cima, R. F. F., Joore, M., Maes, I., Scheyen, D., El Refaie, A., Baguley, D. M., et al. (2009). Cost-effectiveness of multidisciplinary management of Tinnitus at a specialized Tinnitus centre. *BMC Health Serv. Res.* 9:29. doi: 10.1186/1472-6963-9-29

Cima, R. F. F., Maes, I. H., Joore, M. A., Scheyen, D. J. W. M., El Refaie, A., Baguley, D. M., et al. (2012). Specialised treatment based on cognitive behavior therapy versus usual care for tinnitus: a randomised controlled trial. *Lancet* 379, 1951–1959. doi: 10.1016/S0140-6736(12)60469-3

Cohen, J. (1992). A power primer. *Psychol. Bull.* 112, 155–159. doi: 10.1037/0033-2909.112.1.155

Coles, R. R. A. (1995). "Classification of causes, mechanisms of patient disturbance, and associated counseling," in *Mechanisms of Tinnitus*, eds J. Vernon and A. R. Moller (Boston, MA: Allen & Bacon), 11–19.

Davis, A. (1995). *Hearing in Adults.* London: Whurr.

Davis, A., and El Rafaie, A. (2000). "Epidemiology of tinnitus," in *Tinnitus Handbook*, ed R.S. Tyler (San Diego, CA: Singular), 1–23.

Delb, W., D'Amelio, R., and Schonecke, O. (2002). *Tinnitus: ein Manual zur Tinnitus-Retrainingtherapie.* Göttingen: Hogrefe.

De Ridder, D., Elgoyhen, A. B., Romo, R., and Langguth, B. (2011). Phantom percepts: tinnitus and pain as persisting aversive memory networks. *Proc. Natl. Acad. Sci. U.S.A.* 108, 8075–8080. doi: 10.1073/pnas.1018466108

Dobie, R. A., Sullivan, M. D., Katon, W. J., Sakai, C. S., and Russo, J. (1992) Antidepressant treatment of tinnitus patients. *Acta Otolaryngol.* 112, 242–247 doi: 10.1080/00016489.1992.11665412

Ellis, A. (1993). *Grundlagen der Rational-Emotiven Verhaltenstherapie.* München: Pfeiffer.

El Refaie, A., Davis, A., Kayan, A., Baskill, J., Lovell, E., and Owen, V. (2004). A questionnaire study of the quality of life and quality of family life of individuals complaining of tinnitus pre- and post-attendance at a tinnitus clinic. *Int. J. Audiol.* 43, 410–416. doi: 10.1080/14992020400050052

Epp, B., Hots, J., Verhey, J. L., and Schaette, R. (2012). Increased intensity discrimination thresholds in tinnitus subjects with a normal audiogram. *J. Acoust. Soc. Am.* 132, EL196-EL201. doi: 10.1121/1.4740462

Erlandsson, S. I., and Hallberg, L. R. M. (2000). Prediction of quality of life in patients with tinnitus. *Br. J. Audiol.* 34, 11–20. doi: 10.3109/03005364000000114

Erlandsson, S. I., Hallberg, L. R. M., and Axelsson, A. (1992). Psychological and audiological correlates of perceived tinnitus severity. *Audiology* 31, 168–179. doi: 10.3109/00206099209072912

Evans, C., Mellor-Clark, J., Margison, F., Barkham, M., Audin, K., Connell, J., et al. (2000). CORE: Clinical Outcomes in Routine Evaluation. *J. Ment. Health* 9, 247–255. doi: 10.1080/713680250

Fabijanska, A. K. K., Raj-Koziak, D., and Skarzynski, H. (2014). *Tinnitus and Normal Hearing: Searching for Underlying Pathology.* Berlin: International tinnitus seminar.

Feldmann, H. (1992). *Tinnitus.* Stuttgart: Georg Thieme Verlag KG.

Frenzel, A. (1998). *Chronischer Tinnitus: Evaluation Eines Kognitiv-Behavioralen Gruppentrainings und Einer Minimalintervention.* Herdecke: GCA-Verl.

Funk, C., Wohlfeil, J., Jauch, E., and Sorg, R. (2008). *Manual der Terzo®Gehörtherapie.* Unpublished manual.

Galazyuk, A. V., Wenstrup, J. J., and Hamid, M. A. (2012). Tinnitus and underlying brain mechanisms. *Curr. Opin. Otolaryngol. Head Neck Surg.* 20, 409–415. doi: 10.1097/MOO.0b013e3283577b81

German Society of Otorhinolaryngology, Head and Neck Surgery (2015). *German S3 guideline Ol 7/064: Chronic tinnitus.* Available online at: http://www.awmf.org/leitlinien/detail/ll/017-064.html (Accessed November 23, 2016).

Goebel, F. (2008). *Langzeitverlauf des chronischen Tinnitus bei Patienten mit Hörsturz, Lärmschädigung und M.* Meniére. Dissertation, Technische Universität, München.

Goebel, G. (1995). Fortschritte bei der verhaltensmedizinischen Diagnostik und Behandlung quälender chronischer Ohrgeräusche. *Oto Rhino Laryngologia Nova* 5, 178–189. doi: 10.1159/000313202

Goebel, G. (1998). *Therapie des chronischen Tinnitus. Evaluation und Prädiktoranalyse einer multimodalen Verhaltenstherapie. Habilitationsschrift.* Postdoctoral thesis, Technische Universität, München.

Goebel, G., and Hiller, W. (1998). *Tinnitus-Fragebogen (TF): ein Instrument zur Erfassung von Belastung und Schweregrad bei Tinnitus* Göttingen: Hogrefe.

Goebel, G., and Hiller, W. (1999). "Quality management in the therapy of chronic tinnitus" in *Proceedings of the Sixth International Tinnitus Seminar*, ed J.W. Hazell (London: The Tinnitus and Hyperacusis Center Cambridge), 357–363.

Goebel, G., and Hiller, W. (2007). When tinnitus loudness and annoyance are discrepant: audiological characteristics and psychological profile. *Audiol. Neurootol.* 12, 391–400. doi: 10.1159/000106482

Goebel, G., Kahl, M., Arnold, W., and Fichter, M. (2006). 15-year prospective follow-up study of behavioral therapy in a large sample of inpatients with chronic tinnitus. *Acta Otolaryngol. Suppl.* 126, 70–79. doi: 10.1080/03655230600895267

Gulliver, A., Griffiths, K. M., and Christensen, H. (2010). Perceived barriers and facilitators to mental health help-seeking in young people: a systematic review *BMC Psychiatry* 10:113. doi: 10.1186/1471-244X-10-113

Haerkötter, C. (2001). *Kognitive Verhaltenstherapie bei chronischem Tinnitus Evaluation neuer Ansätze. Eine Studie zu Potentiellen Therapieeffekten verbesserter Edukation und Apparativer Versorgung Mit therapeutischen Rauschgeneratoren.* Dissertation, Eberhard-Karls-Universität, Tübingen.

Hall, D. (2016). Interpreting Treatment-Related Changes Using the Tinnitus Questionnaire in Argstatter H, Grapp M, Plinkert PK, Bolay HV. Heidelberg neuro-music therapy for chronic-tonal tinnitus - treatment outline and psychometric evaluation. *Int. Tinnitus J.* 20, 73–75. doi: 10.5935/0946-5448.20160014

Hall, J. W., and Ruth, R. A. (1999). "Outcome for tinnitus patients after consultation with an audiologist," in *Proceedings of the Sixth International Tinnitus Seminar*, ed J.W. Hazell (London: The Tinnitus and Hyperacusis Center Cambridge), 378–80.

Hallam, R. S. (1996). *Manual of the Tinnitus Questionnaire (TQ)*. London: Psychological Corporation.

Hallam, R. S., Rachman, S., and Hinchcliffe, R. (1984). "Psychological aspects of tinnitus" in *Contributions to Medical Psychology*, ed S. Rachman (Oxford: Pergamon Press), 31–53.

Hallam, R. S., and Stephens, S. D. (1985). Vestibular disorder and emotional distress. *J. Psychosom. Res.* 29, 407–413. doi: 10.1016/0022-3999(85)90026-1

Harrop-Griffiths, J., Katon, W., Dobie, R., Sakai, C., and Russo, J. (1987). Chronic tinnitus: association with psychiatric diagnosis. *J. Psychosom. Res.* 31, 613–621. doi: 10.1016/0022-3999(87)90040-7

Hausotter, W. (2004). Neurologische und psychosomatische Aspekte bei der Begutachtung des Tinnitus. *Med. Sach.* 100, 5–10.

Hennig, T. A., Costa, M. J., Urnau, D., Becker, K. T., and Schuster, L. C. (2011). Recognition of speech of normal-hearing individuals with Tinnitus and Hyperacusis. *Intl. Arch. Otorhinolaryngol.* 15, 21–28.

Henry, A., Meikle, M., and Gilbert, A. (1999). "Audiometric correlates of tinnitus pitch: insights from the Tinnitus Data Registry," in *Proceedings of the Sixth International Tinnitus Seminar*, ed J.W. Hazell (London: The Tinnitus and Hyperacusis Center Cambridge), 51–57.

Henry, J. A., Dennis, K. C., and Schechter, M. A. (2005). General review of tinnitus: prevalence, mechanisms, effects and management. *J. Speech Lang. Hear. Res.* 48, 1204–1235. doi: 10.1044/1092-4388(2005/084)

Henry, J. L., and Wilson, P. H. (1996). The psychological management of tinnitus: comparison of a combined cognitive educational program, education alone and a waiting-list control. *Int. Tinnitus J.* 2, 9–20.

Hesse, G., and Schaaf, H. (2015). *Manual der Hörtherapie: Schwerhörigkeit, Tinnitus und Hyperakusis*. Göttingen: Hogrefe.

Hesse, G., and Schaaf, H. (2007). Musiktherapie bei Tinnitus. Wirkungsvolle Ergänzung *zur Habituations- und Hörtherapie.* HNO 55, 328–330. doi: 10.1007/s00106-007-1570-4

Hesser, H., Gustafsson, T., Lundén, C., Henrikson, O., Fattahi, K., Johnsson, E., et al. (2012). A randomized controlled trial of Internet-delivered cognitive behavior therapy and acceptance and commitment therapy in the treatment of tinnitus. *J. Consult. Clin. Psychol.* 80, 649–661. doi: 10.1037/a0027021

Hesser, H., Weise, C., Rief, W., and Andersson, G. (2011a). The effect of waiting: a meta-analysis of wait-list control groups in trials for tinnitus distress. *J. Psychosom. Res.* 70, 378–384. doi: 10.1016/j.jpsychores.2010.12.006

Hesser, H., Weise, C., Westin, V. Z., and Andersson, G. (2011b). A systematic review and meta-analysis of randomized controlled trials of cognitive-behavioral therapy for tinnitus distress. *Clin. Psychol. Rev.* 31, 545–553. doi: 10.1016/j.cpr.2010.12.006

Hiller, W., and Goebel, G. (1999). Assessing audiological, pathophysiological, and psychological variables in chronic tinnitus: a study of reliability and search for prognostic factors. *Int. J. Behav. Med.* 6, 312–330. doi: 10.1207/s15327558ijbm0604_2

Hiller, W., and Haerkötter, C. (2005). Does sound stimulation have additive effects on cognitive-behavioral treatment of chronic tinnitus? *Behav. Res. Ther.* 43, 595–612. doi: 10.1016/j.brat.2004.03.012

Hoare, D. J., Gander, P. E., Collins, L., Smith, S., and Hall, D. A. (2012). Management of tinnitus in English NHS audiology departments: an evaluation of current practice. *J. Eval. Clin. Pract.* 18, 326–334. doi: 10.1111/j.1365-2753.2010.01566.x

Hoare, D. J., Kowalkowski, V. L., Kang, S., and Hall, D. A. (2011). Systematic review and meta-analyses of randomized controlled trials examining tinnitus management. *Laryngoscope* 121, 1555–1564. doi: 10.1002/lary.21825

Hoffman, H. J., and Reed, G. W. (2004). "Epidemiology of tinnitus" in *Tinnitus: Theory and Management*, ed J. B. Snow (Lewiston, NY: BC Decker Inc), 16–41.

International Bureau for Audiophonology (2017). *BIAP Recommendation 02/1: Audiometric Classification of Hearing Impairments*. Available online at: https://www.biap.org/de/empfehlungen/empfehlungen/ct-02-classification-des-deficiences-auditives-1/55-02-1-audiometric-classification-of-hearing-impairments/file (Accessed May 15,2017).

Ivansic-Blau, D. (2012). *Wirksamkeit von ambulanten Gruppentherapien bei chronischem Tinnitus. Eine Psychotherapie-Vergleichsstudie*. Dissertation, Universität Koblenz-Landau, Landau.

Jacobson, E. (2006). *Entspannung als Therapie*. Progressive Relaxation in Theorie und Praxis. Stuttgart: Klett-Cotta.

Jakes, S. C., Hallam, R. S., McKenna, L., and Hinchcliffe, R. (1992). Group cognitive therapy for medical patients: an application to tinnitus. *Cognit. Ther. Res.* 16, 67–82. doi: 10.1007/BF01172957

Jasper, K., Weise, C., Conrad, I., Andersson, G., Hiller, W., and Kleinstauber, M. (2014). Internet-based guided self-help versus groupcognitive behavioral therapy for chronic tinnitus: a randomized controlled trial. *Psychother. Psychosom.* 83, 234–246. doi: 10.1159/000360705

Jastreboff, P. J., Gray, W. C., and Gold, S. L. (1996). Neurophysiological approach to tinnitus patients. *Am. J. Otol.* 17, 236–240.

Kaldo,V. (2008). *Cognitive Behavioural Therapy as Guided Self-Help to Reduce Tinnitus Distress*. Dissertation, Uppsala Universitet, Uppsala.

Kaldo, V., Haak, T., Buhrman, M., Alfonsson, S., Larsen, H. C., and Andersson, G. (2013). Internet-based cognitive behaviour therapy for tinnitus patients delivered in a regular clinical setting: outcome and analysis of treatment dropout. *Cogn. Behav. Ther.* 42, 146–158. doi: 10.1080/16506073.2013.769622

Kaldo, V., Levin, S., Widarsson, J., Buhrman, M., Larsen, H. C., and Andersson, G. (2008). Internet versus group cognitive-behavioral treatment of distress associated with tinnitus: a randomized controlled trial. *Behav. Ther.* 39, 348–359. doi: 10.1016/j.beth.2007.10.003

Koffmann, A. (2017). Has growth mixture modeling improved our understanding of how early change predicts psychotherapy outcome? *Psychother. Res.* 2, 1–13. doi: 10.1080/10503307.2017.1294771

Konzag, T. A., Rübler, D., Bloching, M., Bandemer-Greulich, U., Fikentscher, E., and Frommer, J. (2006). Counselling versus Selbsthilfemanual bei ambulanten Tinnituspatienten. *HNO* 54, 599–604. doi: 10.1007/s00106-005-1350-y

Kröner-Herwig, B., Zachriat, C., and Weigand, D. (2006). Do patient characteristics predict outcome in the outpatient treatment of chronic tinnitus? *Psychosoc. Med.* 3, Doc07.

Lambert, M. J., Morton, J. J., Hatfield, D., Harmon, C., Hamilton, S., Reid, R. C., et al. (2004). *Administration and scoring manual for the Outcome Questionnaire (OQ-45.2)*. Orem, UT: American Professional Credentialing Service.

Lambert, M. J., and Ogles, B. (2003). "The efficacy and effectiveness of psychotherapie," in *Bergin and Garfield's Handbook of Psychotherapy and Behavior Change*, ed M. J. Lambert (New York, NY: John Wiley & Sons), 139–93.

Langenbach, M., Olderog, M., Michel, O., Albus, C., and Köhle, K. (2005). Psychosocial and personality predictors of tinnitus-related distress. *Gen. Hosp. Psychiatry* 27, 73–77. doi: 10.1016/j.genhosppsych.2004.08.008

Langguth, B., Landgrebe, M., Frank, E., Schecklmann, M., Sand, P. G., Vielsmeier, V., et al. (2014). Efficacy of different protocols of transcranial magnetic stimulation for the treatment of tinnitus: pooled analysis of two randomized controlled studies. *World J. Biol. Psychiatry* 15, 276–285. doi: 10.3109/15622975.2012.708438

Lenarz, T. (1992). "Chirurgische Therapie," in *Tinnitus*, ed H. Feldmann (Stuttgart: Thieme), 112–115.

Martines-Devesa, P., Perera, R., Theodoulou, M., and Waddell, A. (2010). Cognitive behavioural therapy for tinnitus (Review): an update. *Cochrane Database Syst. Rev.* 9: CD005233. doi: 10.1002/14651858.CD005233.pub3

Mazurek, B., Fischer, F., Haupt, H., Georgiewa, P., Reisshauer, A., and Klapp, B. F. (2006). A modified version of tinnitus retraining therapy: observing long-term outcome and predictors. *Audiol Neurotol.* 11, 276–286. doi: 10.1159/0000 93526

Mazurek, B., Georgiewa, P., Seydel, C., Haupt, H., Scherer, H., Klapp, B. F., et al. (2005). Integrierte Tinnitusintensivbehandlung: konzept und erste praktische Erfahrungen. *Gesundheitswesen* 67, 485–491. doi: 10.1055/s-2005-858379

Mazurek, B., Seydel, C., Haupt, H., Szczepek, A., Klapp, B. F., and Schrom, T. (2009). Integrierte Tinnitusintensivbehandlung: verringerung der tinnitusbedingten Belastung während einer 1-Jahres-Katamnese. *Gesundheitswesen* 71, 35–40. doi: 10.1055/s-0028-1082303

Michiels, S., De Hertogh, W., Truijen, S., and Van de Heyning, P. (2015). Cervical spine dysfunctions in patients with chronic subjective tinnitus. *Otol. Neurotol.* 36, 741–745. doi: 10.1097/MAO.0000000000000670

Noreña, A., Micheyl, C., Chery-Croze, S., and Collet, L. (2002). Psychoacoustic characterization of the tinnitus spectrum: implications for the underlying mechanisms of tinnitus. *Audiol. Neurootol.* 7, 358–369. doi: 10.1159/000066156

Olderog, M. (1999). Metaanalyse zur Wirksamkeit psychologisch fundierter Behandlungskonzepte des chronischen dekompensierten Tinnitus. *Zeitschrift für Medizinische Psychologie* 1, 5–18.

Olderog, M., Langenbach, M., Michel, O., Brusis, T., and Köhle, K. (2004). Prädiktoren und Mechanismen der ausblendenden Tinnitus-Toleranzentwicklung - eine Längsschnittstudie. *Laryngo Rhino Otol.* 83, 5–13. doi: 10.1055/s-2004-814235

Ostermann, K. T. M., Vincent, Y., Debaty, M. E., Cotton, P., and Lurquin, P. (2014) *Incidence of Somatic Tinnitus in Current ENT Practice*. Berlin: International tinnitus seminar.

Richter, K., Acker, J., Miloseva, L., Peter, L., and Niklewski, G. (2017). Management of chronic tinnitus and insomnia with repetitive transcranial magnetic stimulation and cognitive behavioral therapy – a combined approach. *Front. Psychol.* 8:575. doi: 10.3389/fpsyg.2017.00575

Rief, W., Weise, C., Kley, N., and Martin, A. (2005). Psychophysiologic treatment of chronic tinnitus: a randomized clinical trial. *Psychosom. Med.* 67, 833–838. doi: 10.1097/01.psy.0000174174.38908.c6

Rübler, D. (1997). *Psychosoziale Belastungsfaktoren und Komorbidität bei Tinnituspatienten - Wie effektiv ist Counselling?* Dissertation, Martin-Luther-Universität, Halle-Wittenberg.

Savastano, M. (2008). Tinnitus with or without hearing loss: are its characteristics different? *Eur. Arch. Otorhinolaryngol.* 265 1295–1300. doi: 10.1007/s00405-008-0630-z

Schaaf, H., Weiß, S., and Hesse, G. (2017). Catamnesis results of an inpatient neuro-otologic and psychosomatic tinnitus therapy 1-5 years after discharge. *Eur. Arch. Otorhinolaryngol.* 274, 701–710. doi: 10.1007/s00405-016-4316-7

Schaette, R., and McAlpine, D. (2011). Tinnitus with a normal audiogram: physiological evidence for hidden hearing loss and computational model. *J. Neurosci.* 31, 13452–13457. doi: 10.1523/JNEUROSCI.2156-11.2011

Schibbye, P., Ghaderi, A., Ljótsson, B., Hedman, E., Lindefors, N., Rück, C., et al. (2014). Using early change to predict outcome in cognitive behaviour therapy: exploring timeframe, calculation method, and differences of disorder-specific versus general measures. *PLoS ONE* 9:e100614. doi: 10.1371/journal.pone.0100614

Scott, B., Lindberg, P., Melin, L., and Lyttkens, L. (1990). Predictors of tinnitus discomfort, adaptation and subjective loudness. *Br. J. Audiol.* 24, 51–62. doi: 10.3109/03005369009077842

Seydel, C., Haupt, H., Szczepek, A. J., Hartmann, A., Rose, M., and Mazurek, B. (2015). Three years later: report on the state of well-being of patients with chronic tinnitus who underwent modified tinnitus retraining therapy. *Audiol. Neurotol.* 20, 26–38. doi: 10.1159/000363728

Spitzer, R. L., Williams, J., and Kroenke, K. (1999). *Prime MD Today. Evaluation of Mental Disorders. Manual.* New York, NY: Pfizer.

Stein, A., Engell, A., Okamoto, H., Wollbrink, A., Lau, P., Wunderlich, R., et al. (2013). Modulatory effects of spectral energy contrasts on lateral inhibition in the human auditory cortex: an MEG study. *PLoS ONE* 8:80899. doi: 10.1371/journal.pone.0080899

Stein, A., Wunderlich, R., Lau, P., Engell, A., Wollbrink, A. Shaykevich, A., et al (2016). Clinical trial on tonal tinnitus with tailor-made notched music training. *BMC Neurol.* 16:38. doi: 10.1186/s12883-016-0558-7

Stobik, C., Weber, R. K., Münte, T. F., and Frommer, J. (2003). Psychosomatic stress factors in compensated and decompensated tinnitus. *Psychother. Psychosom. Med. Psychol.* 53, 344–352. doi: 10.1055/s-2003-40947

Stobik, C., Weber, R. K., Münte, T. F., Walter, M., and Frommer, J. (2005). Evidence of psychosomatic influences in compensated and decompensated tinnitus. *Int. J. Audiol.* 44, 370–378. doi: 10.1080/14992020500147557

Sullivan, M. D., Katon, W., Dobie, R. A., Saskai, C., Russo, J., and Harrop-Griffiths, J. (1988). Disabling tinnitus: association with affective disorder. *Gen. Hosp. Psychiatry* 10, 285–291. doi: 10.1016/0163-8343(88)90037-0

Tan, C. M., Lecluyse, W., McFerran, D., and Meddis, R. (2013). Tinnitus and patterns of hearing loss. *J. Assoc. Res. Otolaryngol.* 14, 275–282. doi: 10.1007/s10162-013-0371-6

Tyler, R. S., and Baker, L. J. (1983). Difficulties experienced by tinnitus suffers. *J. Speech Hear. Disord.* 48, 150–154. doi: 10.1044/jshd.4802.150

Von Wedel, H., and von Wedel, U. (2000). Eine Bestandsaufnahme zur Tinnitus-Retraining-Therapie. *HNO* 48, 887–901. doi: 10.1007/s001060050685

Weise, C. (2008). *Biofeedback als Chance für die Tinnitusbehandlung.* Dissertation, Philipps-Universität, Marburg.

Weise, C., Heinecke, K., and Rief, W. (2007). Biofeedback bei chronischem Tinnitus – Behandlungsleitfaden und vorläufige ergebnisse zu wirksamkeit und Akzeptanz. *Verhaltenstherapie* 17, 220–230 doi: 10.1159/0001 11462

Weise, C., Kleinstäuber, M., and Andersson, G. (2016). Internet-Delivered cognitive-behavior therapy for tinnitus: a randomized controlled trial. *Psychosom. Med.* 78, 501–510. doi: 10.1097/PSY.00000000000 00310

Weisz, N., Hartmann, T., Dohrmann, K., Schlee, W., and Norena, A. (2006). High-frequency tinnitus without hearing loss does not mean absence of deafferentation. *Hear. Res.* 222, 108–114. doi: 10.1016/j.heares.2006. 09.003

Wilson, P. H., Henry, J., Bowen, M., and Haralambous, G. (1991). Tinnitus reaction questionnaire: psychometric properties of a measure of distress associated with tinnitus. *J. Speech Hear. Res.* 34, 197–201. doi: 10.1044/jshr.3401.197

Yalom, I. D. (1995). *The Theory and Practice of Group Psychotherapy.* New York, NY: Basic Books.

Zenner, H. P., Delb, W., Kröner-Herwig, B., Jäger, B., Peroz, I., Hesse, G., et al. (2015). On the interdisciplinary S3 guidelines for the treatment of chronic idiopathic tinnitus. *HNO* 63, 419. doi: 10.1007/s00106-015-0011-z

Zenner, H. P., Delb, W., Kröner-Herwig, B., Jäger, B., Peroz, I., Hesse G., et al. (2016). A multidisciplinary systematic review of the treatment for chronic idiopathic tinnitus. *Eur. Arch. Otorhinolaryngol.* 274, 2079–2091. doi: 10.1007/s00405-016-4401-y

Zöger, S., Svedlund, J., and Holgers, K. M. (2001). Psychiatric disorders in tinnitus patients without severe hearing impairment: 24 months follow- up of patients at an audiological clinic. *Audiology* 40, 133–140. doi: 10.3109/0020609001090 73108

11

Identification of Candidate Allosteric Modulators of the M1 Muscarinic Acetylcholine Receptor Which May Improve Vagus Nerve Stimulation in Chronic Tinnitus

Tijana Bojić [1], Vladimir R. Perović [2], Milan Senćanski [2] and Sanja Glišić [2]*

[1] *Laboratory of Radiobiology and Molecular Genetics, Institute of Nuclear Sciences Vin ˇca, University of Belgrade, Belgrade, Serbia,*

[2] *Center for Multidisciplinary Research, Institute of Nuclear Sciences Vin ˇca, University of Belgrade, Belgrade, Serbia*

Correspondence:
Tijana Bojić
tijanabojic@vinca.rs;
bojictijana@gmail.com

Chronic tinnitus is characterized by neuroplastic changes of the auditory cortex. A promising method for therapy of chronic tinnitus is vagus nerve stimulation (VNS) combined with auditory stimulation. The principle of VNS is reversal of pathological neuroplastic changes of the auditory cortex toward physiological neural activity and synchronicity. The VNS mechanism of action in chronic tinnitus patients is prevailingly through the muscarinic neuromodulation of the auditory cortex by the activation of nc. basalis Meynerti. The aim of this study is to propose potential pharmaceutics which may improve the neuromodulatory effects of VNS. The working hypothesis is that M1 receptors have a dominant role in the neural plasticity of the auditory cortex. We propose that allosteric agonists of the muscarinic receptor type 1 (M1) receptor could improve specificity and selectivity of the neuromodulatory effect of VNS on the auditory cortex of chronic tinnitus patients even in the circumstances of lower acetylcholine brain concentration. This intervention would also reinforce the re-learning process of tinnitus (sub)networks by acting on cholinergic memory and learning mechanisms. We performed *in silico* screening of drug space using the EIIP/AQVN filter and selected 50 drugs as candidates for allosteric modulators of muscarinic receptors. Further filtering of these compounds by means of 3D QSAR and docking revealed 3 approved drugs—bromazepam, estazolam and flumazenil as the most promising candidates for combined chronic tinnitus therapy. These drugs should be further evaluated by biological tests and clinical trials.

Keywords: tinnitus, muscarinic allosteric agonists, M1 receptor, vagus nerve stimulation, *in silico* analysis, information spectrum method

INTRODUCTION

Tinnitus, the perception of phantom sound, is a debilitating condition with notable prevalence: approximately 10–15% of the general population experience tinnitus and for 7 million this is a debilitating condition (Geven et al., 2014). The Royal National Institute for Deaf People estimates that 13 million people in Western Europe and USA seek medical assistance for their tinnitus symptoms (Vio and Holme, 2005). Demographic development and increase of occupational and ambient noise support the view that this problem will be even more prevalent in the future. In spite of the fact that more than 4 million prescriptions are written for the treatment of tinnitus, there is not a single drug approved by the FDA specific for the treatment of tinnitus. The estimates are that a potential tinnitus drug could have a product value of more than $600 million in the first year after its release (https://www.ata.org/understanding-facts).

The problem of chronic tinnitus is mainly of central origin. The pathophysiological substrate of chronic tinnitus is still a matter of intense debate (De Ridder et al., 2014b; Norena, 2015). The majority of chronic states of tinnitus begin with the functional damage of the cochlea (i.e., noise or hearing loss) and consequent abnormal input to the higher level neural structures of the auditory pathway (Eggermont and Roberts, 2004; Guitton, 2012; Chen et al., 2013; Wu et al., 2016). When tinnitus stabilizes as a chronic condition (not less than 1 year, Malinvaud et al., 2016), then numerous functional disarrangements occur, like the hyperpolarization of thalamic relay cells (Llinas et al., 2005), the changes in the central neural sensitivity or gain (Norena, 2011) and the functional coupling of different parallel brain networks (Kalauzi et al., 2012, 2014) into the "tinnitus (sub)network" (De Ridder et al., 2014b). This finally results also with the functional and anatomical disarrangement of the auditory cortex tonotopic map (Norena and Eggermont, 2005; Guitton, 2012).

The central (Zoccoli et al., 2005; Bojić et al., 2016) and peripheral components of the autonomic nervous system (Bojić, 2003; Silvani et al., 2003; Platiša et al., 2016) play crucial roles in the stabilization and manifestations of chronic tinnitus (Jastreboff, 2011). Cholinergic innervation plays a major role in the development and plasticity of the auditory cortex (Shideler and Yan, 2010). The growth and functional coupling of cholinergic innervations with auditory cortical cells goes in parallel with the forming of thalamocortical connections during embryological development and in the early stage after the birth. The presence of muscarinic acetylcholine receptors plays a crucial role in this process: muscarinic receptor type 1 (M1) regulates the expression of different neurotrophins (brain-derived neurotrophic factor and nerve growth factor; Da Penha Berzaghi et al., 1993; Betancourt et al., 2006), determines the structure of neurons by promoting cell survival (Tobin and Budd, 2003) and stimulates the neural (VanDeMark et al., 2009) and dendritic outgrowth (Zhang et al., 2005). Finally, muscarinic antagonists decrease the frequency specific plasticity of the auditory cortex in the paradigm of auditory fear conditioning (Ji et al., 2005; Ji and Suga, 2009) and, importantly for this concept, the stimulation of nc. basalis Meynerti (Bakin and Weinberger, 1996; Weinberger, 2003). Nc. basalis Meynerti electrical stimulation paired with tones acutely enhances cortical neural plasticity and reverses the neurological and perceptual correlates of tinnitus in adult animals (Nichols et al., 2011). M1 impacts also the processes of learning and memory (Zhang et al., 2006; Butcher et al., 2016) which are crucially important for the genesis and maintenance of tinnitus (De Ridder et al., 2014b; Eggermont and Kral, 2016; Vanneste and De Ridder, 2016).

Different techniques, both noninvasive and invasive, were tested in order to reverse the pathological neuroplastic changes of the auditory cortex toward the physiological state (Vanneste and De Ridder, 2012). Vagus nerve stimulation paired with tone stimulation is among the most promising tools for treatment of chronic tinnitus (Engineer et al., 2011; Shetake et al., 2012; De Ridder et al., 2014a). It is based on the principle of provoking the central neuromodulatory responses by stimulation of vagal afferent fibers and nc. basalis Meynerti which abundantly innervate the auditory cortex. Vagus stimulation paired with tone stimulation has an effect of targeted plasticity, the phenomenon of reversing the map changes in individuals with tinnitus. The area of tinnitus specific cortical neurons is consequently diminished (Engineer et al., 2011). In human studies the efficiency of this method to reduce tinnitus severity was around 40%, and interestingly, all the patients who did not experience an improvement were on drug therapy that included, among others, muscarinic antagonists (De Ridder et al., 2014a). More, it is well-documented in the literature that M1 receptors have a crucial role in the experience-dependent plasticity of the auditory cortex (Shideler and Yan, 2010). Our hypothesis is that *in silico* identification of M1 receptor allosteric agonists would propose a new line for the clinical research for modulated vagus nerve stimulation (VNS) paired with tones, potentially more targeted and more efficient. In addition, by agonizing the cholinergic mechanisms of learning and memory, attention, stress response, wakefulness and sleep and sensory information processing (Ferreira-Vieira et al., 2016), M1 allosteric agonists would stabilize the process of re-learning of neural networks involved in tinnitus perception. In order to choose the best candidates for these drugs we applied *in silico* strategies that resulted with three candidates for M1 allosteric modulators.

METHODS

In this paper, we implemented a virtual screening protocol that includes both short and long-range interactions between interacting molecules. The long-range interactions are denoted by the parameters—the average quasi valence number (AQVN) and the electron-ion interaction potential (EIIP).

First, the EIIP/AQVN filter was applied for *in silico* screening of the DrugBank (http://www.drugbank.ca) (Wishart et al., 2006) and then followed by 3D QSAR and molecular docking for identification of candidate allosteric modulators of M1.

EIIP/AQVN

The EIIP for organic molecules can be determined by the following simple equation derived from the "general model pseudopotential" (Veljkovic et al., 2011)

$$\text{EIIP} = 0.25\, Z^* \sin(1.04\, \pi\, Z^*)/2\pi \quad (1)$$

where Z^* is the average quasi valence number (AQVN) determined by

$$Z^* = \sum^{m} (niZi/N) \quad (2)$$

where *Zi* is the valence number of the *i*th atomic component, *ni* is the number of atoms of the *i*th component, *m* is the number of atomic components in the molecule, and *N* is the total number of atoms. EIIP values calculated according to Equations (1, 2) are expressed in Rydberg units (Ry).

Further filtering of these compounds was performed by means of 3D QSAR(quantitative structure–activity relationships) in Pentacle software and followed by docking.

3D QSAR

In order to build a pharmacophoric model and select compounds based on their pharmacophoric similarity, 12 literature M1 modulators (Target ID CHEMBL216) were downloaded from the ChEMBL database. All compounds were converted into the SDF format and then imported, along with candidate compounds into the Pentacle QSAR software, protonated at pH 7.4, and oriented according to the principal moments of inertia. Standard GRIND descriptors were calculated and the PCA model was built. From PCA scores that included the first two major components, PC1 and PC2, the most similar drug molecules to literature allosteric modulators were selected for further filtering.

Molecular Docking

Molecular docking of selected candidates was performed into the built homology model of the M1 receptor. The binding site of allosteric modulators was identified from the 4MQT structure and was placed in between extracellular loops of the 2 and 3 region. The grid box for docking, with dimensions 20 × 20 × 20 Å was placed to occupy this space. The receptor and ligands were prepared in Autodock Tools 1.5.6. Docking was carried out in AutodockVina (Trott and Olson, 2010). Exhaustiveness was set to 250.

RESULTS

EIIP/AQVN Filter

The virtual screening (VS) protocol in this study was based on the application of consecutive filters to select candidate allosteric modulators of M1. Previously it was shown for molecular targets in diverse pathological states that small molecules with similar AQVN and EIIP values interact with the common therapeutic agent (Veljkovic et al., 2011, 2013). This resulted in determining criteria for virtual screening of molecular libraries for compounds with similar therapeutic properties (Veljkovic et al., 2013). The selected learning set consisted of allosteric agonists and positive allosteric modulators of M1, reported in literature (Conn et al., 2009). The compounds from the learning set were inside the active domain with AQVN and EIIP values within the intervals of (3–3.08) and (0.004–0.073), respectively, and this domain was selected as a criterion for the selection of compounds representing candidate allosteric modulators of M1 (**Figure 1**). By applying the EIIP/AQVN-based virtual screening criterion, 50 drugs were chosen out of 1463 approved drugs from the DrugBank (http://www.drugbank.ca) (Wishart et al., 2006).

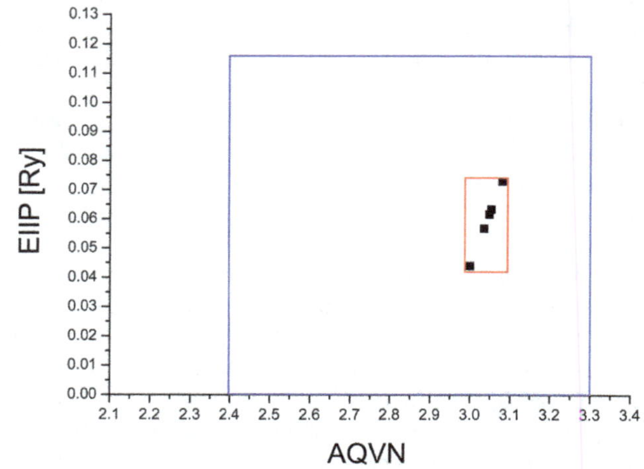

FIGURE 1 | Schematic presentation of the EIIP/AQVN criterion for selection of candidate allosteric modulators of muscarinic receptor M1. Active domain (red): AQVN (3–3.08), EIIP (0.004–0.073). Chemical space (blue) AQVN (2.40–3.30) EIIP (0.000–0.116) EIIP/AQVN domain of homologous distribution of >90% compounds from PubChem Compound Database.

QSAR Selection

The 103 molecules after EIIP filtering were subjected to pharmacophoring modeling and selection. Twelve literature M1 modulators were converted into 3D structures, along with drug candidates and GRIND descriptors for all compounds were calculated, from which a PCA model was built (**Table 1**).

From PCA scores that included the first two major components, PC1 and PC2, based on their vicinity in the PC1-PC2 space to literature M1 modulators, the most pharmacologically similar drug molecules were selected. The QSAR filtering was carried in Pentacle software (Duran et al., 2009). Finally, 10 compounds were selected for molecular docking (**Table 2**).

M1 Muscarinic Receptor Homology Modeling

In order to obtain the relevant structure of the M1 receptor active state, the crystal structure of the M2 muscarinic receptor in the active state with the agonist and allosteric modulator (PDB ID 4MQT) was used as a template for homology modeling. The P11229 sequence of the Homo sapiens muscarinic acetylcholine receptor M1 was used. The modeling was carried out on the Protein Homology/analogY Recognition Engine V 2.0 (Phyre) server (Kelley et al., 2015).

Molecular Docking

Ten selected compounds after 3D QSAR were further subjected to molecular docking into the M1 receptor model. Three compounds with the lowest binding energy values (**Table 2**) and identified hydrophilic and hydrophobic interactions with allosteric binding site amino acid residues (Tyr 82, Tyr 85, Tyr 106, Tyr 179, Trp 400, Glu 401) were selected to be the best candidates, along with considerations of drug side effects and purpose. Finally, BROMAZEPAM, ESTAZOLAM,

TABLE 1 | PCA models for M1 alosteric modulators and candidates.

Component	SSX	SSXacc	VarX	VarXacc
1	44.48	44.48	43.92	43.92
2	11.32	55.8	10.98	54.9
3	5.48	61.29	5.19	60.09
4	4.97	66.26	4.77	64.86
5	4.09	70.35	3.94	68.8

SSX, Percentage of the X sum of squares; SSXacc, accumulative percentage of the X sum of squares; VarX, percentage of the X variance; VarXaac, accumulative percentage of the X variance.

TABLE 2 | QSAR selection of 10 compounds for molecular docking, with docking energies.

Compound	VINA docking energy, kcal mol-1
Estazolam	−9.9
Diloxanide	−9
Flumazenil	−9.2
Rosoxacin	−9.6
Bromazepam	−9.3
Penicilin V	−9
Sulfamethazine	−8.4
Fluconasole	−8.7
Dapsone	−8
Bromfenac	−9.4
Raltegravir	−10.3

and FLUMAZENIL were found to be the best promising candidates (**Figures 2–4**, respectively).

DISCUSSION

We hypothesized that allosteric activation of M1 receptors in the circumstances of increased cholinergic neurotransmission to the auditory cortex by targeted VNS, will provoke an increase of M1 mediated effects:

(1) Neuromodulatory action of BDGF and NGF (Da Penha Berzaghi et al., 1993) in neuronal zones adjacent to the tinnitus;
(2) Neuromodulatory action on frequency specific neuronal zones enabling the recruitment of pathologically active neurons back to the physiological pattern of activity;
(3) Regaining the physiological tonotopy (Zhang et al., 2006) of the auditory cortex;
(4) Recruitment of novel neurons from undifferentiated neuronal pools in the hippocampus (VanDeMark et al., 2009) and
(5) The dendritic and axonal "rewiring" of the tinnitus "subnetwork" (De Ridder et al., 2014b).

The AQVN/EIIP approach was applied previously for the selection of new candidates in pharmacotherapy of the vasovagal syncope (VVS) revealing that the majority of antimuscarinic drugs might have a therapeutical potential for VVS. In this study sequential virtual screening criteria were applied, first the AQVN/EIIP based filter for the selection of candidate allosteric agonists of the M1 receptor selecting 50 drugs out of 1463 approved drugs from the DrugBank (http://www.drugbank.ca; Wishart et al., 2006). This step was followed by 3DQSAR analysis and finally docking. The screening identified bromazepam, estazolam, and flumazenil as the most promising drugs which could be repurposed as allosteric agonists of the M1 receptor.

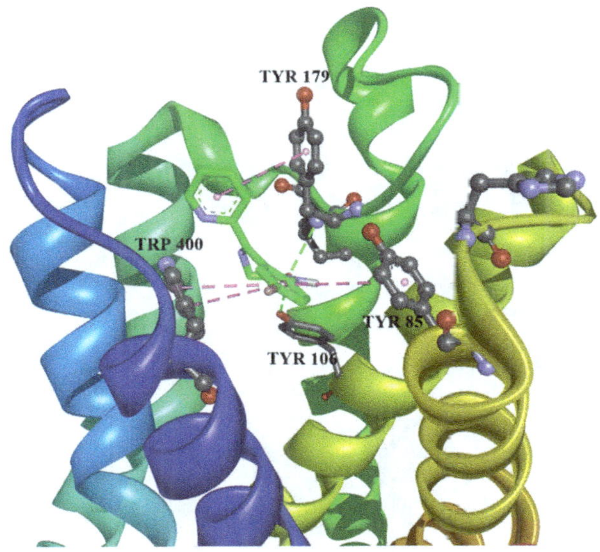

FIGURE 2 | Bromazepam in allosteric modulator binding region of M1 acetylcholine receptor, with marked aminoacids, and intermolecular interactions. Green: hydrogen bonds, purple: hydrophobic interactions.

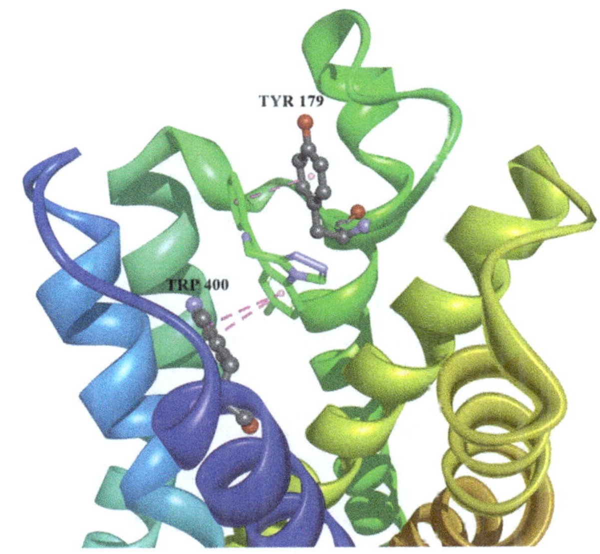

FIGURE 3 | Estazolam in allosteric modulator binding region of M1 acetylcholine receptor, with marked aminoacids, and intermolecular interactions. Green: hydrogen bonds, purple: hydrophobic interactions.

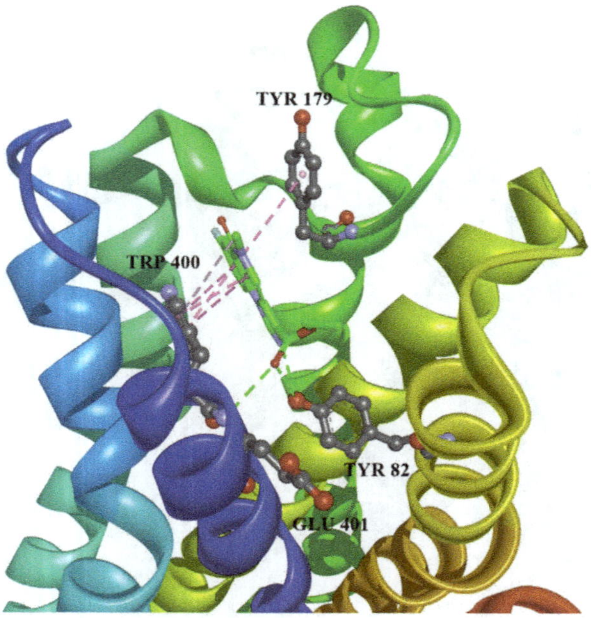

FIGURE 4 | Flumazenil in allosteric modulator binding region of M1 acetylcholine receptor, with marked aminoacids, and intermolecular interactions. Green: hydrogen bonds, purple: hydrophobic interactions.

Bromazepam and estazolam are known anti-anxiety agents with a hypnotic effect. Flumazenil has specific antibenzodiazepine action and is used as an antihypnotic agent in circumstances where the benzodiazepine and nonbenzodizepine hypnotic effect has to be reduced.

If we expand the concept to other methods of treatment of tinnitus (invasive or noninvasive; Vanneste and De Ridder, 2012), it is reasonable to propose that pharmacological facilitation of neuromodulatory changes by the *in silico* identified drugs in our investigation in tinnitus network structures would be beneficial even in these treatments. Future clinical studies of the combined M1 allosteric agonist therapy with VNS and potentially other invasive and noninvasive methods of chronic tinnitus treatment will reveal the final answer regarding their synergistic action.

Learning during wakefulness induces neural plasticity changes. Their stabilization occurs during sleep (Tononi and Cirelli, 2005). The process of sleep selects the synaptic weights of the neural synapses on the basis of their engagement during wakefulness: if the synapses are more used, the sleep process will make them more stabile while the less used synapses during wakefulness will not be strengthened. This is at least partially due to the intensity of cholinergic neurotransmission that increases from wakefulness toward NREM and REM sleep (Hobson and Friston, 2012). The last phase, REM, also known as a dream state, is the state of consciousness where tinnitus is not perceived (De Ridder et al., 2014b). The sleep process in this way supports the mechanisms of learning and memory acquired during wakefulness. If we presume that VNS paired with tones is also the process of re-learning of the cortical networks pathologically changed in tinnitus, then the quality of sleep in chronic tinnitus patients is essential for stabilization of daily acquired neuroplastic changes by the VNS therapy. In line with that, the cholinergic effect together with the hypnotic effect of the proposed drugs could be beneficial and their application justified before bedtime. The caveat that has to be taken into consideration is the feature of benzodiazepines to promote or to reinforce already existing sleep apnea by increased miorelaxation. This effect could diminish the amount of both NREM and REM sleep and potentially prevent the beneficial effect of the sleep on the process of the recovery in tinnitus patients. Biological experiments will address the question of concentration applied to the treatment of tinnitus and the question if sleep apnea as the contraindication for application of the proposed M1 allosteric agonists.

In conclusion, the results presented here suggest a potential novel approach in treatment of chronic tinnitus by VNS paired with tones with *in silico* repurposed drugs as therapeutic candidates that may target M1 and prospectively improve the treatment.

AUTHOR CONTRIBUTIONS

TB, VP, MS, and SG contributed equally to the conception of the work, acquisition, analysis, and interpretation of data. TB, VP, and SG participated in drafting the manuscript, revisiting it critically and gave final approval of the version to be published. The authors reached the agreement to be accountable for all the aspects of the work in ensuring that questions related to the accuracy or integrity of any part of the work are appropriately investigated and resolved.

ACKNOWLEDGMENTS

This work was financed by the Ministry of Education, Science and Technological Development of the Republic of Serbia, project III 41028 and 173001. The preliminary results of this article presented at 10th International Tinnitus Research Initiative Conference and 1st EU COST action (TINNET) Conference. Tinnitus: subtypes, mechanisms and interventions, 16–18th March 2016, Nottingham, UK were awarded by MRC Institute of Hearing Research Early Career Award.

REFERENCES

Bakin, J. S., and Weinberger, N. M. (1996). Induction of a physiological memory in the cerebral cortex by stimulation of the nucleus basalis. *Proc. Natl. Acad. Sci. U.S.A.* 93, 11219–11224. doi: 10.1073/pnas.93.20.11219

Betancourt, A. M., Burgess, S. C., and Carr, R. L. (2006). Effect of developmental exposure to chlorpyrifos on the expression of neurotrophin growth factors and cell-specific markers in neonatal rat brain. *Toxicol. Sci.* 92, 500–506. doi: 10.1093/toxsci/kfl004

Bojić, T. (2003). *Mechanisms Of Cardiovascular Control And Effects Of Acoustic Stimulation On Cardiovascular System During The Wake-Sleep Cycle*. Ph.D. Dissertation, Alma Mater Università di Bologna.

Bojić, T., Perović, V., and Glišić, S. (2016). *In silico* therapeutics for neurogenic hypertension and vasovagal syncope. *Front. Neurosci.* 9:520. doi: 10.3389/fnins.2015.00520

Butcher, A. J., Bradley, S. J., Prihandoko, R., Brooke, S. M., Mogg, A., Bourgognon, J. M., et al. (2016). An antibody biosensor establishes the activation of the M1 muscarinic acetylcholine receptor during learning and memory. *J. Biol. Chem.* 291, 8862–8875. doi: 10.1074/jbc.M115.681726

Chen, G. D., Stolzberg, D., Lobarinas, E., Sun, W., Ding, D., and Salvi, R. (2013). Salicylate-induced cochlear impairments, cortical hyperactivity and re-tuning, and tinnitus. *Hear. Res.* 295, 100–113. doi: 10.1016/j.heares.2012.11.016

Conn, P. J., Jones, C. K., and Lindsley, C. W. (2009). Subtype-selective allosteric modulators of muscarinic receptors for the treatment of CNS disorders. *Trends Pharmacol. Sci.* 30, 148–155. doi: 10.1016/j.tips.2008.12.002

Da Penha Berzaghi, M., Cooper, J., Castren, E., Zafra, F., Sofroniew, M., Thoenen, H., et al. (1993). Cholinergic regulation of brain-derived neurotrophic factor (BDNF) and nerve growth factor (NGF) but not neurotrophin-3 (NT-3) mRNA levels in the developing rat hippocampus. *J. Neurosci.* 13, 3818–3826.

De Ridder, D., Vanneste, S., Engineer, N. D., and Kilgard, M. P. (2014a). Safety and efficacy of vagus nerve stimulation paired with tones for the treatment of tinnitus: a case series. *Neuromodulation* 17, 170–179. doi: 10.1111/ner.12127

De Ridder, D., Vanneste, S., Weisz, N., Londero, A., Schlee, W., Elgoyhen, A. B., et al. (2014b). An integrative model of auditory phantom perception: tinnitus as a unified percept of interacting separable subnetworks. *Neurosci. Biobihav. Rev.* 44, 16–32. doi: 10.1016/j.neubiorev.2013.03.021

Duran, A., Zamora, I., and Pastor, M. (2009). Suitability of GRIND-based principal properties for the description of molecular similarity and ligand-based virtual screening. *J. Chem. Inf. Model.* 49, 2129–2138. doi: 10.1021/ci900228x

Eggermont, J. J., and Kral, A. (2016). Somatic memory and gain increase as preconditions for tinnitus: insights from congenital deafness. *Hear. Res.* 333, 37–48. doi: 10.1016/j.heares.2015.12.018

Eggermont, J. J., and Roberts, L. E. (2004). The neuroscience of tinnitus. *Trends Neurosci.* 27, 676–682. doi: 10.1016/j.tins.2004.08.010

Engineer, N. D., Riley, J. R., Seale, J. D., Vrana, W. A., Shetake, J. A., Sudanagunta, S. P., et al. (2011). Reversing pathological neural activity using targeted plasticity. *Nature* 470, 101–104. doi: 10.1038/nature09656

Ferreira-Vieira, T. H., Guimaraes, I. M., Silva, F. R., and Ribeiro, F. M. (2016). Alzheimer's disease: targeting the cholinergic system. *Curr. Neuropharmacol.* 14, 101–115. doi: 10.2174/1570159X13666150716165726

Geven, L. I., De Kleine, E., Willemsen, A. T., and Van Dijk, P. (2014). Asymmetry in primary auditory cortex activity in tinnitus patients and controls. *Neuroscience* 256, 117–125. doi: 10.1016/j.neuroscience.2013.10.015

Guitton, M. J. (2012). Tinnitus: pathology of synaptic plasticity at the cellular and system levels. *Front. Syst. Neurosci.* 6:12. doi: 10.3389/fnsys.2012.00012

Hobson, J. A., and Friston, K. J. (2012). Waking and dreaming consciousness: neurobiological and functional considerations. *Prog. Neurobiol.* 98, 82–98. doi: 10.1016/j.pneurobio.2012.05.003

Jastreboff, P. (2011). "Tinnitus retraining therapy," in *Textbook of Tinnitus*, eds A. Moller, B. Langguth, D. De Ridder, and T. Kleinjung (New York, NY: Springer), 575–596.

Ji, W., and Suga, N. (2009). Tone-specific and nonspecific plasticity of inferior colliculus elicited by pseudo-conditioning: role of acetylcholine and auditory and somatosensory cortices. *J. Neurophysiol.* 102, 941–952. doi: 10.1152/jn.00222.2009

Ji, W., Suga, N., and Gao, E. (2005). Effects of agonists and antagonists of NMDA and ACh receptors on plasticity of bat auditory system elicited by fear conditioning. *J. Neurophysiol.* 94, 1199–1211. doi: 10.1152/jn.00112.2005

Kalauzi, A., Vuckovic, A., and Bojic, T. (2012). EEG alpha phase shifts during transition from wakefulness to drowsiness. *Int. J. Psychophysiol.* 86, 195–205. doi: 10.1016/j.ijpsycho.2012.04.012

Kalauzi, A., Vuckovic, A., and Bojic, T. (2014). Topographic distribution of EEG alpha attractor correlation dimension values in wake and drowsy states in humans. *Int. J. Psychophysiol.* 95, 278–291. doi: 10.1016/j.ijpsycho.2014.11.008

Kelley, L. A., Mezulis, S., Yates, C. M., Wass, M. N., and Sternberg, M. J. (2015). The phyre2 web portal for protein modeling, prediction and analysis. *Nat. Protoc.* 10, 845–858. doi: 10.1038/nprot.2015.053

Llinas, R., Urbano, F. J., Leznik, E., Ramirez, R. R., and Van Marle, H. J. (2005). Rhythmic and dysrhythmic thalamocortical dynamics: GABA systems and the edge effect. *Trends Neurosci.* 28, 325–333. doi: 10.1016/j.tins.2005.04.006

Malinvaud, D., Londero, A., Niarra, R., Peignard, P., Warusfel, O., Viaud-Delmon, I., et al. (2016). Auditory and visual 3D virtual reality therapy as a new treatment for chronic subjective tinnitus: results of a randomized controlled trial. *Hear Res.* 333, 127–135. doi: 10.1016/j.heares.2015.12.023

Nichols, J. A., Nichols, A. R., Smirnakis, S. M., Engineer, N. D., Kilgard, M. P., and Atzori, M. (2011). Vagus nerve stimulation modulates cortical synchrony and excitability through the activation of muscarinic receptors. *Neuroscience* 189, 207–214. doi: 10.1016/j.neuroscience.2011.05.024

Norena, A. (2011). An integrative model of tinnitus based on a central gain controlling neural sensitivity. *Neurosci. Biobehav. Rev.* 35, 1089–1109. doi: 10.1016/j.neubiorev.2010.11.003

Norena, A. (2015). Revisiting the cochlear and central mechanisms of tinnitus and therapeutic approaches. *Audiol. Neurootol.* 20, 53–59. doi: 10.1159/000380749

Norena, A. J., and Eggermont, J. J. (2005). Enriched acoustic environment after noise trauma reduces hearing loss and prevents cortical map reorganization. *J. Neurosci.* 25, 699–705. doi: 10.1523/JNEUROSCI.2226-04.2005

Platiša, M. M., Bojić, T., Pavlović, S. U., Radovanović, N. N., and Kalauzi, A. (2016). Generalized poincare plots-a new method for evaluation of regimes in cardiac neural control in atrial fibrillation and healthy subjects. *Front. Neurosci.* 10:38. doi: 10.3389/fnins.2016.00038

Shetake, J. A., Engineer, N. D., Vrana, W. A., Wolf, J. T., and Kilgard, M. P. (2012). Pairing tone trains with vagus nerve stimulation induces temporal plasticity in auditory cortex. *Exp. Neurol.* 233, 342–349. doi: 10.1016/j.expneurol.2011.10.026

Shideler, K. K., and Yan, J. (2010). M1 muscarinic receptor for the development of auditory cortical function. *Mol. Brain* 3:29. doi: 10.1186/1756-6606-3-29

Silvani, A., Bojic, T., Cianci, T., Franzini, C., Lodi, C. A., Predieri, S., et al. (2003). Effects of acoustic stimulation on cardiovascular regulation during sleep. *Sleep* 26, 201–205. doi: 10.1093/sleep/26.2.201

Tobin, A. B., and Budd, D. C. (2003). The anti-apoptotic response of the Gq/11-coupled muscarinic receptor family. *Biochem. Soc. Trans.* 31, 1182–1185. doi: 10.1042/bst0311182

Tononi, G., and Cirelli, C. (2005). "A possible role of sleep in synaptic homeostasis," in *The Physiological Nature of Sleep*, eds P. L. Parmeggiani and R. Velluti (London: Imperial College Press), 77–103.

Trott, O., and Olson, A. J. (2010). AutoDock vina: improving the speed and accuracy of docking with a new scoring function, efficient optimization, and multithreading. *J. Comput. Chem.* 31, 455–461. doi: 10.1002/jcc.21334

VanDeMark, K. L., Guizzetti, M., Giordano, G., and Costa, L. G. (2009). The activation of M1 muscarinic receptor signaling induces neuronal differentiation in pyramidal hippocampal neurons. *J. Pharmacol. Exp. Ther.* 329, 532–542. doi: 10.1124/jpet.108.150128

Vanneste, S., and De Ridder, D. (2012). Noninvasive and invasive neuromodulation for the treatment of tinnitus: an overview. *Neuromodulation* 15, 350–360. doi: 10.1111/j.1525-1403.2012.00447.x

Vanneste, S., and De Ridder, D. (2016). Deafferentation-based pathophysiological differences in phantom sound: tinnitus with and without hearing loss. *Neuroimage* 129, 80–94. doi: 10.1016/j.neuroimage.2015.12.002

Veljkovic, N., Glisic, S., Perovic, V., and Veljkovic, V. (2011). The role of long-range intermolecular interactions in discovery of new drugs. *Expert Opin. Drug Discov.* 6, 1263–1270. doi: 10.1517/17460441.2012.638280

Veljkovic, N., Glisic, S., Prljic, J., Perovic, V., and Veljkovic, V. (2013). Simple and general criterion for "*in silico*" screening of candidate HIV drugs. *Curr. Pharm. Biotechnol.* 14, 561–569. doi: 10.2174/138920101405131111105301

Vio, M. M., and Holme, R. H. (2005). Hearing loss and tinnitus: 250 million people and a US$10 billion potential market. *Drug Discov. Tod.* 10, 1263–1265. doi: 10.1016/S1359-6446(05)03594-4

Weinberger, N. M. (2003). The nucleus basalis and memory codes: auditory cortical plasticity and the induction of specific, associative behavioral memory. *Neurobiol. Learn. Mem.* 80, 268–284. doi: 10.1016/S1074-7427(03)00072-8

Wishart, D. S., Knox, C., Guo, A. C., Shrivastava, S. Hassanali, M., Stothard, P., et al. (2006). DrugBank: a comprehensive resource for *in silico* drug discovery and exploration. *Nucleic Acids Res.* 34, D668–D672. doi: 10.1093/nar/gkj067

Wu, C., Stefanescu, R. A., Martel, D. T., and Shore, S. E. (2016). Tinnitus: maladaptive auditory-somatosensory plasticity. *Hear. Res.* 334, 20–29. doi: 10.1016/j.heares.2015.06.005

Zhang, Y., Dyck, R. H., Hamilton, S. E., Nathanson, N. M., and Yan, J. (2005). Disrupted tonotopy of the auditory cortex in mice lacking M1 muscarinic acetylcholine receptor. *Hear. Res.* 201, 145–155. doi: 10.1016/j.heares.2004.10.003

Zhang, Y., Hamilton, S. E., Nathanson, N. M., and Yan, J. (2006). Decreased input-specific plasticity of the auditory cortex in mice lacking M1 muscarinic acetylcholine receptors. *Cereb. Cortex* 16, 1258–1265. doi: 10.1093/cercor/bhj067

Zoccoli, G., Bojić, T., and Franzini, C. (2005). "Regulation of cerebral circulation during sleep," in *The Physiological Nature of Sleep, 1st Edn.*, eds P. L. Parmeggiani and R. Velluti (London: Imperial College Press), 351–369.

12

Excitation of the Auditory System as a Result of Non-Invasive Extra-Cochlear Stimulation in Normal Subjects and Tinnitus Patients

Marzena Mielczarek [1], Arnaud Norena [2], Winfried Schlee [3] and Jurek Olszewski [1]***

[1] *Department of Otolaryngology, Laryngological Oncology, Audiology and Phoniatrics, Medical University of Lodz, Lodz, Poland,* [2] *Laboratoire Neurosciences Intégratives et Adaptatives, Aix-Marseille Université, Marseille, France,* [3] *Department for Psychiatry and Psychotherapy, University of Regensburg, Regensburg, Germany*

Correspondence:
Marzena Mielczarek
marzena.mielczarek@umed.lodz.pl

One of possible approach that may suppress tinnitus is electrical stimulation of the ear. At first invasive techniques were used (promontory or round window stimulation), nowadays a non-invasive method, namely hydrotransmissive electric stimulation (ES) through external acoustic canal, has been developed. The aim of the study is to investigate the effect of applying ES with positive and negative current polarities on the ears of healthy subjects and on the tinnitus ears of patients with tinnitus. This comparison further clarifies the mechanisms of operation of non-invasive extra-cochlear ear ES. A second aim is to assess the effects of ES on tinnitus in tinnitus patients. The material was composed of two groups: tinnitus group—49 patients suffering from tinnitus, and healthy students group—34 healthy individuals. ES was performed with the use of a custom-made apparatus. The active, silver probe–was immersed inside saline filling external ear canal. The passive electrode was placed on the forehead. Positive and next negative DC stimulation was provided with the use following frequencies: 0.25, 1, 2, 3, 4, 5, 6, 7, 8 kHz. We checked for the presence of the auditory percept (AP) and, if AP was present, the minimum current amplitude necessary to produce AP was measured. In our research both positive and negative polarities were efficient to evoke AP in the participants. This effect, however, was more pronounced for positive polarity in no tinnitus and normal hearing individuals (healthy students group). In the tinnitus group, current intensity needed to evoke AP was higher than in the healthy students group. However, comparing normal hearing vs. hearing loss patients within the tinnitus group, we did not observe the relationship between hearing threshold and current intensity evoking AP. Afterwards, we analyzed the effect of multi-frequency ES on tinnitus. It appeared to be effective in 75% of tinnitus ears (with a high score of disappearance–22%). Our study proved that extracochlear ES with positive and negative current was efficient to stimulate the auditory system. Stimulating tinnitus ears with two polarities we obtained a higher ratio of improvement (75%) comparing to positive stimulations.

Keywords: tinnitus, electric stimulation, cathodal stimulation, anodal stimulation, auditory percept, ear, sensorineural hearing loss

INTRODUCTION

Tinnitus, an auditory percept that is not induced by any acoustic stimulation in the environment, is largely prevalent in the general population and can dramatically impair the quality of life. Tinnitus can be classified as peripheral or central: Peripheral tinnitus is defined as resulting from aberrant neural activity in the cochlear nerve propagating all the way up to the auditory centers, while central tinnitus is defined as resulting from aberrant neural activity generated in the auditory centers, when cochlear spontaneous activity is reduced or absent (in the case of severe hearing loss) (Noreña, 2015). However, according to some models of tinnitus, it is possible that tinnitus may have a mixed origin, i.e., peripheral and central (Noreña, 2011, 2015). It has been proposed that this mixed tinnitus can result from an amplification of residual cochlear nerve activity (Mulders and Robertson, 2009; Noreña, 2011). Various approaches to treatment can also be used. Central tinnitus can be treated by interfering with the tinnitus-related central mechanisms (Noreña and Eggermont, 2005; Pantev et al., 2012; Tass and Popovych, 2012); these approaches assume that tinnitus results from the central changes after hearing loss, and that these changes can be reversed by appropriate stimulation. Alternatively, peripheral or mixed tinnitus is treated by suppressing or reducing the spontaneous activity in the cochlea; more precisely, if tinnitus is caused by hyperactivity in the cochlear nerve, then a clinical approach should reduce this activity. This is the rationale for pharmacological treatment using NMDA antagonists (Puel, 2007; Ruel et al., 2008; van de Heyning et al., 2014).

Another approach that may suppress tinnitus-related cochlear activity is electrical stimulation (ES), first used when House reported total tinnitus suppression after cochlear implantation (House, 1976). Invasive techniques have been found to remove tinnitus in 43–60% (Aran and Cazals - transtympanal stimulations of the promontorium and round window respectively), 45% (Rubinstein–round window stimulation) in 69–77% (Ito and Sakakihara–promontory test and cochlear implant respectively) of cases depending on the study (Cazals et al., 1978; Portmann et al., 1979; Ito and Sakakihara, 1994; Rubinstein et al., 2003). Further non- invasive techniques have been developed, with success rates of 62.2% (Lee et al.—transcutaneous ES of the auricle), 50% (Kuk et al.—eardrum) and 40.4% (Maini and Deoganonkar - stimulation of the mastoid) (Portmann et al., 1979; Chouard et al., 1981; Shulman, 1987; Quaranta et al., 2004; Mielczarek and Olszewski, 2014). Nowadays electrical stimulation is used as a test to predict post-operative profits before cochlear implantation. During non-invasive extratympanic ear stimulation (via a ball-shaped electrode dipped in saline in external ear canal) sound perception is considered an evidence of acoustic nerve excitation, also confirming restored function (Bochenek et al., 1989; Skarzynski et al., 1999; Dehmel et al., 2008).

The first experiments with ES at the Medical University of Lodz date back to the 1980s. At first, invasive transtympanic promontory positive DC stimulations were used with a success rate reaching 42% (Konopka et al., 2001). Later, a non-invasive approach was used: hydrotransmissive stimulations through the external acoustic canal with the use of positive DC. Improvement was obtained directly after treatment in 37.8% of cases; however, the follow up after 1 month found the success ratio had increased to 51.3%. A comparison with a placebo group showed statistically significant differences indicating the value of the method (Mielczarek and Olszewski, 2014).

Although many studies have reported tinnitus improvement or tinnitus suppression after ES (Shulman, 1987; Bochenek et al., 1989; Skarzynski et al., 1999), the exact mechanism of this phenomenon remains unclear. It has been suggested that ES works by increasing the transmission of neurotransmitters in the synapses (Latkowski, 1981), modifying the electrical potentials of the hearing organ (Portmann et al., 1979), or by improving the blood flow in the inner ear and synchronizing the spontaneous impulses in the auditory nerve fibers (Watanabe et al., 1997). Another suggested mechanism of action is by stimulation of the C_2 dorsal root. Dehmel et al note that the C_2 fibers, supplying the skin of the retroauricular region and mucosal lining of the tympanic cavity, target cells in the dorsal column nuclei, which then send axons to the dorsal cochlear nuclei (Dehmel et al., 2008). This mechanism may account for the relief of tinnitus experienced after stimulation of the cochlea surface (Møller, 2016).

Despite the fact that ES have been used in tinnitus treatment since the1970s (studies testing different locations of the stimulating electrode and different parameters of the stimulating current) there are no recommendations on the adjustment of the stimulation conditions in tinnitus treatment. Two early studies on peripheral ES suggest that anodic (positive) ES, with an inhibitory potential should be used to suppress tinnitus; however, cathodic (negative) ES, bearing stimulating properties, should be used to excite the auditory nerve, evoking sound perception (Bochenek et al., 1989; Ren and Nuttall, 1995).

The aim of the study is to investigate the effect of applying positive and negative current polarities on the ear of a healthy subject and on the tinnitus ear of a patient with tinnitus. This comparison will further clarify the mechanisms of operation of non-invasive extra-cochlear ear ES. A second aim was to assess the effects of ES on tinnitus in tinnitus patients.

METHODS

The research was approved by Institutional Review Board of the Medical University of Lodz (RNN/251/05/KB) and was in accordance with the declaration of Helsinki. All patients gave their written, informed consent prior to inclusion in the study.

Study Sample

The research was conducted in the Department of Otolaryngology, Laryngological Oncology, Audiology and Phoniatrics, Medical University of Lodz. The material was composed of two groups (**Table 1**). Group I was a tinnitus group comprising 49 patients suffering from tinnitus ($n = 71$ tinnitus ears: 24 normal hearing ears and 47 sensorineural hearing loss ears). Twenty-eight of the participants were females and 21 were males, with an age range of 22–79 years (average = 53.4, SD = 15.6). In the case of unilateral tinnitus, only the tinnitus ear was

TABLE 1 | Patient characteristics.

	Tinnitus group (group I)	Healthy students group (group II)
Number of participants	49 (22 patients with bilateral, 27-unilateral tinnitus)	34 (in 33 students both ears were tested in 1 person - one ear was tested)
Number of tested ears	71	67
Gender	28 F, 21 M	13 F, 21 M
Age in years (mean ± standard deviation), range	53.4 ± 15.6 range: 22–79 year	23.5 ± 2.9 range: 20–35 year
Visual Analog Scale for tinnitus loudness (range 0–10) Mean ± standard deviation	Before ES: 5.52 ± 1.70 After ES: 3.27 ± 2.37	

tested. The allocation to tinnitus group was randomized, done according to the order of admission to our department. Group II was formed of healthy subjects. This group comprised 34 healthy, normal hearing individuals without tinnitus: 13 female and 21 male, mean age 23.5 years, range 20–35 years ($SD = 2.9$) (n–67 ears). The study was not blinded.

Before the beginning of the study, otorhinolaryngological examination, and hearing tests (pure tone audiometry, speech audiometry, impedance audiometry, auditory brainstem responses) were conducted, as well as radiological diagnostics of head and cervical spine if necessary. Pathology in the external and/or the middle ear was an exclusion criterion, together with the presence of a pacemaker, CNS vascular malformation, epilepsy, or any history of head and neck neoplasm. Patients who reported tinnitus in the head but not in the ears were also excluded from the study. The patients from Group I were asked to assess tinnitus in visual analog scale (VAS) for loudness, directly before and directly after electrical stimulation. The scale ranged from 0 – no tinnitus, 1 – very quiet tinnitus to 10 – extremely loud tinnitus.

Experimental Procedure

ES was performed with the use of a custom-made apparatus supplied with four batteries of 1.5 V. The device allows for direct current stimulation within a frequency range of 0.25–8 kHz and an amplitude range of 0.01–2.24 mA. The external ear canal was filled with saline solution. The active silver probe was immersed inside external ear canal, avoiding contact with the skin of the canal. The passive electrode was placed on the forehead (in the midline) after skin abrasion with a suitable sterile abrasive electrode paste and clean gauze. The two electrodes were placed in such a way as to allow current transmission throughout the hypothetical plane (longitudinal axis) of the cochlea.

DC electrical stimulation was provided. The effects of positive current were first assessed. The series of tests with positive currents were completed then the same tests were carried out with negative currents. ES was performed using the following frequencies: 0.25, 1, 2, 3, 4, 5, 6, 7, and 8 kHz. For each stimulation frequency, the presence of an auditory precept (AP) was confirmed and, if AP was present, the minimum current amplitude necessary to produce AP was measured. ES treatment was started with a maximum well tolerated current intensity. If AP was present, the intensity of current was slowly decreased and the patient was asked to indicate the moment when the sound ceased to be audible. The protocol was performed first for positive (anodal), then for negative (cathodal) current in both groups, for each of the abovementioned frequencies.

The duration of the rectangular pulse depended on the frequency, e.g., for 250 Hz, one period lasted 4 ms (2 ms pulse and 2 ms pause). The voltage was constant and equaled 3 V. The maximum intensity was variable (ranged from 0.15 to 2.24 mA) and was applied according to the sensation of the patient. If the patient reported pain or other unpleasant sensation, the intensity of the current was smoothly decreased (with the intensity knob) to a level producing a tolerable sensation.

Next, the pitch of electrically-evoked AP was assessed in a sound proof chamber. A subgroup of 20 patients from the tinnitus group were selected. These perceptions were matched with free field sounds as pure tones from the audiometer. A pair of pure tones was delivered in a free field through the loudspeakers (Martin Audio C115), and the patient was asked to indicate the one which more closely resembled the sound perceived during ES. One tone was similar to the stimulating frequency and the other was next lower tone on the audiometer (Madsen Electronic Orbiter 922). If neither sound was similar, the next pair of tones was given. Matching was performed simultaneously with ES.

Statistical Testing

The numerical data was tested for normality of distribution using the Shapiro-Wilk W-test. Levene's test was performed in order to assess the homogeneity of variances in both compared groups. A p-level of 0.05 was assumed for all tests of significance. All the statistical procedures were conducted as two-tailed ones. Due to the small sample sizes and lack of normality, appropriate non-parametric tests were performed, and also robust standard errors or standard errors allowing for intragroup correlation were estimated when applicable.

Generalized estimating equations with clustered standard errors (i.e., allowing for intragroup correlation) were carried out for a numerical dependent variable (hearing threshold), a set of independent variables comprising current threshold values measured at selected frequencies, and subject hearing (hearing loss vs. normal hearing). All p-values obtained during the analysis approximated to a value of one.

RESULTS

Overall, 1,278 stimulations were conducted in the tinnitus group (71 ears × nine frequencies × two polarities), and 1,206 in

TABLE 2 | Logistic regression estimates for predictors of auditory perception (AP).

Investigated trait	OR (95% CI)	Level of statistical significance (*p*-value)
Type of tinnitus (tone vs. noise vs. tone + noise)	0.42 (0.15–1.13)	= 0.085
Age (1-year step)	0.97 (0.92–1.02)	= 0.172
Hearing level	0.65 (0.09–4.63)	= 0.664

the healthy student group (67 ears × nine frequencies × two polarities).

The Presence of AP During ES

In both groups, in the majority of cases, AP was produced during ES. Overall, it was present in 60 ears in the tinnitus group (84.5%) and in 66 ears in the healthy students group (98.5%). In the tinnitus group, from all the 1,278 stimulations, AP was evoked in 182 (14.24%) stimulations while no sound perception was evoked in the other 1,096 (85.76%). In the healthy students group, out of 1,206 stimulations, AP was evoked in 798 (66.2%) stimulations, while no AP was evoked in the other 408 (33.8%). The analysis showed that sound perception was less likely during ES in the tinnitus group than the healthy students group ($p < 0.001$). During ES temporary pain was reported by persons from both groups: in tinnitus group—by 25 patients (51%), and in healthy subjects group—by 14 individuals (41%). In all cases it was exclusively momentary and it disappeared as soon as current intensity was smoothly decreased, so the procedure was continued.

Furthermore, in the tinnitus group we tested whether the presence of the AP depended on the type of tinnitus (tone vs. noise vs. tone + noise), age or hearing level. Binary logistic regression with robust standard error was performed (**Table 2**). No relationship was confirmed (OR = 0.42; 95% CI: 0.15–1.13; $p = 0.085$). AP was present in 91.1% of ears with tone-like tinnitus, in 70.0% in noise-like tinnitus and 80.0% of ears when tinnitus was a mixture of tone and noise. Within the tinnitus group, the presence of AP did not depend on age (OR = 0.97; 95% CI: 0.92–1.02; $p = 0.172$), nor hearing level (OR = 0.65; 95% CI: 0.09–4.63; $p = 0.664$). It was present in 71.4% of normal hearing ears, and in 71.6% of hearing loss ears. The mean age of patients with AP was 51.5 years ($SD = 15.7$), and the mean age of those without was 60.5 years ($SD = 13.5$). The averaged pure tone audiograms in the tinnitus group (normal hearing and hearing loss subjects) and in the healthy students group are presented in **Figures 1–3**.

Analysis of Current Intensities Needed to Evoke AP

In the tinnitus group, the intensities of current evoking AP ranged from 0.16 to 1.67 mA (mean-0.614 mA), in the healthy students group—from 0.01 to 1.61 mA (mean-0.461 mA). The analysis showed that in the tinnitus group, ES needed higher intensities of current to evoke sound perception ($p < 0.003$). Moreover, in the tinnitus group we analyzed intensities of current evoking sound perception vs. averaged hearing thresholds at 0.25, 1, 2 kHz, respectively. We did not perform this analysis for higher stimulating frequencies since AP was practically absent for 4 kHz (present in five ears) and 8 kHz (present in three ears). There was no correlation between hearing threshold and current intensity needed to evoke AP during electrical stimulation.

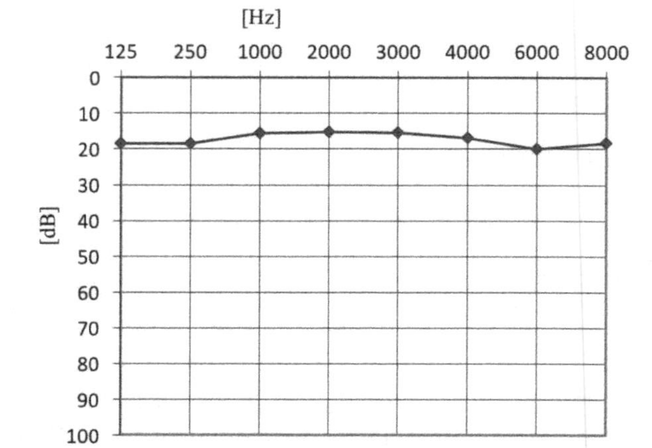

FIGURE 1 | The averaged pure tone audiogram in tinnitus group–normal hearing tinnitus patients.

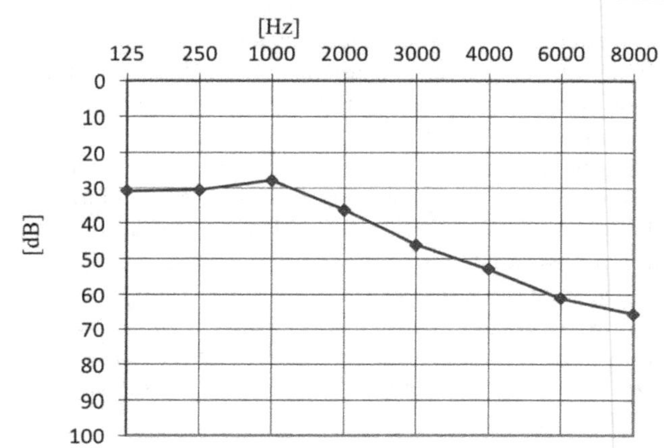

FIGURE 2 | The averaged pure tone audiogram in the tinnitus group–hearing loss tinnitus patients.

Analysis of Current Frequencies Needed to Evoke AP

In the tinnitus group, in the majority of cases (83.1%), AP was present for stimulating frequencies between 0.25 and 2 kHz (**Figure 4**).

In the healthy students group, AP was present for each stimulating frequency—0.25–8 kHz (**Figure 5**).

Correlation Between Frequency and Intensity of Current Needed to Evoke AP

Evaluation of the correlation between stimulating frequency and intensity of current indicated that higher stimulating frequencies needed higher current intensities to evoke AP in the tinnitus group ($p < 0.001$) as well as the healthy students group ($p < 0.001$) (**Figure 6**).

Current Polarity vs. AP vs. Ear

Both current polarities (positive and negative) evoked AP during ES. In the majority of ears AP was evoked by both positive and negative current: in 57.7% of tinnitus ears in the tinnitus group and in 97% of ears in the healthy students group (**Figure 7**).

The binary logistic regression with robust standard error was performed. Furthermore, in tinnitus group, with respect to AP, positive polarity appeared to be significantly more efficient than negative. AP was present in nearly 82% of tinnitus ears when positive current was used, and in 61% during negative stimulations ($p < 0.001$). In healthy students group, both polarities were equally effective, evoking AP in 98.5% of ears ($p > 0.9$).

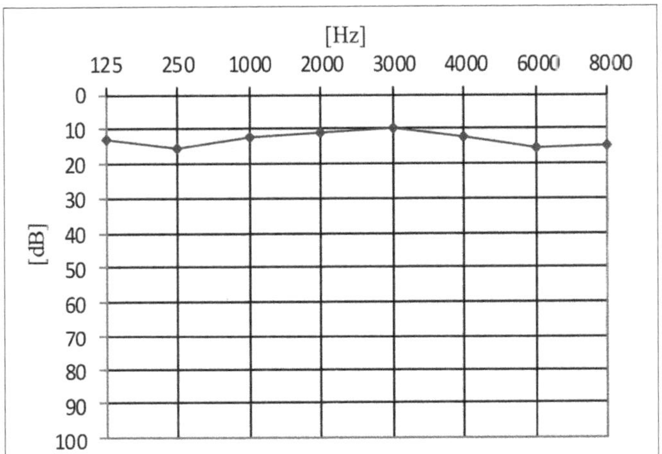

FIGURE 3 | The averaged pure tone audiogram in the healthy students group.

In the tinnitus group, ES needed higher intensities of current to evoke AP for positive polarity and for the left ear compared with negative polarity and the right ear (Pos. left vs. Pos. right: $t = 2.6041$, $p < 0.009$; Pos. left vs. Neg. left: $t = 2.511$, $p = 0.012$). All other comparisons (T-tests) were not significant ($p > 0.05$). In the healthy students group, positive polarity needed higher intensities to evoke AP ($p = 0.001$), without significant differences between left and right ear in this group ($p = 0.92$).

Matching Electrically Evoked AP With Free Field Sounds in Tinnitus Group

The matching was done in tinnitus group in 20 patients. A total of 448 matchings were performed. Electrically-evoked AP were matched with free field sounds (pure tones from the audiometer). The pitch of electrically-evoked AP changed with a change in stimulating current frequency. Sound perceptions evoked by low stimulating frequencies (0.25–2 kHz) had more exact matching to free field sounds. 1 kHz appeared to have the most adequate matchings. 3 and 4 kHz were mainly identified as lower sounds like 2 and 3 kHz, respectively. 6 and 8 kHz were identified as low (1 kHz) sounds (**Figure 8**).

Analysis of Tinnitus After ES in Tinnitus Group

Generalized estimating equations with robust standard errors were carried out for a categorical dependent variable (an

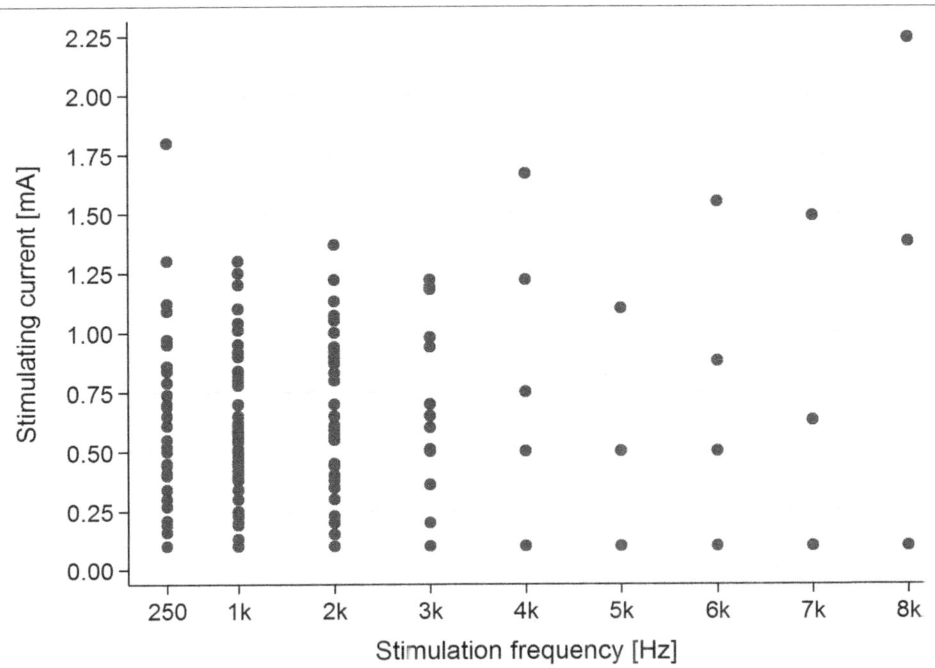

FIGURE 4 | The presence of the AP in the tinnitus group for particular stimulating current parameters (mA/kHz).

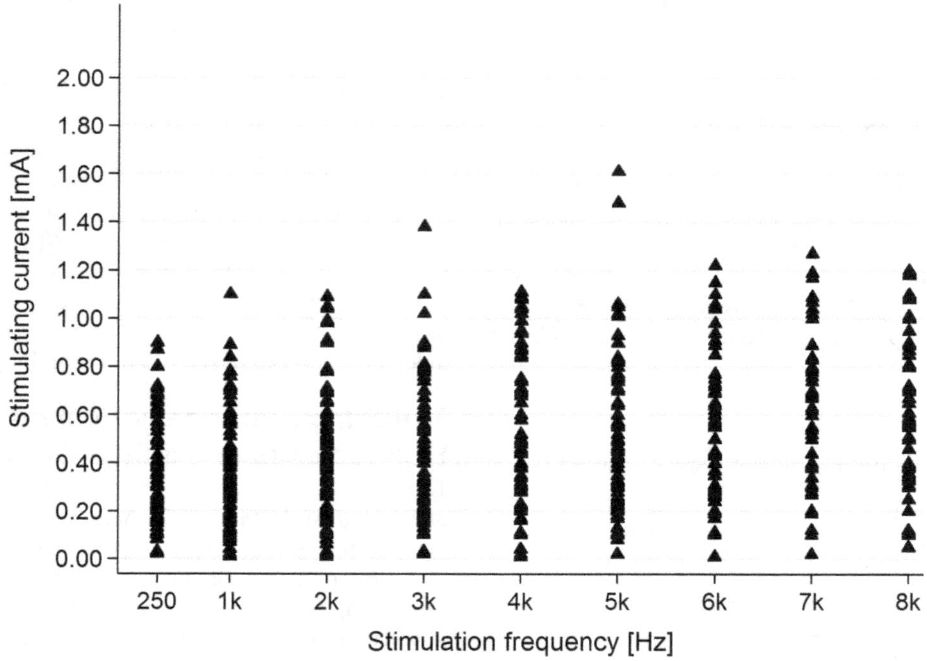

FIGURE 5 | The presence of the AP in the healthy students group for particular stimulating current parameters (mA/kHz).

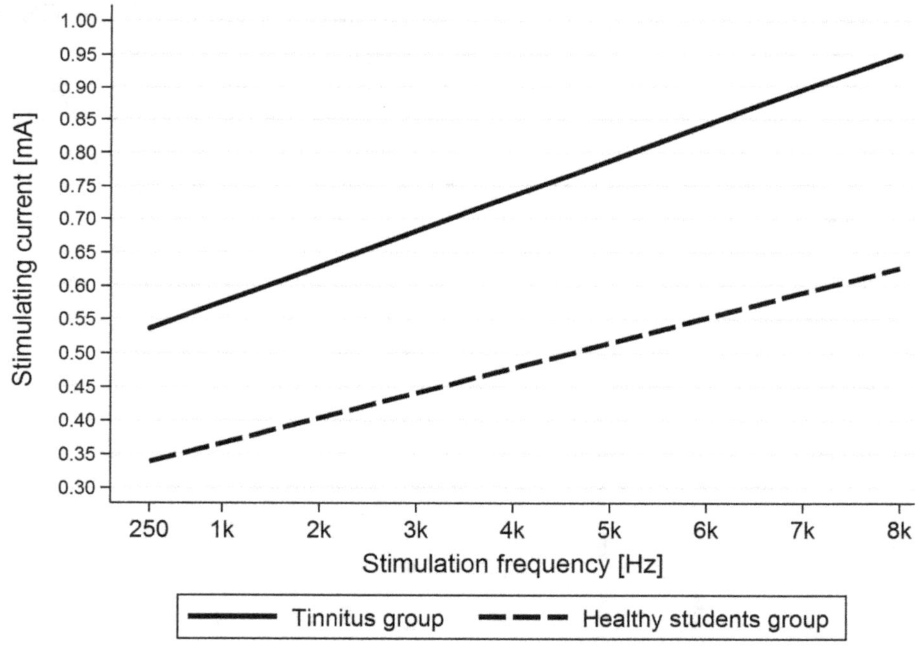

FIGURE 6 | The dependence of stimulating current intensity on stimulating frequency.

improvement in tinnitus) and a set of independent variables comprising sound perception and the subject status before and after stimulation.

Before and directly after ES, we asked 28 patients from the tinnitus group (46 tinnitus ears) to describe the loudness of tinnitus in VAS (visual analog scale for tinnitus loudness). The

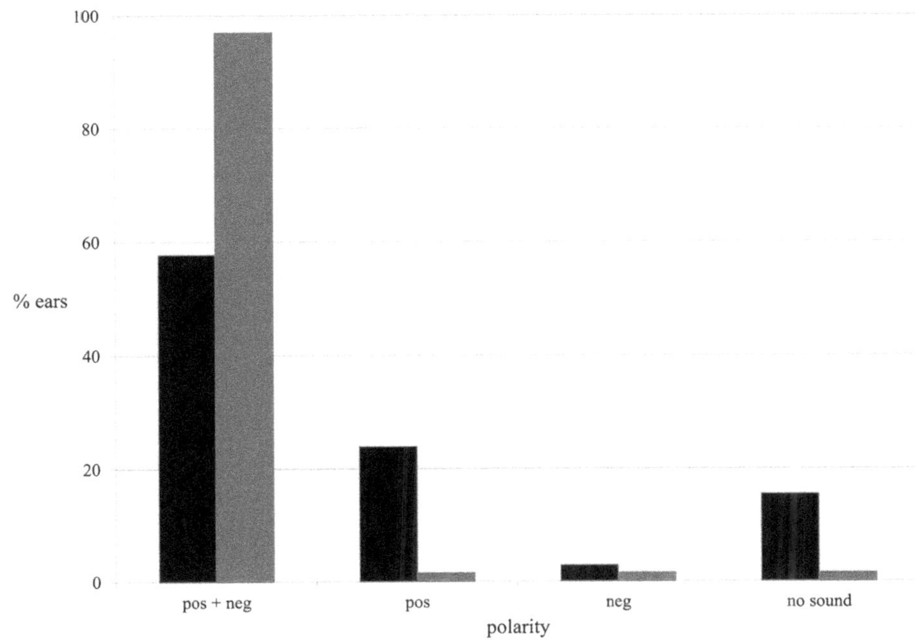

FIGURE 7 | The presence of the AP in terms of current polarity in the tinnitus group (black column) and the healthy students group (gray column)

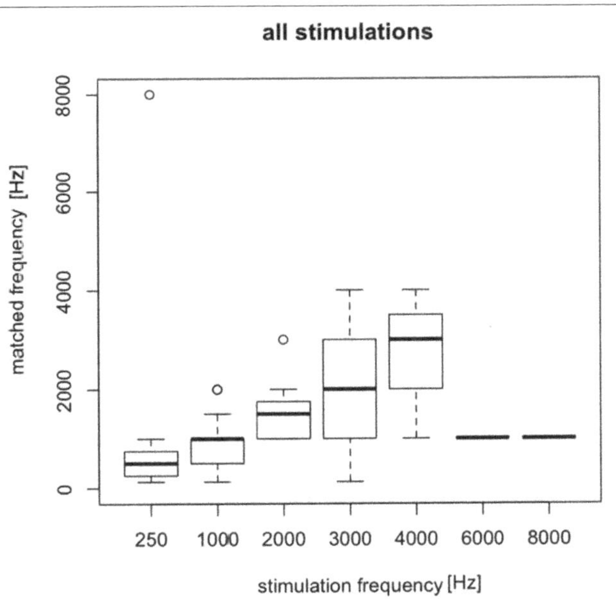

FIGURE 8 | Matching electrically evoked pitch of AP with free field sounds in the tinnitus group.

mean tinnitus loudness before stimulation was 5.52 (*SD* 1.70), and after 3.27 (*SD* 2.37; $p < 0.001$) **Figure 9**.

Directly after ES, there was improvement in 21 ears (75%), no change in five ears (18%), and worsening in two ears (7%). In 10 out of 46 ears (22%), tinnitus disappeared. Interestingly, there was no correlation between the improvement in tinnitus and the presence of electrically evoked AP ($p > 0.5$).

DISCUSSION

In our research both positive and negative polarities excited the auditory system evoking an AP in the study participants. This effect, however, was more pronounced for positive polarity in no tinnitus and normal hearing individuals (healthy students group). In the tinnitus group the AP was present for a much narrower range of stimulating frequencies (0.25–2 kHz) when compared to the no tinnitus and normal hearing healthy students group (0.25–8 kHz).

In the tinnitus group, the current intensity needed to evoke an AP was higher than in the healthy students group, which could suggest the effect of hearing threshold. However, comparing normal hearing vs. hearing loss patients within tinnitus group, again, we did not observe any relationship between hearing threshold and current intensity evoking AP. Furthermore, we matched electrically evoked AP pitch with free field sounds in tinnitus group. We saw that the pitch of AP changed with a change in stimulating frequency. Afterwards, we analyzed the effect of multi-frequency ES on tinnitus. It appeared to be effective in 75% of tinnitus ears (with a high score of disappearance – 22%). The interesting fact was that the improvement in tinnitus was not correlated with the presence of AP during the ES.

Animal studies showed that electrical current influences the micromechanics of the Corti organ. Nuttall and Ren stimulating the round window membrane and cochlear duct in guinea pigs reported movements in the basilar membrane and emission of sound from the cochlea. This phenomenon was possible only when some OHCs were intact so their movements displaced the basilar membrane. The authors indicated that any intra- or

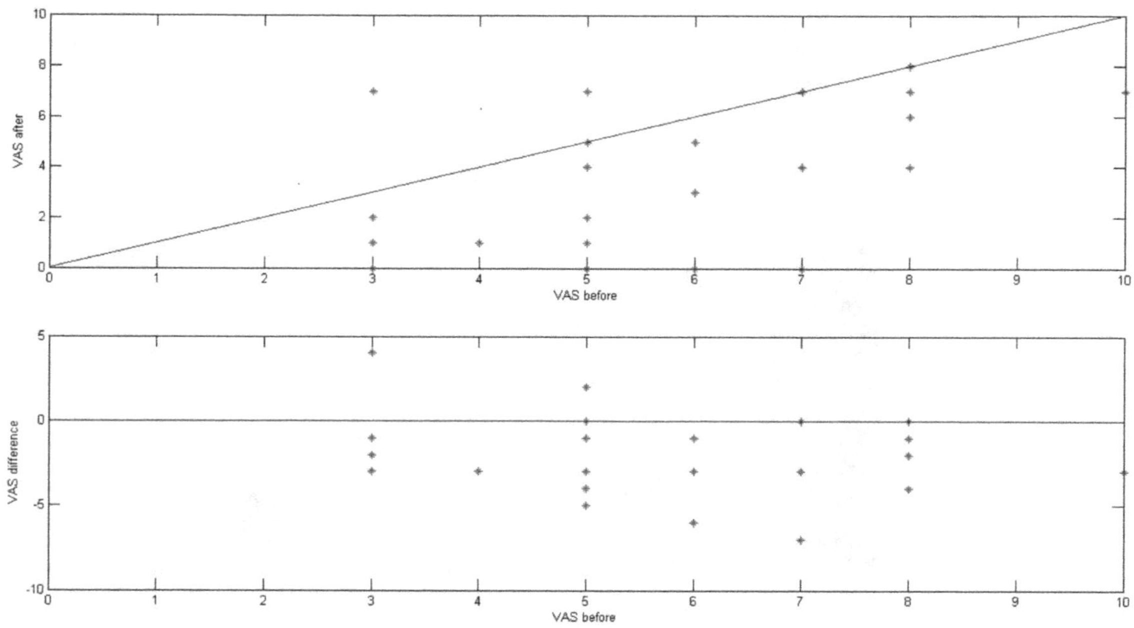

FIGURE 9 | The effect of ES on tinnitus in the tinnitus group presented as a result in VAS for tinnitus loudness (before and after stimulation).

extra-cochlear electric current stimulation affects the polarization of OHCs and could induce a traveling wave in the basilar membrane (Nuttall and Ren, 1995; Ren and Nuttall, 1995).

In our research, this mechanism of ES is also possible. Applying electric current to external ear canal we reach the cochlea (the conduction of the stimulus through the lining of the tympanic cavity and the round window) but since soft tissues have conductive properties, this might not be a single way in which electric impulse affects auditory system. Earlier research on ear ES demonstrated cortical potential alternations after ear ES, so we may alike influence central auditory system directly in the same time (Mielczarek et al., 2016). Furthermore, since the pitch of electrically evoked AP changed with a change of stimulating frequency, it is possible that we stimulate the cochlea (and auditory nerve) selectively, producing a normal traveling wave or directly changing (selectively) the OHC potential. However, the selectivity of the excitation is probably worst comparing to excitation of Corti organ with sound.

By applying negative pulses to the impaired cochlea, Portman et al. elicited auditory sensation, which was regarded as proof of auditory nerve excitation. This response, however, was not based on the stimulating frequency, as auditory sensation remained unchanged when the frequency was altered (Portmann et al., 1979).

Secondly, since in our research the AP was more pronounced in the group of healthy students (no tinnitus normal hearing young individuals) and since there were no differences between normal hearing and hearing loss patients in this regard within the tinnitus group, the authors assume that OHC function is not a determining factor for the AP phenomenon. We hypothesize that the condition of the synapsis and auditory neurons are responsible for these variations (Kujawa and Liberman, 2015; Viana et al., 2015).

Many studies describe the dependence of the ES effect on current polarity. Cazals et al. point to the direction of current flow applied to cochlea suggesting that positive polarity should be used to reduce tinnitus, and a negative polarity to evoke sound perception (Cazals et al., 1978). These findings have been confirmed elsewhere (Sun et al., 2000; Noreña et al., 2015), but the results seem to be inconsistent (Guo, 2001). Furthermore Cazals et al. claimed that when stimulating with negative current, the AP was present in a wider range of frequencies and lower intensities were required to produce auditory sensation. They placed the electrodes on the promontory or round window, and a reference one on the earlobe (Cazals et al., 1978). The results of our study showed that the direction of current flow (the polarity) is not a deciding factor whether ES evokes AP or not. In the healthy students group, AP appeared to be independent from the current polarity; however, in the tinnitus group, negative stimulations were less likely to evoke AP when compared to positive current. Negative stimulations needed lower intensities to evoke sound perception, which was coherent with Cazals et al.

AP evoked during stimulation of the deaf ears seems to be a confirmation that this perception is generated above the cochlea. Chouard et al. stimulating deaf ears (round window) registered auditory brainstem potentials and noticed sound sensation (AP) in almost all deaf ears (Chouard et al., 1979, 1994). These results may be considered proof for the concept that AP depends on auditory nerve function, not on the cochlea, although the cochlea acts as the first effector of the electric stimulus. Some authors evoke AP during ES on deaf ears (before cochlear implantation) to confirm restored function of the acoustic nerve (Gersuni and

Volokhov, 1936; House and Brackmann, 1974; Bochenek et al., 1977; Portmann et al., 1979; Skarzynski et al., 1999). The use of promontory ES in patients labyrinthectomized due to Meniere's disease, resulted in sound percept despite complete loss of inner ear function (Lambert et al., 1990).

Rattay et al. suggest a correlation between polarity sensitivity and the state of degeneration and demyelination of peripheral neurons. According to them degenerated peripheral neurons would require lower anodic thresholds (Rattay et al., 2001). Our results do not confirm any such effect. In our research, in the tinnitus group, the intensity of current needed to evoke AP was higher than in healthy students group—suggesting the effect of neural degeneration due to natural processes in the tinnitus group, and the levels of current were higher for positive stimulation. Interestingly, in the tinnitus group, AP did not depend on hearing threshold. Since the two subgroups (tinnitus patients with normal hearing and tinnitus patients with hearing loss) were similar in terms of age, we can assume that the condition of the auditory nerve was similar, even if the hearing status differed. Viana et al. demonstrated in five "normal" ears, features of cochlear synaptopathy and the degeneration of cochlear nerve peripheral axons, in the presence of a near-normal hair cell population; they suggest that such changes account for human presbyacusis (Viana et al., 2015). Other animal studies showed that in age-related hearing loss, degeneration of cochlear synapses precedes both hair cell loss and hearing threshold elevation (Kujawa and Liberman, 2015).

In early research by Jellinek and Schreiber (1930) it was reported that ES of the ear with alternating current causes AP, which induces a sound perception at the stimulating frequency. The phenomenon was at first explained by vibratory or mechanical forces arising at the electrode, changes in the fluid volume (filling external ear canal) and mechanical excitation of the tympanum or ossicles. Afterwards Arapova et al. (1937) suggested another two possible mechanisms: the first was that AC evokes mechanical forces in the cochlea, thus stimulating the receptors in the usual way, while the second was that AC directly affects the receptor, omitting the stage of transformation from electrical to mechanical forces. For Gersuni and Volokhov, the proof of cochlea excitation was their production of beats by simultaneous electrical and sound stimulation at approximately similar frequencies (Gersuni and Volokhov, 1936).

Lusted and Simmons give two possible explanations for electrically-evoked AP: the OHC stimulation or afferent auditory fiber excitation (Lusted et al., 1984). Stevens et al. accounts for the "electrophonic effect" by direct stimulation of the auditory nerve, and by electromechanical transduction in the inner ear or tympanum (Stevens and Jones, 1939). Kellaway argues in favor of cochlear structure excitation: sound sensation was always a pure tone, never noise, the change in the polarity of current did not change the character of the sound effect, the absence of tympanic membrane did not influence the perceived sound (Kellaway, 1946). In our research, the AP was a pure tone sound, never noise, suggesting the involvement of sensory elements rather than mechanical. Furthermore, it did not depend on current polarity, since it was present for both.

Many papers have confirmed the value of ES of the ear in tinnitus treatment (Cazals et al., 1978; Portmann et al., 1979; Rubinstein et al., 2003; Arts et al., 2015). Our study proved that extracochlear ES with positive and negative current was efficient to stimulate the auditory system. The auditory nerve appeared to be the most probable place of AP generation. Stimulating tinnitus ears with two polarities, we obtained a higher ratio of improvement (75%) comparing to positive stimulation alone (Mielczarek and Olszewski, 2014). However, since the presence of AP was not correlated with the improvement in tinnitus, some other mechanisms may account for this effect.

AUTHOR CONTRIBUTIONS

MM, AN, WS, and JO: Substantial contribution to the design of the study and the draft of the manuscript; MM and JO: Data acquisition; WS and MM: Performed statistical testing; MM, WS, and AN: Created figures. All authors revised and approved the manuscript.

ACKNOWLEDGMENTS

This publication is supported by Biomedicine and Molecular Biosciences European Cooperation in Science and Technology COST. Action framework - TINNET BM1306.

REFERENCES

Arapova, A. A., Gersuni, G. V., and Volokhov, A. A. (1937). A further analysis of the action of alternating currents on the auditory apparatus. *J. Physiol.* 89, 122–131. doi: 10.1113/jphysiol.1937.sp003468

Arts, R. A., George, E. L., Chenault, M. N., and Stokroos, R. J. (2015). Optimizing intracochlear electrical stimulation to suppress tinnitus. *Ear Hear.* 36, 125–135. doi: 10.1097/AUD.0000000000000090

Bochenek, W., Chorzempa, A., Hazell, J. W., Kiciak, J., and Kukwa, A. (1989). Non-invasive electrical stimulation of the ear canal as a communication aid in acquired total deafness. *Br. J. Audiol.* 23, 285–291. doi: 10.3109/03005368909076516

Bochenek, Z., Bochenek, W., and Bieniek, J. (1977). Electric stimulation of the human auditory system with transtympanic electrodes. *Otolaryngol. Pol.* 31, 225–228.

Cazals, Y., Negrevergne, M., and Aran, J. M. (1978). Electrical stimulation of the cochlea in man: hearing induction and tinnitus suppression. *J. Am. Aud. Soc.* 3, 209–213.

Chouard, C. H., Koca, E., Meyer, B., and Jacquier, I. (1994). Test of electrical stimulation of the round window. Diagnostic and prognostic value of the rehabilitation of total deafness by cochlear implant. *Ann. Otolaryngol. Chir. Cervicofac.* 111, 75–84.

Chouard, C. H., Meyer, B., and Donadieu, F. (1979). Auditory brainstem potentials in man evoked by electrical stimulation of the round window. *Acta Otolaryngol.* 87, 287–293. doi: 10.3109/00016487909126422

Chouard, C. H., Meyer, B., and Maridat, D. (1981). Transcutaneous electrotherapy for severe tinnitus. *Acta Otolaryngol.* 91, 415–422. doi: 10.3109/00016488109138522

Dehmel, S., Cui, Y. L., and Shore, S. E. (2008). Cross-modal interactions of auditory and somatic inputs in the brainstem and midbrain and their imbalance in tinnitus and deafness. *Am. J. Audiol.* 17, S193–S209. doi: 10.1044/1059-0889(2008/07-0045)

Gersuni, G. V., and Volokhov, A. A. (1936). On the electrical excitability of the auditory organ: on the effect of alternating current on the normal auditory apparatus. *J. Exp. Phychol.* 16, 370–382. doi: 10.1037/h0060771

Guo, M. (2001). Effects of direct current on vibration of cochlear basilar membrane. *Zhonghua Er Bi Yan Hou Ke Za Zhi* 36, 338–341.

House, W. F. (1976). Cochlear implants. *Ann. Otol. Rhinol. Laryngol.* (Suppl. 27), 50–56. doi: 10.1177/00034894760850S303

House, W. F., and Brackmann, D. E. (1974). Electrical promontory testing in differential diagnosis of sensori-neural hearing impairment. *Laryngoscope* 84, 2163–2171. doi: 10.1288/00005537-197412000-00007

Ito, J., and Sakakihara, J. (1994). Tinnitus suppression by electrical stimulation of the cochlear wall and by cochlear implantation. *Laryngoscope* 104(6 Pt 1), 752–754. doi: 10.1288/00005537-199406000-00017

Jellinek, S., and Schreiber, T. (1930). Eine neue methode des Horens. *Wien klin. Wsche.* 43:417.

Kellaway, P. (1946). The mechanism of the electrophonic effect. *J. Neurophysiol.* 9, 23–31. doi: 10.1152/jn.1946.9.1.23

Konopka, W., Zalewski, P., Olszewski, J., Olszewska-Ziaber, A., and Pietkiewicz, P. (2001). Tinnitus suppresion by electrical promontory stimulation (EPS) in patients with sensorineural hearing loss. *Auris Nasus Larynx* 28, 35–40. doi: 10.1016/S0385-8146(00)00086-9

Kujawa, S. G., and Liberman, M. C. (2015). Synaptopathy in the noise-exposed and aging cochlea: primary neural degeneration in acquired sensorineural hearing loss. *Hear. Res.* 330(Pt B), 191–199. doi: 10.1016/j.heares.2015.02.009

Lambert, P. R., Ruth, R. A., and Halpin, C. F. (1990). Promontory electrical stimulation in labyrinthectomized ears. *Arch. Otolaryngol. Head Neck Surg.* 116, 197–201. doi: 10.1001/archotol.1990.01870020073019

Latkowski, B. (1981). Original improvement of the technique of implantation of microelectrodes in cochlear deafness. *Minerva Otolaringol* 1:69

Lusted, H. S., Shelton, C., and Simmons, F. B. (1984). Comparison of electrode sites in electrical stimulation of the cochlea. *Laryngoscope* 94, 878–882. doi: 10.1288/00005537-198407000-00003

Mielczarek, M., Michalska, J., Polatyńska, K., and Olszewski, J. (2016). An increase in alpha band frequency in resting state EEG after electrical stimulation of the ear in tinnitus patients-a pilot study. *Front. Neurosci.* 10:453. doi: 10.3389/fnins.2016.00453

Mielczarek, M., and Olszewski, J. (2014). Direct current stimulation of the ear in tinnitus treatment: a double-blind placebo-controlled study. *Eur. Arch. Otorhinolaryngol.* 271, 1815–1822. doi: 10.1007/s00405-013-2849-6

Møller, A. R. (2016). Sensorineural tinnitus: its pathology and probable therapies. *Int. J. Otolaryngol.* 2016:2830157. doi: 10.1155/2016/2830157

van de Heyning, P., Muehlmeier, G., Cox, T., Lisowska, G., Maier, H., Morawski, K., and Meyer, T. (2014). Efficacy and safety of AM-101 in the treatment of acute inner ear tinnitus–a double-blind, randomized, placebo-controlled phase II study. *Otol. Neurotol.* 35, 589–597. doi: 10.1097/MAO.0000000000000268

Mulders, W. H., and Robertson, D. (2009). Hyperactivity in the auditory midbrain after acoustic trauma: dependence on cochlear activity. *Neuroscience* 164, 733–746. doi: 10.1016/j.neuroscience.2009.08.036

Noreña, A. J. (2011). An integrative model of tinnitus based on a central gain controlling neural sensitivity. *Neurosci. Biobehav. Rev.* 35, 1089–1109. doi: 10.1016/j.neubiorev.2010.11.003

Noreña, A. J. (2015). Revisiting the cochlear and central mechanisms of tinnitus and therapeutic approaches. *Audiol. Neurootol.* 20(Suppl. 1), 53–59. doi: 10.1159/000380749

Noreña, A. J., and Eggermont, J. J. (2005). Enriched acoustic environment after noise trauma reduces hearing loss and prevents cortical map reorganization. *J. Neurosci.* 25, 699–705. doi: 10.1523/JNEUROSCI.2226-04.2005

Noreña, A. J., Mulders, W. H., and Robertson, D. (2015). Suppression of putative tinnitus-related activity by extra-cochlear electrical stimulation. *J. Neurophysiol.* 113, 132–143. doi: 10.1152/jn.00580.2014

Nuttall, A. L., and Ren, T. (1995). Electromotile hearing: evidence from basilar membrane motion and otoacoustic emissions. *Hear. Res.* 92, 170–177. doi: 10.1016/0378-5955(95)00216-2

Pantev, C., Okamoto, H., and Teismann, H. (2012). Tinnitus: the dark side of the auditory cortex plasticity. *Ann. N.Y. Acad. Sci.* 1252, 253–258. doi: 10.1111/j.1749-6632.2012.06452.x

Portmann, M., Cazals, Y., Negrevergne, M., and Aran, J. M. (1979). Temporary tinnitus suppression in man through electrical stimulation of the cochlea. *Acta Otolaryngol.* 87, 294–299. doi: 10.3109/00016487909126423

Puel, J. L. (2007). Cochlear NMDA receptor blockade prevents salicylate-induced tinnitus. *B-ENT* 3 (Suppl. 7), 19–22.

Quaranta, N., Wagstaff, S., and Baguley, D. M. (2004). Tinnitus and cochlear implantation. *Int. J. Audiol.* 43, 245–251. doi: 10.1080/14992020400050033

Rattay, F., Lutter, P., and Felix, H. (2001). A model of the electrically excited human cochlear neuron. I. Contribution of neural substructures to the generation and propagation of spikes. *Hear Res.* 153, 43–63. doi: 10.1016/S0378-5955(00)00256-2

Ren, T., and Nuttall, A. L. (1995). Extracochlear electrically evoked otoacoustic emissions: a model for *in vivo* assessment of outer hair cell electromotility. *Hear. Res.* 92, 178–183. doi: 10.1016/0378-5955(95)00217-0

Rubinstein, J. T., Tyler, R. S., Johnson, A., and Brown, C. J. (2003). Electrical suppression of tinnitus with high-rate pulse trains. *Otol. Neurotol.* 24, 478–485. doi: 10.1097/00129492-200305000-00021

Ruel, J., Chabbert, C., Nouvian, R., Bendris, R., Eybalin, M., Leger, C. L., et al. (2008). Salicylate enables cochlear arachidonic-acid-sensitive NMDA receptor responses. *J. Neurosci.* 28, 7313–7323. doi: 10.1523/JNEUROSCI.5335-07.2008

Shulman, A. (1987). External electrical tinnitus suppression: a review. *Am. J. Otol.* 8, 479–484.

Skarzynski, H., Czyzewski, A., and Kostek, B. (1999). "Prediction of post-operative profits in cochlear implanted patients using the electrostimulation procedure," in *Proceedings of the 1999 Workshop on Applications of Signal to Audio and Acoustics* (New Palts, NY), 17–20.

Stevens, S. S., and Jones, R. C. (1939). The mechanism of hearing by electrical stimulation. *J. Acoust. Soc. Amer* 10, 261–269. doi: 10.1121/1.1915984

Sun, W., Ding, D., Reyes, S., and Salvi, R. J. (2000). Effects of AC and DC stimulation on chinchilla SOAE amplitude and frequency. *Hear. Res.* 150, 137–148. doi: 10.1016/S0378-5955(00)00195-7

Tass, P. A., and Popovych, O. V. (2012). Unlearning tinnitus-related cerebral synchrony with acoustic coordinated reset stimulation: theoretical concept and modelling. *Biol. Cybern.* 106, 27–36. doi: 10.1007/s00422-012-0479-5

Viana, L. M., O'Malley, J. T., Burgess, B. J., Jones, D. D., Oliveira, C. A., Santos, F., et al. (2015). Cochlear neuropathy in human presbycusis: confocal analysis of hidden hearing loss in post-mortem tissue. *Hear. Res.* 327, 78–88. doi: 10.1016/j.heares.2015.04.014

Watanabe, K., Okawara, D., Baba, S., and Yagi, T. (1997). Electrocochleographic analysis of the suppression of tinnitus by electrical promontory stimulation. *Audiology* 36, 147–154. doi: 10.3109/00206099709071968

13

In Patients Undergoing Cochlear Implantation, Psychological Burden Affects Tinnitus and the Overall Outcome of Auditory Rehabilitation

Petra Brüggemann[1†], Agnieszka J. Szczepek[2*†], Katharina Klee[2], Stefan Gräbel[2], Birgit Mazurek[1] and Heidi Olze[2*]

[1] *Tinnitus Center, Charité Universitätsmedizin Berlin, Berlin, Germany,*

[2] *Department of ORL, Head and Neck Surgery, Charité Universitätsmedizin Berlin, Berlin, Germany*

***Correspondence:**
Agnieszka J. Szczepek
agnes.szczepek@charite.de
Heidi Olze
heidi.olze@charite.de

Cochlear implantation (CI) is increasingly being used in the auditory rehabilitation of deaf patients. Here, we investigated whether the auditory rehabilitation can be influenced by the psychological burden caused by mental conditions. Our sample included 47 patients who underwent implantation. All patients were monitored before and 6 months after CI. Auditory performance was assessed using the Oldenburg Inventory (OI) and Freiburg monosyllable (FB MS) speech discrimination test. The health-related quality of life was measured with Nijmegen Cochlear implantation Questionnaire (NCIQ) whereas tinnitus-related distress was measured with the German version of Tinnitus Questionnaire (TQ). We additionally assessed the general perceived quality of life, the perceived stress, coping abilities, anxiety levels and the depressive symptoms. Finally, a structured interview to detect mental conditions (CIDI) was performed before and after surgery. We found that CI led to an overall improvement in auditory performance as well as the anxiety and depression, quality of life, tinnitus distress and coping strategies. CIDI revealed that 81% of patients in our sample had affective, anxiety, and/or somatoform disorders before or after CI. The affective disorders included dysthymia and depression, while anxiety disorders included agoraphobias and unspecified phobias. We also diagnosed cases of somatoform pain disorders and unrecognizable figure somatoform disorders. We found a positive correlation between the auditory performance and the decrease of anxiety and depression, tinnitus-related distress and perceived stress. There was no association between the presence of a mental condition itself and the outcome of auditory rehabilitation. We conclude that the CI candidates exhibit high rates of psychological disorders, and there is a particularly strong association between somatoform disorders and tinnitus. The presence of mental disorders remained unaffected by CI but the degree of psychological burden decreased significantly post-CI. The implants benefitted patients in a number of psychosocial areas, improving the symptoms of depression and anxiety, tinnitus, and their quality of life and coping strategies. The prevalence of mental disorders in patients who are candidates for CI suggests the need for a comprehensive psychological and psychosomatic management of their treatment.

Keywords: tinnitus, cochlear implants, psychological disorders, CIDI, psychological comorbidities

INTRODUCTION

Cochlear implants (CI) make it possible for many people with hearing disorders to regain auditory perception and an acoustic understanding of language. The degree of improvement any particular patient experiences is influenced by complex, individual factors, leading to great variations in outcomes. A better grasp of the causes of this variation would improve our ability to predict the outcome for individual CI candidates.

One area of discussion has been the influence of concurrent psychological conditions on the neuronal plasticity of the auditory cortex. Alongside quantitative improvements in hearing, CI is known to have a positive effect on patients' quality of life (Olze et al., 2011, 2012b, 2016; Blasco and Redleaf, 2014; Ramos-Macias et al., 2016). Other influential factors include the progression of deafness, whether and how effectively hearing aids are used in rehabilitation, and motivational and psychological factors among patients—which can only be determined through a quantitative and qualitative measurement of their psychological burden.

In our earlier study of 43 patients with unilateral deafness who had undergone the cochlear implantation, we showed that tinnitus and concurrent psychological conditions had a significant influence on their quality of life (Olze et al., 2011). This study took into account the need for a qualified assessment of the patients' psychological conditions prior to and following implantation. The following year, we demonstrated that the CI patients with a high level of tinnitus-related distress had low quality of life, experienced more stress and more difficulties in coping with their situation (Olze et al., 2012a,b). From 2,251 language tests carried out on post-lingually deafened adults, Blamey et al. concluded that the level of successful postoperative hearing was negatively correlated with the length of the period of deafness prior to Cl (Blamey et al., 2013). Lin et al. observed a 60% improvement of speech recognition among patients over 60 years of age when assessed 1 year post-implantation. Beyond 60, each additional year was accompanied by a drop in the level of speech understanding of 1.3% (Lin et al., 2012). Several of these studies also employed standardized interviews such as the Composite Diagnostic Interview (CIDI), which revealed a range of psychological disturbances.

Van der Werf et al. described an association between psychological disturbances and limitations in hearing in a study of 3,021 youths and adults ranging from 14 to 24 years of age; the subjects were interviewed at regular intervals over a period of 10 years (van der Werf et al., 2011). The younger members of this group (aged 14–17) exhibited a higher incidence of psychological disturbances than those in the 18–24 age group. Their conclusion was that younger patients were going through a more sensitive period of development and as a result, their deafness had a greater impact on their psychological state and social interactions.

Mance and Edwards showed that a young Cl patient's psychological well-being correlated positively with the degree to which they considered themselves similar to people of their own age with normal hearing (Mance and Edwards, 2012). Fellinger et al. (2005) indicated that deaf patients are more commonly affected by somatic disturbances, fear and stress, than those with normal hearing. The deaf subjects had more social contact with other hearing-impaired people than with the unimpaired. The same group of hearing-impaired individuals generally had poorer social relationships than their deaf counterparts (Fellinger et al., 2007). All the scales that were employed yielded worse scores; in contrast to the truly deaf study participants, they were not simply members of a peer group with similar problems. This indicated that their quality of life depends on the level of contentment and success they feel within a system in which hearing plays an important role. The study concludes that the hearing-impaired are generally more isolated than those who are completely deaf, and that Cl can represent a successful form of assistance for this group.

In the present study, we aim to determine the occurrence of psychosocial burden, including the manifestation of psychological diagnoses, using questionnaires and a standardized interview in a subset of patients scheduled to undergo cochlear implantation. We formulated the following hypotheses:

(H1) that patients undergoing CI would suffer from a higher psychological burden than the general population;

(H2) that psychological burden is significantly reduced by the provision of a Cl;

(H3) that a lower-level of post-operative speech recognition improvement is associated with a higher level of psychological burden;

(H4) that certain dimensions of psychosocial limitations decrease the benefits of Cl.

METHODS

Data Collection

Between October 2010 and January 2012, within the framework of the Cochlear Implant Program of the Charité University Hospital in Berlin, 52 post-lingually, bilaterally deafened adults were interviewed prior to CI; 47 subjects were consecutively included in the study (**Table 1**), approved by a local Ethics Committee. All investigations were conducted according to the principles expressed in the Declaration of Helsinki. All patients gave their informed written consent.

The mean value of FB MS on the implanted ear was for all 47 patients 3.08; $SD = 8.8$. On the contralateral ear, 36 patients were hard of hearing with a mean value of FB MS 16.1; $SD = 24.0$, whereas the remaining 11 patients had a mean value of FB MS 77.3; $SD = 16.9$.

The following procedures were applied to all patients prior to implantation and then half a year after they had received the Cl. The CIDI was carried out on a laptop computer. As questionnaires on paper, patients were administered the Oldenburg Inventory (OI), the Nijmegen Questionnaire (NCIQ), and the general perceived quality of life questionnaire (SF36). The following additional questionnaires were completed using a pocket computer: General- Anxiety Disorder (GAD), General Depression Scale (ADS), the COPE Inventory, the tinnitus questionnaire (TQ), and the Perceived Stress Questionnaire. Audiometric measurements were performed in the Audiometry Unit of the ORL, Head and Neck Surgery Department.

TABLE 1 | Descriptive statistics.

Total number of patients	47	
Gender	Women	Men
	30	17
Mean age (years)	56.09	63.08
Mean duration of deafness* on the implanted side (in years)	15.4 (*SD* = 18.8)	
Side of implantation	21 left and 23 right	
Mean use of CI per day (in hours)	13.1 (*SD* = 3.7)	

*According to subjective patient's reports.

The consent of the Ethics Commission was obtained prior to the study. All patients consented to their participation in the interviews and questionnaires.

Composition of the Patient Sample

The cohort for this study was comprised of 30 women and 17 men who averaged 58.62 years of age and a period of deafness lasting 15.4 years averaged over the group. The cause of deafness varied between the patients: unknown cause of deafness was stated by 19 patients; recurrent otitis media in the childhood was reported by 6 patients; sudden sensorineural hearing loss was reported by 4 patients; noise was reported by 3 patients; meningitis in 2 patients. Meniére's disease, otosclerosis, hypoxia at birth, cholesteatoma, autoimmune diseases, familial hearing loss, and childhood violence were given once as a reason for deafness. Six patients did not answer this question. The period of deafness was determined based on the statement about the time when a patient felt that wearing a hearing aid stopped being of significant benefit. Most of the patients had secondary school education and had completed professional training, they were in a long-term relationship and, as expected given the high average age, were retired. The causes of their hearing loss correspond to the types and distribution generally found in data from literature on this topic.

Composite International Diagnostic Interview

The CIDI was developed in the context of epidemiological studies by the World Health Organization (WHO) (Robins et al., 1988). The interview is used in both a Short Form and the DIA- X/M-CIDI Münchner Composite International Diagnostic Interview (Wittchen, 1994). For this project the latter was used, specifically version 1.2 from 13.08.1999. Its goal is to assess psychological and behavioral disturbances according to ICD-10 and DSM-IV, and its contents are divided into several sections (A through X) and three supplementary sections, listed in **Table 2**. Not all of the sections were employed in this study because to do so would have represented an undue burden on patients' time. Single interviews lasted between 30 and 90 min. Questions covered time frames ranging from the previous 2 weeks to 12 months and extended to the patient's entire lifespan. The interview can be conducted by anyone; no prior clinical or diagnostic expertise is required. The

TABLE 2 | Sections of CIDI.

Section	Description	Included in this study	ICD10 code
A	General questions	X	
B	Disorders resulting from the use of tobacco		F17
C	Somatoform disorders	X	F45
D	Phobic disorders	X	F40- F41
E	Depression (affective disorders F30- F39)	X	F32- F33
F	Manic episode (affective disorders F30)		F30
G	Schizophrenia and schizoaffective disorders		F20- F29
H	Eating disorders	X	F50
I	Psychological and behavioral disorders caused by alcohol	X	F10
K	Obsessive-compulsive disorder	X	F42
L	Disorders resulting from the use of medications other substance abuse	X	F11- F19
M	Organic disorders (including symptomatic mental disorders)		F0- F09
N	Post-traumatic stress disorder	X	F43
ML	Munich task list		
Q	Final questions		
P	Interview observations		
X	Interview judgment		
FR	Family genetics		
SQ	Personal and other questions		
RL	Restless-leg syndrome Questionnaire		

Interrater Reliability of the CIDI lies at 0.81–1.0. The reliability of retesting for single diagnoses of somatic conditions lies between 0.49 and 0.67; for affective disturbances the value lies at 0.77, for single diagnoses between 0.45 and 0.69, and for anxiety diagnoses between 0.57 and 0.72.

Audiometric Testing Procedure: Freiburg Monosyllable Test in Quiet (FB MS)

The Freiburg monosyllable speech discrimination test (Hahlbrock, 1953) involves presenting patients with 2 × 20 monosyllabic words at a volume of 65 dB HL under quiet conditions. The patient's task is to repeat each word. The FB MS can be selected from 10 test lists, here lists 9 and 10 were used. Each correctly repeated word counts for 5% of the comprehension score. The test was carried out on each ear separately prior to the CI procedure (noted as the "ear to be implanted," and "opposite ear"). Following CI implantation measurements were carried out using the same lists of words. As on the ear to be implanted, the average speech comprehension prior to CI was only about 3%, the learning bias was excluded. On the non-CI ear, the average speech comprehension was 16.1% for 36 patients and 77.3% for the remaining 11 patients.

Any patients who wore a hearing aid in the "opposite ear" had to remove it prior to the test. The words were presented *via* speakers and the non-CI ears were plugged.

Testing the Quality of Hearing by Questionnaire

Oldenburg Inventory

The OI (Kollmeier and Holube, 1991) originally consisted of 21 items with 5 subscales. The current study used the shortened version of the questionnaire with 12 questions and 3 scales: Listening in a quiet setting (Questions 1, 3, 5, 7), listening with noise interference (4, 6, 8, 11, 12) and directional listening (2, 9, 10). The 12 closed questions about everyday situations were marked with points from 1 to 5. The range for each item of the 3 subscales of the Ol was chosen from 1 to 5 which adds up to a total range from 12 to 60 for the 12 questions. Average scores for each subscale was used as well as the overall result ranging from 1 to 5. The higher the score, the better the subjective hearing.

Nijmegen Cochlear Implantation Questionnaire

The purpose of the NCIQ (Hinderink et al., 2000) is to establish the quality of a patient's life prior to being outfitted with a CI and again afterwards. It is based on 6 scales and consists of 60 items, listed in **Table 3**. The NCIQ scores of the subscales as well as the total score are normalized to percentages. When used in studies of patients with CI, questions about contentment and the time the device has been worn are added to the NCIQ.

TABLE 3 | Domains of the Nijmegen Cochlear Implant Questionnaire (NCIQ).

Domains	Content	
Basic sound perception	Background sounds	NCIQ1
Advanced sound perception	Ability to communicate	NCIQ2
Speech production	Voice monitoring	NCIQ3
Self-esteem (psychological domain	Communicative skills	NCIQ4
activity	Personal and professional	NCIQ5
Social interactions	Communication with family, friends, peer groups	NCIQ6
NCIQ total	Score for health-related quality of life	NCIQ total

Psychometric Questionnaire to Establish Psychological Burden

SF36: Questions Regarding General Health

SF36 (Piehlmeier et al., 1996) is a German translation of the American SF36 Health Survey (Jenkinson et al., 1993) and consists of 8 scales. The questions relate to a patient's state of health and query an individual's overall perception of his or her state of health for the period of 1 week. Estimations of psychological and bodily health are scored separately and appear as individual values in the results provided here.

Tinnitus Questionnaire

The German version of TQ (Goebel and Hiller, 1994) aims to establish the degree of severity of a patient's tinnitus and consists of 52 items distributed in 6 scales. Scores can range from 0 to 84 and are evaluated as follows: a 1st degree burden falls within the range 0–30; 2nd degree, 31–46; 3rd degree, 47–59; and 4th degree from 60 to 84. Scores under 47 are considered "compensated" tinnitus and all higher scores are termed "decompensated." The compensatory type represents a form of tinnitus that is chronic and yet does not impose grave restrictions on a patient's life.

Perceived Stress Questionnaire

The German version of PSQ (Fliege et al., 2005) delivers a patient's subjective perception of stress factors. It comprises 30 items grouped into 7 scales designated as the following: Harassment, Overload, Fatigue/Irritability, Lack of Joy, Worries, and Tension. This study relies on the shortened version of the scale. Every scale can have values from 0 to 1. A score above 0.45 is considered to represent a moderate level of stress; anything above 0.6 is termed high stress.

COPE Inventory

COPE (Carver et al., 1989) is intended to investigate a patient's personal resources and modes of coping with stress. The shortened German Brief-COPE version used in this study contains 4 scales: avoidance, active problem solving, positive thinking, support-seeking behavior (compare with Knoll et al., 2005), whereas the answer scores may range between 0 and 30.

General Anxiety Disorder 7 Questionnaire

GAD-7 (Spitzer et al., 2006) investigates the frequency and degree to which a patient has experienced fear within the 2-week period preceding the questionnaire. Seven items are measured and scored based on patients' responses, using the following scale: 0 = not at all; 1 = on some days; 2 = more often than every other day; 3 = almost every day. A sum of the scores provides a value for estimating the degree of the burden presented by fear (small, mild, medium or strong). The answer scores range between 0 and 21.

General Depression Scale

The ADS (Mohiyeddini et al., 2002) aims to determine the presence, degree, and length of depression a person has experienced within week immediately prior to the questionnaire. 20 items are covered. The points are added to achieve a total score that ranges from 0 to 60. A score over 23 is considered to describe a condition of serious depression. When the ADS is administered to members of the general public, the average score is 14.30 (SD 9.7). The median score achieved by patients diagnosed with depression is 36.70 (SD 8.4), compared to those who experience states of fear or social phobias, who have on the average a median score of 36.60 (SD 8.71).

Statistical Procedure

Forty-seven patients were included in this study. The statistical evaluation was carried out with the software program SPSS (IBM Corp. Released 2015. IBM SPSS Statistics for Windows, Version 23.0.0.2, Armonk, NY: IBM Corp.). Frequency tables, mean values and standard deviations were calculated descriptively (**Table 2**). The questionnaires and CIDI were evaluated using a nonparametric ANOVA (Friedman Test of relevant samples), once the requirements for the *t*-test of samples were achieved, to test the significance of differences before and following implantation (H2). To clarify the type of association and the influence of various parameters on progressive hearing ability, regression models were calculated, in which the performance in pre- and post-language audiograms were defined as dependent variables.

RESULTS

Hypothesis 1: That Patients Undergoing CI Would Suffer from a Higher Psychological Burden than the General Population (As Measured with CIDI)

Eighty one percent of patients had psychological disturbances before and/or after CI, which is in contrast to the incidence of psychological disturbances in general German population (32.1% in people between 18 and 65 years). In 13% of the cases, patients were diagnosed with a disturbance only prior to CI but not afterwards, while 11% received this diagnosis only afterwards (**Figure 1**).

Prior to implantation, 11% were diagnosed with affective disturbances, 32% suffered from anxiety and 53% from psychosomatic disturbances. Following CI, 11% of the patients exhibited one or more affective disturbances, 30% had anxiety and 34% a psychosomatic illness (**Figure 2**). One patient was diagnosed with obsessive-compulsive disorder before and after CI. Another exhibited a post-traumatic stress disorder prior to CI that was no longer apparent post-implantation based on the CIDI diagnosis.

Hypothesis 1 is regarded as confirmed based on the overall higher psychological comorbidity of relevant diagnoses in the patient group for the areas of anxiety and psychosomatic disturbances, when compared to the general population. These values change only marginally after cochlear implantation. A moderate decrease of psychosomatic disturbances is observed, although it does not reach significance.

Hypothesis 2: That the Psychological Burden Is Significantly Reduced by the Provision of a CI

Here we do not present results related to social data and age, sex, length of wearing the device, contentment, or length of deafness that fail to reach significance, with the exception of the stress level (PSQ). Descriptive results for all of the significant changes in the variables that were evaluated are summarized in **Table 4**.

All of the results related to hearing capacity show a highly significant degree of improvement. They include improvements of the auditory abilities measured by objective (audiometry in quiet and noise and directional hearing) and subjective evaluations (NCIQ, Ol).

All subscores of the Tinnitus Questionnaire and thus the combined total score indicating tinnitus-related distress (TQ) showed significant improvement. The average TQ score decreased significantly from 27.66 prior to CI to 18.70 post-CI ($p > 0.01$; for the subscales see **Table 4**). No significant changes were seen in overall stress perception (PSQ), or in its subscores. The coping mechanisms in COPE changed in the direction of a lower utilization of health care resources. Anxiety (GAD7) and depression (ADS) revealed significant statistical improvement.

All of the self-evaluated and audiometrically measured parameters exhibited significant improvements following CI. Accordingly, we regard hypothesis 2 as confirmed.

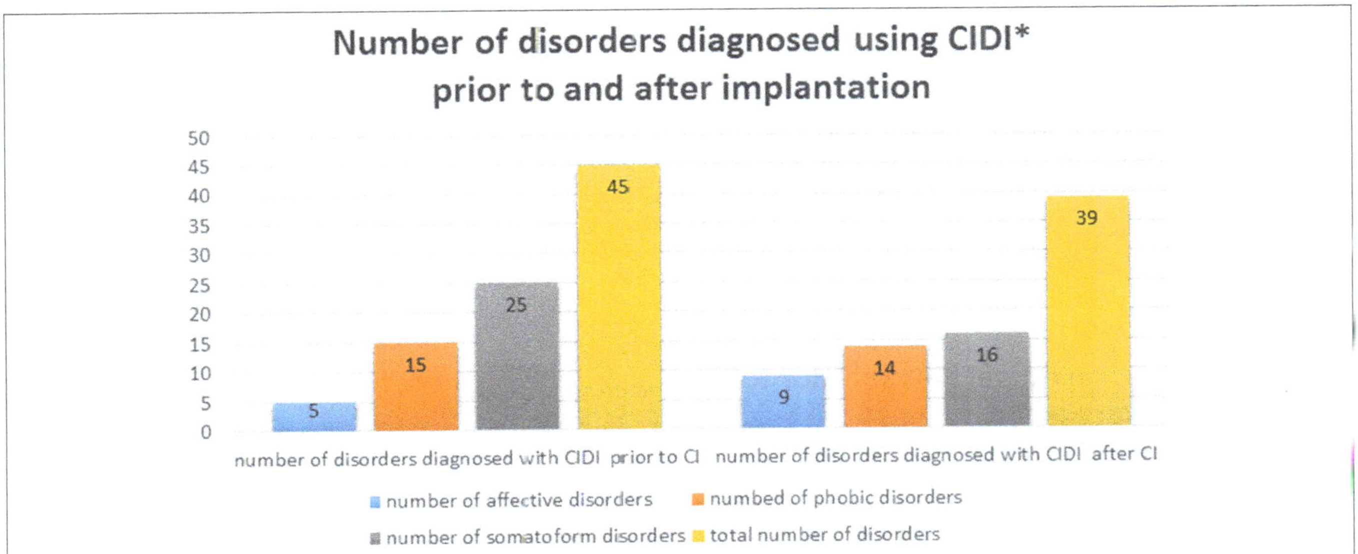

FIGURE 1 | Absolute number of psychological disorders diagnosed in our sample of implanted patients before and after CI, as determined through CIDI. *One subject can be diagnosed with more than one disorder.

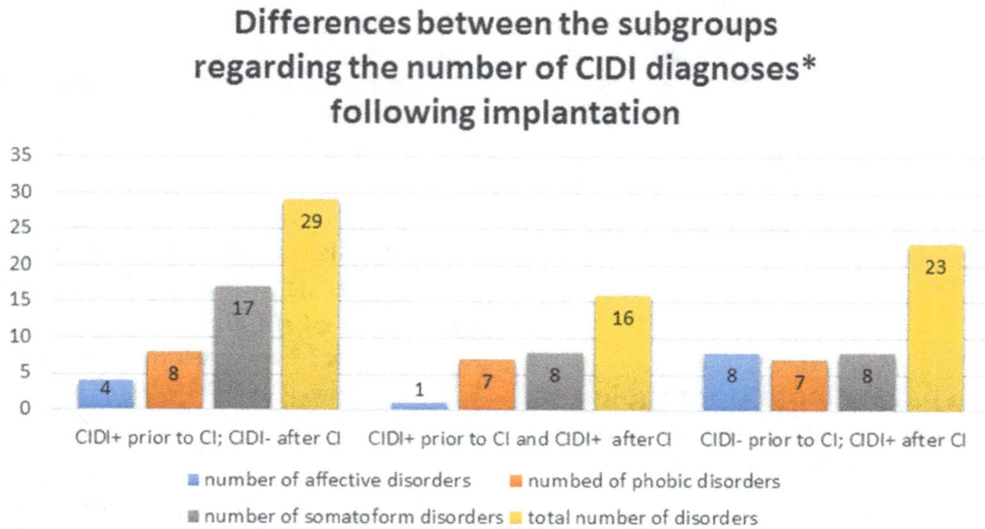

FIGURE 2 | Differences between the numbers of diagnoses occurring in three subgroups of patients. First subgroup represents positive diagnoses of psychological disorders prior to CI and their disappearance after CI. Second subgroup represents positive diagnoses prior to and after CI. The third subgroup represents presence of diagnoses following CI. *One subject can be diagnosed with more than one disorder.

Hypothesis 3: That a Lower-Level of Post-operative Speech Recognition Improvement Is Associated with a Higher Level of Psychological Burden

The analysis of how the psychological disturbances affect the measured parameters, revealed that the patients *without* psychosomatic, anxious or depressive illnesses had significantly better scores in almost all subcategories of the questionnaires before and after cochlear implantations. Across the board in these groups, there was significant improvement in speech comprehension.

Independently of the presence of psychosomatic conditions, changes in the TQ scores indicated significant effect of CI on the emotional burden, hearing problems, sleep disorders or psychosomatic complaints related to tinnitus. Their experience of stress underwent no significant change, with the exception of a significant drop in their level of concern (PSQ). No significant changes were noticed in any subscore of the COPE. Patients without an affective disturbance did not experience a significant change as measured either PSQ or COPE scores between their preoperative and postoperative measurements. This was also the case for patients with anxiety.

Group with Psychological Illness Prior to CI but None Afterwards

Patients who exhibited a psychological disturbance prior to CI but none after implantation could be characterized as follows. Those who were relieved of a psychosomatic illness had better results in FB MS, on all subscores of the OI, basic sound perception (NCIQ1), advanced sound perception (NCIQ2), activity (NCIQ5), emotional and cognitive burden through tinnitus with a significantly poorer performance in SF36 KSS. Patients with anxiety whose condition vanished after CI achieved better scores in directional hearing (OI), active behavior (NCIQ5), the establishment of social interactions (NCIQ6) and active stress management (COPEac).

Group with Psychological Illness before and after CI (Including New Conditions)

Patients whose psychological illness remained after CI, or who exhibited a new condition following the procedure, exhibited notably fewer significant changes overall in the parameters that were measured. The psychosomatic patients improved only in the parameters of hearing accompanied by distracting noise (OI), the establishment of social interactions (NCIQ6), psychological well-being (SF36 PSS), avoidance behavior (COPE ec) and assistance-seeking (COPE sc). The group with anxiety before and after CI showed significant improvement only in hearing accompanied by distracting noise (OI) and in basic sound perception (NCIQ1). This group had, however, significantly poorer results in measurements of physical well-being (SF 36 KSS) and experience of joy (PSQ joy).

The group in which new psychosomatic disturbances appeared had significantly better scores in the subareas: hearing accompanied by distracting noise (OI), speech production (NCIQ3), self-esteem (NCIQ4), activity (NCIQ5), social interactions (NCIQ6), and assistance-seeking behavior (COPEsc), while at the same time achieving significantly lower results for total bodily health (SF36 KSS).

Patients who exhibited new affective illnesses after CI had better results in the Freiburg monosyllable test, hearing against a quiet background (OI), advanced sound perception (NCIQ2), active behavior (NCIQ5) and social interactions (NCIQ6). They had significantly poorer results in total physical scores in SF36.

TABLE 4 | Test scores prior to and following CI (means, significance levels).

	N	Range	mean before CI	Standard deviation	mean after CI	Standard deviation	*Z*	*p* (<0.05)
FB MS	47	0–87.5	3.08	8.81	28.27	28.72	4.394	0.00001
OI quiet setting	45	1.0–4.6	2.56	0.77	3.34	0.85	4.114	0.00004
OI noise interference	45	1.0–4.4	1.93	0.65	2.74	0.80	4.939	0.000001
OI directional listening	45	1.0–4.5	2.10	0.73	2.78	0.95	3.749	0.0002
OI total	45	1.0–4.6	2.22	0.62	3.07	0.70	5.246	0.000000
NCIQ 1	46	0–92.5	45.32	20.95	61.23	17.44	3.74	0.0002
NCIQ 2	47	12.5–78	45.48	16.62	58.26	17.14	4.19	0.00003
NCIQ 3	47	25–82.5	64.02	18.11	71.51	15.86	2.912	0.004
NCIQ 4	46	20–82.5	43.79	16.94	51.54	18.12	2.68	0.007
NCIQ 5	47	0–94.2	41.56	18.29	53.57	18.27	4.342	0.000014
NCIQ 6	46	10–100	44.42	19.37	57.58	22.46	3.960	0.00008
NCIQ total	46	11.4–94	47.28	13.43	59.00	14.94	4.518	0.000006
SF36 physical health	46	21.5–64	52.07	7.48	45.21	10.51	4.357	0.00001
SF36 psychological health	46	15.5–62	42.91	10.72	48.33	9.87	3.414	0.0006
TQ emotional distress	47	0–20	7.19	6.11	5.15	5.77	2.414	0.016
TQ cognitive distress	47	0–14	5.19	4.86	3.808	4.84	3.472	0.0005
TQ intrusiveness	47	0–15	6.34	4.74	4.49	4.53	2.738	0.06
TQ auditory perceptual difficulties	47	0–14	5.70	4.91	3.85	4.26	2.451	0.01
TQ sleep disturbance	47	0–6	1.70	2.21	0.97	1.79	2.259	0.02
TQ somatic complaints	47	0–5	1.00	1.47	0.62	1.21	1.980	0.04
TQ total	47	0–72	27.66	22.01	18.70	19.34	3.001	0.002
PSQ worries	47	0–0.67	0.31	0.18	0.28	0.18	1.87	0.06
PSQ tension	47	0–0.93	0.36	0.22	0.34	0.23	0.726	0.468
PSQ joy	47	0.07–1	0.62	0.23	0.58	0.27	1.400	0.161
PSQ demands	47	0–0.8	0.28	0.18	0.27	0.20	0.570	0.569
PSQ total	47	0–0.69	0.34	0.17	0.33	0.18	0.638	0.524
COPE avoidance	43	7–22	11.74	2.74	10.21	2.97	2.346	0.02
COPE seeking support	43	7–21	13.93	3.4	12.74	3.62	2.718	0.007
COPE positive thinking	43	6–22	13.85	3.04	13.40	3.82	0.705	0.481
COPE active problem solving	43	4–16	10.53	2.59	9.33	2.80	2.056	0.04
Depression (ADSL)	47	5–41	17.93	10.84	14.40	9.24	2.336	0.02
GAD7	47	0–21	5.64	4.69	3.81	4.01	3.057	0.002

Patients diagnosed with anxiety disorders after but not prior to CI, showed significant improvement only in directional hearing (OI), social interactions (NCIQ6) and psychosomatic complaints through tinnitus (TQ SO).

Associations between Psychological Burden and Effects of CI in the Group as a Whole

Overall our work shows that the high-grade anxiety or depression present before (and after) CI lead to poorer estimates of acoustic perception (OI and NCIQ) than in patients who had low-grade of anxiety or depression (**Table 5**). Subjective estimates of a good quality of life (SF36) correlate positively with estimates regarding auditory perception. The benefits of speech recognition (FB MS) demonstrate a negative correlation with the length of deafness. The physical aspects of quality of life are initially reported at a lower level than these benefits, but over time this trend seems to reverse itself. Overall, older patients don't seem to profit as quickly as younger patients with regard to the perception of the quality of hearing, and they estimate their physical quality of life at lower levels before the implantation; the same is true of their estimates of contentment.

We were able to partially confirm hypothesis 3: that the level of psychological burden is accompanied by a decrease in the profit perceived/obtained from CI. This is particularly true in cases of symptoms of anxiety and depression, which potentially influence the target improvement in hearing capacity through their effects on quality of life.

Hypothesis 4: That Certain Dimensions of Psychosocial Limitations Decrease the Benefits of CI

To determine what influence CIDI-diagnosed conditions have on the effects of CI in terms of audiometrically determined speech recognition, we calculated a linear regression. As predictors, the

TABLE 5 | Correlations for pre- and post-implantation results.

	N	Pearson's correlation	Significance (<0.05)
DELTA MS (changes language hearing) and SF 36 psychological	45	−0.394	0.021
DELTA MS (changes language hearing) and duration deafness	45	−0.308	0.059
age and NCIQ (acoustic aspects quality of life) pre	46	−0.321	0.051
age and NCIQ (acoustic aspects quality of life) post	46	−0.321	0.051
age und satisfaction with CI	45	−0.488	0.005
age und SF 36 (bodily health) pre	46	−0.671	0.013
time after implantation and SF 36 PSS (psychological health) pre	45	0.275	0.030
NCIQ total (acoustic QOL) pre and satisfaction	46	0.468	0.007
NCIQ total (acoustic QOL) pre und OL (hearing quality) pre CI	46	0.441	0.011
NCIQ total (acoustic QOL) pre und OL(hearing quality) post CI	46	0.565	0.001
NCIQ total (acoustic QOL) pre and GAD pre CI	46	−0.434	0.012
NCIQ total (acoustic QOL) pre and ADS pre CI	46	−0.357	0.034
NCIQ total (acoustic QOL) post and satisfaction with CI	46	0.453	0.009
NCIQ total (acoustic QOL) post and duration deafness r	46	0.429	0.013
NCIQ total (acoustic QOL) post und OL (hearing quality) pre CI	46	0.549	0.002
NCIQ total (acoustic QOL) post und OL (hearing quality) post CI	46	0.440	0.011
NCIQ total (acoustic QOL) post and GAD (anxiety) pre CI	46	−0.368	0.030
NCIQ total (acoustic QOL) post and ADS (depression) post CI	46	−0.317	0.053
NCIQ total (acoustic QOL) post and SF 36 KSS (somatic aspects quality of life) post	46	0.388	0.013
NCIQ total (acoustic QOL) post and SF 36 PSS (psychological aspects quality of life) post	46	0.521	0.002
Ol (hearing quality) pre CI and duration of deafness	46	0.406	0.018
Ol (hearing quality) pre CI and satisfaction	46	0.385	0.024
Ol (hearing quality) post CI and duration of deafness	46	0.390	0.022
Ol (hearing quality) post CI and satisfaction	46	0.399	0.019
Ol (hearing quality) post CI and ADS (depression) post CI	46	−0.327	0.048
Ol (hearing quality) post CI and TF pre CI	46	0.418	0.015
Ol (hearing quality) post CI and time after implantation	46	0.312	0.057
TQ (tinnitus distress) post and duration of deafness	47	0.316	0.054
TQ (tinnitus distress) post and satisfaction	47	−0.313	0.056
TQ (tinnitus distress) post and GAD (anxiety) post CI	47	0.638	0.000
TQ (tinnitus distress) post and ADS (depression) pre CI	47	0.393	0.021
TQ(tinnitus distress) post and ADS (depression) post CI	47	0.406	0.018
GAD (anxiety) pre CI and ADS (depression) pre CI	47	0.650	0.000
GAD (anxiety) pre CI and ADS (depression) post CI	47	0.357	0.034
GAD (anxiety) pre CI and SF 36 KSS (bodily health)	47	−0.364	0.026
GAD (anxiety) pre CI and SF 36 PSS (psychological health)	47	−0.426	0.010
GAD (anxiety) pre CI and stress pre CI	47	0.800	0.000
GAD (anxiety) pre CI and stress post CI	47	0.678	0.000
GAD (anxiety) post CI and duration deafness	47	0.444	0.010
GAD (anxiety) post CI and TQ(tinnitus distress) post	47	0.638	0.000
GAD (anxiety) post CI and stress post CI	47	0.535	0.002
GAD (anxiety) post CI and depression post CI	47	0.589	0.001
ADS (depression) pre CI and stress pre CI	47	0.787	0.000
ADS (depression) pre CI and stress post CI	47	0.744	0.000
ADS (depression) pre CI and SF 36 PSS (psychological aspects quality of life)	47	−0.620	0.002
ADS (depression) post CI and stress pre CI	47	10.53	0.04
ADS (depression) post CI and stress post CI	47	17.93	0.02
ADS (depression) post CI and SF 36 PSS (psychological health)	47	5.64	0.002

Shown are only significant results, with no correlations between tests.

TABLE 6 | Regression model: coefficients of predictors for speech perception after CI.

Model		Unstandardized coefficients		Standardized Coefficients	*t*	Significance
		B	Std. Error	Beta		
1	(Constant)	28.834	24.786		1.163	0.254
	Satisfaction	0.002	0.203	0.002	0.011	0.991
	Compliance (duration of CI per day)	1.116	1.559	0.123	0.716	0.479
	Affective disorder before but not after CI	20.601	19.737	0.197	1.044	0.305
	No affective disorder before but after CI	21.656	15.895	0.247	1.362	0.183
	Phobic disorder before but not after CI	−25.313	15.896	−0.373	−1.592	0.121
	No phobic disorder before but after CI	−25.820	14.500	−0.313	−1.781	0.085
	Phobic disorder before and after CI	28.958	24.032	0.306	1.205	0.237
	Somatoform Disorder before but not after CI	−14.527	12.848	−0.230	−1.131	0.267
	No somatoform disorder before but after CI	−31.122	18.030	−0.378	−1.726	0.094
	Somatoform disorder before and after CI	−28.909	18.616	−0.330	−1.553	0.131

Dependent Variable: Delta in speech perception (Freiburg monosyllable speech perception test).

presence of symptoms of affective, psychosomatic and anxiety disturbances were considered; the time of wearing a hearing aid and level of contentment were used as controls. The overall regression model was determined not to be significant ($F = 1.175$, $p < 0.344$).

Post-operative statistics reveal a tendency toward effects related to psychosomatic and anxiety disturbances. Patients who suffered from these types of conditions before and after the implantation exhibited less of a gain in audiometrically measured speech recognition. This effect was already evident in correlations related to the questionnaires (see **Table 6**), but only shows a tendency toward significance. Overall, in explaining the significant improvements in all areas of auditory perception and particularly language perception of the group of patients who underwent cochlear implantation, the presence of a psychological disturbance does not appear to be relevant.

Hypothesis 4 regarding the influence of diagnoses related to psychological factors cannot be confirmed, but psychosomatic effects and anxiety before the surgery seem to have an influence on the negative effect hearing specifics after CI.

DISCUSSION

Psychological Diagnosis and Hearing Deficiencies

In Germany, approximately 32.1% of the population aged 18–65 is affected by psychological disturbances. Figures from the Federal German Retirement Insurance system state that in the year 2014, 43% of the population reported having been affected by such problems at least once in their lives; the results are a reduction in performance and a retreat from social life. These disturbances are the most common reason for work-related disabilities in Germany, which is a key motivation to develop effective diagnoses and treatment. In our survey of 47 deaf patients, 31 had a psychological diagnosis before the implantation, a figure which is significantly higher than the average in the general population. Following the intervention, 25 patients (over half of the measured group) had such a diagnosis, which is still much higher than the standard reference. We regard this as relevant despite methodological criticisms which have been raised concerning the form of the interview that was used.

It is impossible to say how reliable and valid the results of the diagnoses captured with CIDI are in relation to clinical diagnoses. Becker et al. regard the use of CIDI as insufficient; in a study of the degree of consistency between clinical diagnoses and the use of CIDIs, they found Kappa values between 0.0 and 0.33 for all diagnoses (Becker et al., 2006). Such unsatisfactory values for the validity and reliability of the CIDI are partially confirmed by the literature (Semler et al., 1987). The important coping disturbances in deaf patients are not covered in these estimates (Hund et al., 2014). Kessler et al. reported good rates of correspondence between clinical diagnoses and standard interviews (Kessler et al., 2009). Knappe et al. consider the use of standardized interviews such as CIDI the "gold standard" (Knappe et al., 2008). In spite of these methodological issues, in agreement with data, we believe that the higher level of psychological diagnoses in our sample is an accurate representation of the patients' situation. In this context, we do not consider the burden of biopsychological and social factors related to deafness and potential side effects of the treatment to be the only causes of the higher level of psychological diagnoses. Some of the problems may be neurological; animal experiments have shown that there are direct connections between the acoustic cortex and the limbic system, and these also may play a role (Kraus and Canlon, 2012).

Our results are in agreement with data from the literature. In the current patient cohort, CIDI diagnoses could be broken down into three major groups: affective, anxiety-related, and psychosomatic disturbances. The diagnoses were commonly the following: for affective disturbance, dysthymia (coping disturbances); in anxiety: agoraphobia and other phobias of an indistinct nature; psychosomatic disturbances: pain and undefined psychosomatic conditions (possibly including tinnitus). Using CIDIs, we diagnosed frequent affective, psychosomatic and anxiety disorders in patients with chronic tinnitus (Zirke et al., 2013). This is in agreement with high prevalence of psychological disorders diagnosed in patients with other chronic somatic diseases, such as cardiovascular diseases (Baumeister and Harter, 2011) or kidney dysfunction (McClellan et al., 2010).

Improvement of Burden Following CI

The loss of binaural hearing is associated with a decreased speech comprehension in noise and problems with sound localization, even when the unaffected ear is healthy. Additionally, in CI patients diagnosed with unilateral hearing loss and tinnitus, they showed improvement in speech understanding in noise following implantation (Blasco and Redleaf, 2014). Our study revealed a significant improvement in speech discrimination following CI (measured with FB MS, which is a standard component of measuring the speech recognition). Subjective hearing abilities increased in all subscales (OI), as was the case for all the subdomains of the NCIQ. Parallel use of audiometric and psychometric evaluations leads to consistent measurement of the CI effects.

Today, the improvement of speech recognition that is achieved through CI is presumed to be linked at least in part to the neuronal plasticity of the cortex. The ultrastructural organization of each component of the auditory system (periphery, cochlear nucleus and auditory midbrain and the auditory cortex) undergoes degradation if it is not stimulated (Baizer et al., 2015). Anatomical and physiological changes have all been shown to be at least partly reversible with renewed stimulation of the cochlear nerve, even considering that certain periods are more sensitive than others. This reorganization occurs in many areas: those that are directly connected to the cochlear nerve, those anatomically linked to it, more distant regions, and in homologically related areas of the other brain hemisphere (Hotting and Roder, 2013). In a review, Kral also addressed the issue of sensitive periods and visual/auditory cross-modal reorganization in adults who become deaf post-lingually (Kral, 2007). In imaging studies, a hypometabolism of the auditory cortex was predictive of better speech perception following CI (Lee et al., 2007). Our present study deals with the connectivity between the auditory cortex (possibly undergoing plastic changes) with other cortical areas like limbic system or the cortical areas responsible for attention.

Here TQ, COP, PSQ, ADS, and GAD7 revealed significant improvements, also confirming the results of previous studies. All of the subscales of the TQ achieved better scores. Earlier we reported a 39.2% drop in the burden of tinnitus after 2 years, and none of the patients without tinnitus exhibited worsening in this area (Olze et al., 2012b, 2016).

The effects of tinnitus are also considered highly connected to basic principles of synaptic and cortical plasticity (Mazurek et al., 2010; Georgiewa et al., 2016). Synaptic plasticity is defined as the degree to which the strength of synaptic transmission changes through activity. The repeated stimulation of afferent processes can lead to changes through long-term potentiation (LTP), whereas decreases in stimulation can cause long-term depression (LTD). Damage to the central or peripheral auditory systems can lead to an imbalance between LTP and LTD, and consequently to changes in the activity of ion channels, receptors, and neuronal transmission. Cellular hyperactivity may induce hyperactivation of the central auditory pathways and change cortical plasticity in ways that lead to tinnitus. A restoration of acoustic stimulation can be achieved through cochlear implants, and in the best-case-scenario this may lead to a reorganization of synaptic plasticity in ways that are accompanied by a reduction in tinnitus, which we observed in our sample using the TQ.

The COPE Inventory revealed a decrease in the degree to which patients rely on coping strategies following CI. In other words, a significant drop in efforts required to master a situation was observed after CI. This finding is consistent with Kobosko et al. (2012), who found that 78 post-lingually deafened adult patients employed less active coping strategies and more avoidance following CI.

The values we obtained here for HRQoL (SF-36) showed significant drops in total scores for physical factors, whereas psychological scores rose. However, our overall results suggest general improvements in the quality of life, corroborating similar findings of Arnoldner et al., who also reported inconsistencies in SF 36 with regard to the quality of life in a 10-year study following cochlear implantations (Arnoldner et al., 2014).

Perceived stress (PSQ) revealed no significant changes following CI but the scores of depression (ADS) and anxiety (GAD7) demonstrated statistically significant improvements. We speculate that this could reflect stronger connectivity between the auditory and limbic systems (amygdala) than this between the auditory system and HPA axis. At both measurement time points, ADS scores lay higher than those for the general population ($M =$ 14.30), but clearly below the cut-off of 23, which is considered the level at which a patient is considered manifestly depressive. The scores we obtained were 17.93 ± 10.84 (prior to CI) and 14.40 ± 9.24 (post-CI).

The Effects of Psychological Disturbances on the Success of Treatment

The significant improvements in auditory and psychosocial parameters that we measured were higher for patients without psychological disturbances than for those who had been diagnosed. The former group enjoyed greater benefits in terms of the quality of life, their perception of tinnitus and speech recognition. This does not, however, seem to be directly related to the presence of preexisting psychological diagnoses. We were unable to confirm hypothesis 4 using a regression model to account for changes in speech comprehension. We interpret the correlative data in **Table 6** as potential evidence for an indirect link between the degree of psychological burden and the success of treatment. One factor to consider in this regard is that the neuronal plasticity of the auditory cortex permits an improvement of hearing after CI even in patients with high levels of burden. The degree of improvement is clearly lower, however, in patients suffering from depression or anxiety. This too, in our opinion, may be due to connectivity within the hearing networks of the brain, which are thought to directly link the auditory cortex with the amygdala (Kraus and Canlon, 2012). Existing emotional burdens could lead to defects in this network. Another issue that will require further reflection is whether affective disorders—or the limitations in learning and memory that accompany them—have a direct impact on the mechanisms underlying neuronal plasticity.

Clinicians have long recognized that patients burdened by both a physical illness and a psychological disturbance have a lower life expectancy, poorer compliance, and poorer quality of life than those who exhibit only physical symptoms. The identification of accompanying psychological disturbances is a basic requirement in establishing a patient's right to rehabilitative care and is also crucial in predicting the likely effect of therapies on individuals (Blasco and Redleaf, 2014). Past observations by our group also indicate that patients with chronic tinnitus achieved significantly better scores not only for the burden brought by tinnitus, but also for stress, anxiety and other parameters if there was no indication of an accompanying psychological disorder (Zirke et al., 2013).

A diagnosis of anxiety or psychosomatic disturbances seems to have a particularly negative effect on the degree to which speech recognition improves from the pre- to postoperative stages of CI. The effects of therapy are modulated by mechanisms of neuronal plasticity, as described above, but also by behavioral patterns and dysfunctional coping strategies. Anxiety promotes avoidance behavior and a tendency to withdraw, which can result in a failure to engage in essential types of communication. The trends seen in our psychosomatic observations suggest that a focus on models and therapies related to the physical causes of these conditions places a stronger emphasis on external factors in accounting for the benefits of therapy, while making patients less aware of and less likely to draw on their resources to influence the outcome. For instance, patients should be psychologically encouraged and supported in their use of CI. We assumed that some CI recipients are simply highly focused on the degree of their disability before the implantation, whether or not they are affected by a psychological disturbance (Olze et al., 2011). As their hearing improves, psychological and other types of burdens, which may have been masked by auditory and communication problems, move into the foreground.

Study Limitations

The major limitations of this study are small size and lack of homogeneity in our sample. Of 47 patients, 36 were bilaterally deaf. The remaining 11 patients had a significant hearing loss on the non-CI ear that could not be classified as deafness. This might have affected some of our results, for instance it could have lowered the average scores of anxiety post-implantation. In addition, there may be differences between the bilaterally- and single sided deafened patients with significant hearing loss on non-CI ear, in terms of CIDI psychological diagnoses. Future focus on homogenous groups and increasing the sample number will clarify this issue. The next limitation of our study is the heterogeneity of our sample regarding the duration of hearing loss. The last limitation is the known hypersensitivity of disease detection by CIDI, when compared to classical diagnostic process (Becker et al., 2006; Terber et al., 2010). Despite this fact, this is the first work when CIDI is used to diagnose the patients undergoing cochlear implantation.

Clinical Significance

Since deaf patients have been shown to suffer from a higher psychological stress than the normal-hearing people, psychometric diagnosis and a patient history extended by psychosomatic aspects are indispensable when planning CI. In the presence of manifest psychological disorder (depression, anxiety, somatization disorder) appropriate therapeutic co-operation should be initiated even before the implantation. Apart from establishing the psychological status of a patient before the CI, psychosomatic monitoring should also be carried out after the implantation because of possible occurrence of psychological disorders after the CI, which could make the auditory rehabilitation process more difficult. Over the entire course of treatment, close cooperation of the ORL, head and neck surgeons and audiologists with therapists specialized in psychosomatic medicine is indispensable in order to achieve an optimal result of cochlear rehabilitation.

SUMMARY

In general, patients suffering from deafness have higher levels of psychological burden than the population as a whole. The standardized tools of psychiatric diagnosis reveal that they are particularly subject to affective disorders and anxiety, as well as psychosomatic illnesses, which are strongly associated with tinnitus. Conditions diagnosed before the surgery do not directly change through the implantation—this can only occur through targeted therapies. According to the sample description (age, sex, and other social variables) none of these factors significantly correlated with the significant improvement in all aspects of hearing abilities measured during this study. However, duration of deafness correlated significantly with the hearing quality (measured by OI) pre- and post-CI. In addition, CI did have positive influence extending beyond hearing, particularly in many psychosocial aspects of their lives, including self-evaluations of their levels of depression and anxiety, tinnitus, quality of life, and coping strategies, as measured through the questionnaires.

Our results align with current models of the mechanisms that underlie neuronal plasticity, which at least partially account for post-CI improvements in the auditory processing of patients, including reductions in the symptoms of tinnitus independent of a person's degree of psychological burden While here the influence of concurrent psychological illnesses and various aspects of a patient's quality of life seem to have a rather indirect effect, it will be crucial to collect further data, such as the degree of hearing loss in the contralateral ear, to capture a better picture of how these factors, which vary highly between individuals, should be integrated into predictions about the potential effectiveness of therapies. This strongly suggests that through the entire process of cochlear implantation, from the original diagnosis through rehabilitation and follow-up care, there is a particular need to provide comprehensive psychosomatic care for patients, especially considering the negative effects that anxiety and other psychosomatic conditions have on the ultimate value of the therapy in their lives.

AUTHOR CONTRIBUTIONS

PB: study design; analysis and interpretation of data; drafting of manuscript. AS: analysis and interpretation of data; drafting of manuscript. KK: data acquisition; analysis and interpretation of data. SG: data acquisition; data analysis. BM: critical revision; HO: study conception and design; analysis and interpretation of data.

REFERENCES

Arnoldner, C., Lin, V. Y., Honeder, C., Shipp, D., Nedzelski, J., and Chen, J. (2014). Ten-year health-related quality of life in cochlear implant recipients: prospective SF-36 data with SF-6D conversion. *Laryngoscope* 124, 278–282. doi: 10.1002/lary.24387

Baizer, J. S., Wong, K. M., Manohar, S., Hayes, S. H., Ding, D., Dingman, R., et al. (2015). Effects of acoustic trauma on the auditory system of the rat: the role of microglia. *Neuroscience* 303, 299–311. doi: 10.1016/j.neuroscience.2015.07.004

Baumeister, H., and Harter, M. (2011). [Psychological comorbidity in patients with musculoskeletal diseases]. *Bundesgesundheitsblatt Gesundheitsforschung Gesundheitsschutz* 54, 52–58. doi: 10.1007/s00103-010-1185-x

Becker, J., Kocalevent, R. D., Rose, M., Walter, O. B., Frommer, J., and Klapp, B. F. (2006). Standardized diagnosing: computer-assisted (CIDI) diagnoses compared to clinically-judged diagnoses in a psychosomatic setting. *Psychotherapie Psychosomatik Medizinische Psychologie* 56, 5–14. doi: 10.1055/s-2005-866997

Blamey, P., Artieres, F., Baskent, D., Bergeron, F., Beynon, A., Burke, E., et al. (2013). Factors affecting auditory performance of postlinguistically deaf adults using cochlear implants: an update with 2251 patients. *Audiol. Neurootol.* 18, 36–47. doi: 10.1159/000343189

Blasco, M. A., and Redleaf, M. I. (2014). Cochlear implantation in unilateral sudden deafness improves tinnitus and speech comprehension: meta-analysis and systematic review. *Otol. Neurotol.* 35, 1426–1432. doi: 10.1097/MAO.0000000000000431

Carver, C. S., Scheier, M. F., and Weintraub, J. K. (1989). Assessing coping strategies: a theoretically based approach. *J. Pers. Soc. Psychol.* 56, 267–283. doi: 10.1037/0022-3514.56.2.267

Fellinger, J., Holzinger, D., Gerich, J., and Goldberg, D. (2007). Mental distress and quality of life in the hard of hearing. *Acta Psychiatr. Scand.* 115, 243–245. doi: 10.1111/j.1600-0447.2006.00976.x

Fellinger, J., Holzinger, D., Schoberberger, R., and Lenz, G. (2005). [Psychosocial characteristics of deaf people: evaluation of data from a special outpatient clinic for the deaf]. *Nervenarzt* 76, 43–51. doi: 10.1007/s00115-004-1708-5

Fliege, H., Rose, M., Arck, P., Walter, O. B., Kocalevent, R. D., Weber, C., et al. (2005). The Perceived Stress Questionnaire (PSQ) reconsidered: validation and reference values from different clinical and healthy adult samples. *Psychosom. Med.* 67, 78–88. doi: 10.1097/01.psy.0000151491.80178.78

Georgiewa, P., Szczepek, A. J., Rose, M., Klapp, B. F., and Mazurek, B. (2016). Cerebral processing of emotionally loaded acoustic signals by tinnitus patients. *Audiol. Neurootol.* 21, 80–87. doi: 10.1159/000443364

Goebel, G., and Hiller, W. (1994). [The tinnitus questionnaire. A standard instrument for grading the degree of tinnitus. Results of a multicenter study with the tinnitus questionnaire]. *HNO* 42, 166–172.

Hahlbrock, K. H. (1953). [Speech audiometry and new word-tests]. *Arch. Ohren Nasen Kehlkopfheilkd.* 162, 394–431. doi: 10.1007/BF02105664

Hinderink, J. B., Krabbe, P. F., and Van Den Broek, P. (2000). Development and application of a health-related quality-of-life instrument for adults with cochlear implants: the Nijmegen cochlear implant questionnaire. *Otolaryngol. Head Neck Surg.* 123, 756–765. doi: 10.1067/mhn.2000.108203

Hotting, K., and Roder, B. (2013). Beneficial effects of physical exercise on neuroplasticity and cognition. *Neurosci. Biobehav. Rev.* 37, 2243–2257. doi: 10.1016/j.neubiorev.2013.04.005

Hund, B., Reuter, K., Jacobi, F., Siegert, J., Wittchen, H.-U., Härter, M., et al. (2014). Adaptation of the composite international diagnostic interview (CIDI) for the assessment of comorbid mental disorders in oncology patients: the CIDI-O. *Psychother Psych. Med.* 64, 101–107. doi: 10.1055/s-0033-1357174

Jenkinson, C., Coulter, A., and Wright, L. (1993). Short form 36 (SF36) health survey questionnaire: normative data for adults of working age. *BMJ* 306, 1437–1440. doi: 10.1136/bmj.306.6890.1437

Kessler, R. C., Avenevoli, S., Green, J., Gruber, M. J., Guyer, M., He, Y., et al. (2009). National comorbidity survey replication adolescent supplement (NCS-A): III. Concordance of DSM-IV/CIDI diagnoses with clinical reassessments. *J. Am. Acad. Child Adolesc. Psychiatry* 48, 386–399. doi: 10.1097/CHI.0b013e31819a1cbc

Knappe, S., Runge, J., Beesdo, K., Jacobi, F., and Wittchen, H. U. (2008). [Diagnosing mental disorders: gold or tin standard?–Critical comments on standardized diagnostic interviews and clinical routine diagnoses]. *Psychother. Psychosom. Med. Psychol.* 58, 72–75. doi: 10.1055/s-2007-986197

Knoll, N., Rieckmann, N., and Schwarzer, R. (2005). Coping as a mediator between personality and stress outcomes: a longitudinal study with cataract surgery patients. *Eur. J. Pers.* 19, 229–247. doi: 10.1002/per.546

Kobosko, J., Pankowska, A., and Skarżyński, H. (2012). Coping strategies in postlingually deafened adult cochlear implant users in comparison to the hearing population. *Otolaryngol. Pol.* 66, 132–137. doi: 10.1016/S0030-6657(12)70761-8

Kollmeier, B., and Holube, I. (1991). Ein Fragebogen zur Erfassung des subjektiven Hörvermögens: erstellung der Fragen und Beziehungen zum Tonschwellenaudiogramm. *Audiologische Akustik* 30, 48–64.

Kral, A. (2007). Unimodal and cross-modal plasticity in the 'deaf' auditory cortex. *Int. J. Audiol.* 46, 479–493. doi: 10.1080/14992020701383027

Kraus, K. S., and Canlon, B. (2012). Neuronal connectivity and interactions between the auditory and limbic systems. Effects of noise and tinnitus. *Hear. Res.* 288, 34–46. doi: 10.1016/j.heares.2012.02.009

Lee, J. C., Yoo, M. H., Ahn, J. H., and Lee, K. S. (2007). Value of the promontory stimulation test in predicting speech perception after cochlear implantation. *Laryngoscope* 117, 1988–1992. doi: 10.1097/MLG.0b013e318 13437e6

Lin, F. R., Chien, W. W., Li, L., Clarrett, D. M., Niparko, J. K., and Francis, H. W. (2012). Cochlear implantation in older adults. *Medicine (Baltimore).* 91, 229–241. doi: 10.1097/MD.0b013e31826b145a

Mance, J., and Edwards, L. (2012). Deafness-related self-perceptions and psychological well-being in deaf adolescents with cochlear implants. *Cochlear Implants Int.* 13, 93–104. doi: 10.1179/1754762811Y.0000000017

Mazurek, B., Olze, H., Haupt, H., Klapp, B. F., Adli, M., Gross, J., et al. (2010). [Molecular biological aspects of neuroplasticity: approaches for treating tinnitus and hearing disorders]. *HNO* 58, 973–982. doi: 10.1007/s00106-010-2177-8

McClellan, W. M., Abramson, J., Newsome, B., Temple, E., Wadley, V. G., Audhya, P., et al. (2010). Physical and psychological burden of chronic kidney disease among older adults. *Am. J. Nephrol.* 31, 309–317. doi: 10.1159/000285113

Mohiyeddini, C., Hautzinger, M., and Bauer, S. (2002). A latent state-trait analysis on assessing trait and state components of three instruments for measuring depression: ADS, BDI, and SDS. *Diagnostica* 48, 12–18. doi: 10.1026//0012-1924.48.1.12

Olze, H., Grabel, S., Forster, U., Zirke, N., Huhnd, L. E., Haupt, H., et al. (2012a). Elderly patients benefit from cochlear implantation regarding auditory rehabilitation, quality of life, tinnitus, and stress. *Laryngoscope* 122, 196–203. doi: 10.1002/lary.22356

Olze, H., Knopke, S., Grabel, S., and Szczepek, A. J. (2016). Rapid positive influence of cochlear implantation on the quality of life in adults 70 years and older. *Audiol. Neurootol.* 21(Suppl. 1), 43–47. doi: 10.1159/000448354

Olze, H., Szczepek, A. J., Haupt, H., Forster, U., Zirke, N., Grabel, S., et al. (2011). Cochlear implantation has a positive influence on quality of life, tinnitus, and psychological comorbidity. *Laryngoscope* 121, 2220–2227. doi: 10.1002/lary.22145

Olze, H., Szczepek, A. J., Haupt, H., Zirke, N., Graebel, S., and Mazurek, B. (2012b). The impact of cochlear implantation on tinnitus, stress and quality of life in postlingually deafened patients. *Audiol. Neurootol.* 17, 2–11. doi: 10.1159/000323847

Piehlmeier, W., Bullinger, M., Kirchberger, I., Land, W., and Landgraf, R. (1996). Evaluation of the quality of life of patients with insulin-dependent diabetes mellitus before and after organ transplantation with the SF 36 health survey. *Eur. J. Surg.* 162, 933–940.

Ramos-Macias, A., Falcon Gonzalez, J. C., Borkoski-Barreiro, S. A., Ramos De Miguel, A., Batista, D. S., and Perez Plasencia, D. (2016). Health-related quality of life in adult cochlear implant users: a descriptive observational study. *Audiol. Neurootol.* 21(Suppl. 1), 36–42. doi: 10.1159/000448353

Robins, L. N., Wing, J., Wittchen, H. U., Helzer, J. E., Babor, T. F., Burke, J., et al. (1988). The composite international diagnostic interview. An epidemiologic instrument suitable for use in conjunction with different diagnostic systems and in different cultures. *Arch. Gen. Psychiatry* 45, 1069–1077.

Semler, G., Wittchen, H. U., Joschke, K., Zaudig, M., Von Geiso, T., Kaiser, S., et al. (1987). Test-retest reliability of a standardized psychiatric interview (DIS/CIDI). *Eur. Arch. Psychiatry Neurol. Sci.* 236, 214–222. doi: 10.1007/BF00383851

Spitzer, R. L., Kroenke, K., Williams, J. B. W., and Lowe, B. (2006). A brief measure for assessing generalized anxiety disorder - The GAD-7. *Arch. Intern. Med.* 166 1092–1097. doi: 10.1001/archinte.166.10.1092

Terber, S., Bernardy, K., Philippe, J., Untersinger, I., and Kollner, V. (2010). Clinical diagnosis adjustment disorder: what does a structured interview reveal? *J. Psychosom. Res.* 68, 669.

van der Werf, M., Thewissen, V., Dominguez, M. D., Lieb, R., Wittchen, H., and Van Os, J. (2011). Adolescent development of psychosis as an outcome of hearing impairment: a 10-year longitudinal study. *Psychol. Med.* 41, 477–485. doi: 10.1017/S0033291710000978

Wittchen, H. U. (1994). Reliability and validity studies of the WHO-composite international diagnostic interview (CIDI): a critical review. *J. Psychiatr. Res.* 28, 57–84. doi: 10.1016/0022-3956(94)90036-1

Zirke, N., Seydel, C., Szczepek, A. J., Olze, H., Haupt, H., and Mazurek, B. (2013). Psychological comorbidity in patients with chronic tinnitus: analysis and comparison with chronic pain, asthma or atopic dermatitis patients. *Qual. Life Res.* 22, 263–272. doi: 10.1007/s11136-012-0156-0

14

Comparison of the Long-Term Effect of Positioning the Cathode in tDCS in Tinnitus Patients

Sarah Rabau[1,2], Giriraj S. Shekhawat[3,4,5], Mohamed Aboseria[6], Daniel Griepp[6], Vincent Van Rompaey[1,2], Marom Bikson[6] and Paul Van de Heyning[1,2]*

[1]University Department of Otorhinolaryngology and Head and Neck Surgery, Antwerp University Hospital, Edegem, Belgium, [2]Faculty of Medicine, Campus Drie Eiken, University of Antwerp, Antwerp, Belgium, [3]Section of Audiology/Health Systems, University of Auckland, Auckland, New Zealand, [4]Centre for Brain Research, University of Auckland, Auckland, New Zealand, [5]Tinnitus Research Initiative, Regensburg, Germany , [6]Department of Biomedical Engineering, City College of New York, The City University of New York, New York, NY, United States

***Correspondence:**
Sarah Rabau
sarah.rabau@uantwerpen.be

Objective: Transcranial direct current stimulation (tDCS) is one of the methods described in the literature to decrease the perceived loudness and distress caused by tinnitus. However, the main effect is not clear and the number of responders to the treatment is variable. The objective of the present study was to investigate the effect of the placement of the cathode on the outcome measurements.

Methods: Patients considered for the trial were chronic non-pulsatile tinnitus patients with complaints for more than 3 months and a Tinnitus Functional Index (TFI) score that exceeded 25. The anode was placed on the right dorsolateral prefrontal cortex (DLPFC). In the first group—"bifrontal"—the cathode was placed on the left DLPFC, while in the second group—"shoulder"—the cathode was placed on the shoulder. Each patient received two sessions of tDCS weekly and eight sessions in total. Evaluations took place on the first visit for an ENT consultation, at the start of therapy, after eight sessions of tDCS and at the follow-up visit, which took place 84 days after the start of the therapy. Subjective outcome measures such as TFI, Visual Analog Scales (VAS) for loudness and percentage of consciousness of tinnitus were administered in every patient.

Results: There was no difference in the results for tinnitus loudness and the distress experienced between the placement of the cathode on the left DLPFC or on the shoulder. In addition, no statistically significant overall effect was found between the four test points. However, up to 39.1% of the patients experienced a decrease in loudness, measured by the VAS for loudness. Moreover, 72% of those in the bifrontal group, but only 46.2% of those in the shoulder group reported some improvement in distress.

Conclusion: While some improvement was noted, this was not statistically significant. Both electrode placements stimulated the right side of the hippocampus, which could be responsible for the effect found in both groups. Further research should rule out the placebo effect and investigate alternative electrode positions.

Keywords: neuromodulation, tDCS, electrode placement

INTRODUCTION

Tinnitus is the perception of sound in the absence of a corresponding external sound source (Eggermont and Roberts, 2004) and is a very common problem. Approximately 25.3% of the US population reports having tinnitus, while 7.9% experience tinnitus frequently (Shargorodsky et al., 2010). Tinnitus affects daily activities and can lead to a high level of distress. The literature describes several mechanisms and structures that could be involved in tinnitus. However, the findings reported cannot always be repeated and the proposed brain structures do not always match. However, it is certain that it is not only the auditory system which is responsible for inducing tinnitus (Jastreboff, 1990). Multiple non-auditory systems involved in cognition, emotion and memory play an important role (De Ridder et al., 2014).

Currently, no treatment is available that eliminates tinnitus completely. Most researchers and clinicians focus on diminishing the level of disturbance experienced and/or the loudness of the tinnitus. One method that can be used is neuromodulation, namely transcranial Direct Current Stimulation (tDCS). In the case of tDCS, the current is applied to the brain by means of two electrodes. The goal of tDCS is to influence those regions involved in tinnitus and consequently lessen the distress caused by, or the loudness of, tinnitus. Previous research has shown that bifrontal tDCS strengthens deficient inhibitory top-down mechanisms in tinnitus and interferes with the emotional processing of tinnitus (Tanaka et al., 2008; Vanneste et al., 2010). However, in the literature tDCS is reported as having a variable effect, with the percentage of responders ranging from 0% to almost 47% (Fregni et al., 2006; Vanneste et al., 2011; Song et al., 2012). The difference in outcomes might be due to different factors such as orientation of the current field, electrode positions, electrode size, stimulation duration and current intensity (Nitsche et al., 2008). Depending on the orientation of the current field, tDCS can either increase or decrease the excitability. Under the cathode, excitability is decreased due to neural hyperpolarization. However, under the anode, excitability is enhanced due to neural depolarization (Nitsche and Paulus, 2000).

The literature also reports the use of different electrode positions to treat tinnitus, with bifrontal tDCS and left temporoparietal area (LTA) tDCS most frequently applied in tinnitus patients. In bifrontal tDCS, the anode and cathode are placed on the right and left dorsolateral prefrontal cortex (DLPFC), respectively. In LTA tDCS, the anode is placed on the left temporal area. Song et al. (2012) found that LTA and bifrontal positioning produced similar results with respect to the percentage of responders and a reduction in tinnitus intensity (Song et al., 2012). Furthermore, the current intensity and duration can also play an important role. Shekhawat et al. (2013) concluded that 2 mA anodal tDCS at LTA for 20 min was the most effective setting for transient tinnitus suppression (Shekhawat et al., 2013).

Concluding, more research is needed towards parameters of tDCS to optimize the effect of it. In that interest, a computational model was calculated to predict differences in the current pathway of two placement montages, namely the "bifrontal" montage and the "shoulder" montage. The "bifrontal" group had the anode and cathode positioned over the F4 (right DLPFC) and F3 (left DLPFC) positions respectively; in the "shoulder" group, the anode electrode was placed over F4 and the cathode on the left shoulder Considering these differences, interest was raised towards the difference in the perception outcome of the tinnitus patients undergoing tDCS using these two different montages. The objective of the present study was to compare the outcomes of the placement of the cathode on the left DLPFC vs. the shoulder.

MATERIALS AND METHODS

Subjects

Patients considered for the trial were chronic non-pulsatile tinnitus patients who had complaints for more than 3 months and a Tinnitus Functional Index (TFI) score that exceeded 25. Written informed consent was obtained from every patient (n = 65). The study protocol was approved by the ethical committee of Antwerp University Hospital. Of the 65 subjects, six were lost to follow-up for various reasons. The median age of the subjects was 52 years, within a range of 23 years to 70 years. The median duration of tinnitus was 28 months and fluctuated between 3 months and 264 months. In total 59 subjects—41 men and 18 women were included and randomized based on the parameters of age, TFI score, etiology, gender and degree of hearing loss. In order to create two equal groups, the MS-DOS program MINIM (by S. Evans, P. Royston and S. Day) was used to allocate the subjects by minimization. A flow diagram is presented in **Figure 1**.

Transcranial Direct Current Stimulation

In the first group—"bifrontal"—the anode and the cathode were placed on the right and left DLPFC, respectively (F4 and F3), while in the second group—"shoulder"—the cathode was placed on the left upper arm, according to the 10–20 international system for EEG electrode placement. Each patient received two sessions of tDCS weekly and a total of eight sessions. The direct current was transferred by means of two saline-soaked pairs of surface sponge electrodes (35 cm^2) and delivered by a specially developed, battery-driven constant current Neuroconn stimulator (neuroConn, Ilmenau, Germany), with a maximum output of 10 mA. A constant current of 2 mA was applied for 20 min with a fade-in and fade-out of 10 s. **Figure 2** shows the current pattern in both cathode placements. In the bifrontal group, the DLPFC and the hippocampus are stimulated, but not the cingulate cortex. In contrast, in the shoulder placement, the temporal lobe is stimulated, in addition to the cingulate cortex and the right side of the hippocampus.

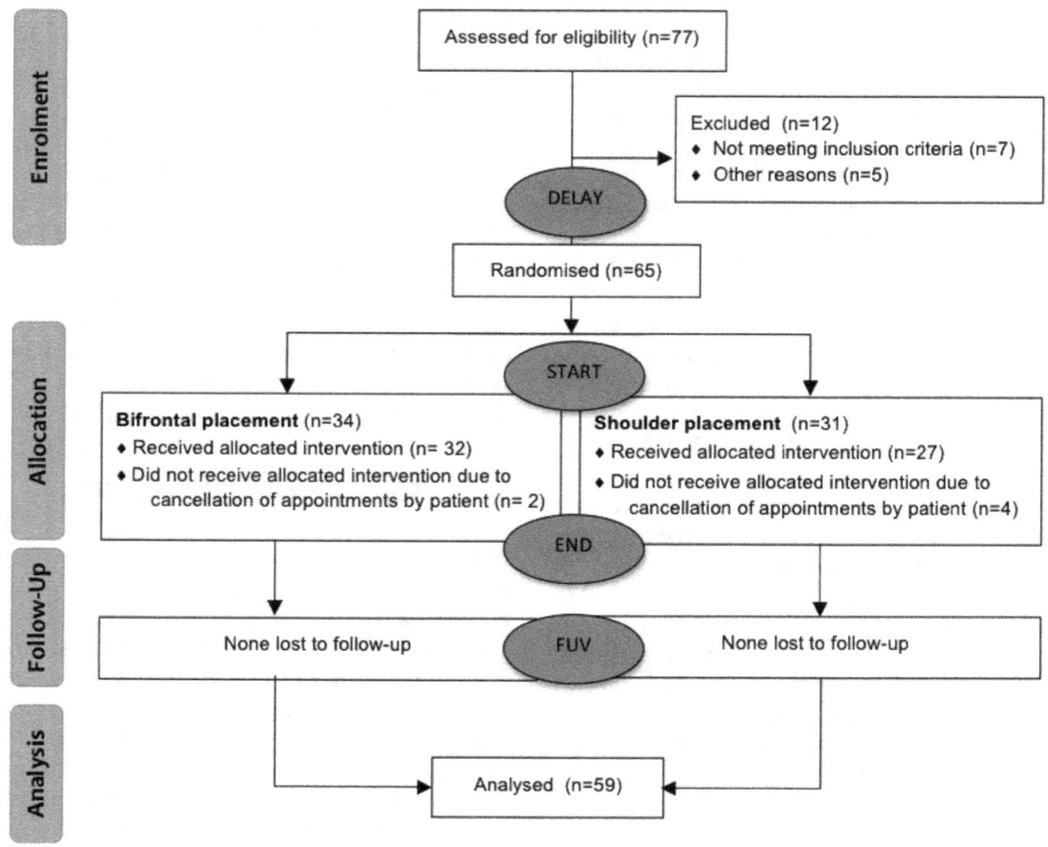

FIGURE 1 | Flow chart.

Outcome Measures

Evaluations took place on the first visit for an ENT consultation (Delay), at the start of therapy (Start), after eight sessions of tDCS (End) and 84 days after the start of the therapy (FUV). The delay was added to test spontaneous recovery after visiting an ENT-specialist. The FUV was added to measure the long-term effect of tDCS. The flow diagram is presented in **Figure 1**.

The subjective outcome measures of TFI (Meikle et al., 2012; Rabau et al., 2014), Visual Analog Scales (VAS) for loudness and the Hyperacusis Questionnaire (HQ; Khalfa et al., 2002) were completed for every patient. The Dutch version of the TFI, a self-report questionnaire consisting of 25 questions, was chosen as the primary outcome measurement. A reduction of 13 points on the TFI is considered a meaningful reduction in annoyance experienced by the patient. In addition to a total score, scores of the subscales of intrusiveness, reduced sense of control, cognitive interference, sleep disturbance, auditory difficulties attributed to tinnitus, interference with relaxation, reduced quality of life and emotional distress can also be calculated (Meikle et al., 2012).

The secondary outcome measures were the VAS for loudness and the HQ. On the VAS the patient had to rate the maximum and mean loudness of their tinnitus on a scale of 0–10, with 0 indicating a very soft sound that is not audible and 10 meaning as loud as possible—the tinnitus could not be any louder. The HQ surveys the over-sensitivity to sounds, and consists of 14 items with four answer possibilities: no (0 points); yes, a little (1 point); yes, quite a lot (2 points) and yes, a lot (3 points). The maximum score is 42, with Khalfa et al. (2002) suggesting a cut-off score of 28. Patients scoring more than 28 are considered to have hyperacusis (Khalfa et al., 2002).

Statistical Analysis

Statistical analyses were performed on the data to determine whether one placement was preferable to the other. The data were analyzed using SPSS statistical software version 22 MAC OS X (IBM; Armonk, NY, USA). Normal distribution of the data was checked using the Shapiro-Wilk test and Q-Q plots. For each of the outcome measurements, a repeated measures ANOVA was performed with test moment as within subject and group (bifrontal vs. shoulder) as between subject variable. The interaction between test moment and group were added to the model. To assess the impact of the demographic details, covariants (hearing loss and age) were added into the model. The significance level was set at $p < 0.05$. Descriptive statistics was used to compare the characteristics of the subjects.

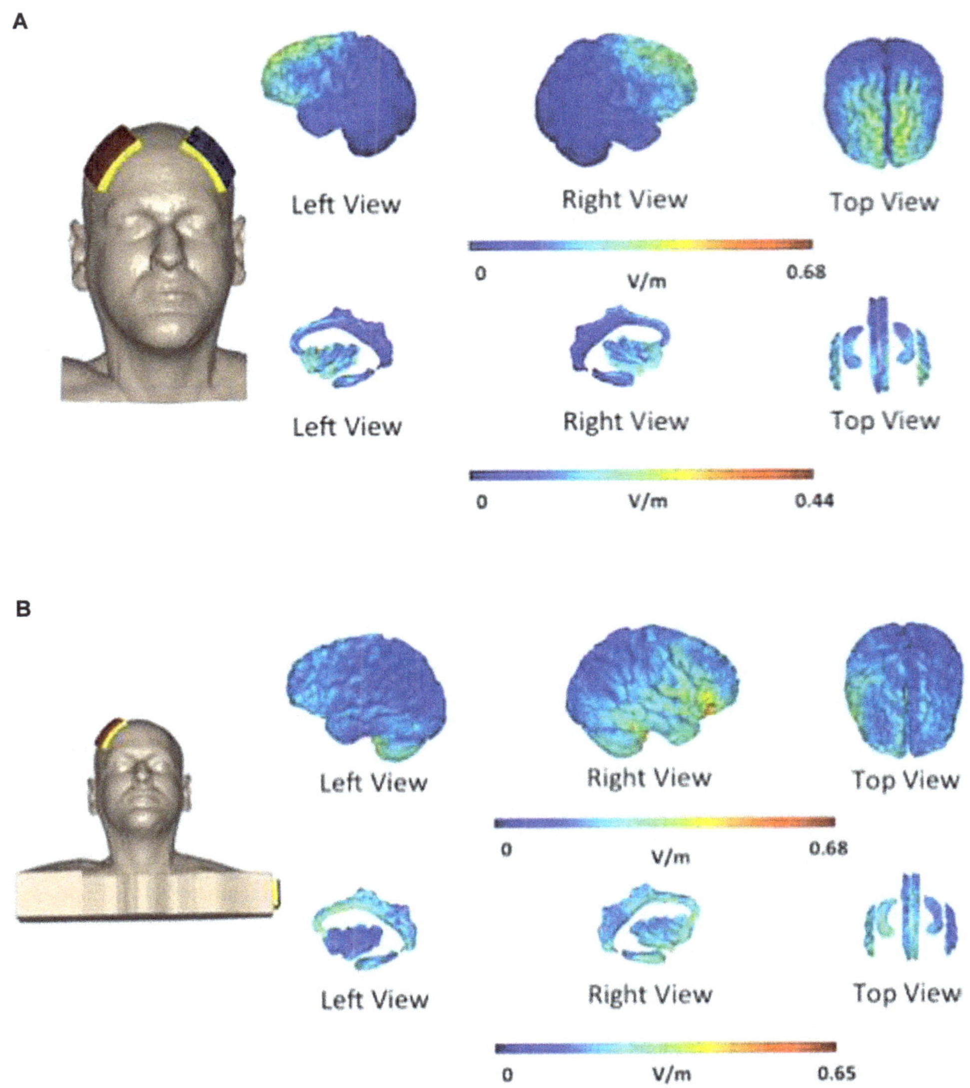

FIGURE 2 | Distribution of electric field during transcranial direct current stimulation (tDCS). The electric field is shown as electric field/current density magnitude (V/m). The cathode placed on the left dorsolateral prefrontal cortex (DLPFC) **(A)** vs. the cathode placed on the shoulder **(B)**. In the bifrontal group **(A)** the DLPFC and hippocampus are stimulated. In the shoulder placement group **(B)**, the temporal lobe is stimulated in addition to the cingulate cortex and the right side of the hippocampus.

Computational Model

A finite element montages were generated in COMSOL multi physics 4.2 for analysis based on previous procedures (Truong et al., 2012a,b). Briefly, initially, a 3-D 1 mm*1 mm*1 mm T1 MRI of an adult male was segmented into different head regions using both automated segmentation algorithms and manual segmentation techniques available in the ScanIP software (Simpleware, Ltd., Exeter, UK) to correct for segmentation errors from the automated algorithms, add fat, segment a number of brain deep structures. 5 × 7 cm sponge pads were then placed on F4 and F3 for the "bifrontal" montage, and F4 and the left shoulder for the "shoulder" montage using ScanCAD (Simpleware, Ltd., Exeter, UK). The mesh was then generated and imported into COMSOL multi physics 4.2 (COMSOL, Inc., Burlington, MA, USA). In COMSOL, the segmented regions were assigned a conductivity (S/m): air, 10^{-15}; skin, 0.465; fat, 0.025; skull, 0.01; CSF, 1.65; gray matter, 0.276; or white matter, 0.126. The electrodes were assigned a conductivity of 5.99×10^{7} S/m and the sponges were modeled using the conductivity of saline which is 1.4 S/m. Boundary conditions were set such that the cathode (F3 for "bifrontal"; left shoulder electrode for "shoulder") was the ground and a total of 2 mA of current was applied from the F4 anode. The model was solved and cortical electric field magnitude was plotted for

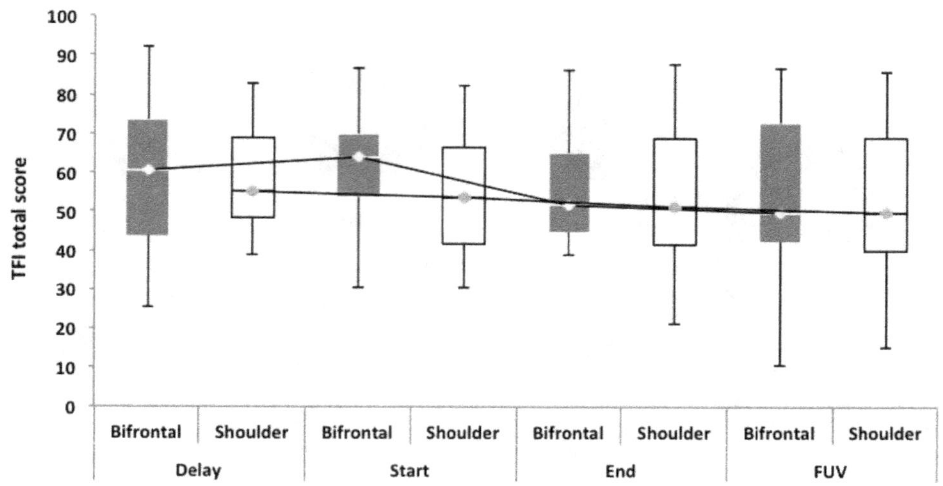

FIGURE 3 | Tinnitus functional index (TFI) total score. No significant effect was found between either cathode placement and the test moments for the TFI total score.

each montage to analyze the differences between the two montages.

RESULTS

Repeated measures showed no statistically significant difference between both groups with regard to the TFI, the subscales of the TFI, the VAS for maximum and mean loudness, the percentage of consciousness, or problems experienced falling asleep and waking up during the night ($p > 0.05$). Looking at the overall effect, no significant effect was found between the test moments for the TFI total score (**Figure 3**), the TFI subscales of intrusiveness, cognitive interference, sleep disturbance, auditory difficulties, quality of life and emotional distress, or with the maximum (**Figure 4**) and mean VAS for loudness and percentage of consciousness ($p > 0.05$). For the subscale of sleep disturbance ($p = 0.048$), a statistically significant effect was found between the Start (mean = 64.03) and the FUV (mean = 52.50) test moments in the bifrontal group (**Figure 5**). Concerning the shoulder group, a statistically significant effect was found for the subscale of intrusiveness ($p = 0.040$) between the Delay (mean = 72.50) and the FUV (mean = 62.50) test moments. The results are shown in **Figure 6**. No statistically significant effect of the demographic details age and hearing loss was found on the outcome measurements ($p > 0.05$).

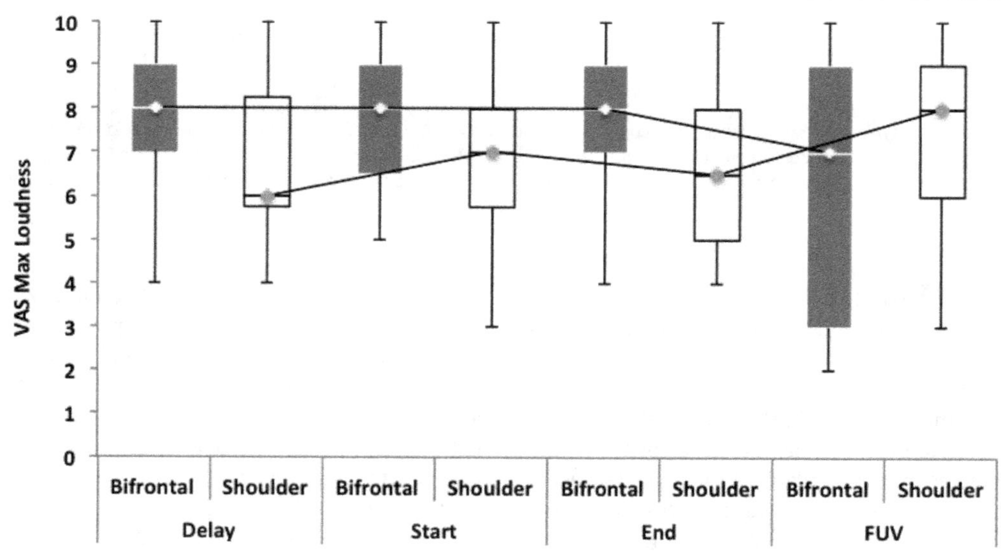

FIGURE 4 | Visual analog scales (VAS) for maximum loudness. No significant effect was found between groups and the test moments for the VAS for maximum loudness.

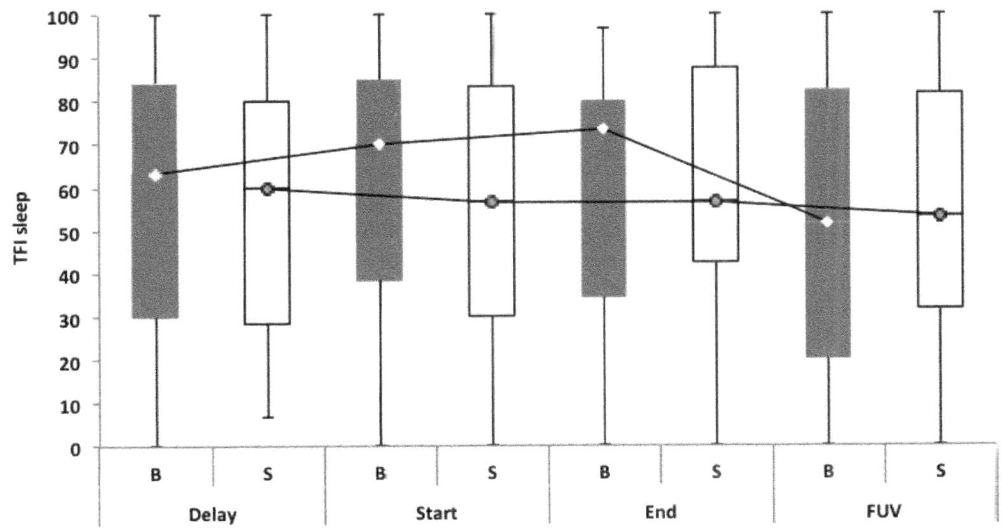

FIGURE 5 | TFI subscale of sleep disturbance. In the bifrontal group, a statistically significant effect ($p = 0.048$) was found for the subscale of sleep disturbance between the Start (mean = 64.03) and the FUV (mean = 52.50) test moments.

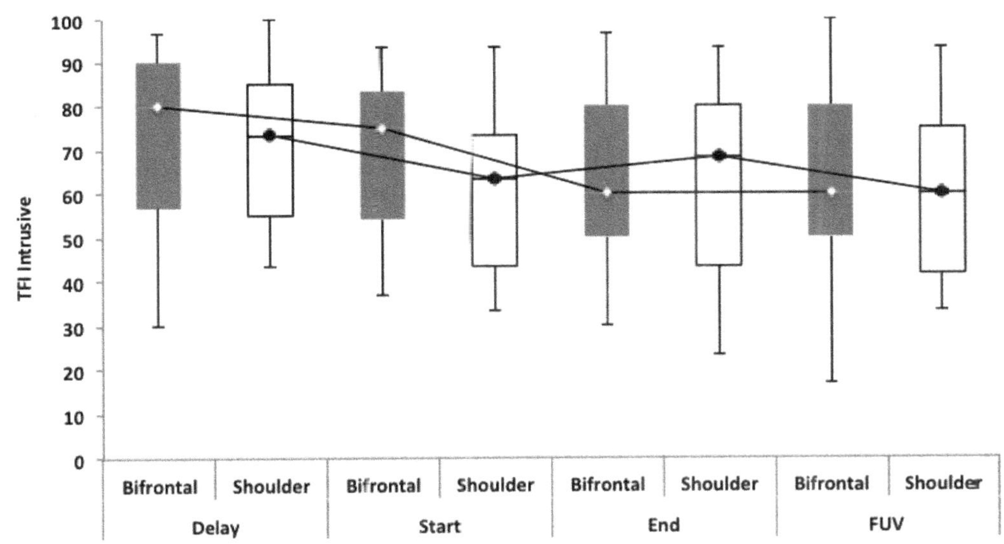

FIGURE 6 | TFI subscale of intrusiveness. Concerning the shoulder group, a statistically significant effect was found for the subscale of intrusiveness ($p = 0.040$) between the Delay (mean = 72.50) and the FUV (mean = 62.50) test moments. The effect found cannot be attributed to the tDCS therapy, but to the spontaneous recovery or placebo effect found between the Delay (median = 73.30) and Start (median = 63.33) test moments.

Focusing on the measurements before and after the eight sessions of tDCS, we found that 26.8% ($n = 7$) of the bifrontal group and 37.5% ($n = 9$) of the shoulder group experienced an improvement of 1 or more on the VAS for maximum loudness, while 30.6% ($n = 8$) of the subjects in the bifrontal group and 39.1% ($n = 9$) of the subjects in the shoulder group showed an improvement on the VAS for mean loudness. With respect to the change in TFI scores, 16% ($n = 4$) of the bifrontal group and 8.4% ($n = 2$) of the shoulder group showed a clinically significant improvement of more than 13 points, while 56% ($n = 14$) of the bifrontal group and 37.8% ($n = 9$) of the shoulder group showed an improvement of less than 13 points on the TFI.

DISCUSSION

The present study failed to find any difference between the electrode placements with respect to their effects on tinnitus distress and tinnitus loudness. One possible explanation for this may be the limited focus of the tDCS, due to the large electrodes used (Nitsche et al., 2008). The lack of focus prevents the stimulation of a specific area of the brain. Moliadze et al. (2010) have suggested that an extracephalic reference electrode has the potential to better focus stimulation (Moliadze et al., 2010), but direct proof is lacking. In contrast, Parazzini et al. (2012) argued that if the anode and cathode are placed on the far sides of the brain this results in a more widely spread current/electric field (Parazzini et al., 2012). Bikson has studied the role of the position of the return electrode, finding that the repositioning of the return electrode from the contralateral forehead to the upper arm caused the relocation of the current from the frontal regions to the more posterior regions of the brain (Bikson et al., 2010). This finding is consistent with our current pattern, as presented in **Figure 2**. Tissue resistance and altered current flow can also play an important role (Nitsche and Paulus, 2011). Moliadze et al. (2010) claimed that higher current intensity is required to induce identical aftereffects in comparison to bicephalic electrode placement (Moliadze et al., 2010). In relation to bicephalic electrode placement, Shekhawat et al. (2013) concluded that 2 mA anodal tDCS at the LTA for 20 min was sufficient (Shekhawat et al., 2013). Further research should determine whether 2 mA is sufficient to induce aftereffects in the case of extracephalic reference electrode placement and the best dose-response ratio with this electrode position.

No statistically significant overall effect was found between the four test moments. Only for the TFI subscale of sleep disturbance in the bifrontal group was a significant effect found between the Start (median = 70.00) and FUV (median = 51.67) test moments. The statistically significant difference found for the subscale of intrusiveness in the shoulder group cannot be attributed to the tDCS therapy, but to spontaneous recovery or a placebo effect between the Delay (median = 73.30) and Start (median = 63.33) test moments. To rule out a placebo effect, we recommend including a control group in the study protocol for further research. The percentage of responders varied from 26.8% to 39.1% for tinnitus loudness. For the outcome measurement of distress, a clinically significant effect was only found in 16% and 8.4% of the subjects in the bifrontal and shoulder groups respectively. None of these results were statistically significant. The results confirm previous findings reported in the literature, which suggest no long-term effects on distress. However, a positive transient effect of bifrontal tDCS has been reported for tinnitus intensity (Garin et al., 2011; Frank et al., 2012). The present study failed to repeat these results. Most studies have reported a positive effect of tDCS on tinnitus loudness and distress immediately after a tDCS session (Vanneste et al., 2010; Vanneste and De Ridder, 2011; Joos et al., 2014); however, in this study, we focused on the long-term effect.

Another explanation for the lack of statistically significant results may be related to the factors that cause the variance of responders. For tDCS to be considered useful in a clinical setting, it would be interesting to know what causes this variance in the percentage of responders. Further research should also determine what might improve the administration of tDCS to attain clinically significant outcomes. High definition tDCS seems to be a promising alternative in this respect (Shekhawat et al., 2016).

While some improvement was found in both groups, the difference was not statistically significant. This finding would suggest that the area that was stimulated in both groups can be hold responsible for this improvement, namely the right side of the hippocampus, which is the part of the brain that is involved in learning and memory processes. Jastreboff (1990) has pointed out that in addition to the auditory system, the limbic system, including the hippocampus, is responsible for the preseverance of tinnitus. The gating model proposed by Rauschecker et al. (2010) also makes predictions about the structures involved in tinnitus. Although the hippocampus is not a part of the model presented, this structure may be involved in tinnitus but not sufficient to cause tinnitus on its own (Rauschecker et al., 2010; Adjamian et al., 2014). The positioning of an electrode such that it influences the structures involved in the proposed gating model would be an interesting topic for further research. In this study we did not investigate the underlying structures activated during the tDCS stimulation during the two montages (cathode on L DLPFC and shoulder). However, in future it would be insightful to incorporate MRI scans to investigate the neurophysiological structures involved during the tDCS. Another possible explanation is that the effect found can be attributed to a placebo effect. Further research should include a control group to rule out the placebo effect and reveal the real effect of tDCS.

CONCLUSION

There was no significant difference in outcomes between the electrode placements. Both placements stimulated the right side of the hippocampus, which could be responsible for the effect found in both groups. Further research should rule out a placebo effect, while alternative electrode positions, as well as high definition tDCS, could reveal the effects of stimulating brain structures that are involved in the gating model proposed by Rauschecker et al. (2010).

AUTHOR CONTRIBUTIONS

SR, VVR and PV designed and set up the study protocol. SR collected and analyzed the data. SR and MB wrote the manuscript. MA and DG designed the model of the distribution of the electric field of tDCS. GSS, VVR, DG, MA and MB reviewed the manuscript.

FUNDING

The study was supported by a grant from the TOP-BOF project of the University of Antwerp.

REFERENCES

Adjamian, P., Hall, D. A., Palmer, A. R., Allan, T. W., and Langers, D. R. (2014). Neuroanatomical abnormalities in chronic tinnitus in the human brain. *Neurosci. Biobehav. Rev.* 45, 119–133. doi: 10.1016/j.neubiorev.2014.05.013

Bikson, M., Datta, A., Rahman, A., and Scaturro, J. (2010). Electrode montages for tDCS and weak transcranial electrical stimulation: role of "return" electrode's position and size. *Clin. Neurophysiol.* 121, 1976–1978. doi: 10.1016/j.clinph.2010.05.020

De Ridder, D., Vanneste, S., Weisz, N., Londero, A., Schlee, W., Elgoyhen, A. B., et al. (2014). An integrative model of auditory phantom perception: tinnitus as a unified percept of interacting separable subnetworks. *Neurosci. Biobehav. Rev.* 44, 16–32. doi: 10.1016/j.neubiorev.2013.03.021

Eggermont, J. J., and Roberts, L. E. (2004). The neuroscience of tinnitus. *Trends Neurosci.* 27, 676–682. doi: 10.1016/j.tins.2004.08.010

Frank, E., Schecklmann, M., Landgrebe, M., Burger, J., Kreuzer, P., Poeppl, T. B., et al. (2012). Treatment of chronic tinnitus with repeated sessions of prefrontal transcranial direct current stimulation: outcomes from an open-label pilot study. *J. Neurol.* 259, 327–333. doi: 10.1007/s00415-011-6189-4

Fregni, F., Marcondes, R., Boggio, P. S., Marcolin, M. A., Rigonatti, S. P. Sanchez, T. G., et al. (2006). Transient tinnitus suppression induced by repetitive transcranial magnetic stimulation and transcranial direct current stimulation. *Eur. J. Neurol.* 13, 996–1001. doi: 10.1111/j.1468-1331 2006.01414.x

Garin, P., Gilain, C., Van Damme, J. P., De Fays, K., Jamart, J., Ossemann, M., et al. (2011). Short- and long-lasting tinnitus relief induced by transcranial direct current stimulation. *J. Neurol.* 258, 1940–1948. doi: 10.1007/s00415-011-6037-6

Jastreboff, P. J. (1990). Phantom auditory perception (tinnitus): mechanisms of generation and perception. *Neurosci. Res.* 8, 221–254. doi: 10.1016/0168-0102(90)90031-9

Joos, K., De Ridder, D., Van de Heyning, P., and Vanneste, S. (2014). Polarity specific suppression effects of transcranial direct current stimulation for tinnitus. *Neural Plast.* 2014:930860. doi: 10.1155/2014/930860

Khalfa, S., Dubal, S., Veuillet, E., Perez-Diaz, F., Jouvent, R., and Collet, L. (2002). Psychometric normalization of a hyperacusis questionnaire. *ORL J. Otorhinolaryngol. Relat. Spec.* 64, 436–442. doi: 10.1159/000067570

Meikle, M. B., Henry, J. A., Griest, S. E., Stewart, B. J., Abrams, H. B., Mcardle, R., et al. (2012). The tinnitus functional index: development of a new clinical measure for chronic, intrusive tinnitus. *Ear Hear.* 33, 153–176. doi: 10.1097/AUD.0b013e3182597b3e

Moliadze, V., Antal, A., and Paulus, W. (2010). Electrode-distance dependent after-effects of transcranial direct and random noise stimulation with extracephalic reference electrodes. *Clin. Neurophysiol.* 121, 2165–2171. doi: 10.1016/j.clinph.2010.04.033

Nitsche, M. A., and Paulus, W. (2000). Excitability changes induced in the human motor cortex by weak transcranial direct current stimulation. *J. Physiol.* 527, 633–639. doi: 10.1111/j.1469-7793.2000.t01-1-00633.x

Nitsche, M. A., and Paulus, W. (2011). Transcranial direct current stimulation—update 2011. *Restor. Neurol. Neurosci.* 29, 463–492. doi: 10.3233/RNN-2011-0618

Nitsche, M. A., Cohen, L. G., Wassermann, E. M., Priori, A., Lang, N., Antal, A., et al. (2008). Transcranial direct current stimulation: state of the art 2008. *Brain Stimul.* 1, 206–223. doi: 10.1016/j.brs.2008.06.004

Parazzini, M., Fiocchi, S., and Ravazzani, P. (2012). Electric field and current density distribution in an anatomical head model during transcranial direct current stimulation for tinnitus treatment. *Bioelectromagnetics* 33, 476–487. doi: 10.1002/bem.21708

Rabau, S., Wouters, K., and Van de Heyning, P. (2014). Validation and translation of the dutch version of the tinnitus functional index. *B-ENT* 10, 251–258.

Rauschecker, J. P., Leaver, A. M., and Mühlau, M. (2010). Tuning out the noise: limbic-auditory interactions in tinnitus. *Neuron* 66, 819–826. doi: 10.1016/j.neuron.2010.04.032

Shargorodsky, J., Curhan, G. C., and Farwell, W. R. (2010). Prevalence and characteristics of tinnitus among US adults. *Am. J. Med.* 123, 711–718 doi: 10.1016/j.amjmed.2010.02.015

Shekhawat, G. S., Stinear, C. M., and Searchfield, G. D. (2013). Transcranial direct current stimulation intensity and duration effects on tinnitus suppression. *Neurorehabil. Neural Repair* 27, 164–172. doi: 10.1177/1545968312459908

Shekhawat, G. S., Sundram, F., Bikson, M., Truong, D., De Ridder, D., Stinear, C. M., et al. (2016). Intensity, duration and location of high-definition transcranial direct current stimulation for tinnitus relief. *Neurorehabil. Neural Repair* 30, 349–359. doi: 10.1177/1545968315595286

Song, J. J., Vanneste, S., Van de Heyning, P., and De Ridder, D. (2012). Transcranial direct current stimulation in tinnitus patients: a systemic review and meta-analysis. *ScientificWorldJournal* 2012:427941. doi: 10.1100/2012/427941

Tanaka, E., Inui, K., Kida, T., Miyazaki, T., Takeshima, Y., and Kakigi, R. (2008). A transition from unimodal to multimodal activations in four sensory modalities in humans: an electrophysiological study. *BMC Neurosci.* 9:116. doi: 10.1186/1471-2202-9-116

Truong, D. Q., Datta, A., Xu, J., Fregni, F., and Bikson, M. (2012a). "Prefrontal cortex transcranial direct current stimulation via a combined high definition and conventional electrode montage: a FEM modeling studying," in *34th Annual International Conference of the IEEE Engineering in Medicine and Biology Society (EMBS)*, (San Diego, CA), 6608-6611.

Truong, D. Q., Magerowski, G., Pascual-Leone, A., Alonso-Alonso, M., and Bikson, M. (2012b). "Finite element study of skin and fat delineation in an obese subject for transcranial direct current stimulation," in *34th Annual International Conference of the IEEE Engineering in Medicine and Biology Society (EMBS)*, (San Diego, CA), 6587-6590.

Vanneste, S., and De Ridder, D. (2011). Bifrontal transcranial direct current stimulation modulates tinnitus intensity and tinnitus-distress-related brain activity. *Eur. J. Neurosci.* 34, 605–614. doi: 10 1111/j.1460-9568.2011.07778.x

Vanneste, S., Focquaert, F., Van de Heyning, P., and De Ridder, D. (2011). Different resting state brain activity and functional connectivity in patients who respond and not respond to bifrontal tDCS for tinnitus suppression. *Exp. Brain Res.* 210, 217–227. doi: 10.1007/s00221-011-2617-z

Vanneste, S., Plazier, M., Ost, J., van der Loo, E., Van de Heyning, P., and De Ridder, D. (2010). Bilateral dorsolateral prefrontal cortex modulation for tinnitus by transcranial direct current stimulation: a preliminary clinical study. *Exp. Brain Res.* 202, 779–785. doi: 10.1007/s00221-010-2183-9

15

Measuring the Moment-to-Moment Variability of Tinnitus: The "TrackYourTinnitus" Smart Phone App

Winfried Schlee[1], Rüdiger C. Pryss[2], Thomas Probst[3,4], Johannes Schobel[2], Alexander Bachmeier[2], Manfred Reichert[2] and Berthold Langguth[1]*

[1]Department of Psychiatry and Psychotherapy, University of Regensburg, Regensburg, Germany, [2]Institute of Databases and Information Systems, Ulm University, Ulm, Germany, [3]Department of Psychology, University of Regensburg, Regensburg, Germany, [4]Department of Psychology and Psychotherapy, University of Witten/Herdecke, Witten, Germany

Correspondence:
Winfried Schlee
winfried.schlee@gmail.com

Tinnitus, the phantom perception of sound without a corresponding external sound, is a frequent disorder which causes significant morbidity. So far there is no treatment available that reliably reduces the tinnitus perception. The research is hampered by the large heterogeneity of tinnitus and the fact that the tinnitus perception fluctuates over time. It is therefore necessary to develop tools for measuring fluctuations of tinnitus perception over time and for analyzing data on single subject basis. However, this type of longitudinal measurement is difficult to perform using the traditional research methods such as paper-and-pencil questionnaires or clinical interviews. Ecological momentary assessment (EMA) represents a research concept that allows the assessment of subjective measurements under real-life conditions using portable electronic devices and thereby enables the researcher to collect longitudinal data under real-life conditions and high cost efficiency. Here we present a new method for recording the longitudinal development of tinnitus perception using a modern smartphone application available for iOS and Android devices with no costs for the users. The TrackYourTinnitus (TYT) app is available and maintained since April 2014. A number of 857 volunteers with an average age of 44.1 years participated in the data collection between April 2014 and February 2016. The mean tinnitus distress at the initial measurement was rated on average 13.9 points on the Mini-Tinnitus Questionnaire (Mini-TQ; max. 24 points). Importantly, we could demonstrate that the regular use of the TYT app has no significant negative influence on the perception of the tinnitus loudness nor on the tinnitus distress. The TYT app can therefore be proposed as a safe instrument for the longitudinal assessment of tinnitus perception in the everyday life of the patient.

Keywords: chronic tinnitus, smartphone application, ecological momentary assessment, moment-to-moment analysis, crowd sourcing, ecological validity

INTRODUCTION

Tinnitus is the perception of a sound when no corresponding external sound is present. The severity of tinnitus varies largely between tinnitus sufferers. While a large percentage of cases is only minimally impaired during their daily routing, the severe cases of tinnitus are affected by anxiety, depression, insomnia and concentration problems all of which can impair their quality of life (Dobie, 2003; Heller, 2003; Kreuzer et al., 2013).

Epidemiological studies of tinnitus indicate a prevalence between 6%–26% with 1.2%–1.6% reporting severely annoying tinnitus (Davis and Rafaie, 2000; Hasson et al., 2010; Gallus et al., 2015). There is currently little evidence for an effective treatment of tinnitus loudness and no pharmacological treatment approved by the US Food and Drug Administration (FDA) or the European Medicines Evaluation Agency (EMEA; Langguth and Elgoyhen, 2012). Among other factors the large heterogeneity of the tinnitus patient population represents a major barrier for the development of effective tinnitus treatments (for a review see e.g., Elgoyhen et al., 2015). A recent review of tinnitus identified at least 13 different types of causal factors for tinnitus (Baguley et al., 2013) that can be described on various dimensions such as its etiology, perceptual characteristics of the sound (i.e., pitch and loudness), time since onset, continuous or intermittent levels of conscious awareness and perceived distress and comorbidities.

As tinnitus is a purely subjective phenomenon, its assessment is not trivial (Langguth et al., 2007). For the assessment of tinnitus severity standardized questionnaires have been developed, whereas tinnitus loudness can be assessed either by visual analog scale (VAS; Adamchic et al., 2012) or by psychoacoustic measurements. All these measurements are based on the assumption that tinnitus is a rather static phenomenon. However recent data demonstrates that tinnitus loudness and annoyance fluctuate significantly from moment to moment (Henry et al., 2012; Wilson et al., 2015). Henry et al. (2012) conducted a pilot study in which tinnitus symptoms were measured in 24 participants over 2-weeks at four random time points per day using a personal digital assistant (PDA) device. They presented results, which suggest a large between-days variability of tinnitus distress for some study participants. Notably, the frequent measurement of tinnitus over the 2 weeks period had no negative impact on the perceived tinnitus distress as measured by the tinnitus handicap inventory (THI, Newman et al., 1996) indicating that directing the attention on tinnitus several times per day does not worsen the tinnitus (Henry et al., 2012). Using a similar study design (4 assessments per day for 2 weeks), Wilson et al. (2015) also investigated the intra-individual variability of tinnitus distress using smart phone notifications. Likewise, to the study by Henry et al. (2012) they showed that tinnitus fluctuations vary strongly across individuals. Some individuals report strong fluctuations of their tinnitus distress while others report relatively low fluctuations. A coefficient of variation (CV) calculated over the tinnitus self-reports of each participant ranged between 11.5% and 109.9% with a median of 48.4% (Wilson et al., 2015). So far it is not understood why tinnitus fluctuates in some cases and what are the underlying mechanisms for the fluctuations of tinnitus from one moment to the other. Better assessment of the fluctuations of tinnitus is of highest importance for many different reasons: (1) exact assessment of tinnitus fluctuations are of diagnostic importance as intra-individual fluctuations may be an important characteristic feature of an individual's tinnitus; (2) exact measurement of perceptual fluctuations is a precondition for investigating the neurobiological mechanisms of tinnitus changes over time; (3) knowledge of tinnitus fluctuations over time is important for patient management (e.g., for tinnitus counselling); and (4) information of tinnitus fluctuations is highly relevant for clinical studies, e.g., when effects of specific therapeutic interventions are assessed.

In this article, we want to present a conceptual and technical framework for an ecologically momentary assessment (EMA: Stone and Shiffman, 1994), which allows to systematically assess the moments of different tinnitus symptom severity. The method of EMA (also called Experience sampling method, e.g., Csikszentmihalyi and Larson, 2014) was originally developed for the collection of self-reports of behavior, cognition or emotions in the daily lives of the participants. In the context of tinnitus, we extend this framework to also collect self-reports about the perception of the phantom tinnitus sound and objective measurements of contextual variables (here: sound pressure of the environmental sounds to discover tinnitus masking). The EMA method offers several benefits for the assessment of tinnitus.

First, the EMA approach minimizes the retrospective bias. Several studies from multiple disciplines have demonstrated that multiple biases may jeopardize the retrospective data collection, e.g., in pain reports (Erskine et al., 1990) or for coping strategies (Todd et al., 2004). The retrospective recall is based on a process of mental reconstruction rather than a correct retrieval whereby the current circumstances and the peak of symptoms are emphasized (for a review see e.g., Fredrickson, 2000 on this peak-and-end rule). EMA approaches with momentary assessments of the tinnitus symptoms allow the measurements with exact time stamps in real life and should thereby be well suited for minimizing this retrospective bias.

Second, longitudinal assessment can reveal dynamic processes and temporal relationships. Even though it has been shown that tinnitus symptoms fluctuate from one moment to the other (Henry et al., 2012; Wilson et al., 2015), many questions about this dynamic process are still open: how much varies the extent of fluctuations from one person to the other? How strong are the fluctuations within and between days? Is there a temporal pattern (e.g., tinnitus symptoms are higher/lower in the morning compared to the evening)? Is there a temporal relationship with other factors like stress, emotion, concentration, sleep etc. which can suggest a causal relationship (e.g., emotional arousal increases lead to an increase of tinnitus or vice versa)? Are there context-specific factors for tinnitus improvement or worsening? All these questions can be systematically addressed by the EMA approach at the level of individual subjects (for a review see e.g., Wichers, 2013 about EMA assessment in mental disorders). With this manuscript, we want to introduce the technical platform of the TrackYourTinnitus (TYT) app that will be able to answer a large number of these questions. Some work using TYT has already been published investigating the relationships between tinnitus and emotional states (Probst et al., 2016a) as well as between tinnitus and emotion dynamics (Probst et al., 2016b). Further analyses are currently under preparation.

Third, assessment in real-life situations is characterized by large ecological validity. There are multiple examples in clinical research where a large discrepancy can be observed between the measurements in the clinic (or laboratory) and the measurements in everyday life. For instance, blood pressure readings made by a physician in the clinical context are often higher than the ambulatory blood pressure recordings done outside the clinic—typically described as the "white coat effect" (Hansen et al., 2006). On the other side, measurements of clinical symptoms outside the clinical or laboratory settings are hampered by low controllability, which can lead to noisy signals. An adequate item selection (items should measure the respective moment, should be short and can be answered in a view seconds) with respect to the research question is a key element for using the EMA approach. We consider both types of measurements, in the clinical/laboratory context and in real life, as important for both comprehensive diagnostic assessment and evaluation of treatment effects. While there is already a rich collection of tinnitus research tools than can be used in the laboratory or clinical context, the research tools for assessing tinnitus in real life are still limited and shall be improved by the EMA approach presented here.

Fourth, the technical integration of additional sensor data allows the objective measurement of contextual and biological variables. With the current development, we are using the microphone of the smart phone to measure the environmental sound pressure level for assessing the effect of external sounds on perceived tinnitus loudness and distress. This goes beyond earlier developments where this integration was not possible (Henry et al., 2012; Wilson et al., 2015). In this manuscript we only want to mention this option of the technical platform. Detailed analyses will be reported elsewhere and will also take into account the variance of these measures in the different types of smartphones. Further implementation in the future might also integrate biosensors for objective assessment of biological parameters (e.g., heart rate).

Fifth, the TYT is a non-commercial product and is available all over the world for no costs and without advertisements. To ensure the longitudinal assessment, the technical framework is constantly maintained and updated by the team. Furthermore, the technical implementation allows offline use to ensure that permits the use even in areas without internet connection.

MATERIALS AND METHODS

"TYT"[1] was implemented as a technical realization of the envisaged EMA approach. The TYT platform will be outlined below. A detailed description of the technical aspects is published elsewhere (Pryss et al., 2015a,b; Schickler et al., 2015).

Recruitment

TYT is an open-access platform at no costs for the users. Upon registration, the users have to agree with the terms of the smartphone app use, which includes that the anonymized data can be used for scientific purposes. The analysis of anonymized data from the smart phone app has been approved by the Ethics Committee of the University Clinic of Regensburg. Before the start of the study, all volunteers agreed with informed consent and no vulnerable populations were involved. To recruit the patients, the TYT app was advertised at the webpages and Facebook pages of the Tinnitus Research Initiative, the TINNET COST Action and the webpage of the participating research groups.

Data Collection

There are three types of data collected by the TYT platform:

1. The "registration questionnaires" consists of three questionnaires that were completed by the app-user upon registration. The registration questionnaires include the Tinnitus Sample Case History Questionnaire (TSCHQ, Langguth et al., 2007), the short Version of the Tinnitus Questionnaire (miniTQ, Hiller and Goebel, 2004) and a short questionnaire asking for the individually most disturbing tinnitus related aspect.
2. The "state questionnaire" is designed to assess tinnitus and situation-specific variables with eight short questions during everyday life. The state questionnaires constitute the main part of this EMA study. The smartphone app will notify the user at several time points during the day to fill out the state questionnaire. The state questionnaires are delivered randomly within a time frame that can be set by the user (see the "Technical Realization" Section for more details). We decided to give the user more freedom for this setting in order to enhance the usability of the app and allow adaptation to the individual needs. This, however, also enhances the variability in the number of sampling points and the time lag between them. The selection of data analysis methods need to take this into account.

   The state questionnaire consists of eight questions. With the first question we ask the patient if she/he perceives the tinnitus at this moment (answer with yes or no). The second and third question ask about the loudness of the tinnitus and how stressful the tinnitus is. The patients can give their answers on a VAS by moving a slider between the endpoints. Technically, the VAS was implemented as a slider without pre-set values to avoid anchoring affects (Tversky and Kahneman, 1974). The endpoints are "not audible" (question 2) or "not stressful" (question 3) on the left side and "maximal loudness" (question 2) or "maximal stressful" (question 3). The questions 4 and 5 ask for the emotional valence and arousal respectively, using the self-assessment manikins (SAM) developed by Bradley and Lang (1994). Question 6 asks if the person feels currently stressed on a VAS (endpoints "not stressed" and "maximal stressed"). Question 7 asks how much the user concentrated on the task that she/he was doing at the moment (VAS with the endpoints "not at all" and "fully concentrated"). Question 8 asked if the user was irritated at this moment (answer with yes/no).

[1] www.trackyourtinnitus.org

The state questionnaire was implemented to allow fast answering by the user. Typically, it takes less than a minute to complete the state questionnaire.

3. The sound pressure of environmental sounds was measured using the built-in microphone of the smartphone while the user was answering the state questionnaire. The microphone recordings were set to record with a resolution of 16 bit for both, the Android and the iOS devices. While inter-subject comparison of the sound pressure measures is limited because of the different smartphone manufacturers, an intra-subject comparison between different moments will be possible. The sound pressure measurements are not reported in this manuscript and is subject to further analyses.

Technical Realization

The Front-End (**Figure 1**) of the TYT includes two smart phone applications for iOS (implemented using Objective C) and Android devices (implemented using Java), and the www.trackyourtinnitus.org website (implemented using the Open-Source PHP-Framework LARAVEL: Code Bright, Otwell, 2016) for the registration and display of the results. Both smart phone apps are freely available for English and German speaking users in the respective app stores. The Back-End consists of a MySQL database running on a Linux Server for the storage of the collected data from all mobile devices. The data on the smart phone devices are stored in the internal SQLite database of the mobile device. If the user is online while he is answering the state questionnaire, the answers between the mobile device and the server will be synchronized immediately. If the user is offline, this synchronization process will be triggered the next time the user is online. In all cases, only anonymized data is transferred and the data transfer is encrypted using the secure sockets layer (SSL) technology. The user has the option to review his own data within the app or download the dataset using the web interface. The anonymized data of all users are stored in a central database maintained by the University of Ulm for research purposes. The user can select between two settings for the state questionnaires: in the "standard settings", the user receives the state questionnaires at random time points between 8 a.m. and 10 p.m. (can be adjusted) following a randomization algorithm described by Pryss et al. (2015b). A maximum number of 12 state questionnaires per day is allowed by system. In the "custom" settings, the user can define an own schedule with time points where she/he wants to receive the state questionnaire. The TYT platform was developed by the authors of the manuscript (RCP, AB, JS, MR) with additional support by several programmers from the University of Ulm (see "Acknowledgments" Section, Jochen Herrmann, Robin Kraft, Robin Zöller, Aliyar Aras, Marc Schickler). The TYT platform is developed for users with chronic tinnitus. No prior knowledge of EMA is required to use the app.

Data Management

High emphasis is placed on data management of the TYT platform. Given the automated procedures, the data collection is highly standardized for all participants. Data entry masks are designed carefully to only allow the entry of meaningful data and minimize the risk of wrong entries (e.g., defined value ranges). The data collection of TYT is continuously ongoing. Therefore, strict rules for data analysis were defined in order to reduce reporting biases: at fixed time points during the year, the database is frozen. Data analysis will always be done using the most recent database freeze. The data reported in this article contains the data collected between April 2014 (start of the TYT platform) and February 2016. Further analysis on the dataset have been published elsewhere (Probst et al., 2016a,b) and additional analyses will be performed in the future. This will also include time-series analyses to explore temporal relationships between the tinnitus loudness or distress and the emotional state or the perceived stress level.

Data Analysis

The influence of the duration of app-use on the perceived tinnitus loudness and distress was tested by means of regression

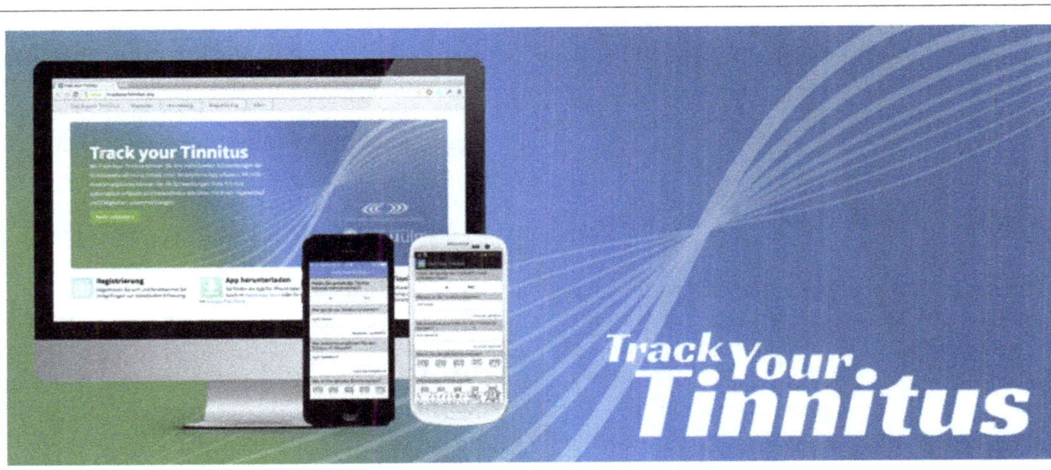

FIGURE 1 | Frontend of the TrackYourTinnitus (TYT) framework including the website and the smart phone applications for iOS and Android.

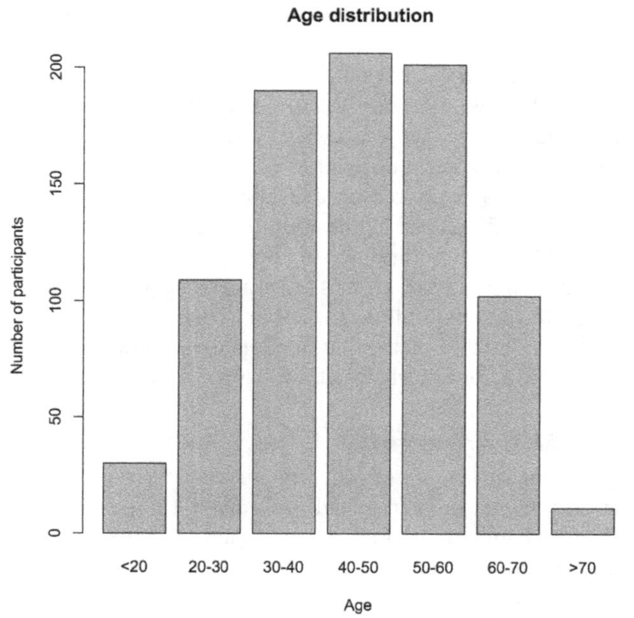

FIGURE 2 | Age distribution of the participants.

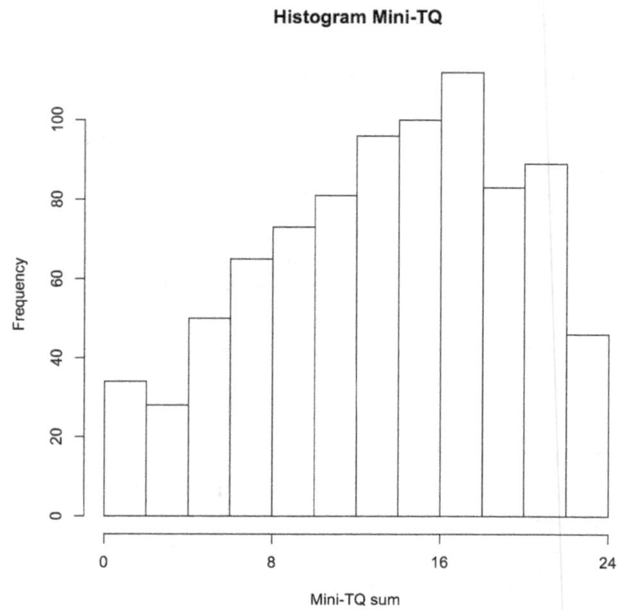

FIGURE 3 | Histogram of the Mini-Tinnitus Questionnaire (Mini-TQ) sum scores of the participants. During the registration process, the participants are required to fill out the Mini-TQ. The Mini-TQ measures the strength of the tinnitus distress on a scale from 0 to 24.

analysis. Statistical analysis was done using the statistical software package R[2].

RESULTS

Study Sample

A number of 857 volunteers (26.9% female, 73.1% male) participated in the data collection between the launch of the app in April 2014 and February 2016. To recruit the patients, the TYT app was advertised at the webpages and Facebook pages of the Tinnitus Research Initiative, the TINNET COST Action and the webpage of the participating research groups. The average age of the participants was 44.1 years (standard deviation: 14.1 years, **Figure 2**). Upon registration, the participants completed the Mini-Tinnitus Questionnaire (Mini-TQ) for the assessment of tinnitus-related distress. The average sum score over all participants was 13.9 points (SD 6.0, **Figure 3**, maximum score of the Mini-TQ is 24 points).

Influence of Study Participation on Tinnitus Symptoms

An important question is whether the continuous participation in the study, with repeated measurements of tinnitus-related symptoms, leads to a worsening or improvement of tinnitus symptoms. To analyze this question, we selected a subgroup of subjects that have used the app regularly for at least a month. Linear regression analysis was calculated for these users (n = 66) in this timeframe to test the influence of the study duration on the tinnitus loudness.

The duration of app-use measured in days was used as a regressor in this model, the tinnitus loudness as regressand (tinnitus loudness $\sim$ app-use duration). Duration of app-use did not predict tinnitus loudness, $\beta < 0.001$, $t_{(6291)} = 1.26$, $p = 0.21$. Furthermore, the duration of the app-use did not explain the variance of the tinnitus loudness significantly, R-squared <0.001, $F_{(1,6291)} = 1.58$, $p = 0.21$. Similarly, we investigated the influence of the duration of app-use on tinnitus distress (tinnitus distress $\sim$ app-use duration). The duration of app-use did not predict tinnitus distress, $\beta < 0.001$, $t_{(6264)} = 1.3$, $p = 0.19$. Also, the duration of the app-use did not explain the variance of the tinnitus distress significantly, R-squared <0.001, $F_{(1,6264)} = 1.7$, $p = 0.19$. Additionally, we calculated a paired t-test comparing the mean of the first 5 sampling state questionnaires against the mean of the last 5 state questionnaires for each user. Again, there was no significant influence of time neither on tinnitus loudness ($t_{(61)} = 1.25$, $p > 0.2$) nor on tinnitus distress ($t_{(61)} = 0.38$, $p > 0.7$), indicating, that app-use did not have a negative impact on the users' tinnitus.

The same type of paired t-test was repeated for the subjects, which used the app for less than 1 month. We selected all users with more than 5 days of app-use and less than 30 days of use. Also for this group of users, there was no significant influence of time neither on tinnitus loudness ($t_{(133)} = 0.53$, $p > 0.5$) nor on tinnitus distress ($t_{(129)} = 0.79$, $p > 0.4$).

To give an impression of the fluctuation of tinnitus loudness and tinnitus distress over time, a random selection of three participants is illustrated in **Figure 4**.

[2]www.r-project.org, version 3.3.1.

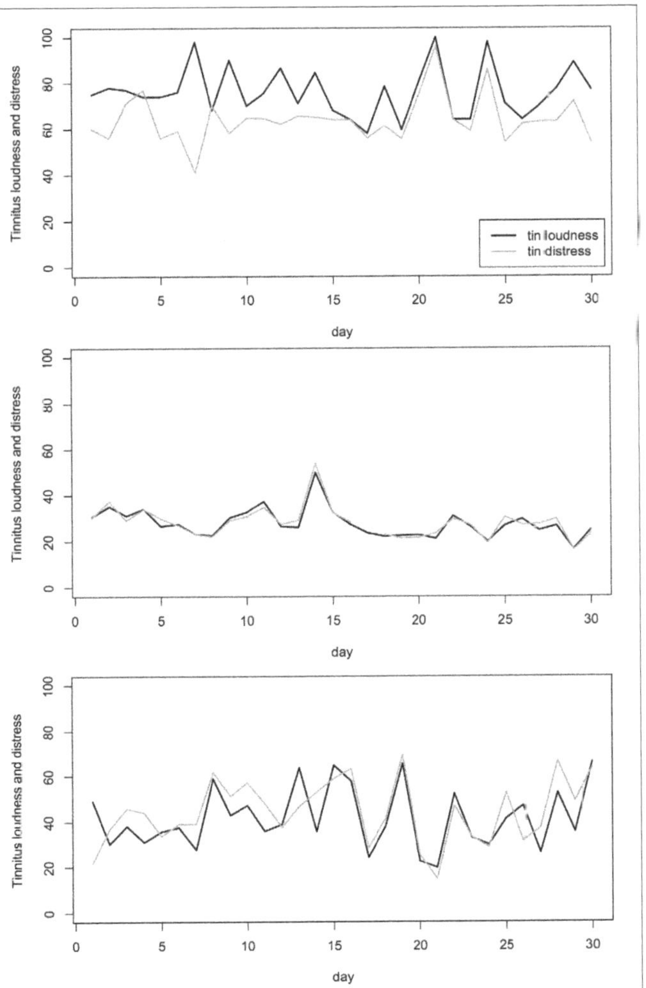

FIGURE 4 | Example of three individual tinnitus patients. Measurements of the tinnitus loudness (black) and tinnitus distress (gray) on 30 consecutive days are shown for the three individuals. The tinnitus loudness and tinnitus distress were both measured on a visual analog scale (VAS) and converted to numerical values in the range of 0 ("not audible"/"not stressful") to 100 ("maximal loudness"/"maximal stressful").

DISCUSSION

We have introduced the TYT app as a new platform that allows the assessment of tinnitus-related symptoms during the everyday life of people with tinnitus. The app is available in the two major app stores for Android and iOS devices. Between April 2014 and February 2016, the app was used by 857 people with tinnitus, with the majority of users between 30 and 60 years old. The amount of tinnitus-related distress as measured with the Mini-TQ covered the full range of the measurement spectrum showing that the app was used by people with various levels of tinnitus distress. However, further studies will need to clarify, whether the population using the app is representative to the general tinnitus population. The recruitment of patients via the internet and the app stores introduces a new way in patient recruitment compared to earlier studies. It is therefore important to mention that our results are in line with the previous studies on mobile assessment of tinnitus (Henry et al., 2012; Wilson et al., 2015). The large amount of sampled data allows the analysis of more specific research questions about tinnitus which are reported elsewhere (Probst et al., 2016a,b).

From a clinical point of view, there could be the concern that the tinnitus increases by the repeated assessment (and therefore a reminder) of the tinnitus perception. It is notable here that the tinnitus perception did not change as a result of repeated sampling, neither tinnitus loudness nor tinnitus distress. This is in line with the study by Henry et al. (2012) in which it was shown that tinnitus did not change during a 2 week assessment period with four measurements each day. Furthermore, we also analyzed the data of users with only a short duration of app-use. In principle it would be possible that users where the app-use has a negative impact on their tinnitus stop using the app, while the users without negative impact use the app for a longer time. This is clearly not the case since the paired *t*-tests on the subgroup of subjects with short app-use duration did not reveal a significant difference between the first and the last state measurements either. These findings further support the notion that assessment of tinnitus symptoms during everyday life is a safe method that is not increasing neither tinnitus loudness nor tinnitus distress.

The aim of the TYT platform is: (1) to enable real-time assessment of tinnitus variations and reduce the effect of recall bias; (2) to investigate the factors influencing the increase and decrease of tinnitus symptoms at the individual subject level; (3) to enable the longitudinal assessment of tinnitus symptoms and their dynamic processes; (4) to introduce tinnitus measurements with higher ecological validity in real-life conditions as opposed to tinnitus measurements in the lab or the clinic, and therefore establish ecological momentary assessment (EMA) methods for tinnitus research; and (5) to implement and validate tinnitus assessment with smart phones as a cost-effective assessment tool that can be applied for large populations.

Future technical implementation will also enable monitoring of clinical treatments. The effects of clinical treatments are currently typically assessed by weekly or monthly questionnaires and can therefore hardly be used to investigate dynamic changes during the treatment phase. Although EMA has been used in other domains to monitor treatment progress, e.g., for antidepressant treatment (Barge-Schaapveld and Nicolson, 2002), it has not been used for the assessment of tinnitus treatments yet. Another benefit of EMA was revealed by the study of Barge-Schaapveld and Nicolson (2002), which demonstrated an increased reporting of side-effects. The side effect of increased dizziness was reported by 35 patients using EMA while only seven patients reported increased dizziness to their general practitioner (Barge-Schaapveld and Nicolson, 2002). This suggests that the recall bias of retrospective assessment not only influences the measurement of treatment related symptom reduction but also the reporting of treatment-related side effects. Additionally, frequent assessment of treatment effects with smart phones could help to learn more about reasons for study drop out by providing more precise data of what has happened immediately before drop out.

However, beside all the excitement about the new opportunities and advantages of EMA, we also want to mention the drawbacks of this method, which mainly arise from the low controllability of our sampling method. Since the assessment with smart phones is not completed under the supervision of clinical staff, the correct usage of the device as well as the identity of the user cannot be guaranteed. Also, there is little control over the situation and circumstances of the app usage, which on one side enhances the ecological validity of the measurement, but on the other side reduces its controllability. It is, therefore, important to mention that EMA should not be considered as a substitute for standard questionnaires used in the clinical routine, but rather be seen as a complementary method with additional value for both clinical practice and for basic as well as clinical research. We are looking forward to a new wave of studies using EMA for its various applications in tinnitus research.

AUTHOR CONTRIBUTIONS

WS: substantial contribution to the design of the study, data analysis, conception and implementation of the TrackYourTinnitus app, drafted and revised the manuscript. RCP: substantial contribution to the design of the study, data analysis, conception, implementation and maintenance of the TrackYourTinnitus app, drafted and revised the manuscript. TP and BL: substantial contribution to the design of the study and data analysis, drafted and revised the manuscript. JS, AB and MR: substantial contribution to the conception, implementation and maintenance of the TrackYourTinnitus app.

ACKNOWLEDGMENTS

We are very thankful for the continuous and reliable support of additional programmers from the University of Ulm that helped to implement and maintain the TrackYourTinnitus app: Jochen Herrmann, Robin Kraft, Robin Zöller, Aliyar Aras, Marc Schickler.

REFERENCES

Adamchic, I., Langguth, B., Hauptmann, C., and Tass, P. A. (2012). Psychometric evaluation of visual analog scale for the assessment of chronic tinnitus. *Am. J. Audiol.* 21, 215–225. doi: 10.1044/1059-0889(2012/12-0010)

Baguley, D., McFerran, D., and Hall, D. (2013). Tinnitus. *Lancet* 382, 1600–1607. doi: 10.1016/S0140-6736(13)60142-7

Barge-Schaapveld, D. Q. C. M., and Nicolson, N. A. (2002). Effects of antidepressant treatment on the quality of daily life: an experience sampling study. *J. Clin. Psychiatry* 63, 477–485. doi: 10.4088/jcp.v63n0603

Bradley, M. M., and Lang, P. J. (1994). Measuring emotion: the self-assessment manikin and the semantic differential. *J. Behav. Ther. Exp. Psychiatry* 25, 49–59. doi: 10.1016/0005-7916(94)90063-9

Csikszentmihalyi, M., and Larson, R. (2014). "Validity and reliability of the experience-sampling method", in *Flow and the Foundations of Positive Psychology*, ed. M. Csikszentmihalyi (Berlin: Springer Netherlands), 35–54.

Davis, A., and Rafaie, E. A. (2000). "Epidemiology of tinnitus," in *Tinnitus Handbook*, ed. R. S. Tyler (San Diego, CA: Singular), 1–24.

Dobie, R. A. (2003). Depression and tinnitus. *Otolaryngol. Clin. North Am.* 36, 383–388. doi: 10.1016/s0030-6665(02)00168-8

Elgoyhen, A. B., Langguth, B., De Ridder, D., and Vanneste, S. (2015). Tinnitus: perspectives from human neuroimaging. *Nat. Rev. Neurosci.* 16, 632–642. doi: 10.1038/nrn4003

Erskine, A., Morley, S., and Pearce, S. (1990). Memory for pain: a review. *Pain* 41, 255–265. doi: 10.1016/0304-3959(90)90002-u

Fredrickson, B. L. (2000). Extracting meaning from past affective experiences: the importance of peaks, ends, and specific emotions. *Cogn. Emot.* 14, 577–606. doi: 10.1080/026999300402808

Gallus, S., Lugo, A., Garavello, W., Bosetti, C., Santoro, E., Colombo, P., et al. (2015). Prevalence and determinants of tinnitus in the italian adult population. *Neuroepidemiology* 45, 12–19. doi: 10.1159/000431376

Hansen, T., Jeppesen, J., Rasmussen, S., Ibsen, H., and Torp-Pederson, C. (2006). Ambulatory blood pressure monitoring and risk of cardiovascular disease: a population based study. *Am. J. Hypertens.* 19, 243–250. doi: 10.1016/j.amjhyper.2005.09.018

Hasson, D., Theorell, T., Westerlund, H., and Canlon, B. (2010). Prevalence and characteristics of hearing problems in a working and non-working Swedish population. *J. Epidemiol. Community Health* 64, 453–460. doi: 10.1136/jech.2009.095430

Heller, A. J. (2003). Classification and epidemiology of tinnitus. *Otolaryngol. Clin. North Am.* 36, 239–248. doi: 10.1016/s0030-6665(02)00160-3

Henry, J. A., Galvez, G., Turbin, M. B., Thielman, E. J., McMillan, G. P., and Istvan, J. A. (2012). Pilot study to evaluate ecological momentary assessment of tinnitus. *Ear Hear.* 33, 179–290. doi: 10.1097/AUD.0b013e31822f6740

Hiller, W., and Goebel, G. (2004). Rapid assessment of tinnitus-related psychological distress using the Mini-TQ. *Int. J. Audiol.* 43, 600–604.

Kreuzer, P. M., Vielsmeier, V., and Langguth, B. (2013). Chronic tinnitus: an interdisciplinary challenge. *Dtsch. Arztebl. Int.* 110, 278–284. doi: 10.3238/arztebl.2013.0278

Langguth, B., and Elgoyhen, A. B. (2012). Current pharmacological treatments for tinnitus. *Expert Opin. Pharmacother.* 13, 2495–2509. doi: 10.1517/14656566.2012.739608

Langguth, B., Goodey, R., Azevedo, A., Bjorne, A., Cacace, A., Crocetti, A., et al. (2007). Consensus for tinnitus patient assessment and treatment outcome measurement: tinnitus research initiative meeting, regensburg, July 2006. *Prog. Brain. Res.* 166, 525–536. doi: 10.1016/S0079-6123(07)66050-6

Newman, C. W., Jacobson, G. P., and Spitzer, J. B. (1996). Development of the tinnitus handicap inventory. *Arch. Otolaryngol. Head Neck Surg.* 122, 143–148. doi: 10.1001/archotol.1996.01890140029007

Otwell, T. (2016). Laravel - The PHP Framework for Web Artisans. Laravel.com. Last accessed 30 November 2016. Available online at: http://www.laravel.com

Probst, T., Pryss, R., Langguth, B., and Schlee, W. (2016a). Emotion dynamics and tinnitus: daily life data from the "TrackYourTinnitus" application. *Sci. Rep.* 6:31166. doi: 10.1038/srep31166

Probst, T., Pryss, R., Langguth, B., and Schlee, W. (2016b). Emotional states as mediators between tinnitus loudness and tinnitus distress in daily life: Results from the "TrackYourTinnitus" application. *Sci. Rep.* 6:20382. doi: 10.1038/srep20382

Pryss, R., Reichert, M., Herrmann, J., and Langguth, B. (2015a). "Mobile crowd sensing in clinical and psychological trials–A case study," in *28th IEEE International Symposium on Computer-Based Medical Systems* (Sao Carlos, Brazil).

Pryss, R., Reichert, M., Langguth, B., and Schlee, W. (2015b). "Mobile crowd sensing services for tinnitus assessment, therapy and research," in *IEEE 4th International Conference on Mobile Services (MS)* (New York, NY).

Schickler, M., Reichert, M., Pryss, R., Schobel, J. Schlee, W., and Langguth, B. (2015). *Entwicklung Mobiler Apps: Konzepte, Anwendungsbausteine und Werkzeuge im Business und E-Health.* Berlin: Springer Vieweg.

Stone, A. A., and Shiffman, S. (1994). Ecological momentary assessment (EMA) in behavorial medicine. *Ann. Behav. Med.* 16, 199–202.

Todd, M., Tennen, H., Carney, M. A., Armeli, S., and Affleck, G. (2004). Do we know how we cope? Relating daily coping reports to global and time-limited retrospective assessments. *J. Pers. Soc. Psychol.* 86, 310–319. doi: 10.1037/0022-3514.86.2.310

Tversky, A., and Kahneman, D. (1974). Judgement under uncertainty: heuristics and biaises. *Sciences* 185, 1124–1131. doi: 10.126/science.185

Wichers, M. (2013). The dynamic nature of depression: a new micro-level perspective of mental disorder that meets current challenges. *Psychol. Med.* 44, 1349–1360. doi: 10.1017/S0033291713001979

Wilson, M. B., Kallogjeri, D., Joplin, C. N., Gorman, M. D., Krings, J. G., Lenze, E. J., et al. (2015). Ecological momentary assessment of tinnitus using smartphone technology: a pilot study. *Otolaryngol. Head Neck Surg.* 152, 897–903. doi: 10.1177/0194599815569692

16

Evaluation of the Acoustic Coordinated Reset (CR®) Neuromodulation Therapy for Tinnitus: Update on Findings and Conclusions

Markus Haller[1] and Deborah A. Hall[2, 3]*

[1] Desyncra Technologies Limited, London, United Kingdom, [2] National Institute for Health Research Nottingham Biomedical Research Centre, Nottingham, United Kingdom, [3] Otology and Hearing Group, Division of Clinical Neuroscience, School of Medicine, University of Nottingham, Nottingham, United Kingdom

Keywords: coordinated reset, neuromodulation, RESET2, clinical trial, tinnitus

***Correspondence:**
Markus Haller
markus.haller@desyncra.com

BACKGROUND

The therapeutic effects of Coordinated Reset (CR®) Neuromodulation were originally discovered by researchers at the Forschungzentrum Juelich GmbH (FZJ) in Germany, under the supervision of Tass et al. (2012a).

Based on confirmatory research in primates, initial results of Prof. Tass' research suggested that the plastic modification of the behavior of neuron populations by induced desynchronization (i.e., a process of "unlearning" of both pathological neuronal synchrony and pathological synaptic connectivity) results in a substantial and long-lasting reduction of disease symptoms (Tass et al., 2012b; Adamchic et al., 2014a).

In this set of experiments, Parkinson's-induced monkey models were treated in independent laboratories with Coordinated Reset (CR®) Neuromodulation through the well-established deep brain stimulation (DBS) technique. Standard high frequency DBS was used as a control condition. The stimulation lasted 2 h a day for 5 consecutive days. In both experiments the primates remained symptom-free for over 30 days after CR stimulation was ceased (Tass et al., 2012b; Wang et al., 2016).

Subsequent trials in human patients showed alleviation of Parkinson's symptoms such as tremor, akinesia, dystonia, etc., for many hours after only short periods of CR® Neuromodulation (4 h for 3 consecutive days) (Adamchic et al., 2014a).

These results led to an expansion and further development of the CR® Neuromodulation program in different research centers worldwide. Additional focus was given to the application of CR® via other sensory inputs, e.g., acoustic, tactile, visual, etc. That eventually led to the development of a treatment program for tinnitus.

There is a general consensus that the percept of tinnitus is triggered by cochlear damage, which degrades the auditory input to central neural pathways. This initiates physiological and electrical changes within the auditory areas that result in aberrant patterns of neuronal activity interpreted as sound.

Acoustic CR® Neuromodulation is designed as a patient specific targeted sound therapy. The treatment has been provided to over 3,000 patients worldwide to date. Several peer-reviewed papers have reported reduction of tinnitus symptoms (from baseline) in populations of tinnitus sufferers by using a portable acoustic neurostimulator providing Acoustic CR® Neuromodulation; including tinnitus loudness measured using a visual analog scale (Tass et al., 2012a; Williams et al., 2015), tinnitus annoyance measured using a visual analog scale (Tass et al., 2012a; Bencsik et al., 2015; Williams et al., 2015), and various multi-attribute scales used to measure tinnitus symptom severity, i.e., Tinnitus Questionnaire (Tass et al., 2012a), Tinnitus Handicap Questionnaire (Williams et al., 2015), and Tinnitus Handicap Inventory (Bencsik et al., 2015; Hauptmann et al., 2015).

Both accurate tone "location" of the tinnitus percept on the auditory cortex, as well as the timing and sequence of the tone based impulses have been reported to be important factors in effective inducement of neuronal desynchronization. In the studies referred to above, such neural desynchronization led to a reduction of tinnitus symptoms. Because accurate tone location in the auditory cortex was found to be important, a proprietary tinnitus pitch matching procedure was developed and deployed in order to calibrate the patient specific sound therapy tones.

Because tinnitus is a highly subjective pathology, it has been proven to be difficult to assess with objective and standardized tests. In these circumstances, any placebo effects can have a great impact on treatment of tinnitus, as well as its personal percept.

In October 2011, Nottingham University Hospitals NHS Trust agreed to conduct an investigator-led evaluation of acoustic CR neuromodulation versus placebo effects, recruiting 100 participants with a 1:1 allocation ratio (Hoare et al., 2013) (ClinicalTrials.gov NCT01541969). Participants were adults aged ≥18 years of age, chronic subjective tinnitus for more than 3months with a minimum score of 18 points measured using the Tinnitus Handicap Inventory and a dominant tinnitus pitch corresponding to a frequency between 0.2 and 10 kHz, and with an average hearing loss no greater than 60 dB (0.5, 1, 2, and 4 kHz).

MAIN TRIAL RESULTS AND POTENTIAL EXPLANATION OF THE OBSERVATIONS

The formal results of the RESET2 trial (ClinicalTrials.gov identifier: NCT01541969) were non-conclusive, which was not expected, considering the past and current volumes of observational data showing substantial benefit (Hoare et al., 2013).

In Tass et al. (2012a) and in a number of later publications (Hauptmann et al., 2015; Williams et al., 2015) statistically and clinically significant improvements have been reported in visual analog scales, in tinnitus loudness and annoyance scores (reduction of 53 and 49% after 12 weeks of therapy, respectively, on stimulation), and in tinnitus questionnaire results (reduction of 29% after 12 weeks of therapy) results (Adamchic et al., 2012b, 2014b; Tass et al., 2012a). Furthermore, the measured tinnitus pitch was reduced by 28.5% in the first 12 weeks of treatment (Tass et al., 2012a), and the observed tinnitus pitch change was correlated with a treatment-induced reduction of tinnitus loudness and/or annoyance and changes in oscillatory brain activity (Adamchic et al., 2012a; Tass et al., 2012a). The EEG results indicated a substantial, CR-induced reduction of tinnitus-related auditory binding in a pitch-processing network associated with the therapeutic procedure, where a readjustment of stimulation parameters was performed at each visit, provided the matched tinnitus frequency had changed (Adamchic et al., 2012a).

Whilst the RESET2 trial at NHS did not observe a significant difference between treatment and placebo in experimental conditions, all the more recent above mentioned clinical studies report significant improvements in patient populations.

Tinnitus questionnaires could have reduced responsiveness to treatment-related change when a large proportion of participants respond at baseline at either extreme of the response scale. The so-called "floor effects" (scores at the minimum of the response scale) reduce sensitivity to detecting group-level improvement, while "ceiling effects" (scores at the maximum of the response scale) reduce sensitivity to detecting group-level worsening (Terwee et al., 2007). In a more recent analysis of the baseline TFI (Tinnitus Functional Index; Meikle et al., 2012) data from RESET2, Fackrell et al. (2016) found over 50% of questionnaire items scored at either floor or ceiling. This evidence certainly warrants caution in future studies with similar use of these tinnitus assessment questionnaires.

The exact application as defined of the proprietary tinnitus pitch matching procedure is paramount in order to observe any beneficial effect. Sub-optimal pitch matching will potentially lead to incorrectly computed patient specific therapy tones, which may not have any more effect than a placebo. The study-specific pitch matching procedure used in RESET2 differed from manufacturer's recommendations (Hall et al., 2016).

Professor Tass' team has since validated and launched an automated adaptive pitch-matching method (Hauptmann et al., 2016) to prevent deviations from a recommended pitch-matching procedure, which has since been utilized in all commercial applications of Acoustic CR® as well as in current and future clinical trials. The authors concluded that this new procedure offers more guidance to the audiologist and patient which is seen as of particular importance for a uniform and standardized application of pitch-matching in clinical trials. Such standardization is expected to improve the quality of measures in tinnitus therapy effectiveness.

It is reasonable to question whether only 12-weeks of device usage is sufficient for the benefit of therapy to accrue. It is noted that more recent clinical studies report alleviation of tinnitus after 6 and 12 months of therapy (Hauptmann et al., 2015; Williams et al., 2015), and data on tinnitus status at 3-, 6- and 12-months post-fitting indicate a gradual decline in mean self-reported tinnitus severity measured using a shortened version of the Tinnitus Handicap Inventory (Hauptmann et al., 2015). The RESET2 trial design does not permit anything more than mere speculation, because all participants exited the RCT at 3 months and were unblinded to the intervention.

Abbreviations: CR®, coordinated reset; DBS, deep brain stimulation; TFI, Tinnitus Functional Index.

CONCLUSIONS

Recommendation

The authors therefore consider that controlled trials to test clinical effectiveness of Acoustic CR Neuromodulation for tinnitus are worthwhile. With the knowledge gained from the RESET2 trial, it is suggested that future trials should include a placebo or "usual standard of care" control group that is well characterized, should follow a well-defined and trained pitch matching protocol, should assess the status of tinnitus for longer than 12 weeks (we suggest at least 6 months), should better control the baseline characteristics to avoid floor and ceiling effects and should use an outcome instrument with known measurement properties for the target population.

What Else Could Be Learned from the RESET2 Trial?

Among the many other aspects learned another key fact was demonstrated by the RESET2 results:

During the trial 50 patients received stimulation from tones delivered at frequencies very different from the tinnitus frequency perceived by the patient and were therefore independent of used pitch-matching procedure. These stimulating tones were intended to be placebo control tones, as the trial was designed to be a double blind trial. The frequency of these tones was very different from the frequency of the tones which would have been deployed had these patients been receiving Acoustic CR® Neuromodulation treatment. Only a small "placebo-" benefit, i.e., <7.5% of an improvement in THQ (Tinnitus Handicap Questionnaire) was observed in these patients receiving the placebo treatments.

ETHICS, CONSENT, AND PERMISSIONS

Permission to conduct the study was granted by the National Research Ethics Service (NRES) Committee, East Midlands–Nottingham 1, Nottingham, UK. Written informed consent was obtained from each participant in accordance with the permissions granted. For further details see Hoare et al. (2013).

AUTHOR CONTRIBUTIONS

Both authors read and approved the final manuscript. DH planned and conducted the trial. MH and DH performed analysis and discussed the results. Both authors drafted the manuscript and were involved in final editing.

ACKNOWLEDGMENTS

DH is funded by the National Institute for Health Research (NIHR) Biomedical Research Centre Program. The views expressed are those of the author and not necessarily those of the National Health Service (NHS), the NIHR, or the Department of Health (DH).

REFERENCES

Adamchic, I., Hauptmann, C., Barnikol, U. B., Pawelczyk, N., Popovych, O., Barnikol, T. T., et al. (2014a). Coordinated reset neuromodulation for Parkinson's disease: proof-of-concept study. *Mov. Disord.* 29, 1679–1684. doi: 10.1002/mds.25923

Adamchic, I., Hauptmann, C., and Tass, P. A. (2012a). Changes of oscillatory activity in pitch processing network and related tinnitus relief induced by acoustic CR neuromodulation. *Front. Sys. Neurosci.* 6:18. doi: 10.3389/fnsys.2012.00018

Adamchic, I., Langguth, B., Hauptmann, C., and Tass, P. A. (2014b). Abnormal cross-frequency coupling in the tinnitus network. *Front. Neurosci.* 8:284. doi: 10.3389/fnins.2014.00284

Adamchic, I., Tass, P. A., Langguth, B., Hauptmann, C., Koller, M., Schecklmann, M., et al. (2012b). Linking the tinnitus questionnaire and the subjective clinical global impression: which differences are clinically important? *Health Qual. Life Outcomes.* 10:79. doi: 10.1186/1477-7525-10-79

Bencsik, B., Gáborján, A., Harnos, A., László, K., Végso, P., and Tamás, L. (2015). Acoustic CR®-Neuromodulation-First experiences in Hungary with a novel method in the therapy of chronic subjective tinnitus. *Ideggyogy. Sz.* 68, 189–198. doi: 10.18071/isz.68.0189

Fackrell, K., Hall, D. A., Barry, J. G., and Hoare, D. J. (2016). Psychometric properties of the Tinnitus Functional Index (TFI): assessment in a UK research volunteer population. *Hear. Res.* 335, 220–235. doi: 10.1016/j.heares.2015.09.009

Hall, D. A., Pierzycki, R. H., Thomas, H., and Hoare, D. J. (2016). Designing and conducting a double-blind randomized placebo-controlled trial of a novel sound therapy for tinnitus: a commentary on medical device trials in ENT and Audiology. *Ann. Oto Rhinol.* 3:1101. Available online at: www.jscimedcentral.com/Otolaryngology/otolaryngology-3-1101.pdf

Hauptmann, C., Ströbel, A., Williams, M., Patel, N., Wurzer, H., von Stackelberg, T., et al. (2015). Acoustic coordinated reset neuromodulation in a real life patient population with chronic tonal tinnitus. *Biomed Res. Int.* 2015:569052. doi: 10.1155/2015/569052

Hauptmann, C., Wegener, A., Poppe, H., Williams, M., Popelka, G., and Tass, P. A. (2016). Validation of a mobile device for Acoustic Coordinated Reset Neuromodulation tinnitus therapy. *J. Am. Acad. Audiol.* 27, 720–731. doi: 10.3766/jaaa.15082

Hoare, D. J., Pierzycki, R. H., Thomas, H., McAlpine, D., and Hall, D. A. (2013). Evaluation of the acoustic coordinated reset (CR®) neuromodulation therapy for tinnitus: study protocol for a double-blind randomized placebo-controlled trial. *Trials* 14:207. doi: 10.1186/1745-6215-14-207

Meikle, M. B., Henry, J. A., Griest, S. E., Stewart, B. J., Abrams, H. B., McArdle, R., et al. (2012). The tinnitus functional index: development of a new clinical measure for chronic, intrusive tinnitus. *Ear. Hear.* 33, 153–176. doi: 10.1097/AUD.0b013e31822f67c0

Tass, P. A., Adamchic, I., Freund, H. J., von Stackelberg, T., and Hauptmann, C. (2012a). Counteracting tinnitus by acoustic coordinated reset neuromodulation. *Restor. Neurol. Neurosci.* 30, 137–159. doi: 10.3233/RNN-2012-110218

Tass, P. A., Qin, L., Hauptmann, C., Dovero, S., Bezard, E., Boraud T., et al. (2012b). Coordinated reset has sustained aftereffects in Parkinsonian monkeys. *Ann Neurol.* 72, 816–820. doi: 10.1002/ana.23663

Terwee, C. B., Bot, S. D., de Boer, M. R., van der Windt, D. A., Knol, D. L., Dekker, J., et al. (2007). Quality criteria were proposed for measurement properties of health status questionnaires. *J. Clin. Epidemiol.* 60, 34–42. doi: 10.1016/j.jclinepi.2006.03.012

Wang, J., Nebeck, S., Muralidharan, A., Johnson, M. D., Vitek, J. L., and Baker, K. B. (2016). Coordinated Reset deep brain stimulation of subthalamic nucleus produces long-lasting, dose-dependent motor improvements in the 1-methyl-4-phenyl-1, 2, 3, 6-tetrahydropyridine non-human primate model of parkinsonism. *Brain Stimul.* 9, 609–617. doi: 10.1016/j.brs.2016.03.014

Williams, M., Hauptmann, C., and Patel, N. (2015). Acoustic CR neuromodulation therapy for subjective tonal tinnitus: a review of clinical outcomes in an independent audiology practice setting. *Front. Neurol.* 6:54 doi: 10.3389/fneur.2015.00054

17

Review of Smart Services for Tinnitus Self-Help, Diagnostics and Treatments

*Sven Kalle[1,2], Winfried Schlee[2], Rüdiger C. Pryss[3], Thomas Probst[4], Manfred Reichert[3], Berthold Langguth[2] and Myra Spiliopoulou[1]**

[1] Faculty of Computer Science, Otto-von-Guericke-University Magdeburg, Magdeburg, Germany, [2] Department of Psychiatry and Psychotherapy of Regensburg University, Regensburg, Germany, [3] Institute of Databases and Information Systems, Ulm University, Ulm, Germany, [4] Department for Psychotherapy and Biopsychosocial Health, Danube University Krems, Krems an der Donau, Austria

***Correspondence:**
Myra Spiliopoulou
myra@ovgu.de

In the recent years, there has been an increasing interest in the potential of internet- and smartphone-based technologies for the support of tinnitus patients. A broad spectrum of relevant approaches, some in the form of studies, others in the form of market products, have been mentioned in literature. They include auditory treatments, internet-based Cognitive Behavioral Therapy (iCBT), serious games, and questionnaires for tinnitus monitoring. The goal of this study is to highlight the role of existing internet-based and smart technologies for the advancement of tinnitus clinical practice: we consider contributions that refer to treatments and diagnostics, and we include contributions refering to self-help measures. We elaborate on the potential and challenges of such solutions and identify constraints associated to their deployment, such as the demand for familiarity with internet-based services and the need to re-design interactive services so that they fit on the small surface of a smartwatch.

Keywords: tinnitus treatment, tinnitus monitoring, smart technologies, internet-based treatments, iCBT, tinnitus masking, tinnitus, mobile crowd sensing

1. INTRODUCTION

Tinnitus is defined as the perception of a sound with a lack of an evident external stimulus to that sound. About 10–15% of the general population is affected by tinnitus, whereas for 1–2% the tinnitus is so severe that it directly affects their quality of life, according to Baguley et al. (2013). Modern technologies, including internet-based services and smart devices, are in principle appropriate for reaching and assisting those patients.

In this work, we survey internet- and smartphone-based solutions for tinnitus treatment as well as for everyday monitoring of tinnitus severity. Two earlier reviews have addressed the role of such technologies for tinnitus therapy, namely the works of Nyenhuis et al. (2013) and Greenwell et al. (2016a), which investigate the efficacy of self-help interventions. Since the technologies of relevance in the context of our study lend themselves to self-help measures, there is an overlap between our materials and theirs. As opposed to these reviews however, our aim is not to discern the efficacy of such solutions, but rather to assess the coverage of this technology in scientific literature with respect to treatments, diagnostics and self-help. The secondary aim reported by Greenwell et al. (2016a), namely "identifying what intervention techniques are used within the interventions" (page 83), relates more to our primary goal. However, our emphasis is not on "identify[ing] and describ[ing] the 'active ingredients' of the interventions" (page 83), but rather on identifying the types of treatment and the types of self-help being offered, the particular challenges that have been addressed in order to make such services as accessible and useful as possible, and the technical limitations that have not been solved yet.

The recent review of Lui et al. (2017) shows some similarities to our approach as well. Lui et al. (2017) study mobile applications for mental health, concentrating on evidence-based apps in the psychotherapeutic context and investigating their efficacy. Tinnitus is not among the conditions they investigate, albeit they discuss apps that support cognitive behavioral therapy (CBT), which belongs to the widespread tinnitus treatments. Accordingly, they do not address the issue of effectiveness of such treatments with respect to tinnitus nor the design of studies involving the use of smartphones and similar technologies among tinnitus patients, as we do here.

2. REVIEW DESIGN

2.1. Specific Aims of the Review

We investigate how internet-based and smart services are taken up clinically for tinnitus diagnostics and treatments, including self-help measures. We aim to identify key findings, key contributors and key challenges.

We solely include scientific articles that report on treatments, diagnostics and self-help for tinnitus, but no gray literature. In addition to the main review, we performed a market overview, on which we report in section 2.3.5. Note that in this market overview it has not been possible to distinguish between services intended exclusively for treatment and those concerning well-being in general.

Internet- or smartphone based treatments for tinnitus can be mainly differentiated into auditory and psychological treatments. *Auditory treatments* encompass (i) environmental sound generators, (ii) tinnitus maskers that generate low-level broad-band noise, (iii) hearing aids, and (iv) devices that combine some of the above, all aiming to reduce or mask the tinnitus percept. *Psychological treatments/interventions*, especially Cognitive Behavioral Therapy (CBT), are also investigated in our search, because earlier studies (e.g., by Martinez-Devesa et al., 2010; Cima et al., 2012) have shown significant effects of CBT on the quality of life and on the depression scores of tinnitus patients. Medications are not considered, since we expect that internet-based and smartphone technologies are used for tinnitus medications in the same way as for medications of other chronical diseases (like diabetes or hypertension), namely to acquire information about the medication, as well as its effects and side-effects, to set reminders about taking the medication and to monitor live signals.

Internet- and smartphone based Diagnostics encompass the use of questionnaires to collect patient assessments and further information, as well as crowdsensing with the help of hardware, e.g., for tinnitus matching. It should be stressed that diagnostics are often linked to treatments. Finally, *Self-help* refers to both helping the patients to cope with tinnitus as well as helping the patients in diagnostics, e.g., by tinnitus matching.

2.2. Approach for the Collection and Selection of Contributions

Our search approach encompasses a broad keyword-based search in Google Scholar using the top-20 results for each keyword, the identification of key authors, a targeted search in selected journals using keywords and key authors, a second search in Google Scholar following the same method as the first one, to update our document collections with more recent publications, and a search for mobile apps released for different smart phones

2.2.1. Broad Keyword-Based Search in Two Runs

We used Google Scholar to collect articles on the following keywords: "tinnitus smart," "tinnitus smart phone," "tinnitus smartphone," "tinnitus internet based," "tinnitus internet based cbt," "tinnitus icbt," "tinnitus sound therapy smart," "tinnitus mobile," "tinnitus online based," and "tinnitus internet acceptance" (excluding citations and patents). We performed one run on August 1, 2016, and a complementary one on June 11, 2017 to add more recent publications.

To decide which articles we should finally include, we first inspected title and abstract. During this inspection, we excluded articles that had reported on how the internet was used to recruit study participants as well as articles investigating the impact of internet usage (e.g., excessive usage) on the well being of patients. In some cases, it has become necessary to also inspect the contents of the articles themselves.

In the first run, out of the 45 articles that potentially seemed to be relevant, actually, 19 were considered as relevant and were thus included in our study.

The second run delivered 27 new articles that were possibly relevant to this work. Of these 27 articles, 11 were indeed relevant to this review. Moreover, there was another study not being traced by the described search procedure, but being added to the present review as the authors consider it as essential (Henry et al., 2012).

2.2.2. Targeted Search in Scopus and in PubMed Using Keywords

As next step, we performed a more targeted journal search in PubMed, focussing on medical advances, and in Scopus. The search on these platforms was performed on February 27, 2017. For both collections we used the same keywords as before, and we acquired 18, respectively 19 papers we marked as potentially relevant. After inspection and duplicate removal, 26 papers remained, of which 11 were considered to be relevant.

2.2.3. Search for Relevant Mobile Apps

We performed a manual search through the most popular stores for smartphone applications. Apps were searched in the browser version of Google's PlayStore, Apple's AppStore by using their software iTunes, and Microsoft's store included in the Windows 10 Mobile OS, using the keyword "tinnitus." The search run was performed on February 28, 2017. We then inspected the textual descriptions of the apps and removed those not related to tinnitus, e.g., wellness apps, as well as packages composed of multiple apps for different purposes. The results are discussed in section 2.3.5.

2.3. Overview of the Collected Contributions

We have organized the studies we found in the five areas described hereafter. Further, we have used the article collection to draw the co-authorship network depicted in **Figure 1**. The larger the node of an author, the more publications he or she has in the collection. Thick edges indicate authors that publish intensively together. Accordingly, the co-authorship network gives a fast overview of the author teams found in the specific field of this review.

2.3.1. Articles on Psychological Intervention Programs

Internet-based CBT (iCBT) is an approach that delivers Cognitive Behavioral Therapy via the internet. With 28 articles found, this method currently is the best documented and most researched treatment option when it comes to internet-based services. Of these, 15 articles providing an overview of the main findings are discussed in section 3.

Acceptance and Commitment Therapy (ACT) can be delivered in a self-help format via the internet as well (Westin

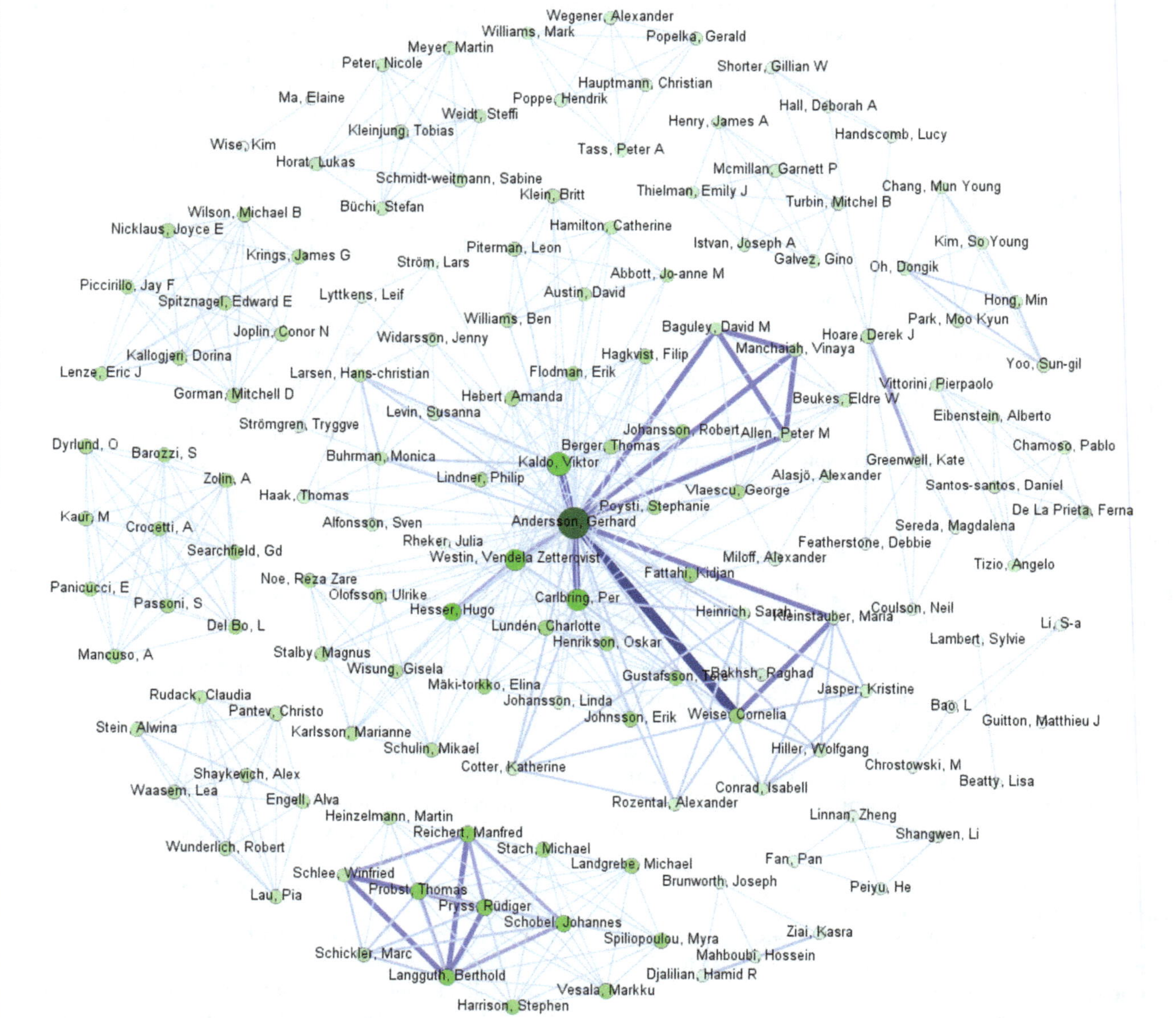

FIGURE 1 | Co-Authorship network: (i) Node size and node color intensity reflect the number of articles that this author wrote and were found relevant for our review; the larger and darker, the higher the number (e.g., Gerhard Andersson has the most works with 21, next is Viktor Kaldo with 7) (ii) Edge thickness and edge color intensity reflect the number of articles co-authored by the nodes linked through the edge; the thicker and darker, the higher the number (e.g., the thickest edge connects Gerhard Andersson and Cornelia Weise, who have co-authored 7 articles). We used the Sci2 Tool [https://sci2.cns.iu.edu/] to extract the network from the bibtex file containing all papers that were identified as relevant. After extracting the network, we used Gephi [https://gephi.org/] (which can be directly called through the Sci2 Tool), to draw the graph. After picking parameters for the colors and size of nodes and edges, we used the layout algorithm "Fruchterman Reingold," which is implemented in Gephi, for achieving a more visually appealing graph-layout.

et al., 2011). One article was found that examined and discussed this in the context of tinnitus treatment.

In another study (Hesser et al., 2012), internet-based ACT (iACT) was compared with iCBT and a moderated online discussion forum. The study revealed substantial improvements for both iCBT and iACT, with no significant difference between the two treatments.

2.3.2. Articles About the Tinnitus E-Programme

The Tinnitus E-Programme (TEP) is an internet-based intervention program that was developed in 2009 and evaluated using the Tinnitus Handicap Inventory (THI) (Newman et al., 1996). The program mainly consists of educational contents (i.e., about tinnitus or "the role of psychological mechanisms in tinnitus" (Greenwell et al., 2015), and relaxation- and attentional-focus exercises. The contents are provided as PDF sheets or mp3 audio files. All of the files are accessible for free on a website created for this intervention program [http://www.tinnituseprogramme.org/]. Two articles dealing with TEP were found: in Greenwell et al. (2015) the program is presented, while in Greenwell et al. (2016b) users' reactions and their daily use of relaxation techniques are reported.

2.3.3. Articles on Smartphone-Delivered Sound Therapy

With technological advances in the development of smartphones, sound therapy is an easily accessible treatment option. There are smartphone applications that claim to reduce tinnitus loudness by the usage of tailor-made notched music (e.g., Tinnitracks [www.tinnitracks.com] or Tinnitus Pro: Music Therapy [www.promedicalaudio.com]) or other forms of sound therapy (Linnan et al., 2015). Two studies provided the patients with tinnitus masking technologies: Yoo et al. (2015) and Mahboubi et al. (2012b).

Another usage of smartphones related to sound therapy are hearing aids that can be controlled via the smartphone via bluetooth. Further, they include volume-control functions as well as tinnitus maskers. An example of this usage is presented in Sauer et al. (2014). A study that further investigates this technology is provided by Barozzi et al. (2016).

2.3.4. Studies About Smartphone-Based Tinnitus Assessment

Diagnosis and assessment of tinnitus are important for a successful treatment. The articles of this category encompass: (1) internet-based hearing tests, namely Mahboubi et al. (2012a), Wunderlich et al. (2015), and Hauptmann et al. (2016), which investigate the potential of internet-based tests in comparison to tests run in the lab; (2) ecological momentary assessments, namely Henry et al. (2012); Pryss et al. (2015a), Schlee et al. (2016); Schickler et al. (2016a), and Wilson et al. (2015); (3) summarizations of the self-measures done by the patients, namely Peter et al. (2016), (4) serious games, namely in Schickler et al. (2016b), and Wise et al. (2015, 2016), (5) a comparison of online vs. paper-based collection of questionnaire data, namely Handscomb et al. (2016) and (6) a study on response times for a web-based emotional Stroop task for tinnitus patients Andersson et al. (2005).

2.3.5. Smartphone Apps Related to Tinnitus

As explained in the last part of section 2.2, three different stores for smartphone applications were searched for tinnitus-related content.

The amount of apps excluded from the initial results vary between the different stores. While there was not much discrepancy between excluded apps from Google's PlayStore (2 of 146 results) and Apple's AppStore (1 of 100 results for iPhone, 4 of 90 results for iPad), Microsoft's Windows 10 Mobile Store displayed a greater number of unrelated applications (58 of 61 results). Most of the irrelevant results in Microsoft's Store included the word "status," which has the same word ending as "tinnitus." This leads to the assumption that search was automatically expanded by similar keywords.

Aside from the amount, we investigated all of the apps in greater detail to count the apps that claim to have a tinnitus masker functionality. This analysis revealed that a large number of apps (104 of 144 in the PlayStore, 66 of 99 in the AppStore for iPhones, 48 of 86 in the AppStore for iPad and 3 of 3 in the Windows 10 Mobile Store) included a masker function in their feature set. Other than maskers, many apps were designed to provide information to the user via news articles, videos or photos. Many apps that were included in the results might be appropriate for tinnitus matching, others require specific kinds of hearing aids, functioning as a control unit for said devices. Very few apps included exercises aiming to treat the tinnitus via hypnosis.

3. DISCUSSION

As shown in section 2.3, internet-based and smartphone-based technologies are used in intervention programs, whereupon iCBT is the most widespread intervention form, as well as for the recording of assessments, whereupon the recordings are often used for diagnostic purposes (e.g., to match the tinnitus frequency) and for self-help support. As discussed below, the new technologies affect (a) the indicators, symptoms and assessments being collected during an intervention or for diagnostic purposes, and (b) the form and intensity of patient involvement.

3.1. Influence of Technologies on the Amount and Form of Collected Patient Information

3.1.1. Assignments and Assessments

Similarly to Lui et al. (2017), we found that CBT and its variants like ACT play a central role among the psychotherapeutic treatments for tinnitus. After the publication of the core article of Andersson and Kaldo (2004) on internet-based CBT (iCBT) for tinnitus, there has been a proliferation of studies on enriching CBT with internet-based functionalities: individual weekly treatment plans are considered by Rheker et al. (2015), homework assignments are suggested by Abbott et al. (2009), while patient chats are presented by the aforementioned authors and by Hesser et al. (2012).

Next to assignments, internet technologies and smart devices are used to record patient assessments. Peter et al. (2016) propose PRISM (Pictorial Representation of Illness and Self Measure), a two-dimensional pictorial method for assessing the "burden of suffering" of tinnitus patients. PRISM has been designed for interactive self-assessment with help of an iPad. Whilst the aforementioned iCBT studies put emphasis in the *nature and purpose* of the assignments given to the patients (treatment plans, homework assignments), Peter et al. (2016) also elaborate on the modalities for *patient-app-interaction*, i.e., on the utilities for showing and filling the questionnaire.

Ecological Momentary Assessments (EMAs) for tinnitus patients are investigated by Probst et al. (2016a,b); Schlee et al. (2016) and Wilson et al. (2015) with the goal of understanding tinnitus physiology and moment-to-moment evolution. All these studies used smartphone technology. The EMA analyzed by Probst et al. (2016a,b), and Schlee et al. (2016) are recorded with a dedicated mHealth app, i.e., Track Your Tinnitus. Similarly to the study of (Peter et al., 2016) on PRISM, many studies on EMA under Track Your Tinnitus investigate the patient-app-interaction, aiming at usability and minimal cognitive patient effort (Pryss et al., 2015b; Schlee et al., 2016; Schickler et al., 2016a). Among them, Schickler et al. (2016b) investigate the potential of serious games, while Schickler et al. (2016a) focus on smartwatches, which are less obtrusive than smartphones and can further introduce additional functionality, e.g., monitor vital signs. These studies indicate the importance of enhancing personal experience in the interaction between the tinnitus patient and the mechanism recording assessments or delivering tasks.

3.1.2. Patient Recordings for Diagnosis and Intervention

Hauptmann et al. (2016) present a review of mobile apps that are used for measuring tinnitus pitch. The studies of Mahboubi et al. (2012a) and Yoo et al. (2015) investigate tinnitus masking and consider smart technologies with which the patients themselves can identify the tinnitus frequency they are experiencing. Wunderlich et al. (2015) consider ipod-based tinnitus pitch matching. In the study of Mahboubi et al. (2012a), the patients were asked to match their tinnitus frequency using a web-based protocol. Furthermore, they were subsequently provided with a "customized Harmonic Sound Therapy file" Mahboubi et al. (2012b), the patients listened for 1 h[1]. These studies demonstrate the potential of internet-based and smart technologies for tinnitus matching, but also stress the need for a reliable interaction between patient and technology.

[1] Mahboubi et al. (2012a) showed a temporary reduction in tinnitus loudness in 26 of their 32 participants, and in tinnitus annoyance in 27 of 32 participants, leading to the conclusion that internet-based, customized sound therapy can be effective in reducing tinnitus annoyance and loudness.

3.2. Influence of Technologies on the Extent and Form of Patient Participation

Internet-based technologies and smartphones allow for a personalized interaction between patient and eHealth/mHealth application. In the literature we investigated, this led to questions about the role of the therapist and the effect of self-help, and about patient involvement and attrition, as described hereafter.

3.2.1. Therapist Assistance and Self-Help

The role of the therapist has been investigated in the context of iCBT by Kaldo et al. (2008), Hesser et al. (2012), and Rheker et al. (2015) among others, while Jasper et al. (2014) juxtaposed self-help to group-based CBT. A remarkable finding is reported by Rheker et al. (2015), who studied the alternatives of "support-on-demand" and "no-support" and found no differences between the two options.

As opposed to iCBT and similar forms of treatment, self-help apps rely entirely on active patient involvement, whereupon the response rate, once and over a long range of time, is used as indicator of success: Wilson et al. (2015) report a response rate of 79.4% for ECA (889 out of 1120 questionnaires were returned), while Pryss et al. (2015b) report that 90% of the questionnaires filled under Track Your Tinnitus come from 18% of the users and thus, incentives for patient involvement need to be established. Advances in that domain include serious games (Schickler et al., 2016b) and passive forms of crowdsensing, as used for other diseases (e.g., diabetes) to monitor vital signals.

3.2.2. Patient Participation and Attrition

An aspect of substantial interest in the identified literature concerns participation and attrition. Number of participants and percentage of dropouts are used as key indicators of iCBT efficancy: in the studies of Abbott et al. (2009), Hesser et al. (2012), Weise et al. (2012, 2016), Kaldo et al. (2013), Jasper et al. (2014), Beukes et al. (2015, 2016), Rheker et al. (2015), and Heinrich et al. (2016), the number of participants ranges between 44 and 293 (average:113). The drop-outs are depicted in the rightmost column of **Table 1**.

As can be seen in the last two columns of **Table 1**, the variance is substantial. This is in agreement with the findings in the review of Greenwell et al. (2016a, p. 84), where large differences are reported among the surveyed studies as well.

Self-help apps like (Pryss et al., 2015b) and Wilson et al. (2015) do not have an explicit notion of dropout, the patient decides whether or not to use the app. However, patient involvement is not less mission-critical. The observation of Pryss et al. (2015b) that 90% of the Track Your Tinnitus questionnaires come from 18% of the app users indicates a very skewed distribution. However, this does not directly imply patient dissatisfaction; patients would most likely give up the app if they do not need it anymore. Hence, the response rates of self-help apps call for further investigation of the factors modulating attrition.

3.3. Technical Challenges

3.3.1. Platform Diversity

As with many smartphone applications, software for tinnitus monitoring, delivery of information materials, and data

TABLE 1 | Participation and attrition (number of dropouts) in the inspected iCBT studies.

Literature source	#Participants	#drop-outs
Hesser et al., 2012	99	10
Rheker et al., 2015	112	9 in the support-on-demand group (out of 56), 11 in the no-support group (out of 56)
Weise et al., 2012	124	5
Jasper et al., 2014	128	7
Beukes et al., 2016	44 (of which 37 completed the screening questionnaire)	15
Weise et al., 2016	124	5
Heinrich et al., 2016	112	14

collection need to take the platform and application interfaces into account. Compatibility with each smartphone operating system translates into additional costs for software development and maintenance. Interaction with hearing aids, sensors, smartwatches and other devices causes further costs and requires expertise. Furthermore, the user interfaces vary substantially: the design of fill-in forms, especially of those requiring free-text, must be re-considered when input is acquired through smartphones and smartwatches.

3.3.2. Non-obtrusive Data Acquisition

Smart technology is appropriate for the acquisition of data without active user involvement, e.g., from the microphone, camera, gyro-sensors, and accelerometers. Such data can be used for tinnitus monitoring without the need to increase user participation. However, data protection and anonymization of the data needs to be addressed.

For the monitoring of other chronical diseases, such as diabetes, the use of non-obtrusive data acquisition technologies is widespread as reported by Brzan et al. (2016). Tinnitus monitoring is less widespread, but gains momentum, as our findings show. Moreover, the collection of data about sleep, social interaction, and behavioral patterns are relevant as well, as reported e.g., by Wang et al. (2014) and Lane et al. (2011): the findings from such initiatives are also of relevance for the support of tinnitus patients, since tinnitus has been found to ".. [be] engendering the sense of cognitive and emotional reactions" as pointed out by Ghodratitoostani et al. (2016), who also list insomnia among the consequences.

4. SUMMARY, LIMITATIONS AND OUTLOOK

Our review has shown that internet-based and smart technologies are intensively investigated for the potential to support tinnitus patients. The technologies are used during treatment, e.g., to assign tasks to the patients, but also to collect patient assessments, including Ecological Momentary Assessments. The technologies are also used for diagnostic purposes, e.g., for tinnitus matching or to monitor tinnitus evolution over time.

We found that these new technologies influence the amount of collected patient information but also the form of the interaction. There is a thread of studies on internet-based and smart technologies as part of a physician-supervised tinnitus therapy, and a younger thread on self-help solutions for patients. In both threads, there is awareness about the need for dedicated questionnaire designs (in the context of tinnitus monitoring) and to a more limited extent, awareness about the need to cope with diversity of platforms and user interfaces.

The use of internet-based and smart technologies also affects the extent and form of patient participation. We identified studies that investigate the role of therapist assistance and that juxtapose therapy design with and without therapist. The role of patient participation is naturally a central subject in these studies. There are research contributions that simply report on the number of drop-outs from a conducted field study, whereby the variance is high. But the new technologies are also used outside the scope of typical clinical studies: research papers that report on such technology use are mainly concentrating on self-help eHealth/mHealth apps; they measure response rate of the patients rather than drop-outs, and identify also a high variance.

The co-authorship network of **Figure 1** highlights the teams of authors that work intensively on the potential of new technologies for tinnitus. The graph shows that teams build clusters with strong links (thick and intensively colored) among the members, indicating intensive joint publication activity, while there are only few and weak links between clusters. These clusters seems to correspond to the topics being investigated, according to our findings. In particular, the cluster with the strongest links corresponds to the most intensive thread of research; the authors in this cluster work together to investigate the role of internet-based and smart technologies for tinnitus treatment, with emphasis on iCBT. The cluster with the second-strongest links (bottom of the figure) contains authors that work together to understand tinnitus through EMA but at the same time investigate the patient-app-interaction.

A limitation of our review lays in the use of Google Scholar as primary source, whereupon only the top-20 articles were considered. It is possible that relevant articles were overlooked, because they were not in the top-20 positions or because they were not indexed in that query engine. The focus on keyword-based retrieval of scientific works implies that our review did not cover studies on smart technologies for chronical diseases with resemblance to tinnitus nor for comorbidities of tinnitus (like depression), but without explicit reference to the keyword "tinnitus." Research articles that investigate the potential of dedicated devices are underrepresented: studies that consider dedicated hardware next to smart technology, e.g., for tinnitus masking, are covered in our work, but studies that only consider dedicated hardware are not.

Our market overview is biased by our inclusion criterion, namely the keyword "tinnitus": we did not consider mobile apps that can be used for tinnitus masking and for relaxation but do not refer explicitly to tinnitus. At the same time, our overview did not address the veracity of the texts we acquired. We took the perspective of the non-expert, potential customer for those apps, and did not verify the claims made in the app description. We strongly believe that certification of such apps is necessary to protect patients from misleading statements, but such a task was beyond the scope of our study.

We plan to extend our work by investigating how smart technologies are used in other chronical diseases that show resemblances to tinnitus. The notion of resemblance has to be specified crisply, but our first focus will be on diseases that require patients to fill-in questionnaires frequently (e.g., diabetes) and diseases for which ambient recordings are collected and exploited in a non-obtrusive way (e.g., dementia).

AUTHOR CONTRIBUTIONS

SK and MS created the search strategies. SK created the networks-graphics and drafted the initial manuscript. All authors contributed equally to all other stages of the manuscript development, produced, and approved the manuscript.

REFERENCES

Abbott, J.-A. M., Kaldo, V., Klein, B., Austin, D., Hamilton, C., Piterman, L., et al. (2009). A cluster randomised trial of an internet-based intervention program for tinnitus distress in an industrial setting. *Cogn. Behav. Ther.* 38, 162–173. doi: 10.1080/16506070902763174

Andersson, G., Bakhsh, R., Johansson, L., Kaldo, V., and Carlbring, P. (2005). Stroop facilitation in tinnitus patients: an experiment conducted via the world wide web. *Cyberpsychol. Behav.* 8, 32–38. doi: 10.1089/cpb.2005.8.32

Andersson, G., and Kaldo, V. (2004). Internet-based cognitive behavioral therapy for tinnitus. *J. Clin. Psychol.* 60, 171–178. doi: 10.1002/jclp.10243

Baguley, D., McFerran, D., and Hall, D. (2013). Tinnitus. *Lancet* 382, 1600–1607. doi: 10.1016/S0140-6736(13)60142-7

Barozzi, S., Del Bo, L., Crocetti, A., Dyrlund, O., Passoni, S., Zolin, A., et al. (2016). A comparison of nature and technical sounds for tinnitus therapy. *Acta Acust. United Acust.* 102, 540–546. doi: 10.3813/AAA.918971

Beukes, E. W., Manchaiah, V., Allen, P. M., Baguley, D. M., and Andersson, G. (2015). Internet-based cognitive behavioural therapy for adults with tinnitus in the uk: study protocol for a randomised controlled trial. *BMJ Open* 5:e008241. doi: 10.1136/bmjopen-2015-008241

Beukes, E. W., Vlaescu, G., Manchaiah, V., Baguley, D. M., Allen, P. M., Kaldo, V., et al. (2016). Development and technical functionality of an internet-based intervention for tinnitus in the uk. *Int. Intervent.* 6, 6–15. doi: 10.1016/j.invent.2016.08.002

Brzan, P. P., Rotman, E., Pajnkihar, M., and Klanjsek, P. (2016). Mobile applications for control and self management of diabetes: a systematic review. *J. Med. Syst.* 40:210. doi: 10.1007/s10916-016-0564-8

Cima, R. F., Maes, I. H., Joore, M. A., Scheyen, D. J., El Refaie, A., Baguley, D. M., et al. (2012). Specialised treatment based on cognitive behaviour therapy versus usual care for tinnitus: a randomised controlled trial. *Lancet* 379, 1951–1959. doi: 10.1016/S0140-6736(12)60469-3

Ghodratitoostani, I., Zana, Y., Delbem, A. C., Sani, S. S., Ekhtiari, H., and Sanchez, T. G. (2016). Theoretical tinnitus framework: a neurofunctional model. *Front. Neurosci.* 10:370. doi: 10.3389/fnins.2016.00370

Greenwell, K., Featherstone, D., and Hoare, D. J. (2015). The application of intervention coding methodology to describe the tinnitus e-programme, an internet-delivered self-help intervention for tinnitus. *Amer. J. Audiol.* 24, 311–315. doi: 10.1044/2015_AJA-14-0089

Greenwell, K., Sereda, M., Coulson, N., El Refaie, A., and Hoare, D. J. (2016a). A systematic review of techniques and effects of self-help interventions for tinnitus: application of taxonomies from health psychology. *Int. J. Audiol.* 55(Suppl. 3), S79–S89. doi: 10.3109/14992027.2015.1137363

Greenwell, K., Sereda, M., Coulson, N., and Hoare, D. J. (2016b). Understanding user reactions and interactions with an internet-based intervention for tinnitus self-management: mixed-methods process evaluation protocol. *JMIR Res. Protoc.* 5:e49. doi: 10.2196/resprot.5008

Handscomb, L., Hall, D. A., Shorter, G. W., and Hoare, D. J. (2016). Online data collection to evaluate a theoretical cognitive model of tinnitus. *Amer. J. Audiol.* 25, 313–317. doi: 10.1044/2016_AJA-16-0007

Hauptmann, C., Wegener, A., Poppe, H., Williams, M., Popelka, G., and Tass, P. A. (2016). Validation of a mobile device for acoustic coordinated reset neuromodulation tinnitus therapy. *J. Amer. Acad. Audiol.* 27, 720–731. doi: 10.3766/jaaa.15082

Heinrich, S., Rozental, A., Carlbring, P., Andersson, G., Cotter, K., and Weise, C. (2016). Treating tinnitus distress via the internet: a mixed methods approach of what makes patients seek help and stay motivated during internet-based cognitive behavior therapy. *Int. Intervent.* 4, 120–130. doi: 10.1016/j.invent.2016.04.001

Henry, J. A., Galvez, G., Turbin, M. B., Thielman, E. J., McMillan, G. P., and Istvan, J. A. (2012). Pilot study to evaluate ecological momentary assessment of tinnitus. *Ear Hear.* 32:179. doi: 10.1097/AUD.0b013e31822f6740

Hesser, H., Gustafsson, T., Lundén, C., Henrikson, O., Fattahi, K., Johnsson, E., et al. (2012). A randomized controlled trial of internet-delivered cognitive behavior therapy and acceptance and commitment therapy in the treatment of tinnitus. *J. Consult. Clin. Psychol.* 80:649. doi: 10.1037/a0027021

Jasper, K., Weise, C., Conrad, I., Andersson, G., Hiller, W., and Kleinstaeuber, M. (2014). Internet-based guided self-help versus group cognitive behavioral therapy for chronic tinnitus: a randomized controlled trial. *Psychother. Psychosomat.* 83, 234–246. doi: 10.1159/000360705

Kaldo, V., Haak, T., Buhrman, M., Alfonsson, S., Larsen, H.-C., and Andersson, G. (2013). Internet-based cognitive behaviour therapy for tinnitus patients delivered in a regular clinical setting: Outcome and analysis of treatment dropout. *Cogn. Behav. Ther.* 42, 146–158. doi: 10.1080/16506073.2013.769622

Kaldo, V., Levin, S., Widarsson, J., Buhrman, M., Larsen, H.-C., and Andersson, G. (2008). Internet vs. group cognitive-behavioral treatment of distress associated with tinnitus: a randomized controlled trial. *Behav. Ther.* 39, 348–359. doi: 10.1016/j.beth.2007.10.003

Lane, N. D., Mohammod, M., Lin, M., Yang, X., Lu, H., Ali, S., et al. (2011). "Bewell: a smartphone application to monitor, model and promote wellbeing," in *5th International ICST Conference on Pervasive Computing Technologies for Healthcare* (Dublin), 23–26.

Linnan, Z., Peiyu, H., Fan, P., and Shangwen, L. (2015). "Design and implementation of a new tinnitus treatment method based on android," in *2015 IEEE International Conference on Digital Signal Processing (DSP)* (Singapore: IEEE), 263–267.

Lui, J. H., Marcus, D. K., and Barry, C. T. (2017). Evidence-based apps? A review of mental health mobile applications in a psychotherapy context. *Prof. Psychol. Res. Pract.* 48:199. doi: 10.1037/pro0000122

Mahboubi, H., Ziai, K., Brunworth, J., and Djalilian, H. R. (2012a). Accuracy of tinnitus pitch matching using a web-based protocol. *Ann. Otol. Rhinol. Laryngol.* 121, 671–674. doi: 10.1177/000348941212101008

Mahboubi, H., Ziai, K., and Djalilian, H. R. (2012b). Customized web-based sound therapy for tinnitus. *Int. Tinnitus J.* 17, 26–30.

Martinez-Devesa, P., Perera, R., Theodoulou, M., and Waddell, A. (2010). Cognitive behavioural therapy for tinnitus. *Cochr. Library.* 9:CD005233. doi: 10.1002/14651858.CD005233.pub3

Newman, C. W., Jacobson, G. P., and Spitzer, J. B. (1996). Development of the tinnitus handicap inventory. *Arch. Otolaryngol. Head Neck Surg.* 122, 143–148. doi: 10.1001/archotol.1996.01890140029007

Nyenhuis, N., Golm, D., and Kröner-Herwig, B. (2013). A systematic review and meta-analysis on the efficacy of self-help interventions in tinnitus. *Cogn. Behav. Ther.* 42, 159–169. doi: 10.1080/16506073.2013.803496

Peter, N., Kleinjung, T., Horat, L., Schmidt-Weitmann, S., Meyer, M., Büchi, S., et al. (2016). Validation of prism (pictorial representation of illness and self measure) as a novel visual assessment tool for the burden of suffering in tinnitus patients. *Health Qual. Life Outcomes* 14, 1–9. doi: 10.1186/s12955-016-0454-2

Probst, T., Pryss, R., Langguth, B., and Schlee, W. (2016a). Emotion dynamics and tinnitus: daily life data from the "trackyourtinnitus" application. *Sci. Rep.* 6:31166. doi: 10.1038/srep31166

Probst, T., Pryss, R., Langguth, B., and Schlee, W. (2016b). Emotional states as mediators between tinnitus loudness and tinnitus distress in daily life: results from the "trackyourtinnitus" application. *Sci. Rep.* 6:20382 doi: 10.1038/srep20382

Pryss, R., Reichert, M., Langguth, B., and Schlee, W. (2015a). "Mobile crowd sensing in clinical and psychological trials–a case study," in *Computer-Based Medical Systems (CBMS), 2015 IEEE 28th International Symposium on* (Sao Carlos: IEEE), 23–24.

Pryss, R., Reichert, M., Langguth, B., and Schlee, W. (2015b). "Mobile crowd sensing services for tinnitus assessment, therapy, and research," in *Mobile Services (MS), 2015 IEEE International Conference on* (New York, NY: IEEE), 352–359.

Rheker, J., Andersson, G., and Weise, C. (2015). The role of "on demand" therapist guidance vs. no support in the treatment of tinnitus via the internet: a randomized controlled trial. *Int. Intervent.* 2, 189–199. doi: 10.1016/j.invent.2015.03.007

Sauer, G., Dickel, T., and Lotter, T. (2014). "Acoustic wireless control–connecting smart phones to hearing instruments," in *Siemens Whitepaper*. Available online at: https://media.sivantos.com/siemens-website/media/2014/11/2014_11_Acoustic-Wireless-Control.pdf

Schickler, M., Pryss, R., Reichert, M., Heinzelmann, M., Schobel, J., Langguth, B., et al. (2016a). "Using wearables in the context of chronic disorders: results of a pre-study," in *Computer-Based Medical Systems (CBMS), 2016 IEEE 29th International Symposium on* (Dublin; Belfast, UK: IEEE), 68–69.

Schickler, M., Pryss, R., Reichert, M., Schobel, J., Langguth, B., and Schlee, W. (2016b). "Using mobile serious games in the context of chronic disorders: a mobile game concept for the treatment of tinnitus," in *Computer-Based Medical Systems (CBMS), 2016 IEEE 29th International Symposium on* (Dublin; Belfast, UK: IEEE), 343–348.

Schlee, W., Pryss, R. C., Probst, T., Schobel, J., Bachmeier, A., Reichert, M., et al. (2016). Measuring the moment-to-moment variability of tinnitus: the trackyourtinnitus smart phone app. *Front. Aging Neurosci.* 8:294. doi: 10.3389/fnagi.2016.00294

Wang, R., Chen, F., Chen, Z., Li, T., Harari, G., Tignor, S., et al. (2014). "Studentlife: assessing mental health, academic performance and behavioral trends of college students using smartphones," in *Proceedings of the 2014 ACM International Joint Conference on Pervasive and Ubiquitous Computing* (Seattle, WA: ACM), 3–14.

Weise, C., Kleinstäuber, M., and Andersson, G. (2012). "Internet-based cognitive-behavioural treatment of chronic tinnitus," in *12th International Congress of Behavioral Medicine (ICBM), 29 August-1 September 2012* (Budapest).

Weise, C., Kleinstäuber, M., and Andersson, G. (2016). Internet-delivered cognitive-behavior therapy for tinnitus: a randomized controlled trial. *Psychosomat. Med.* 78, 501–510. doi: 10.1097/PSY.0000000000000310

Westin, V. Z., Schulin, M., Hesser, H., Karlsson, M., Noe, R. Z., Olofsson, U. et al. (2011). Acceptance and commitment therapy vs. tinnitus retraining therapy in the treatment of tinnitus: a randomised controlled trial. *Behav. Res. Ther.* 49, 737–747. doi: 10.1016/j.brat.2011.08.001

Wilson, M. B., Kallogjeri, D., Joplin, C. N., Gorman, M. D., Krings, J. G., Lenze, E. J., et al. (2015). Ecological momentary assessment of tinnitus using smartphone technology a pilot study. *Otolaryngol. Head Neck Surg.* 152, 897–903. doi: 10.1177/0194599815569692

Wise, K., Kobayashi, K., Magnusson, J., Welch, D., and Searchfield, G. D. (2016). Randomized controlled trial of a perceptual training game for tinnitus therapy. *Games Health J.* 5, 141–149. doi: 10.1089/g4h.2015.0068

Wise, K., Kobayashi, K., and Searchfield, G. (2015). Feasibility study of a game integrating assessment and therapy of tinnitus. *J. Neurosci. Methods* 249, 1–7. doi: 10.1016/j.jneumeth.2015.04.002

Wunderlich, R., Stein, A., Engell, A., Lau, P., Waasem, L. Shaykevich, A., et al. (2015). Evaluation of ipod-based automated tinnitus pitch matching. *J. Amer. Acad. Audiol.* 26, 205–212. doi: 10.3766/jaaa.26.2.9

Yoo, S.-G., Oh, D., Hong, M., and Park, M. (2015). Study on a user-friendly acoustic therapeutic sound source-based mobile application for tinnitus patients. *Adv. Sci. Lett.* 21, 332–336. doi: 10.1166/asl.2015.5777

18

Cochlear Implantation of Bilaterally Deafened Patients with Tinnitus Induces Sustained Decrease of Tinnitus-Related Distress

Steffen Knopke[1], Agnieszka J. Szczepek[2], Sophia Marie Häussler[1], Stefan Gräbel[1] and Heidi Olze[1]**

[1] Department of Otorhinolaryngology, Head and Neck Surgery, Charité – University Hospital Berlin, Campus Virchow-Klinikum, Berlin, Germany, [2] Department of Otorhinolaryngology, Head and Neck Surgery, Charité – University Hospital Berlin, Campus Charité Mitte, Berlin, Germany

***Correspondence:**
Agnieszka J. Szczepek
agnes.szczepek@charite.de;
Heidi Olze
heidi.olze@charite.de

Objective: Tinnitus is a common symptom of hearing impairment. Patients who are bilaterally hard of hearing are often affected by tinnitus. However, they cannot undergo any of the standard tinnitus therapies, since they rely on hearing. Cochlear implantation (CI) used to treat severe hearing disabilities, such as bilateral hearing loss, was also shown to reduce tinnitus. Our goal was to determine if CI induces sustained reduction of tinnitus. We performed prospective, longitudinal analyses of tinnitus-related distress in a uniform group of bilaterally deafened patients after CI.

Patients and Methods: The homogenous sample consisted of 41 patients who met the inclusion criteria and were consecutively included in this study. The impact of unilateral CI on tinnitus-related distress, health-related quality of life (HRQoL), and hearing abilities was studied with validated instruments. The follow-up appointments were scheduled at 6, 12, and 24 months after CI surgery. During the appointments, hearing abilities were estimated with monosyllabic Freiburg test, whereas the tinnitus-related distress, the HRQoL, and the subjective hearing were measured with standard questionnaires [Tinnitus Questionnaire (TQ), Nijmegen Cochlear Implantation Questionnaire, and Oldenburg Inventory, respectively].

Results: Tinnitus-related distress decreased significantly from the mean TQ score of 35.0 (SD = 19.6) prior to surgery to the mean TQ = 27.54 (SD = 20.0) 6 months after surgery and remained sustained low until the end of follow-up period. In addition, CI significantly improved the hearing abilities and the HRQoL of all patients.

Conclusion: The results from our prospective study suggest that in a homogenous sample of bilaterally deafened, implanted patients who report having tinnitus prior to surgery, CI alone not only improves the hearing abilities but also significantly reduces the tinnitus-related distress and improves the HRQoL in a sustained way.

Keywords: cochlear implantation, hearing impairment, health-related quality of life, tinnitus-related distress, depressive symptoms, anxiety

INTRODUCTION

Tinnitus is a common symptom of hearing impairment (1–3). Therapeutic use of hearing aids to treat mild-to moderate hearing loss was demonstrated to correlate with a decrease of tinnitus (4), although the data generated by clinical research neither support nor dismiss the use of hearing aids in tinnitus treatment (5). Of all types of hearing impairment, the most cumbersome is the severe bilateral hearing loss, which is often treated with cochlear implantation (CI) (6–10). Bilateral hearing impairment affects 12.7% (30 million) of the US Americans above 12 years of age, and the prevalence of bilateral hearing impairment increases with age (11). We and others have previously reported the incidence of tinnitus among the bilaterally hearing-impaired patients ranging between 70 and 90% (12–14) and making tinnitus a serious complaint in this particular group of patients.

Already decades ago, clinical observations linked the CI-mediated hearing recovery with the reduction in tinnitus (15–17). Ever since, various studies addressed the relationship between cochlear implants and tinnitus (12); however, the outcomes of the studies were somewhat conflicting. There are three main reasons for this: the first is varying sample size (from 1 to 26); the second is using different follow-up times (from 1 to 24 months) (18, 19); and the third is that despite recent recommendations to measure tinnitus-related distress before and after CI (10), the methods and the domains vary extremely from study to study (20). Furthermore, the design of clinical trials is often retrospective and the patients included have various types of hearing impairment (21–23). Moreover, the methods of treatment are frequently dissimilar and include unilateral hearing impairment treated with unilateral CI to bilateral hearing impairment treated with bilateral CI.

In our earlier studies, we concentrated on measuring the influence of CI on the quality of life (24), tinnitus-related distress, and psychological comorbidities (13, 14). We have demonstrated significant improvement of all domains measured following the CI. However, the follow-up time was rather short (13) and the patient sample was not homogenous (14).

The outstanding question in the field is how the cochlear implants affect tinnitus and tinnitus-related distress. The full answer to this question will be possible upon accumulation of high-quality evidence. This, in turn, can only be achieved by using specific batch of standardized validated instruments and by applying prospective longitudinal design to the studies.

Our present aim was to study tinnitus-related distress in a relatively homogenous group of patients over a longer period after CI. Our main question was if in this defined cohort, tinnitus-related distress improves solely upon auditory rehabilitation, and if yes, if this improvement is sustained over longer period.

PATIENTS AND METHODS

Inclusion Criteria

The patients of both genders were consecutively included in the study upon signing written consent. Following inclusion criteria were used:

- diagnosis of bilateral severe or profound hearing loss with speech recognition ≤40% in the Freiburg Monosyllabic Test in quiet and with hearing aid; 65-dB sound pressure level
- tinnitus
- meeting of the clinical criteria for CI:
  - possibility to use general anesthesia
  - exclusion of retrocochlear disorder (e.g., vestibular schwannoma)
  - unremarkable cochlear anatomy
  - motivation for postoperative audiological rehabilitation
  - post-lingual deafness.

Description of Study

Forty-one patients met the inclusion criteria and were followed for 2 years after CI. The data were collected between 2009 and 2016; the patients were admitted to the hospital between April 2009 and May 2014 for unilateral CI, and their last follow-up appointment was scheduled between July 2011 and February 2016. The appointments were scheduled at 6, 12, and 24 months after the surgery (see **Figure 1**). There were 22 women and 20 men in the sample—descriptive statistics are presented in **Table 1**.

Test Performed

All patients were audiologically examined. In addition, they were asked to complete psychometric questionnaires before surgery and during each consecutive appointment. The audiological tests and psychometric questionnaires used were previously described in detail (14, 25) and are presented in **Table 2**.

Statistical Evaluation

For the statistical analyses, SPSS version 23 was used. Normal distribution was tested prior to statistical analysis using the Shapiro–Wilk test and a histogram. Because of lack of normal distribution in the majority of dataset, the Wilcoxon signed-rank test was used to compare the scores before and after CI. Correlations between Tinnitus Questionnaire (TQ) and Nijmegen Cochlear Implantation Questionnaire (NCIQ) scores were performed by computing the Spearman's rank correlation coefficient.

RESULTS

Postimplantation Sustained Decrease of Tinnitus-Related Distress

Tinnitus was the main inclusion criterion. Prior to CI, the mean TQ score reflecting tinnitus-related distress was 35 (**Table 3**). TQ score decreased significantly already 6 months after CI, and this improvement was sustained over the 24-month follow-up period (**Figure 2**). Significant improvement of tinnitus-related distress was noted in 64.5% of all patients in the cohort. Regarding the individual TQ subscales, the emotional and cognitive distress were significantly reduced 12 and 24 months after implantation but the intrusiveness of tinnitus-related distress decreased already 6 months after surgery and stayed on a significantly lower level as compared to that before CI (**Table 3**). There was a trend in improvement regarding the subscales "auditory perception difficulties" and "somatic complaints," but this trend has not reached the statistical significance.

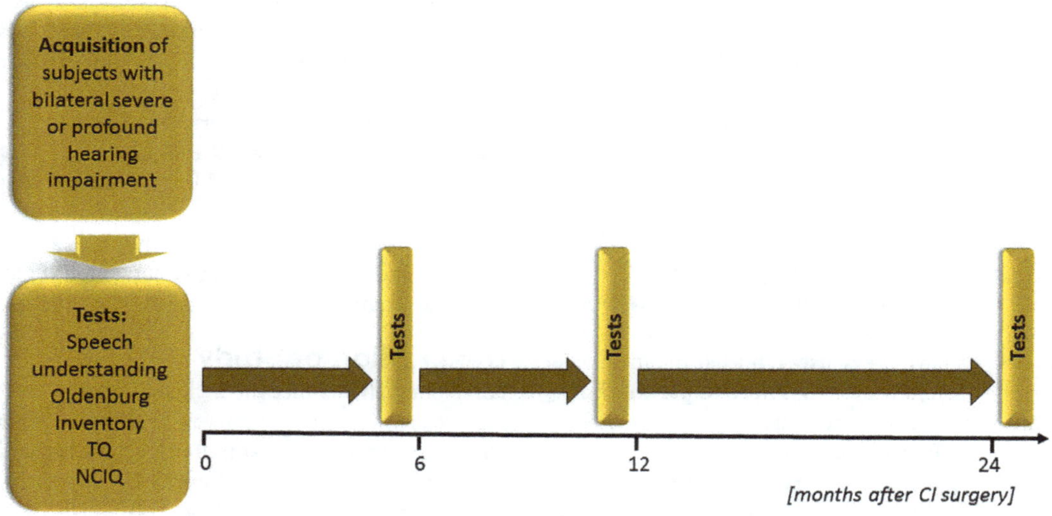

FIGURE 1 | Study design.

TABLE 1 | General patients' characteristics.

	Mean	Minimum	Maximum	SD
Age	61	25	81	13.45
Duration of hearing impairment (years)	18.82	1	67	18.84
Percent of speech recognition using monosyllabic Freiburg test 65-dB sound pressure level on the ear scheduled for implantation	7.86	0	40	13.21

TABLE 2 | Questionnaires used in this study.

Health-related quality of life (HRQoL): Nijmegen Cochlear Implantation Questionnaire (NCIQ)	NCIQ is a validated tool designed to determine the HRQoL of implanted patients. The three main domains "physical," "psychological," and "social" are derived from six subdomains: 1 Basic sound perception 2 Advanced sound perception 3 Speech production 4 Self-esteem 5 Activity 6 Social interactions. The score ranges from 0 (very bad) to 100 (optimal).
Speech perception: Freiburg Monosyllabic Test	The Freiburg Monosyllabic Test was used to determine the preoperative speech recognition in silence at 65-dB sound pressure level with optimized hearing aid and postoperative with cochlear implant again as well
Subjective audiological assessment: Oldenburg Inventory (OI)	Data were collected preoperatively and postoperatively about the subjective hearing with the OI. The OI additionally includes a total score in 3 categories: "hearing in quiet," "hearing with background noise," and "localization." The 12 closed questions about everyday situations were marked with points from 1 to 5. The higher the score, the better the subjective hearing
Tinnitus distress: Tinnitus Questionnaire (TQ)	The tinnitus distress can be determined with TQ (26). Collected data represent 6 subdomains: emotional and cognitive distress, intrusiveness, auditory perceptual difficulties, sleeping disturbances, somatic complaints. The mean value is used to determine tinnitus grade: light (0–30 points), average (31–46 points), high (47–59 points), and very high (60–84 points). In addition, separation into compensated (≤46 points) and decompensated (47–84 points) tinnitus can be done based on the total score. The test–retest reliability is 0.94 for the total value and between 0.86 and 0.92 for the subscales. Cronbach's α is 0.94 for the total value of the TQ and between 0.74 and 0.92 for the subscales

Prior to CI, 13 patients were affected by a severe, decompensated, tinnitus-related distress (TQ score = 47 or more). Six months after surgery, four patients had TQ scores on the compensated level, 12 months after surgery, five patients were compensated, and 24 months later, seven patients were compensated. In two patients with compensated TQ scores prior to surgery, tinnitus-related distress progressed further to the severe, decompensated form after CI (**Figure 3**).

Post-Surgery Improvement of the Health-Related Quality of Life (HRQoL), Speech Perception, and Auditory Performance

The HRQoL measured by NCIQ also improved significantly, and the improvement was sustained over the period of study (**Figure 4**). In detail, the scales measuring basic sound perception, advanced sound perception, self-esteem, activity, and social interactions improved significantly 6 months after CI and remained so over the 24 months of the follow-up period. The only scale without statistically significant changes but with a trend toward improvement was "speech production" (**Table 3**).

Six months after CI, Oldenburg Inventory (**Figure 5**) demonstrated significant improvement in speech understanding in quiet and noise, as well speech localization at all measured time points of the follow-up period (**Table 3**). Similarly, monosyllabic Freiburg test indicated significant recovery of the hearing abilities by the implanted ear (**Table 3**). The speech recognition improved rapidly after surgery and was stable during the observation period of 2 years.

TABLE 3 | Changes in parameters measured as compared to their values prior to cochlear implantation.

	Prior to surgery			6 months after surgery			12 months after surgery			24 months after surgery		
	Mean	Median	SD	Mean	Median	SD	Mean	Median	SD	Mean	Median	SD
SR 65-dB sound pressure level (SPL)	7.9	0.0	13.2	40.4**	43.8	35.9	41.6**	35.0	34.2	43.2**	46.3	25.2
NCIQ 1	40.1	39.4	20.9	59.6**	60.0	20.0	62.1**	65.0	22.4	57.6**	60.0	18.1
NCIQ 2	42.4	40.0	19.2	56.1**	55.0	20.5	54.9**	55.0	21.0	53.2**	52.5	19.4
NCIQ 3	64.4	67.5	22.6	72.1	75.0	20.4	66.9	72.2	20.6	71.7	71.9	24.0
NCIQ 4	42.6	41.7	17.5	50.9**	45.0	19.7	52.9**	52.5	18.9	53.8**	50.0	21.4
NCIQ 5	37.9	37.5	18.2	49.1**	47.5	22.8	49.3**	47.5	23.0	47.5**	43.8	18.6
NCIQ 6	41.5	40.0	22.5	51.2**	50.0	25.7	53.0**	52.8	23.3	50.3**	50.0	18.9
NCIQ total	53.8	43.2	58.7	56.6**	55.1	18.5	57.5**	55.5	19.8	55.8**	56.8	15.2
TQ E	9.0	8.0	6.0	7.4	4.0	6.8	7.1*	5.0	6.6	7.2	7.0	6.4
TQ C	6.9	7.5	4.5	5.7	4.0	5.0	5.4*	4.5	4.4	5.6	4.5	4.5
TQ E + C	15.9	14.0	10.0	13.1	9.0	11.5	12.3*	9.5	10.9	12.7*	13.0	10.6
TQ I	8.2	9.0	4.1	6.1**	5.0	5.2	5.6**	5.5	4.7	5.8**	6.0	4.3
TQ A	6.6	6.0	4.8	5.2	5.0	4.9	5.1	5.5	4.7	5.2	5.5	4.5
TQ SI	2.5	2.0	2.4	1.8*	0.0	2.5	1.9	1.0	2.3	2.3	1.5	2.7
TQ SO	1.8	1.5	1.7	1.3	0.0	2.0	1.8	0.5	2.4	1.5	1.0	1.9
TQ total	35.0	33.5	19.6	27.5*	23.0	24.0	26.7**	26.5	22.8	27.6*	30.0	22.3
OI quiet	2.4	2.4	0.9	3.4**	3.6	1.0	3.4**	3.4	0.8	3.4**	3.4	0.9
OI noise	1.8	1.6	0.6	2.7**	2.6	1.0	2.7**	2.5	0.9	2.6**	2.4	0.8
OI localization	1.9	2.0	0.8	2.8**	3.0	1.0	2.7**	2.5	1.0	2.7**	2.5	1.0
OI total	2.1	1.9	0.7	3.0**	2.9	0.9	3.0**	2.9	0.8	2.9**	2.8	0.8

*Asterisks indicate significant differences between respective variables when compared to their values prior to surgery as per Wilcoxon signed-rank test; *$p \leq 0.05$, **$p \leq 0.01$.*
SR, speech recognition (Freiburg Monosyllabic Test, 65-dB SPL); NCIQ, German version of Nijmegen Cochlear Implantation Questionnaire (1 basic sound perception; 2 advanced sound perception; 3 speech production; 4 self-esteem; 5 activity; and 6 social interactions); TQ, Tinnitus Questionnaire (E, emotional distress; C, cognitive distress; E + C, combined psychological distress; I, intrusiveness; A, auditory perception difficulties; SI, sleep disturbances; SO, somatic complaints; total, total score); OI, Oldenburg Inventory.

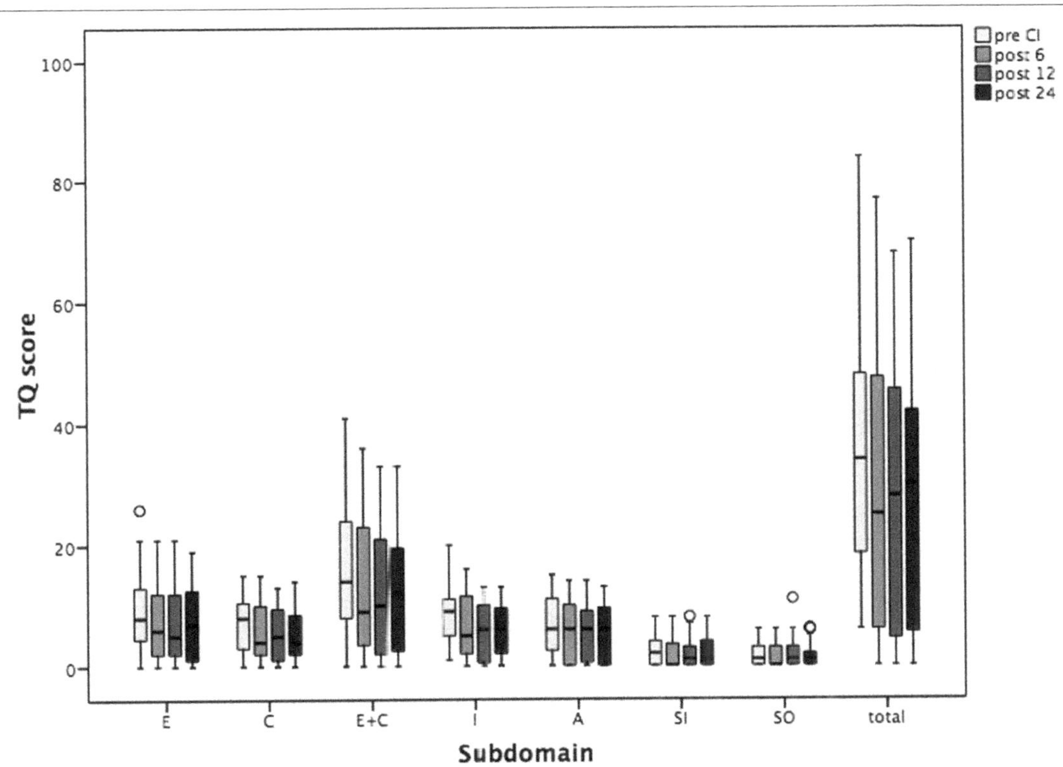

FIGURE 2 | Changes in tinnitus distress [Tinnitus Questionnaire (TQ)] and its subscales over the period of 2 years following cochlear implantation (CI). Shown are mean values and the range. Shown are mean values and the 95% CI. Pre CI, before CI; post 6, post 12, and post 24, 6, 12, and 24 months after surgery. E, emotional distress; C, cognitive distress; I, intrusiveness; A, auditory perceptual difficulties; SI, sleeping disturbances; SO, somatic complaints; total, total value.

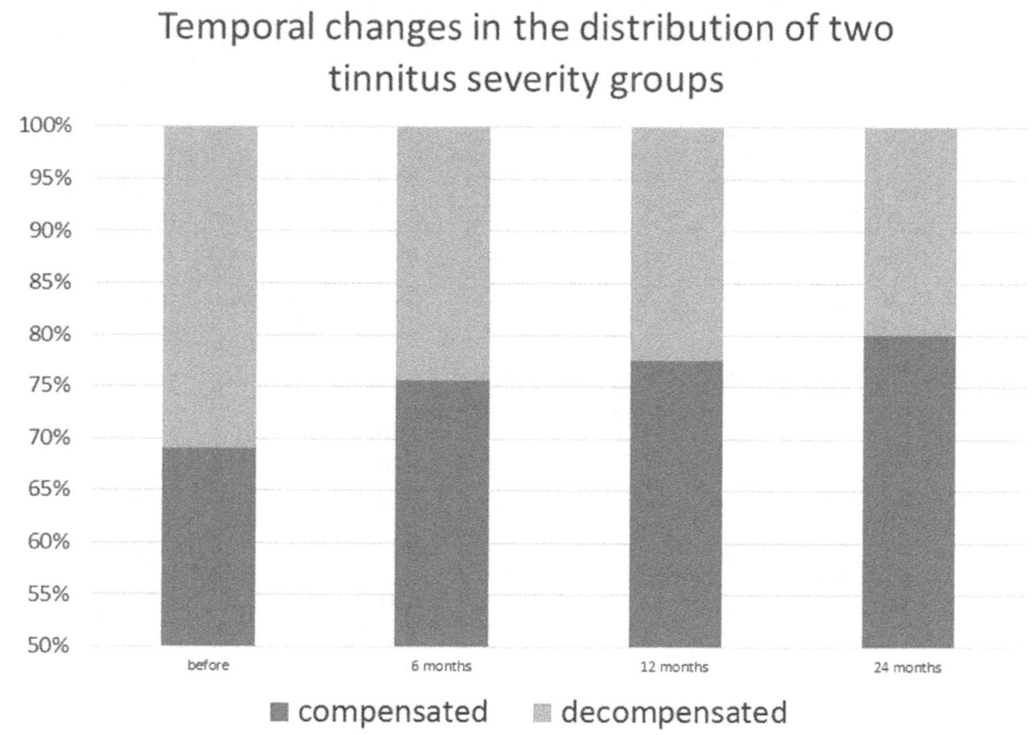

FIGURE 3 | Post-cochlear implantation decrease in decompensated, severe form of tinnitus among implanted patients.

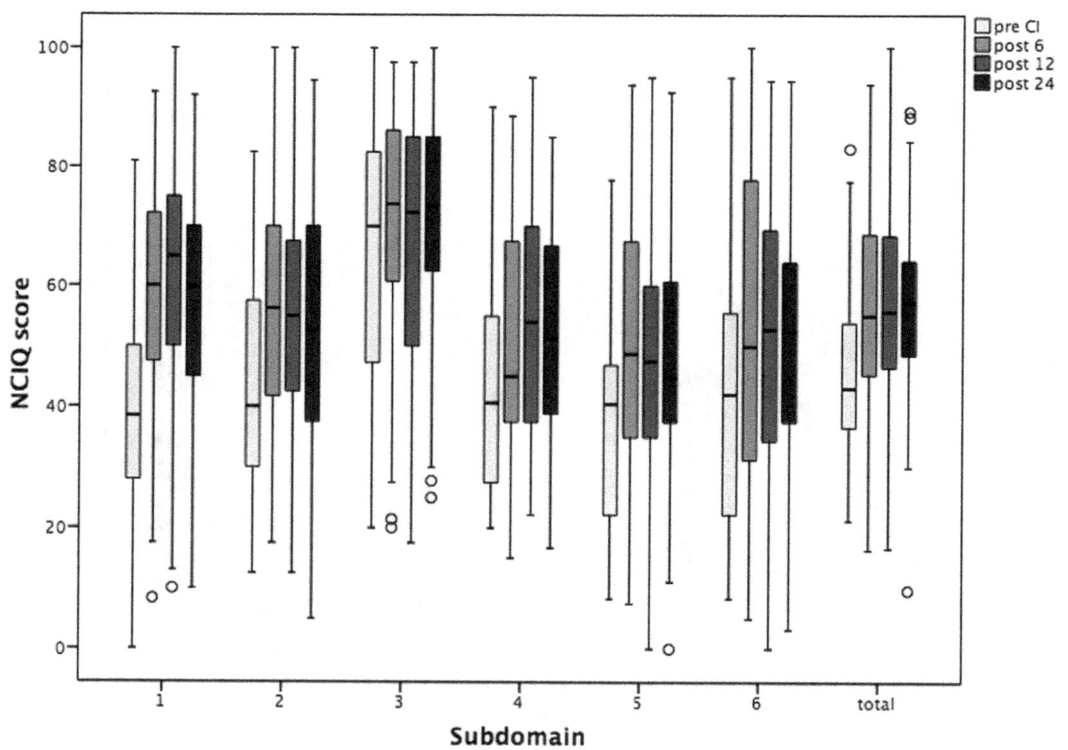

FIGURE 4 | Changes in the health-related quality of life Nijmegen Cochlear Implantation Questionnaire (NCIQ) and its subdomains over the period of 2 years following cochlear implantation (CI). Shown are mean values and the 95% CI. Pre CI, before CI; post 6, post 12, and post 24, 6, 12, and 24 months after surgery. 1 basic speech perception; 2 advanced speech perception; 3 speech production; 4 self-esteem; 5 activity; and 6 social interactions.

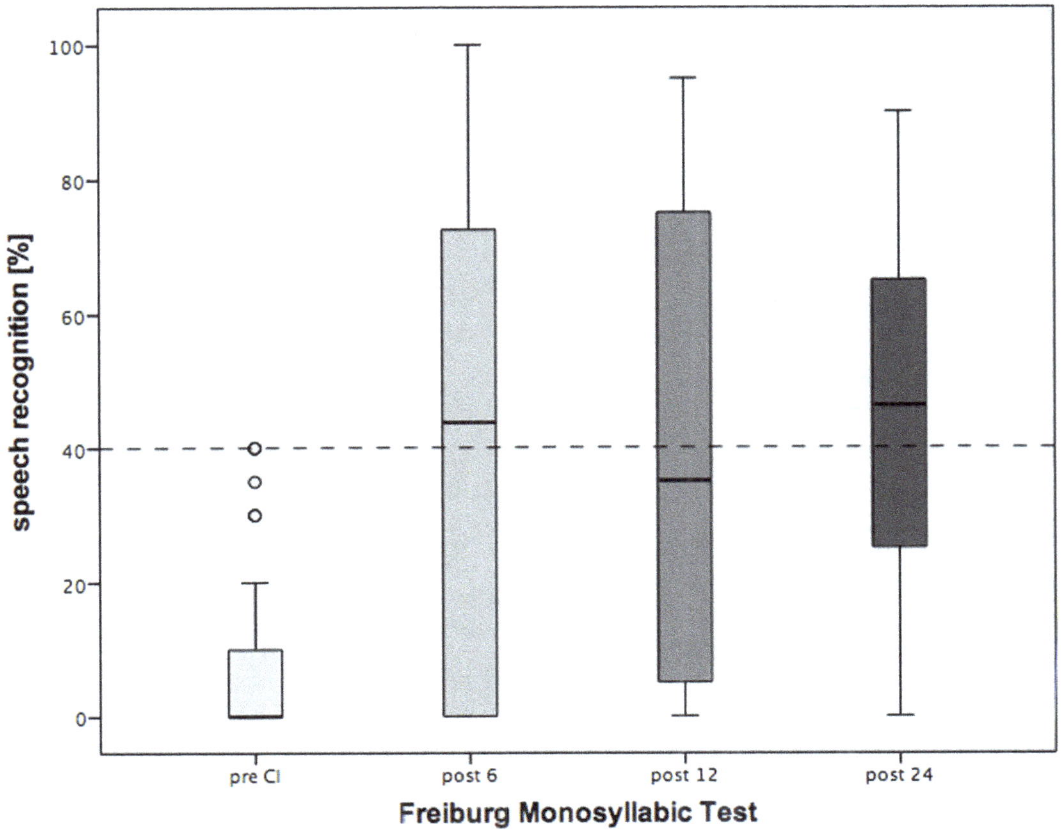

FIGURE 5 | Changes in speech recognition over the period of 2 years following cochlear implantation (CI). Shown are mean values and the range. Shown are mean values and the 95% CI. Dotted line: clinical criteria for CI.

Relationship between TQ and NCIQ

To determine if and how tinnitus-related distress affects the HRQoL, we computed the Spearman correlation coefficient for the respective variables. First, we analyzed the data obtained before CI (**Table 4**). We observed negative correlation between total TQ score and speech production (NCIQ3). The subscales indicating cognitive and emotional subscales as well as auditory difficulties reported by TQ were particularly affected. In addition, somatic complains correlated negatively with the background—and advanced sound perception as well as with self-esteem and social interactions (**Table 4**). Six months after CI, we found significant negative correlations between the total TQ score and all subdomains of NCIQ (**Table 5**), and 12 months after the CI, this was also the case (**Table 6**). Interestingly, 24 months after the CI, the correlations between total TQ score and NCIQ subscales "self-esteem" and "social interaction" were no longer significant (**Table 7**).

Compliance

Of 42 subjects originally included in this study, 41 patients filled the NCIQ questionnaire at the study onset, 39 patients after 12 months, and 40 patients after 2 years.

DISCUSSION

Tinnitus is often a symptom of hearing loss. Here, we demonstrated that in the bilaterally hearing-impaired patients with tinnitus, CI not only restores the auditory abilities but also reduces tinnitus-related distress and that this reduction was sustained for 2 years following surgery. To the best of our knowledge, our present study demonstrates for the first time the course of tinnitus-related distress in a homogenous cohort of bilaterally hard of hearing and tinnitus-positive patients, before and after CI. In addition, we show the relationship between tinnitus-related distress and the HRQoL and the postoperative auditory improvement over the 2-year course.

Prior to CI, the TQ score (total and subscales "emotional and cognitive distress" and "auditory difficulties") correlated significantly with the third subscale of the HRQoL NCIQ "speech production," whereas the total score of NCIQ correlated significantly (negative correlation) with the TQ subscale "somatic complaints" (**Table 4**). All correlations between NCIQ and TQ were negative, meaning that the decrease of tinnitus-related distress correlated with improvement of the quality of life and *vice versa*. Although these correlations decreased with time, they remained significant throughout the 24 months of the follow-up period (**Tables 5–7**),

TABLE 4 | Correlation between tinnitus and health-related quality of life *before* cochlear implantation.

			NCIQ1	NCIQ2	NCIQ3	NCIQ4	NCIQ5	NCIQ6	NCIQ total
Spearman-Rho	TQ E	Correlation coefficient	−0.202	−0.093	−0.313*	−0.097	−0.174	−0.146	−0.162
		Significance	0.205	0.561	0.046	0.548	0.276	0.362	0.313
		N	41	41	41	41	41	41	41
	TQ C	Correlation coefficient *t*	−0.118	−0.113	−0.315*	−0.144	−0.257	−0.240	−0.187
		Significance	0.464	0.483	0.045	0.370	0.105	0.131	0.241
		N	41	41	41	41	41	41	41
	TQ E + C	Correlation coefficient	−0.172	−0.108	−0.324*	−0.130	−0.232	−0.204	−0.191
		Significance	0.281	0.500	0.039	0.417	0.145	0.202	0.233
		N	41	41	41	41	41	41	41
	TQ I	Correlation coefficient	−0.287	−0.074	−0.300	−0.104	−0.210	−0.159	−0.199
		Sig. (2-seitig)	0.069	0.647	0.057	0.516	0.187	0.322	0.212
		N	41	41	41	41	41	41	41
	TQ A	Correlation coefficient	−0.258	−0.210	−0.437**	0.031	−0.044	0.043	−0.142
		Significance	0.104	0.187	0.004	0.849	0.784	0.791	0.378
		N	41	41	41	41	41	41	41
	TQ SI	Correlation coefficient	−0.354*	−0.315*	−0.263	−0.124	−0.279	−0.140	−0.259
		Significance	0.023	0.045	0.097	0.440	0.077	0.384	0.102
		N	41	41	41	41	41	41	41
	TQ SO	Correlation coefficient	−0.408**	−0.407**	−0.253	−0.274	−0.432**	−0.278	−0.413**
		Significance	0.008	0.008	0.111	0.083	0.005	0.078	0.007
		N	41	41	41	41	41	41	41
	TQ total	Correlation coefficient	−0.299	−0.205	−0.405**	−0.126	−0.243	−0.173	−0.260
		Significance	0.057	0.199	0.009	0.434	0.126	0.280	0.101
		N	41	41	41	41	41	41	41

*$p \leq 0.05$.

**$p \leq 0.01$.

Subscales of Nijmegen Cochlear Implantation Questionnaire (NCIQ): 1 basic sound perception; 2 advanced sound perception; 3 speech production; 4 self-esteem; 5 activity; and 6 social interactions.

Subscales of Tinnitus Questionnaire (TQ): E, emotional distress; C, cognitive distress; E + C, combined psychological distress; I, intrusiveness; A, auditory perception difficulties; SI, sleep disturbances; SO, somatic complaints.

TABLE 5 | Correlation between tinnitus and health-related quality of life *6 months after* cochlear implantation.

			NCIQ1	NCIQ2	NCIQ3	NCIQ4	NCIQ5	NCIQ6	NCIQ total
Spearman-Rho	TQ E	Correlation coefficient	−0.308	−0.397*	−0.421**	−0.331*	−0.553**	−0.365*	−0.462**
		Significance	0.050	0.010	0.006	0.034	0.000	0.019	0.002
		N	41	41	41	41	41	41	41
	TQ C	Correlation coefficient *t*	−0.347*	−0.399**	−0.446**	−0.421**	−0.586**	−0.413**	−0.524**
		Significance	0.026	0.010	0.003	0.006	0.000	0.007	0.000
		N	41	41	41	41	41	41	41
	TQ E + C	Correlation coefficient	−0.335*	−0.417**	−0.461**	−0.384*	−0.581**	−0.394*	−0.502**
		Significance	0.032	0.007	0.002	0.013	0.000	0.011	0.001
		N	41	41	41	41	41	41	41
	TQ I	Correlation coefficient	−0.378*	−0.466**	−0.486**	−0.368*	−0.613**	−0.444**	−0.535**
		Sig. (2-seitig)	0.015	0.002	0.001	0.018	0.000	0.004	0.000
		N	41	41	41	41	41	41	41
	TQ A	Correlation coefficient	−0.320*	−0.476**	−0.396*	−0.327*	−0.510**	−0.425**	−0.449**
		Significance	0.041	0.002	0.010	0.037	0.001	0.006	0.003
		N	41	41	41	41	41	41	41
	TQ SI	Correlation coefficient	−0.145	−0.185	−0.191	−0.357*	−0.527**	−0.240	−0.344*
		Significance	0.365	0.246	0.231	0.022	0.000	0.131	0.028
		N	41	41	41	41	41	41	41
	TQ SO	Correlation coefficient	−0.381*	−0.398**	−0.390*	−0.294	−0.457**	−0.413**	−0.449**
		Significance	0.014	0.010	0.012	0.062	0.003	0.007	0.003
		N	41	41	41	41	41	41	41
	TQ Total	Correlation coefficient	−0.331*	−0.435**	−0.430**	−0.359*	−0.589**	−0.404**	−0.497**
		Significance	0.035	0.004	0.005	0.021	0.000	0.009	0.001
		N	41	41	41	41	41	41	41

*$p \leq 0.05$.

**$p \leq 0.01$.

Subscales of Nijmegen Cochlear Implantation Questionnaire (NCIQ): 1 basic sound perception; 2 advanced sound perception; 3 speech production; 4 self-esteem; 5 activity; and 6 social interactions.

Subscales of Tinnitus Questionnaire (TQ): E, emotional distress; C, cognitive distress; E + C, combined psychological distress; I, intrusiveness; A, auditory perception difficulties; SI, sleep disturbances; SO, somatic complaints.

TABLE 6 | Correlation between tinnitus and health-related quality of life *12 months after* cochlear implantation.

			NCIQ1	NCIQ2	NCIQ3	NCIQ4	NCIQ5	NCIQ6	NCIQ total
Spearman-Rho	TQ E	Correlation coefficient	−0.377*	−0.545**	−0.362*	−0.329*	−0.409**	−0.386*	−0.400*
		Significance	0.018	0.000	0.024	0.041	0.010	0.015	0.010
		N	39	39	39	39	39	39	40
	TQ C	Correlation coefficient *t*	−0.505**	−0.593**	−0.372*	−0.408**	−0.477**	−0.447**	−0.488**
		Significance	0.001	0.000	0.020	0.010	0.002	0.004	0.001
		N	39	39	39	39	39	39	40
	TQ E + C	Correlation coefficient	−0.424**	−0.558**	−0.368*	−0.340*	−0.414**	−0.402*	−0.424**
		Significance	0.007	0.000	0.021	0.034	0.009	0.011	0.006
		N	39	39	39	39	39	39	40
	TQ I	Correlation coefficient	−0.454**	−0.598**	−0.490**	−0.332*	−0.472**	−0.446**	−0.490**
		Sig. (2-seitig)	0.004	0.000	0.002	0.039	0.002	0.004	0.001
		N	39	39	39	39	39	39	40
	TQ A	Correlation coefficient	−0.345*	−0.456**	−0.414**	−0.308	−0.348*	−0.306	−0.385*
		Significance	0.032	0.004	0.009	0.056	0.030	0.058	0.014
		N	39	39	39	39	39	39	40
	TQ SI	Correlation coefficient	−0.339*	−0.401*	−0.332*	−0.254	−0.350*	−0.307	−0.314*
		Significance	0.035	0.011	0.039	0.119	0.029	0.057	0.048
		N	39	39	39	39	39	39	40
	TQ SO	Correlation coefficient	−0.309	−0.356*	−0.331*	−0.323*	−0.358*	−0.433**	−0.312*
		Significance	0.056	0.026	0.039	0.045	0.025	0.006	0.050
		N	39	39	39	39	39	39	40
	TQ total	Correlation coefficient	−0.404*	−0.531**	−0.408**	−0.323*	−0.411**	−0.403*	−0.417**
		Significance	0.011	0.001	0.010	0.045	0.009	0.011	0.007
		N	39	39	39	39	39	39	40

$^*p \leq 0.05$.
$^{**}p \leq 0.01$.
Subscales of Nijmegen Cochlear Implantation Questionnaire (NCIQ): 1 basic sound perception; 2 advanced sound perception; 3 speech production; 4 self-esteem; 5 activity; and 6 social interactions.
Subscales of Tinnitus Questionnaire (TQ): E, emotional distress; C, cognitive distress; E + C, combined psychological distress; I, intrusiveness; A, auditory perception difficulties; SI, sleep disturbances; SO, somatic complaints.

TABLE 7 | Correlation between tinnitus and health-related quality of life *24 months after* cochlear implantation.

			NCIQ1	NCIQ2	NCIQ3	NCIQ4	NCIQ5	NCIQ6	NCIQ total
Spearman-Rho	TQ E	Correlation coefficient	−0.416**	−0.499**	−0.358*	−0.174	−0.384*	−0.346*	−0.328*
		Significance	0.008	0.001	0.023	0.282	0.014	0.029	0.039
		N	40	40	40	40	40	40	40
	TQ C	Correlation coefficient *t*	−0.408**	−0.452**	−0.359*	−0.170	−0.341*	−0.277	−0.353*
		Significance	0.009	0.003	0.023	0.296	0.031	0.084	0.026
		N	40	40	40	40	40	40	40
	TQ E + C	Correlation coefficient	−0.406**	−0.474**	−0.362*	−0.165	−0.351*	−0.308	−0.327*
		Significance	0.009	0.002	0.022	0.308	0.026	0.053	0.039
		N	40	40	40	40	40	40	40
	TQ I	Correlation coefficient	−0.434**	−0.496**	−0.357*	−0.215	−0.411**	−0.351*	−0.339*
		Sig. (2-seitig)	0.005	0.001	0.024	0.183	0.008	0.026	0.032
		N	40	40	40	40	40	40	40
	TQ A	Correlation coefficient	−0.301	−0.462**	−0.439**	−0.135	−0.393*	−0.280	−0.257
		Significance	0.060	0.003	0.005	0.405	0.012	0.080	0.109
		N	40	40	40	40	40	40	40
	TQ SI	Correlation coefficient	−0.415**	−0.434**	−0.522**	−0.176	−0.385*	−0.277	−0.396*
		Significance	0.008	0.005	0.001	0.278	0.014	0.083	0.011
		N	40	40	40	40	40	40	40
	TQ SO	Correlation coefficient	−0.413**	−0.460**	−0.357*	−0.210	−0.409**	−0.355*	−0.371*
		Significance	0.008	0.003	0.024	0.194	0.009	0.025	0.019
		N	40	40	40	40	40	40	40
	TQ total	Correlation coefficient	−0.419**	−0.526**	−0.416**	−0.169	−0.372*	−0.311	−0.334*
		Significance	0.007	0.000	0.008	0.297	0.018	0.051	0.035
		N	40	40	40	40	40	40	40

$^*p \leq 0.05$.
$^{**}p \leq 0.01$.
Subscales of Nijmegen Cochlear Implantation Questionnaire (NCIQ): 1 basic sound perception; 2 advanced sound perception; 3 speech production; 4 self-esteem; 5 activity; and 6 social interactions.
Subscales of Tinnitus Questionnaire (TQ): E, emotional distress; C, cognitive distress; E + C, combined psychological distress; I, intrusiveness; A, auditory perception difficulties; SI, sleep disturbances; SO, somatic complaints.

suggesting that the tinnitus-related emotional and cognitive distress as well as tinnitus-related auditory difficulties negatively influenced the life quality of the CI patients. Longer follow-up time should clarify if these correlations decay completely with time.

Before the CI, patients' quality of life (total score) was not affected by the tinnitus-induced auditory difficulties (**Table 4**) confirming our earlier observations (13). Six months after implantation, there was a large (Rho = −0.449) and significant (p = 0.003) negative correlation between these two variables (**Table 5**), very likely reflecting the fact that the process of regaining auditory abilities can be negatively affected by the tinnitus percept. In fact, this correlation and its significance declined 12 months after CI (Rho = −0.385, p = 0.014) (**Table 6**) and were no longer of significance 24 months after the surgery (**Table 7**).

Tinnitus is a complaint of 70–90% of hearing-impaired patients (12–14). In cases of patients who are bilaterally hard of hearing, tinnitus percept is a particularly disturbing symptom, because it is the only auditory input perceived by patients. In such cases, diverting the auditory attention from tinnitus to other sounds is problematic, making the therapeutic approaches difficult if not impossible. The two major therapies globally used for tinnitus treatment are tinnitus retraining therapy (TRT) and cognitive behavioral therapy (CBT). The neurophysiological model proposed by Jastreboff (27, 28) suggests the existence of auditory–limbic–sympathetic network responsible for negative effects of tinnitus sound and inducing the distress and inability to divert the attention of patients from the tinnitus sound. TRT, designed by Jastreboff based on the above theory, has since years been a frequent therapeutic choice of many clinicians (29–31). The second method widely used for tinnitus is the CBT, which was developed to treat anxiety disorders, depression, eating disorders, chronic low back pain, personality disorders, depression, and anxiety and successfully applied in the treatment for tinnitus (32–35). TRT, CBT, or a combination of both require at least some hearing abilities and can only be used to treat the patients who are hard of hearing *and* have tinnitus following successful auditory rehabilitation with CI.

The first positive effect of CI on tinnitus was reported in 1976 by House (15). Ever since, various studies with different sample sizes and inclusion criteria were performed. Corroborating our present results, the decrease of tinnitus-related distress after CI ranging from 46 to 95% was observed previously by others (12, 36, 37). In our present study, we also observed the reduction of tinnitus-related distress in half of the patients who had severe (decompensated) tinnitus prior to CI.

The central question addressing the mechanism in which CI reduces tinnitus-related distress remains open. The evidence collected in our present study suggests following possible scenarios:

- Following CI, the auditory abilities improve to the degree where the patients can focus their auditory attention on sounds other than tinnitus.
- Following CI, the improved auditory abilities increase the quality of life, thus decrease overall stress and positively affect the loop "stress-tinnitus."
- Following CI, the direct electrical stimulation of the auditory nerve induces plastic changes in the auditory reducing the tinnitus percept.

More quality evidence needs to be accumulated to determine, which of the presented scenarios is essential for tinnitus reduction after CI. It can also not be excluded that all three mechanisms play a role in tinnitus reduction and habituation. Future trials with specific tinnitus-oriented fitting of cochlear implants could shed more light on that topic.

While until recently, the clinical research involving cochlear implants was focused mainly on the audiological gain; at present, many authors are increasingly interested in changes of the quality of life and tinnitus-related distress (12, 38, 39). Quaranta et al. reported bilateral disappearance of tinnitus after unilateral CI in 65.8% of the patients (40), as measured by the Tinnitus Handicap Inventory—an instrument that is similar—but not identical—to TQ (41). Also, we have demonstrated earlier that the CI, in addition to having positive effect on hearing abilities, improves the life quality and decreases the tinnitus-related distress and psychological comorbidities (13, 42–45). There are several psychometric instruments measuring various parameters and domains used in tinnitus research and clinical routine. These instruments vary depending on the clinical orientation of the treating unit (audiology, ORL, clinical psychology or psychosomatic medicine) and on the country. Here, we propose creation of a specific set of standardized, validated, and internationally available instruments to measure CI-specific outcomes, which would include various aspects of tinnitus percept and tinnitus-related distress. In our present work, we used instruments that are widely available in the German-speaking countries. The Nijmegen Cochlear Implant Questionnaire NCIQ is an internationally validated, disease-specific instrument created for the assessment of the quality of life in patients with cochlear implants. OI is a popular, standardized instrument measuring perceived benefit of hearing aids. Also, the German version of TQ, which measures the tinnitus-related distress, is frequently used in the inpatient and outpatient settings to monitor the severity of tinnitus and its response to treatment. In order to study the influence of tinnitus on the outcome of CI, we suggest designing prospective, longitudinal clinical trials and using defined monitoring batch. Despite using such design, our present study is not free of pitfalls, as it could have included larger sample, and it was neither double blinded nor randomized. In addition, an appropriate control group is lacking. However, blinded and randomized design in the field of cochlear implant is difficult to be implemented because of specific features of the CI treatment, preventing the design of high-level evidence studies (19). Control group, which for instance could comprise patients who were implanted but their cochlear implants remain switched off, cannot be used because of obvious ethical reasons.

Previously reported high prevalence of tinnitus in the hearing-impaired patients puts the choice of tinnitus treatment in these patients up for discussion (12). In particular, the task of developing appropriate approach for the tinnitus treatment in bilaterally hearing-impaired patients remains open. The increasing incidence of hearing impairments, including the age-related hearing loss in context of demographic changes in our society, emphasizes the need for improvement in the therapy guidelines (46).

In addition, although we observed the most pronounced decrease of tinnitus-related distress 12 months after the implantation, the maximal correlation between TQ score and speech recognition (**Table 3**) occurred 6 months after implantation. These results do not contradict each other; rather, they point at the dependence of auditory rehabilitation on tinnitus treatment. Since the auditory benefit is patient specific, it is difficult to measure. Speech recognition—a typical parameter that measures hearing improvement—when used alone is not enough to act as an adequate indicator of tinnitus suppression. This is reflected by the results obtained 2 years after CI. Similarly, the TQ scores suggest that a unilateral acoustic stimulation with noticeable postoperative asymmetry does not lead to an unfavorable influence on the tinnitus-related distress, even over several years. The bilateral CI could be an ultimate target of hearing rehabilitation. In fact, sustained improvement of TQ scores was observed in 40 patients subjected to sequential bilateral CI (25).

Final Conclusion

Taken together, our results suggest that patients who are bilaterally hard of hearing and have tinnitus profit from CI not only by regaining their auditory skills but also by a significant and sustained improvement of the HRQoL and reduction of tinnitus-related distress. Moreover, the negative correlation between tinnitus and the HRQoL indicates the importance of tinnitus as an obstacle in auditory rehabilitation of CI patients. It is tempting to speculate that therapy for tinnitus used after CI would further decrease tinnitus-related distress and, therefore, could increase the quality of life in this specific group of patients.

ETHICS STATEMENT

The local Ethics Committee (permit number EA2/030/13) approved this prospective, non-interventional, and longitudinal study. All investigations were conducted according to the principles expressed in the Declaration of Helsinki. All patients have given their informed written consent.

AUTHOR CONTRIBUTIONS

SK and HO designed the study. SK, SG, and SH collected the data. SK, AS, and HO interpreted the data. SK and AS drafted the manuscript. HO critically revised the manuscript.

FUNDING

This study was funded by the internal Charité University Hospital Research Fund.

REFERENCES

Axelsson A, Sandh A. Tinnitus in noise-induced hearing loss. *Br J Audiol* (1985) 19:271–6. doi:10.3109/03005368509078983

Griest SE, Bishop PM. Tinnitus as an early indicator of permanent hearing loss. A 15 year longitudinal study of noise exposed workers. *AAOHN J* (1998) 46:325–9.

Mazurek B, Olze H, Haupt H, Szczepek AJ. The more the worse: the grade of noise-induced hearing loss associates with the severity of tinnitus. *Int J Environ Res Public Health* (2010) 7:3071–9. doi:10.3390/ijerph7083071

Saltzman M, Ersner MS. A hearing aid for the relief of tinnitus aurium. *Laryngoscope* (1947) 57:358–66. doi:10.1288/00005537-194705000-00005

Hoare DJ, Edmondson-Jones M, Sereda M, Akeroyd MA, Hall D. Amplification with hearing aids for patients with tinnitus and co-existing hearing loss. *Cochrane Database Syst Rev* (2014) (1):CD010151. doi:10.1002/14651858.CD010151.pub2

Fujimoto C, Ito K, Takano S, Karino S, Iwasaki S. Successful cochlear implantation in a patient with bilateral progressive sensorineural hearing loss after traumatic subarachnoid hemorrhage and brain contusion. *Ann Otol Rhinol Laryngol* (2007) 116:897–901. doi:10.1177/000348940711601205

Suzuki Y, Ogawa H, Baba Y, Suzuki T, Yamada N, Omori K. Cochlear implantation in a case of bilateral sensorineural hearing loss due to mumps. *Fukushima J Med Sci* (2009) 55:32–8. doi:10.5387/fms.55.32

Greenberg SL, Shipp D, Lin VY, Chen JM, Nedzelski JM. Cochlear implantation in patients with bilateral severe sensorineural hearing loss after major blunt head trauma. *Otol Neurotol* (2011) 32:48–54. doi:10.1097/MAO.0b013e3181ff73fd

Aoki M, Tanahashi S, Mizuta K, Kato H. Treatment for progressive hearing loss due to Paget's disease of bone – a case report and literature review. *J Int Adv Otol* (2015) 11:267–70. doi:10.5152/iao.2015.1572

Ramakers GG, Van Zon A, Stegeman I, Grolman W. The effect of cochlear implantation on tinnitus in patients with bilateral hearing loss: a systematic review. *Laryngoscope* (2015) 125:2584–92. doi:10.1002/lary.25370

Lin FR, Niparko JK, Ferrucci L. Hearing loss prevalence in the United States. *Arch Intern Med* (2011) 171:1851–2. doi:10.1001/archinternmed.2011.506

Baguley DM, Atlas MD. Cochlear implants and tinnitus. *Prog Brain Res* (2007) 166:347–55. doi:10.1016/S0079-6123(07)66033-6

Olze H, Szczepek AJ, Haupt H, Forster U, Zirke N, Grabel S, et al. Cochlear implantation has a positive influence on quality of life, tinnitus, and psychological comorbidity. *Laryngoscope* (2011) 121:2220–7. doi:10.1002/lary.22145

Olze H, Szczepek AJ, Haupt H, Zirke N, Graebel S, Mazurek B. The impact of cochlear implantation on tinnitus, stress and quality of life in postlingually deafened patients. *Audiol Neurootol* (2012) 17:2–11. doi:10.1159/000323847

House WF. Cochlear implants. *Ann Otol Rhinol Laryngol* (1976) 85:3–93. doi:10.1177/00034894760850S303

Thedinger B, House WF, Edgerton BJ. Cochlear implant for tinnitus. Case reports. *Ann Otol Rhinol Laryngol* (1985) 94:10–3. doi:10.1177/000348948509400102

House D. Tinnitus suppression via cochlear implants: review and remarks. *Int Tinnitus J* (1999) 5:27–9.

Arts RA, George EL, Stokroos RJ, Vermeire K. Review: cochlear implants as a treatment of tinnitus in single-sided deafness. *Curr Opin Otolaryngol Head Neck Surg* (2012) 20:398–403. doi:10.1097/MOO.0b013e3283577b66

Van Zon A, Peters JP, Stegeman I, Smit AL, Grolman W. Cochlear implantation for patients with single-sided deafness or asymmetrical hearing loss: a systematic review of the evidence. *Otol Neurotol* (2015) 36:209–19. doi:10.1097/MAO.0000000000000681

Hall DA, Haider H, Szczepek AJ, Lau P, Rabau S, Jones-Diette J, et al. Systematic review of outcome domains and instruments used in clinical trials of tinnitus treatments in adults. *Trials* (2016) 17:270. doi:10.1186/s13063-016-1399-9

Gordon KA, Jiwani S, Papsin BC. Benefits and detriments of unilateral cochlear implant use on bilateral auditory development in children who are deaf. *Front Psychol* (2013) 4:719. doi:10.3389/fpsyg.2013.00719

Gartrell BC, Jones HG, Kan A, Buhr-Lawler M, Gubbels SP, Litovsky RY. Investigating long-term effects of cochlear implantation in single-sided deafness: a best practice model for longitudinal assessment of spatial hearing abilities and tinnitus handicap. *Otol Neurotol* (2014) 35:1525–32. doi:10.1097/ MAO.0000000000000437

Ramos Macias A, Falcon Gonzalez JC, Manrique M, Morera C, Garcia-Ibanez L, Cenjor C, et al. Cochlear implants as a treatment option for unilateral hearing loss, severe tinnitus and hyperacusis. *Audiol Neurootol* (2015) 20(Suppl 1): 60–6. doi:10.1159/000380750

Hirschfelder A, Grabel S, Olze H. The impact of cochlear implantation on quality of life: the role of audiologic performance and variables. *Otolaryngol Head Neck Surg* (2008) 138:357–62. doi:10.1016/j.otohns.2007.10.019

Olze H, Grabel S, Haupt H, Forster U, Mazurek B. Extra benefit of a second cochlear implant with respect to health-related quality of life and tinnitus. *Otol Neurotol* (2012) 33:1169–75. doi:10.1097/MAO.0b013e31825e799f

Goebel G, Hiller W. [The Tinnitus Questionnaire. A standard instrument for grading the degree of tinnitus. Results of a multicenter study with the Tinnitus Questionnaire]. *HNO* (1994) 42:166–72.

Jastreboff PJ. Phantom auditory perception (tinnitus): mechanisms of generation and perception. *Neurosci Res* (1990) 8:221–54. doi:10.1016/0168-0102(90)90031-9

Jastreboff PJ, Hazell JW, Graham RL. Neurophysiological model of tinnitus: dependence of the minimal masking level on treatment outcome. *Hear Res* (1994) 80:216–32. doi:10.1016/0378-5955(94)90113-9

Kroener-Herwig B, Biesinger E, Gerhards F, Goebel G, Verena Greimel K, Hiller W. Retraining therapy for chronic tinnitus. A critical analysis of its status. *Scand Audiol* (2000) 29:67–78. doi:10.1080/010503900424471

Bartnik G, Fabijańska A, Rogowski M. Effects of tinnitus retraining therapy (TRT) for patients with tinnitus and subjective hearing loss versus tinnitus only. *Scand Audiol* (2001) 30(Suppl 52):206–8. doi:10.1080/010503901300007542

Seydel C, Haupt H, Szczepek AJ, Hartmann A, Rose M, Mazurek B. Three years later: report on the state of well-being of patients with chronic tinnitus who underwent modified tinnitus retraining therapy. *Audiol Neurootol* (2015) 20:26–38. doi:10.1159/000363728

Andersson G. Psychological aspects of tinnitus and the application of cognitive-behavioral therapy. *Clin Psychol Rev* (2002) 22:977–90. doi:10.1016/S0272-7358(01)00124-6

Hesser H, Weise C, Westin VZ, Andersson G. A systematic review and meta-analysis of randomized controlled trials of cognitive-behavioral ther- apy for tinnitus distress. *Clin Psychol Rev* (2011) 31:545–53. doi:10.1016/j.cpr.2010.12.006

Jun HJ, Park MK. Cognitive behavioral therapy for tinnitus: evidence and efficacy. *Korean J Audiol* (2013) 17:101–4. doi:10.7874/kja.2013.17.3.101

Zenner HP, Vonthein R, Zenner B, Leuchtweis R, Plontke SK, Torka W, et al. Standardized tinnitus-specific individual cognitive-behavioral therapy: a controlled outcome study with 286 tinnitus patients. *Hear Res* (2013) 298:117–25. doi:10.1016/j.heares.2012.11.013

Quaranta N, Wagstaff S, Baguley DM. Tinnitus and cochlear implantation. *Int J Audiol* (2004) 43:245–51. doi:10.1080/14992020400050033

Pan T, Tyler RS, Ji H, Coelho C, Gehringer AK, Gogel SA. Changes in the tinnitus handicap questionnaire after cochlear implantation. *Am J Audiol* (2009) 18:144–51. doi:10.1044/1059-0889(2009/07-0042)

Andersson G, Freijd A, Baguley DM, Idrizbegovic E. Tinnitus distress, anxiety, depression, and hearing problems among cochlear implant patients with tinnitus. *J Am Acad Audiol* (2009) 20:315–9. doi:10.3766/jaaa.20.5.5

Contrera KJ, Betz J, Li L, Blake CR, Sung YK, Choi JS, et al. Quality of life after intervention with a cochlear implant or hearing aid. *Laryngoscope* (2016) 126:2110–5. doi:10.1002/lary.25848

Quaranta N, Fernandez-Vega S, D'elia C, Filipo R, Quaranta A. The effect of unilateral multichannel cochlear implant on bilaterally perceived tinnitus. *Acta Otolaryngol* (2008) 128:159–63. doi:10.1080/00016480701387173

Zeman F, Koller M, Schecklmann M, Langguth B, Landgrebe M; TRI Database Study Group. Tinnitus assessment by means of standardized self-report questionnaires: psychometric properties of the Tinnitus Questionnaire (TQ), the Tinnitus Handicap Inventory (THI), and their short versions in an inter- national and multi-lingual sample. *Health Qual Life Outcomes* (2012) 10:128. doi:10.1186/1477-7525-10-128

Olze H, Grabel S, Forster U, Zirke N, Huhnd LE, Haupt H, et al. Elderly patients benefit from cochlear implantation regarding auditory rehabilitation, quality of life, tinnitus, and stress. *Laryngoscope* (2012) 122:196–203. doi:10.1002/lary.22356

Bruggemann P, Szczepek AJ, Rose M, Mckenna L, Olze H, Mazurek B. Impact of multiple factors on the degree of tinnitus distress. *Front Hum Neurosci* (2016) 10:341. doi:10.3389/fnhum.2016.00341

Knopke S, Grabel S, Forster-Ruhrmann U, Mazurek B, Szczepek AJ, Olze H. Impact of cochlear implantation on quality of life and mental comorbidity in patients aged 80 years. *Laryngoscope* (2016) 126:2811–6. doi:10.1002/lary.25993

Olze H, Knopke S, Grabel S, Szczepek AJ. Rapid positive influence of cochlear implantation on the quality of life in adults 70 years and older. *Audiol Neurootol* (2016) 21(Suppl 1):43–7. doi:10.1159/000448354

Davis A, Mcmahon CM, Pichora-Fuller KM, Russ S, Lin F, Olusanya BO, et al. Aging and hearing health: the life-course approach. *Gerontologist* (2016) 56(Suppl 2):S256–67. doi:10.1093/geront/gnw033

19

Innovations in Doctoral Training and Research on Tinnitus: The European School on Interdisciplinary Tinnitus Research (ESIT) Perspective

*Winfried Schlee[1†], Deborah A. Hall[2, 3†], Barbara Canlon[4], Rilana F. F. Cima[5], Emile de Kleine[6], Franz Hauck[7], Alex Huber[8], Silvano Gallus[9], Tobias Kleinjung[8], Theodore Kypraios[2], Berthold Langguth[1], José A. Lopez-Escamez[10, 11], Alessandra Lugo[9], Martin Meyer[12], Marzena Mielczarek[13], Arnaud Norena[14], Flurin Pfiffner[8], Rüdiger C. Pryss[15], Manfred Reichert[15], Teresa Requena[10], Martin Schecklmann[1], Pim van Dijk[6], Paul van de Heyning[16], Nathan Weisz[17] and Christopher R. Cederroth[4]**

[1] Department of Psychiatry and Psychotherapy of the University of Regensburg at Bezirksklinikum Regensburg, University of Regensburg, Regensburg, Germany, [2] NIHR Nottingham Hearing Biomedical Research Centre, Nottingham, United Kingdom, [3] Otology and Hearing Group, Division of Clinical Neuroscience, School of Medicine, University of Nottingham, Nottingham, United Kingdom, [4] Section of Experimental Audiology, Department of Physiology and Pharmacology, Karolinska Institutet, Stockholm, Sweden, [5] Clinical Psychological Science, Faculty of Psychology and Neuroscience, Maastricht University, Maastricht, Netherlands, [6] Department of Otorhinolaryngology/Head and Neck Surgery, University Medical Center Groningen, University of Groningen, Groningen, Netherlands, [7] Institute of Distributed Systems Ulm University, Ulm, Germany, [8] Department of Otorhinolaryngology, Head and Neck Surgery, University Hospital of Zurich, University of Zurich, Zurich, Switzerland, [9] Department of Environmental Health Sciences, IRCCS - Istituto di Ricerche Farmacologiche Mario Negri, Milan, Italy, [10] Otology and Neurotology Group, Department of Genomic Medicine, Centro Pfizer – Universidad de Granada – Junta de Andalucía de Genómica e Investigación Oncológica (GENYO), Granada, Spain, [11] Department of Otolaryngology, Instituto de Investigación Biosanitaria ibs.GRANADA, Hospital Universitario Virgen de las Nieves, Universidad de Granada, Granada, Spain, [12] Neuroplasticity and Learning in the Healthy Aging Brain (HAB LAB), Department of Psychology, University of Zurich, Zurich, Switzerland, [13] Department of Otolaryngology, Laryngological Oncology, Audiology, and Phoniatrics, Medical University of Lodz, Lodz, Poland, [14] Centre National de la Recherche Scientifique, Aix-Marseille University, Marseille, France, [15] Institute of Databases and Information Systems, Ulm University, Ulm, Germany, [16] Department of ORL and Head and Neck Surgery, Antwerp University Hospital, University of Antwerp, Antwerp, Belgium, [17] Division of Physiological Psychology, Centre for Cognitive Neuroscience, University of Salzburg, Salzburg, Austria

***Correspondence:**
Christopher R. Cederroth
christopher.cederroth@ki.se
[†]*Shared first authors.*

Tinnitus is a common medical condition which interfaces many different disciplines, yet it is not a priority for any individual discipline. A change in its scientific understanding and clinical management requires a shift toward multidisciplinary cooperation, not only in research but also in training. The European School for Interdisciplinary Tinnitus research (ESIT) brings together a unique multidisciplinary consortium of clinical practitioners, academic researchers, commercial partners, patient organizations, and public health experts to conduct innovative research and train the next generation of tinnitus researchers. ESIT supports fundamental science and clinical research projects in order to: (1) advancing new treatment solutions for tinnitus, (2) improving existing treatment paradigms, (3) developing innovative research methods, (4) performing genetic studies on, (5) collecting epidemiological data to create new knowledge about prevalence and risk factors, (6) establishing a pan-European data resource. All research projects involve inter-sectoral partnerships through practical training, quite unlike anything that can be offered by any single university alone. Likewise, the postgraduate training curriculum fosters a deep knowledge about tinnitus whilst nurturing transferable competencies in personal qualities and approaches needed to be an effective researcher, knowledge of the standards, requirements and professionalism to do research, and skills to work with others and to ensure the wider impact of research. ESIT is the seed for future generations of creative, entrepreneurial, and innovative researchers, trained to master the upcoming challenges in the tinnitus field, to implement sustained changes in prevention and clinical management of tinnitus, and to shape doctoral education in tinnitus for the future.

Keywords: tinnitus, education, medical, hearing, PhD studentship, heterogeneity of tinnitus

BACKGROUND

Tinnitus is a condition associated with a continuous auditory percept in the ears or head and can arise as a symptom of many different medical disorders. Assuming a conservative tinnitus prevalence of 10% (1% of severe tinnitus; McCormack et al., 2016) for the 425 million adults living within the European Union (EU), tinnitus affects more than 42 million citizens and is experienced as a severe problem by more than 4 million. Moreover, incidence of new cases is expected to grow over the next few decades (Nondahl et al., 2002, 2010). Although much progress has been made in understanding the pathophysiology (Langguth et al., 2013; Elgoyhen et al., 2015), tinnitus remains a scientific and clinical enigma (Baguley et al., 2013). Unfortunately, tinnitus remains an unmet clinical need and complaining patients are often told "to live with it" (Cederroth et al., 2013). The condition is very common and of varying severity, but the fundamental mechanisms of tinnitus are still incompletely understood. Although not all individuals are unduly troubled, many find the disorder life-changing. In cases with severe tinnitus, mental disorders, and symptoms such as anxiety, depression, insomnia, and concentration problems can impair quality of life often to a level that leads to sick leave and disability pension (Friberg et al., 2012). Therefore, severe tinnitus contributes to a substantial cost to health care and to society at large. In the Netherlands alone, the economic burden of tinnitus is estimated at up to €10.8 billion, with the greater impact being related to socio-economic factors (Maes et al., 2013). The health care costs are enormous. In England there are 750,000 medical consultations yearly with the primary complaint of tinnitus (El-Shunnar et al., 2011).

There is no licensed pharmacological therapy and there is little high quality evidence for the success of palliative management strategies. The Cochrane Library currently lists 9 completed systematic reviews on different tinnitus treatments; namely Tinnitus Retraining Therapy (TRT), Cognitive Behavioral Therapy (CBT), hyperbaric oxygen therapy, sound therapy (masking), hearing aids, repetitive transcranial magnetic stimulation (rTMS), ginkgo biloba, anticonvulsants, and antidepressants (Phillips and McFerran, 2010; Hoekstra et al., 2011; Meng et al., 2011; Baldo et al., 2012; Bennett et al., 2012; Hobson et al., 2012; Hilton et al., 2013; Espinosa-Sánchez et al., 2014; Hoare et al., 2014; Person et al., 2016). However, no uniformly effective treatment for tinnitus has yet been identified. Two main reasons have been discussed: (1) methodological limitations in study design with a paucity of Randomized Controlled Trials (RCTs) and no consensus about what and how to measure therapeutic outcome (Hall et al., 2016), and (2) a large heterogeneity in the patient population with respect to etiology, genetic, and clinical phenotype (Elgoyhen et al., 2015).

Tinnitus is a symptom rather than a distinct disease, and its multivariate manifestations can be subtyped according to various dimensions such as its etiology, time since onset, perceptual characteristics (i.e., pitch, loudness, location, and temporal dynamics), perceived emotional distress, and comorbidities. Progress in scientific understanding and clinical management needs to first address this heterogeneity by identifying scientifically and clinically meaningful subtypes of the condition. Subtyping can then guide the definition of relevant inclusion/exclusion criteria in clinical research and of stratification variables for allocating patients to different intervention groups in RCTS. Subtyping can also guide more sophisticated methods of multivariate data analysis than have been applied hitherto. Current knowledge about etiology, perceptual characteristics, and the neurobiological correlates of tinnitus is not sufficient to enable effective subtyping (Lopez-Escamez et al., 2016). These problems are indicating the need for new approaches.

AN INTERDISCIPLINARY APPROACH IS CRITICAL

Across the EU, no single healthcare system, research organization, or commercial enterprise has an adequate coverage of all relevant issues related to tinnitus and this has resulted in a patchwork of approaches without any coherent framework. Clinically speaking, tinnitus is managed by a variety of different practitioners including general practitioners, otologists, audiologists, psychologists, psychiatrists, neurologists, physical therapists, and dentists (Hall et al., 2011). Academically speaking, tinnitus is of interest to animal neurophysiologists, neuroscientists, epidemiologists, geneticists, trialists, biostatisticians, biomedical engineers, software engineers, and data mining experts. The European School on Interdisciplinary Tinnitus Research (ESIT) uniquely fosters an environment where knowledge and ideas are shared beyond current sectoral borders. The ESIT project provides an international interdisciplinary network of experts from these relevant disciplines working toward a coordinated approach to tinnitus research. Such a partnership is an essential part of the project. It will support data sharing and meta-analyses to gain new insights about tinnitus, to develop an evidence-based treatment protocol for effective personalized medicine and to identify new innovative treatment approaches.

ESIT MANAGEMENT AND PROJECT DETAILS

The ESIT project started on April 1, 2017 with an overall duration of 4 years. The 15 PhD start their work in October 2017. Each student receives funding for 3 years to undertake their PhD. In **Figure 1** we outline the work packages of the ESIT project. The first three work packages focus on the scientific goals, while work packages 4–7 concentrate on the effective management of the project (i.e., governance, recruitment and training, communications, and longer-term sustainability). The ESIT office is led by Schlee and based at the department of psychiatry and psychotherapy at the University Clinic Regensburg. More details about the ESIT project and the most recent achievements of the project can be found on the project website (www.esit.tinnitusresearch.net).

ESIT's INNOVATIVE PERSPECTIVE ON TINNITUS RESEARCH

ESIT is an EU-funded Marie Skłodowska-Curie Innovative Training Network with 12 top-level research institutions in 10 European countries, supporting 15 PhD projects. The research performed under ESIT will be geared toward a more personalized medicine approach, with improved diagnosis and selection of the best-suited therapy based on the individual patient profile. The 15 PhD projects will collectively address three major objectives that are managed under three research-specific work packages. In total, 2 clinics, 8 commercial enterprises, 2 patient organizations, 5 partner academic institutions, and 2 non-profit organizations are actively partnering in the projects and will support 2–3 month research secondments. Secondments are research visits or practical trainings with other academic institutions or industry partners to promote inter-sectoral exchange and embed a broader perspective into the research collaboration from the outset. Commercial partners will also share technological innovations for research purposes.

Research-specific work package 1. "meaningful individual differences" Co-ordinated by Lopez-Escamez, work package 1 seeks to determine meaningful individual differences in tinnitus by integrating knowledge and experience from all relevant clinical and scientific disciplines, and combining it with patient-centered and commercial perspectives. This will be achieved through interdisciplinary ESIT partnerships with the Meniere's Disease Society (patient organization), Tinnitus Research Initiative Foundation (non-profit research organization), Sensorion Pharmaceuticals (commercial sector), Julius Maximilian's University Würzburg, and the Knowledge Management and Discovery Laboratory at the Otto von Guericke University. Through this work package:

1a) ESIT will create a conceptual framework, as an end goal, that describes an individual's tinnitus profile. This framework will be based on multi-disciplinary data deposited in a centralized ESIT database that then enables the integration of common data variables gathered from all ESIT projects and data analyses targeted toward informing the tinnitus profile framework.

1b) ESIT will assess the genetic contribution to the development and maintenance of specific subtypes of tinnitus. This work will focus on whole-exome sequencing of people with tinnitus who do not have any detectable otological comorbidities, and of patients with Meniere's Disease and tinnitus.

1c) ESIT will identify factors of the individual tinnitus profile, which affect the general responsiveness to tinnitus treatment.

Research-specific work package 2. "novel personalized treatment solutions" Co-ordinated by Weisz, work package 2 seeks to develop novel personalized treatment solutions that respect each patient profile and integrate them with state-of-the-art technological innovations. This will be achieved through interdisciplinary ESIT partnerships with Sivantos, Cochlear Europe, Bee Group AG and Soterix Medical Inc. (commercial sector), and Del Bo Technologia per l'ascolto (independent clinic). Through this work package:

2a) ESIT takes advantage of recent technical developments to develop new, innovative treatment strategies by assessing the effectiveness of enhanced amplification or notched amplification around the frequency corresponding to the dominant tinnitus pitch, individual tomographic neurofeedback, and pseudo-monophasic extra-cochlear stimulation, and by identifying the best placement for an intracochlear microphone.

2b) ESIT seeks to improve existing, clinically well-established treatments by assessing Cognitive Behavior Therapy modified by classical learning, individualized transcranial electric stimulation, repetitive transcranial stimulation combined with auditory stimulation, and an optimized protocol for extra-cochlear electric stimulation.

2c) Using meta-analysis techniques, ESIT will identify the parameters of the individual tinnitus profile which optimize responsiveness to a particular treatment and will use these findings to develop a treatment guide.

Research-specific work package 3. "comparability of scientific and clinical results" Co-ordinated by Gallus, work package 3 seeks to promote international comparability of findings across all major relevant disciplines. This will be achieved through interdisciplinary ESIT partnerships with the British Tinnitus Association (patient organization), Brain Products (commercial sector), Nottingham University Hospitals NHS Trust (clinic), and the Institute of Computer Science, University of Tartu. Through this work package:

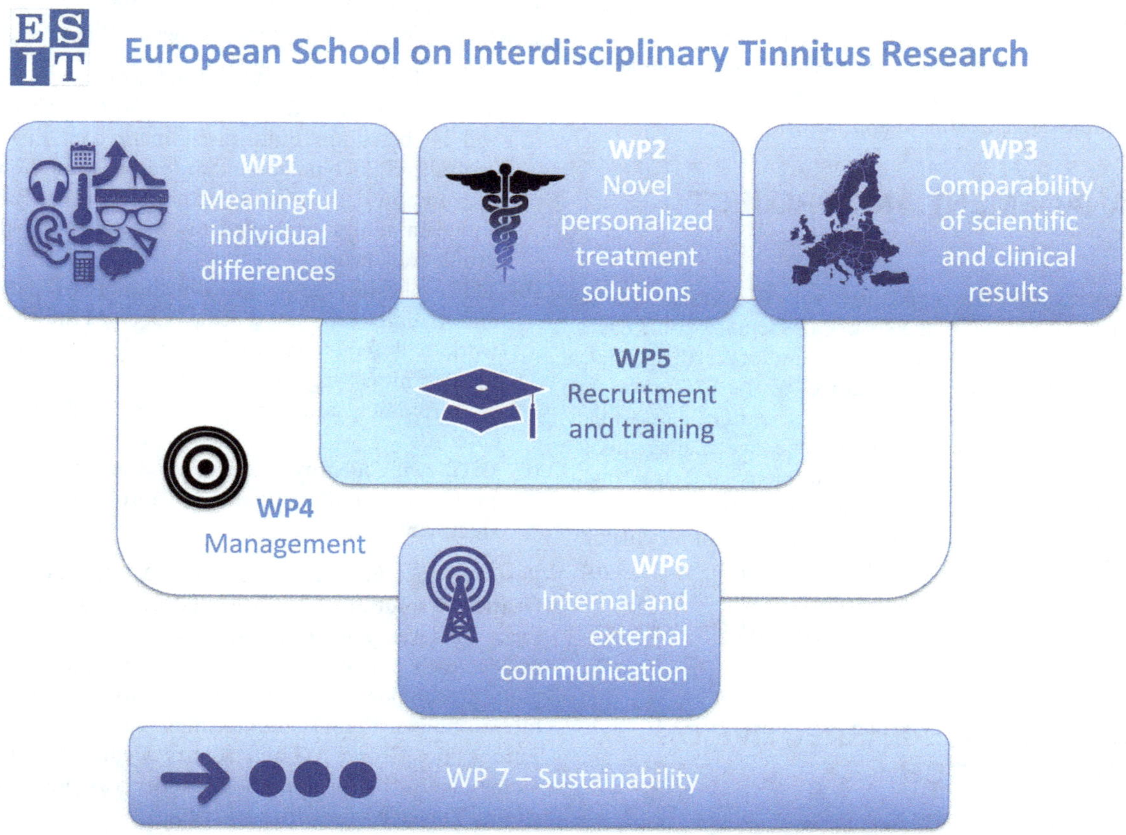

FIGURE 1 | The ESIT structure. Work packages 1–3 deliver the research projects, Work package 4 is to ensure the fluent and effective management of ESIT, Work package 5 is to coordinate the training and recruitment of the students, Work package 6 manages the internal and external communication, and Work package 7 ensures the sustainability of the ESIT achievements. Work packages 4–7 are led by the University of Regensburg, University of Nottingham, Karolinska Institute in Stockholm, and University of Regensburg, respectively.

3a) ESIT will standardize measurements used for diagnostic assessment and inclusion/exclusion criteria for research by developing an evidence-based protocol that will be thoroughly tested using analysis of empirical data, and collecting expert opinions, and patient experiences.
3b) ESIT will integrate large-scale patient data in a central database to support descriptive and inferential analyses.
3c) ESIT will create a standardized framework for collecting longitudinal tinnitus data by implementing novel methods for mobile data collection together with standard assessment tools for validating the crowd-sensing data.
3d) ESIT will collect population-based epidemiological data across many EU countries using the same standardized questions and response options.

This brief overview of the research projects illustrates how the ESIT consortium is characterized by interdisciplinary partnerships both within and across research-specific work packages 1-3. Many projects benefit from the exchange of measurement tools, data sharing, intersectoral knowledge transfer, and dissemination. The overall research program is designed to promote synergies between projects.

ESIT's INNOVATIVE PERSPECTIVE ON TINNITUS TRAINING

ESIT provides the first specialized doctoral curriculum on the topic of tinnitus. Acknowledging that "twenty-first century skills" require more than just knowledge building, ESIT PhD students will develop a balance of transferable competencies, as well as tinnitus-specific knowledge and skills (news feature 2015). In this sense it is unique. Each ESIT PhD student will actively manage his/her own dynamic Personal Career Development Plan. To do this we will promote the Vitae Researcher Development Framework Planner, which is a web-based application for mapping professional development (Vitae, 2017). The planner can be used to keep a unified record of all professional development activities, identify their current expertise and capabilities, record learning and development goals and monitor progress, and upload files such as CVs, conference details, and testimonials to record their personal achievements for lifelong learning. The planner uses the Vitae Researcher Development Framework, which considers four essential domains of learning and development and subdomains which inform the learning objectives of the ESIT training modules (**Figure 2**).

Research governance and organisation	Personal effectiveness
• Legal requirements • Risk management planning • Copyrights and IP Rights • Reporting guidelines and transparency in science • Good practice in publishing and openness in science • Writing successful grants	• Stories of female role models • Cross-cultural aspects, mobility and secondments • International networking • Personal effectiveness/career planning • Personal qualities, personal responsibility and self reflection
Engagement, influence and impact	**Knowledge and intellectual abilities**
• Clinical internship • National tinnitus strategies • What is important to people with tinnitus • Health-care sector engagement • "Keeping it real": Research impact • Public engagement • Mobile platforms for large-scale research • Entrepreneurship	• What is tinnitus? An overview of the state-of-the-art • Challenges for clinical practice • Methodological and technological innovations • Critical evaluation • Intellectual insight and argument construction • Master classes

FIGURE 2 | Overview of the ESIT training curriculum structured according to the Vitae Researcher Development Framework. The four essential domains of learning and development are given in the four squares, with individual training modules arranged below.

1. **Knowledge and intellectual abilities** To be able to work at the highest level, ESIT PhD students will gain a foundation-level, tinnitus-specific knowledge base, as well as exposure to critical evaluation, intellectual insight, and argument construction. All ESIT PhD students will receive scientific training in the structural and functional components of tinnitus, common diagnostic procedures, and the latest developments in technological innovations for tinnitus care.
2. **Personal effectiveness** Action learning opportunities will foster the personal qualities and approach necessary to become an effective researcher.
3. **Engagement, influence, and impact** Interactions with partners from across the clinical, charity, and commercial sectors will enhance the knowledge and skills that are important for working with others and ensure the wider impact of research.
4. **Research governance and organization** A series of lectures and workshops led by experts in the field will inform students about the standards, requirements, and professionalism to do research.

ESIT offers an innovative doctoral training program (see **Figure 2**) for ambitious young researchers and provides those PhD students with a set of unique academic, clinical, charity, and commercial sector experiences as well as learning opportunities that extend far beyond any typical academic training program. In the same way that all beneficiaries and most partner organizations are contributing to the research projects in work packages 1–3, work package 5 co-ordinated by Hall describes the training curriculum and the input from many of the ESIT consortium members. In total, 10 commercial enterprises, 6 patient and non-profit organizations, 6 partner academic institutions, 1 health authority and 11 independent clinics will provide practical training for the 15 ESIT students. Most training will be provided by ESIT training schools, satellite events at annual conferences and internet-based courses. Self-study will be guided by supervisors and coordinated and monitored by a Supervisory Board.

A prerequisite for impactful research is an awareness of real-world challenges in the tinnitus clinic. At the start of the program, all ESIT PhD students will complete a clinical internship whereby they will experience for 1 week the activities within a tinnitus clinic in a European country. They will meet with many tinnitus patients and tinnitus care providers, develop an appreciation of the symptoms and impact of tinnitus on the lives of real people, learn to understand the care system in the respective country, and critically evaluate the challenges in that system.

PLANNED MAJOR DISSEMINATION ACTIVITIES

Real-world development opportunities are afforded through several major dissemination activities. First, ESIT PhD students will write a special commissioned feature for publication in "ENT & Audiology News" magazine aimed at hearing healthcare professionals. Second, the ESIT network aims for a completely revised and updated 2nd edition of the "Textbook of Tinnitus" (Møller et al., 2011). The revised edition will be tailored toward becoming the number one choice as a textbook for doctoral and medical training in tinnitus. Other dissemination activities include an updated version of the Wikipedia page for "Tinnitus" (Wikipedia, 2017Q12), an educational video on tinnitus prepared in the major European languages, and dissemination of activities through social media channels. Dissemination will be coordinated by Cederroth, leader of the work package 6.

IMPACT ON CAREER PROSPECTS

To enable clinical relevance of academic research and its rapid translation into improved tinnitus healthcare, there is an urgent need for closer intersectoral collaboration. In conclusion, ESIT will achieve this by providing high-level training with a multidisciplinary supervisory team. The program will equip ESIT PhD students not only with a comprehensive understanding of the challenges faced by healthcare providers in treating tinnitus and by industry in providing technological healthcare solutions, but also to lay the foundations for leadership positions in the relevant academic and non-academic sectors. The network-integrated training program will ensure that the ESIT PhD student can effectively communicate between disciplines and will have the skills to identify synergistic opportunities, to build bridges between disciplines to exploit these connections, and to interact successfully with the private sector. Exposure across disciplines and sectors is unique and is essential to advance ESIT student personal career development and lead the students into European leadership positions in the future. In this way, ESIT will create a new generation of tinnitus experts who are sensitive to the issues of heterogeneity, have a broad knowledge base and have first-hand experience of the possibilities for inter-sectoral disciplines.

AUTHOR CONTRIBUTIONS

WS, DH, and CC drafted the initial version of the manuscript and created the figures. All authors contributed to the development of the ESIT project and contributed equally to all other stages of the manuscript development. All authors approved the manuscript.

FUNDING

This project has received funding from the European Union's Horizon 2020 research and innovation programme under the Marie Skłodowska-Curie grant agreement No 722046.

ACKNOWLEDGMENTS

ESIT derives from a current EU COST Action BM1306 (TINNET, 2014-2018)[1], whose main ambition is to understand the tinnitus heterogeneity. We thank the current 250 contributors to TINNET (www.tinnet.tinnitusresearch.net), and who made ESIT possible. The Tinnitus Research Initiative (TRI) Foundation financed and founded by Matteo de Nora has laid the groundwork for a multidisciplinary international research network from which the ESIT program developed.

[1] www.cost.eu/COST_Actions/bmbs/BM1306

REFERENCES

Baguley, D., McFerran, D., and Hall, D. (2013). Tinnitus. *Lancet* 382, 1600–1607. doi: 10.1016/S0140-6736(13)60142-7

Baldo, P., Doree, C., Molin, P., McFerran, D., and Cecco, S. (2012). Antidepressants for patients with tinnitus. *Cochrane Database Syst. Rev.* 12:CD003853. doi: 10.1002/14651858.CD003853.pub3

Bennett, M. H., Kertesz, T., Perleth, M., Yeung, P., and Lehm, J. P. (2012). Hyperbaric oxygen for idiopathic sudden sensorineural hearing loss and tinnitus. *Cochrane Database Syst. Rev.* 10:CD004739. doi: 10.1002/14651858.CD004739.pub4

Cederroth, C. R., Canlon, B., and Langguth, B. (2013). Hearing loss and tinnitus–are funders and industry listening? *Nat. Biotechnol.* 31, 972–974. doi: 10.1038/nbt.2736

Elgoyhen, A. B., Langguth, B., De Ridder, D., and Vanneste, S. (2015). Tinnitus: perspectives from human neuroimaging. *Nat. Rev. Neurosci.* 16, 632–642. doi: 10.1038/nrn4003

El-Shunnar, S. K., Hoare, D. J., Smith, S., Gander, P. E., Kang, S., Fackrell, K., et al. (2011). Primary care for tinnitus: practice and opinion among GPs in England. *J. Eval. Clin. Pract.* 17, 684–692. doi: 10.1111/j.1365-2753.2011.01696.x

Espinosa-Sánchez, J. M., Heitzmann-Hernández, T., and López-Escámez, J. A. (2014). [Pharmacotherapy for tinnitus: much ado about nothing]. *Rev. Neurol.* 59, 164–174.

Friberg, E., Jansson, C., Mittendorfer-Rutz, E., Rosenhall, U., and Alexanderson, K. (2012). Sickness absence due to otoaudiological diagnoses and risk of disability pension: a nationwide swedish prospective cohort study. *PLoS ONE* 7:e29966. doi: 10.1371/journal.pone.0029966

Hall, D. A., Haider, H., Szczepek, A. J., Lau, P., Rabau, S., Jones-Diette, J., et al. (2016). Systematic review of outcome domains and instruments used in clinical trials of tinnitus treatments in adults. *Trials* 17:270. doi: 10.1186/s13063-016-1399-9

Hall, D. A., Láinez, M. J., Newman, C. W., Sanchez, T. G., Egler, M., Tennigkeit, F., et al. (2011). Treatment options for subjective tinnitus: self reports from a sample of general practitioners and ENT physicians within Europe and the USA. *BMC Health Serv. Res.* 11:302. doi: 10.1186/1472-6963-11-302

Hilton, M. P., Zimmermann, E. F., and Hunt, W. T. (2013). Ginkgo biloba for tinnitus. *Cochrane Database Syst. Rev.* 28:CD003852. doi: 10.1002/14651858.CD003852.pub3

Hoare, D. J., Edmondson-Jones, M., Sereda, M., Akeroyd, M. A., and Hall, D. (2014). Amplification with hearing aids for patients with tinnitus and co-existing hearing loss. *Cochrane Database Syst. Rev.* 31:CD010151. doi: 10.1002/14651858.CD010151.pub2

Hobson, J., Chisholm, E., and El Refaie, A. (2012). Sound therapy (masking) in the management of tinnitus in adults. *Cochrane Database Syst. Rev.* 11:CD006371. doi: 10.1002/14651858.CD006371.pub3

Hoekstra, C. E., Rynja, S. P., van Zanten, G. A., and Rovers, M. M. (2011). Anticonvulsants for tinnitus. *Cochrane Database Syst. Rev.* 6:CD007960. doi: 10.1002/14651858.CD007960.pub2

Langguth, B., Kreuzer, P. M., Kleinjung, T., and De Ridder, D. (2013). Tinnitus: causes and clinical management. *Lancet Neurol.* 12, 920–930. doi: 10.1016/S1474-4422(13)70160-1

Lopez-Escamez, J. A., Bibas, T., Cima, R. F., Van de Heyning, P., Knipper, M., Mazurek, B., et al. (2016). Genetics of tinnitus: an emerging area for molecular diagnosis and drug development. *Front. Neurosci.* 10:377. doi: 10.3389/fnins.2016.00377

Maes, I. H., Cima, R. F., Vlaeyen, J. W., Anteunis, L. J., and Joore, M. A. (2013). Tinnitus: a cost study. *Ear. Hear.* 34, 508–514. doi: 10.1097/AUD.0b013e31827d113a

McCormack, A., Edmondson-Jones, M., Somerset, S., and Hall, D. (2016). A systematic review of the reporting of tinnitus prevalence and severity. *Hear. Res.* 337, 70–79. doi: 10.1016/j.heares.2016.05.009

Meng, Z., Liu, S., Zheng, Y., and Phillips, J. S. (2011). Repetitive transcranial magnetic stimulation for tinnitus. *Cochrane Database Syst. Rev.* 5:CD007946. doi: 10.1002/14651858.CD007946.pub2

Møller, A. R., Langguth, B., De Ridder, D., and Kleinjung, T. (2011). *Textbook of Tinnitus.* New York, NY: Springer.

Nondahl, D. M., Cruickshanks, K. J., Wiley, T. L., Klein, B. E., Klein, R., Chappell, R., et al. (2010). The ten-year incidence of tinnitus among older adults. *Int. J. Audiol.* 49, 580–585. doi: 10.3109/14992021003753508

Nondahl, D. M., Cruickshanks, K. J., Wiley, T. L., Klein, R., Klein, B. E., and Tweed, T. S. (2002). Prevalence and 5-year incidence of tinnitus among older adults: the epidemiology of hearing loss study. *J. Am. Acad. Audiol.* 13, 323–331.

Person, O. C., Puga, M. E., da Silva, E. M., and Torloni M. R. (2016). Zinc supplementation for tinnitus. *Cochrane Database Syst Rev.* 11:CD009832. doi: 10.1002/14651858.CD009832.pub2

Phillips, J. S., and McFerran, D. (2010). Tinnitus retraining therapy (TRT) for tinnitus. *Cochrane Database Syst. Rev.* 17:CD007330 doi: 10.1002/14651858.CD007330.pub2

Vitae (2017). *About the Vitae Researcher Development Framework Planner - Vitae Website.* Available online at: https://www.vitae.ac.uk/researchers-professional-development/about-the-vitae-researcher-development-framework-planner (Accessed December 31, 2017).

20

Management of Chronic Tinnitus and Insomnia with Repetitive Transcranial Magnetic Stimulation and Cognitive Behavioral Therapy – A Combined Approach

Kneginja Richter[1,2,3†], Jens Acker[4†], Lence Miloseva[3], Lukas Peter[1] and Günter Niklewski[1,3]*

[1] University Clinic for Psychiatry and Psychotherapy, Paracelsus Private Medical University, Nuremberg, Germany, [2] Faculty of Social Sciences, Georg Simon Ohm University of Applied Sciences, Nuremberg, Germany, [3] Faculty of Medicine Sciences, Goce Delcev University, Štip, Macedonia, [4] Clinic for Sleep Medicine Zurzach, Bad Zurzach, Switzerland

***Correspondence:**
Kneginja Richter
kneginja.richter@gmx.de

† These authors have contributed equally to this work.*

It has been estimated that up to 80% of people will experience symptoms of tinnitus over the courses of their lives, with rates of comorbid sleeping problems ranging from 50 to 77%. Because of a potential connection between tinnitus and sleep disorders as well as high rates of comorbid psychiatric disorders, interdisciplinary approaches to treatment seem to be the most efficient option. In this study, we present the case of a 53-year-old male patient, who started to experience symptoms of tinnitus at the age of 49, most likely caused by work-related stress. Over the course of his illness, the patient developed comorbid insomnia. He consulted us for treatment of both conditions and we developed a treatment plan with ten sessions of repetitive transcranial magnetic stimulation (rTMS) followed by 10 sessions of cognitive behavioral therapy (CBT). We used the *Tinnitus Fragebogen* (TF) to assess the severity of the tinnitus, the Beck Depression Inventory (BDI-II) for depressive symptoms, and the WHO Well-being Index (WHO-5) for subjective well-being. Improvements could be achieved with regard to both diagnoses and the patient went from severe (48) to clinically negligible (12) TF scores, from minimal (BDI-II score 10) to no (0) depressive symptoms, and from just above critical (WHO-5 percentile 52) to above average (84) well-being. The combination of technological and psychological approaches to treat tinnitus and insomnia thus proved successful in this case. One may therefore conclude that rTMS may be considered an effective first therapeutic step for tinnitus treatment prior to CBT. To our knowledge this is the first published case in which rTMS and CBT were combined for tinnitus therapy. The approach proved successful since it led to a considerable increase in well-being and everyday functioning. To gauge the effect on a more general level, large-scale studies are still needed to cancel out potential placebo effects. Likewise, the importance of the order of the two treatments, and the possibility of using other therapies in combination with CBT to address certain tinnitus subtypes and different etiologies must be studied in greater detail.

Keywords: tinnitus, insomnia, sleep, rTMS, CBT

INTRODUCTION

When the patient first consulted us for treatment at the interdisciplinary tinnitus clinic at Klinikum Nürnberg, we performed an ear-nose-throat examination, an assessment of his psychological-psychiatric state and a basic sleep examination. These resulted in the diagnosis of an ear noise that had been chronified for 4 years and not been treated in any way yet. The patient reported that he had noticed the ear noise for the first time in connection with high pressure in his job. The ear noise made him feel helpless and caused severe difficulties to fall and stay asleep at night. He could not relax and his ability to work as well as his general well-being were severely impaired.

To deal with this situation, the patient had initially resorted to alcohol consumption in the evening as a first coping strategy (up to 7 servings of beer at a time, 3–4 days a week, at a bodyweight of 120 kg) but had already returned to abstinence when first consulting our clinic. At the time of this first examination, the patient was a non-smoker, working full time, and married.

As part of the initial assessment, we performed conventional audiometry, which showed a discrete sensorineural hearing loss in frequencies higher than 6 kHz. A cranial MRI did not show any anomalies in the patient's brain structure. Blood work revealed no signs of anemia, decreased kidney function or abnormal levels of glucose. Two markers of liver function were slightly above normal ranges (GPT > 50 U/l at 56 U/l; gamma-GT > 55 U/l at 73 U/l), possibly due to the patient's history of alcohol abuse. Levels of triglycerides (>150 mg/dl at 372 mg/dl) and cholesterol (>200 mg/dl at 238 mg/dl) were also increased, corresponding to the patient's diagnosed adiposis. TSH levels were very low (<0.40 mU/l at 0.03 mU/l), indicating possible hyperthyroidism. The patient adhered to the following medication plan: Allopurinol 300 mg, Olmesartan medoxomil – Amlodipin 40 mg/5 mg combination.

The patient's tinnitus symptoms were diagnosed as decompensated and severe according to the German tinnitus questionnaire TF (raw score 48, corresponds to percentile rank 54 and degree of severity 3; Goebel and Hiller, 1998). For tinnitus characterization, we used the TSCHQ (Landgrebe et al., 2010; Müller et al., 2016) in the German translation. The patient himself described the tinnitus as a permanent bilateral buzzing inside the head at very high frequencies, and a loudness level of 70/100 (based on a numerical rating scale from the TSCHQ). Detailed results of the assessment are presented in **Table 1**. An otoscopic examination showed normal, bilaterally intact tympanic membranes. In the Weber test, there was no lateralization at 440 Hz. A PTA test showed mild bilateral sensorineural hearing loss (right ear with a maximum of 30 dB HL at 6 kHz, left ear with a maximum of 40 dB HL at 4 kHz; assessed range: 125 Hz–8 kHz). TOAEs and DPOAEs could not be determined on a repeated basis (Supplementary Figure 1). We did not perform tone matching procedures to characterize "tinnitus pitch."

In his self-anamnesis, the patient listed tension headaches up to three times a week and arthrosis in the shoulder joints. The

TABLE 1 | Tinnitus anamnesis by TSCHQ (Landgrebe et al., 2010; Müller et al., 2016).

Item	Answer
Age	53
Sex	Male
Handedness	Right
Tinnitus occurrence in family	No
Onset of tinnitus	4 years ago
Perceiving the onset of tinnitus	Gradual
Relation of initial onset of tinnitus	None
Pulsation of tinnitus	No
Location of tinnitus	Inside the head
Tinnitus manifestation over time	Constant
Tinnitus loudness variation from day to day	Yes
Loudness of tinnitus (1–100)	70
Description of tinnitus	Buzzing, similar to a defective fluorescent tube
Sound of tinnitus	Noise
Pitch of tinnitus	Very high
Percentage of total awake time of tinnitus awareness	90
Percentage of total awake time being distressed by tinnitus	30
Number of different tinnitus treatments	0
Reduction of tinnitus by music or environmental sounds	Yes
Worsening of tinnitus by loud noise	Do not know
Tinnitus affected by head movement or touch	No
Tinnitus affected by nap	Yes, worsening of Tinnitus
Tinnitus affected by sleep at night	Do not know
Tinnitus affected by stress	Yes, worsening of Tinnitus
Tinnitus affected by medication	No
Hearing problem	Yes
Hearing aids	No
Problems tolerating sounds	Sometimes
Sounds cause pain or physical discomfort	Yes
Headache	Yes
Vertigo or dizziness	Yes
Temporomandibular disorder	No
Neck pain	Yes
Other pain syndromes	Yes (shoulder)
Currently under treatment for psychiatric problems	Yes

Abbreviations: ADANO, Arbeitsgemeinschaft Deutschsprachiger Audiologen, Neurootologen und Otologen German-speaking Audiologists, Neurootologists and Otologists; AHI, apnea–hypopnea index; BDI-II, Beck Depression Inventory (Hautzinger et al., 2006); CBT, cognitive behavioral therapy; DGHNOKHC, Deutsche Gesellschaft für Hals-Nasen-Ohren-Heilkunde, Kopf- und Hals-Chirurgie German Society of Oto-Rhino-Laryngology, Head and Neck Surgery; ESS, Epworth Sleepiness Scale (Johns, 1991); ICD-10, International Classification of Diseases (Dilling et al., 1994); MRI, magnetic resonance imaging; n-CPAP, nasal continuous positive airway pressure; PTA, pure tone audiometry; RDI, respiratory disturbance index; rTMS, repetitive transcranial magnetic stimulation; TEOAE, transiently evoked otoacoustic emissions; TF, Tinnitus Fragebogen (Goebel and Hiller, 1998); TSCHQ, Tinnitus Sample Case History Questionnaire (Landgrebe et al., 2010); WHO-5, WHO-Five Well-Being Index (Brähler et al., 2007).

pain caused by the arthrosis in the left shoulder was treated with conservative forms of therapy in an outpatient setting.

Regarding his sleep quality and daytime alertness, the patient stated to be experiencing considerable daytime sleepiness (Epworth Sleepiness Scale ESS = 14 – severe sleepiness, pre-therapeutic; Johns, 1991), which was aggravated by difficulties to fall and/or stay asleep at night. Here, a clear worsening could be observed over the course of time: while initially it took the patient approximately 30 min to fall asleep, this period gradually extended to times between 30 and 90 min. The patient also reported severe sleep maintenance problems, combined with early morning awakening. This meant that, in general, the patient's overall sleeping time amounted to approximately 4.5 h. A screening with polygraphy showed habitual and at times obstructive snoring as well as a RDI of 7/h. Due to the pauses in respiration found by third-party anamnesis, a polysomnography was performed, in which an upper airway resistance syndrome was diagnosed.

In the consultation sessions, the patient made the impression to be awake, completely oriented, alert and conscious. However, a further psychological exploration showed that he was clearly suffering from inner tension, irritability and an impaired mood and a considerable decrease in drive, both in his private and professional life. The patient tried to counteract his daytime sleepiness by taking several compensatory rests and sleep breaks during the day. With regard to his cognitive and mnestic functions the psychological assessment did not show any signs of an impairment. No suicidal tendencies were observed. Regarding his general mood and possible depressive symptoms, our assessment using the BDI-II (Hautzinger et al., 2006) resulted in a raw score of 10, which corresponds to minimal depressive symptoms.

As to the patient's ear noise, the following diagnoses were made according to ICD-10 research criteria (Dilling et al., 1994): holocephalic, decompensated and chronified Tinnitus aurium (ICD-10 H93.1) with comorbid decompensated insomnia (ICD-10 F51.0) as well as habitual and obstructive snoring (ICD-10 R06.5) and an upper airway resistance syndrome (ICD-10 G47.31). Moreover, arterial hypertonia (ICD-10 I10.0), adipositas (ICD-10 E66.0) and alcohol abuse with current abstinence (ICD 10 F10.1) were diagnosed.

BACKGROUND

Subjective tinnitus is defined as the perception of a sound in absence of an objective source (Møller, 2003). Describing its prevalence can provide a challenge, as numbers vary with age and gender (Møller, 2011). Studies postulate a lifetime prevalence of about 80% (Møller, 2011) and a point prevalence between 1 and 22.2% (Møller, 2011; Langguth et al., 2013; Kim et al., 2015; Kreuzer et al., 2016). It is assumed that between 50 and 77% of all tinnitus patients develop sleeping problems, especially those suffering from more severe forms (Crönlein et al., 2016).

With regard to effective forms of treatment, tinnitus "remains a clinical enigma" (Müller et al., 2016) due to its high levels of heterogeneity and complexity. Tinnitus may appear in various forms, regarding pattern, site, loudness or pitch of the sound, as well as other perceptual characteristics (Langguth et al., 2013). Furthermore, it can relate to several possible etiologies and comorbidities (Müller et al., 2016). A great majority of tinnitus cases do involve sensorineural hearing loss. Central auditory system reorganization is thought to be a prerequisite for chronic tinnitus.

Recent reviews (Langguth et al., 2013; Minen et al., 2014) concluded, that tinnitus may be caused by disturbances in peripheral auditory, central auditory, or non-auditory systems, by temporomandibular joint disorders, as well as by psychological factors. Regarding this last etiology, which, in our opinion, is central in this case, Mazurek et al. (2015) summarize several studies, that demonstrate associations between stress and tinnitus. According to current research, chronic tinnitus may also be triggered by muscular tension (somatosensory tinnitus), specifically in the neck (cervicogenic tinnitus) and can also appear in connection with a cervical pain syndrome, both with and without vertigo (Bechter et al., 2016). We therefore hypothesized, that a multidisciplinary, combinatory approach to treatment targeting multiple blocks could improve the treatment outcome.

When it comes to comorbid sleeping problems, reports on cases like the one discussed above suggest treating tinnitus and insomnia in conjunction: here, psychotherapy (Crönlein et al., 2007), surgery (Chen et al., 2010), as well as non-traditional approaches (Okamoto et al., 2005) may be appropriate means of therapy.

Cognitive behavioral therapy (CBT), relaxation techniques, and rTMS likewise appear to be safe and effective treatments for chronic tinnitus as they have been shown to increase the general quality of life and lower tinnitus symptoms without adverse events (Cima et al., 2012; Soleimani et al., 2016; Zenner et al., 2016). However, rTMS in particular still seems to lack the necessary methodological fine-tuning and has therfore produced moderate to large, but highly variable effects so far (Hesser et al., 2011; Langguth et al., 2013; Kreuzer et al., 2016; Soleimani et al., 2016). Other current forms of treatment were either not feasible in this case due to a lack of time and resources (e.g., notched music therapy (Okamoto et al., 2010), cochlear implantation (Olze et al., 2012) or because of their reported non to mixed-success [e.g., vagus nerve stimulation (De Ridder et al., 2014), AM-101 (van de Heyning et al., 2014), or other drugs (Kingwell, 2016)].

RESULTS

Tinnitus Therapy

Tinnitus Therapy with rTMS

A first treatment attempt was made in October 2010. This initial treatment consisted of 10 sessions of 1 Hz rTMS over 10 consecutive working days with a stimulation intensity of 110% related to the individual resting motor threshold. 2000 stimuli per session were applied, with coil position 10–20 guided over the left primary auditory cortex.

At the time of therapy, our research group had 2 years of clinical experience in treating patients with a chronified tinnitus (Acker et al., 2010). In choosing the stimulation protocol, we followed the experiences by the interdisciplinary Regensburg working group (Kleinjung et al., 2005), who had proven a metabolic activation of the auditory cortex in a series of tinnitus patients with a similar disease process. A placebo-controlled, multicenter study including eight German participant centers on the efficacy of rTMS likewise used the treatment protocol described above (Landgrebe et al., 2008).

The primary therapeutic aim of the rTMS treatment was a favorable modulation of the patient's tinnitus perception. An improvement in the subjective degree of severity of the symptoms could be achieved without any side effects. The main effect of the therapy was a change in the frequency and the subjective intensity of the tinnitus directly after the treatment. The initially very strong effect of the therapy decreased markedly after 3–4 h after the end of each treatment session, though. Limitations in our evaluation are the missing tone matching of tinnitus frequency and the missing high frequency audiometry (>8 kHz).

Figures 1A–C show the development of the patient's raw scores across three different psychometric questionnaires (TF, BDI-II, and WHO-5) assessed at four points in time (Timespans between measurements: pre rTMS to post rTMS: 3 weeks; post TMS to pre CBT: 2 weeks; pre CBT to post CBT: 1 weeks).

The TF questionnaire is an instrument to measure tinnitus severity ($\alpha = 0.94$; range: 0–84; Goebel and Hiller, 1998). Within the approximately 3 weeks of rTMS treatment, TF scores decreased from 48 (degree 3 of 4, decompensated tinnitus) to 38 (degree 2 of 4, compensated tinnitus). The BDI-II was used to measure depressive symptoms ($\alpha = 0.84$–0.94; range: 0–63; Hautzinger et al., 2006). After rTMS treatment, BDI-II scores only slightly changed from 10 to 9 (minimal depressive symptoms). For the measurement of subjective well-being we used the WHO-5 ($\alpha = 0.92$; range: 0–100, critical cut-off: 52, average score: 70; Brähler et al., 2007). WHO-5 scores increased from 52 (critical cut-off) to 76 (normal well-being).

Tinnitus Therapy with CBT

Due to the persistent professional impairment, we continued our treatment with 10 sessions of CBT as recommended by German guidelines for tinnitus management by the ADANO (Society of German-speaking Audiologists, Neurootologists, and Otologists; Lenarz, 1998) and the DGHNOKHC (German Society of Oto-Rhino-Laryngology, Head and Neck Surgery; AWMF, 2015).

The primary therapeutic aim of the behavioral therapy was to develop coping strategies to reduce the subjective impairment caused by the tinnitus as well as the resulting emotional stress. To do so, the following steps were taken: the subjective illness hypothesis was explored and discussed and medical information and explanatory models were provided. Subsequently, a connection between situative stress and tinnitus perception was worked out and, with the help of cognitive restructuring, helpful forms of behavior were successfully transferred to hitherto discouraging situations.

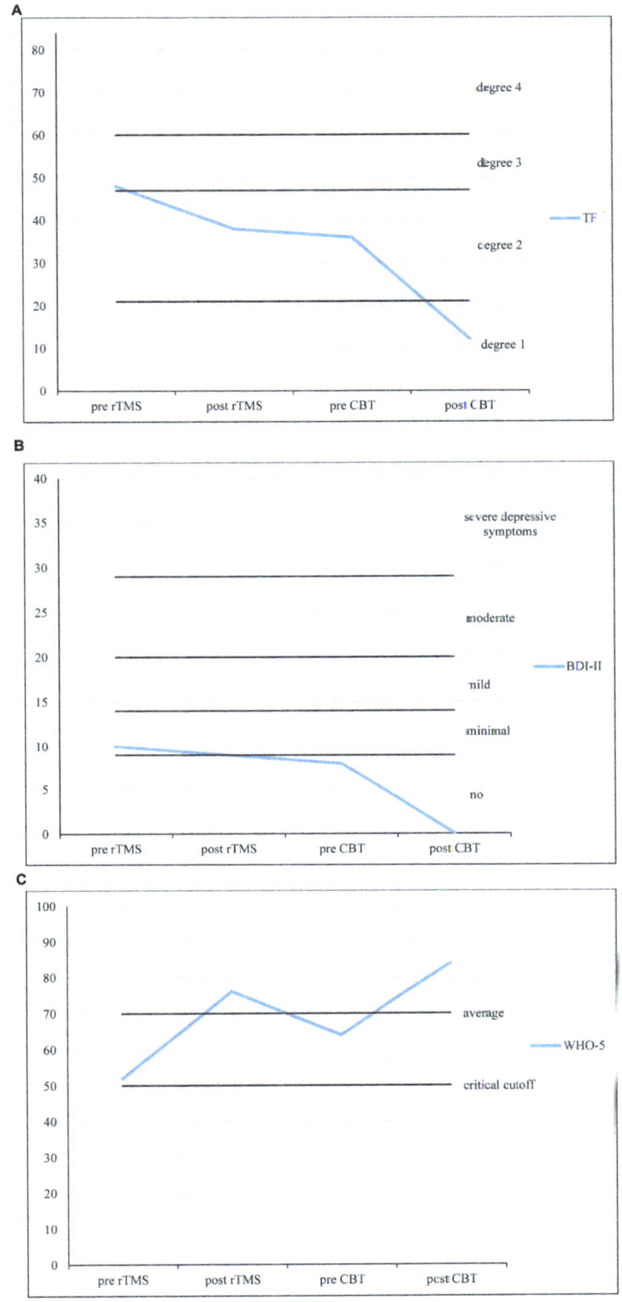

FIGURE 1 | (A) TF scores over the course of treatment. **(B)** BDI-II scores over the course of treatment. **(C)** WHO-5 scores over the course of treatment. Timespans between measurements: pre rTMS to post rTMS: 3 weeks; post TMS to pre CBT: 2 weeks; pre CBT to post CBT: 15 weeks.

The patient particularly profited from practicing progressive muscle relaxation according to Jacobson as well as breathing exercises as a further relaxation method.

Within the approximately 15 weeks of CBT treatment, the patient's TF scores decreased from 36 (degree 2 of 4, compensated tinnitus) to 12 (degree 1 of 4, compensated tinnitus). BDI-II scores had decreased to 8 (no depressive symptoms) within the 2 weeks between the last session of rTMS and the first session of CBT. They stayed at 0 after CBT treatment. WHO-5 scores increased once more, from 64 (average well-being) to 84 (above average well-being).

Therapy of Insomnia

In view of the high subjective affliction, the patient's sleep problems were likewise addressed with behavioral therapeutic means. Here, the main measures employed were sleep restriction and sleep hygiene (Backhaus and Riemann, 1999), as well as psychoeducation regarding sleep, cognitive restructuring of negative thoughts, stimulus control, and relaxation techniques (Piehl et al., 2010; Richter, 2015).

A polysomnography carried out subsequently found an AHI of 8/h and an increased number of respiratory arousal reactions (arousal index 15/h sleep). On diagnosis of an upper airway resistance syndrome (American Academy of Sleep Medicine, 2005) treatment with n-CPAP therapy was initiated. The snoring could be eliminated completely with average application times of 6 h/night. The patient's compliance with CPAP treatment was very good in general.

Further Development

After both courses of treatment (rTMS and CBT) for the tinnitus symptoms had been completed, the patient reported a notable improvement of his general state. GAF scores (global assessment of functioning; range: 0–90; Hall, 1995) increased from 45 (serious symptoms or impairment) to 68 (some mild symptoms). The ear noise and the resulting emotional distress had been reduced considerably. TF scores decreased from 48 (degree 3 of 4, decompensated tinnitus) to 12 (degree 1 of 4, compensated tinnitus). BDI-II scores decreased from 10 (minimal depressive symptoms) to 0 (no depressive symptoms). This 10-point change may be interpreted as moderate and clinically significant (Hautzinger et al., 2006). However, it must be mentioned that a placebo response to r-TMS treatment may be responsible for this change as well as intraindividual variation of subclinical BDI-scores.

WHO-5 scores increased from 52 (critical cut-off 52) to 84 (above average well-being). Likewise, there were great improvements regarding emotional balance, drive, the level of daytime sleepiness, the patient's ability to concentrate and his general mood. Light improvements were reported concerning the ability to relax and the ability to perform.

The patient profited especially from psychoeducation on tinnitus. He could be discharged from treatment with a clearly increased self-efficacy. Throughout the entire course of treatment, the patient's compliance was very good and co-operative. The patient also did not return to alcohol as a coping strategy but stayed abstinent throughout the entire course of treatment.

Summary

The case of our patient demonstrates the complexity of a chronified Tinnitus aurium modulated by comorbidities. Conventional PTA showed a mild notch like sensorineural hearing loss, while high frequency hearing > 8 kHz was not tested.

At the beginning of the therapy, the patient demanded a technical approach to a somatically fixated disease model. After comprehensive information on the neurological nexuses (Tyler, 2006) we agreed to a treatment attempt using rTMS. The treatment protocol follows the experiences of the Regensburg working group led by Kleinjung et al. (2007) and Langguth et al. (2015).

The psychiatric comorbidity of the present case is low for the characteristic tinnitus patient. Other working groups report a high number of afflictions from the depression – anxiety disorders range in their patient collectives (Schaaf et al., 2003; Zirke et al., 2010).

Tinnitus can have a highly negative impact on a person's professional and private life (Zirke et al., 2013) and cause society considerable follow-up costs. Here, the severity of the tinnitus and psychiatric comorbidities are the main factors increasing costs (Maes et al., 2013). For this reason, multimodal therapy up to the point where a stability of symptoms is reached has considerable significance.

A connection between ear noises and sleeping disorders has been reported since the beginning of the 1990s (Alster et al., 1993). In some current reviews, the frequently comorbid sleep problems are conceptualized as an attendant symptom of psychiatric disorders (Mazurek et al., 2005). In contrast, other studies find insomnia-related problems in older tinnitus patients in over 50% of cases (Lasisi and Gureje, 2011). Likewise, there seems to be an increased prevalence of sleep-related respiratory disorders in tinnitus collectives (Fischer et al., 2003; Herold et al., 2010).

Regarding our patient, we hypothesize a modulation of the tinnitus perception by the insomnia understood as a hyperarousal disorder (Crönlein et al., 2016). In the presence of high subjective stress levels the interaction of auditory and limbic brain areas may be disturbed at the thalamic level, leading to a breakdown of an internal "noise-cancelation" mechanism. In this case, the activation by catastrophizing and fear seem to have played a central role (Cima et al., 2011). Potentially, there is also a bi-directional connection between tinnitus and insomnia (Rauschecker et al., 2010).

Our patient did not suffer from cervical pain or vertigo, and the tinnitus did not change after neck inclination. This lead us to exclude the cervical etiology in this case (Bechter et al., 2016).

Modern therapy concepts recommend a tailored approach in planning the therapy (Seydel et al., 2013). Similarly, for an inpatient-setting, evaluated therapy concepts are available by now (Täuber, 2012).

CONCLUDING REMARKS

If healthcare professionals were to choose a standalone treatment for tinnitus symptoms, current evidence suggests selecting validated tinnitus-specific CBT over alternatives, such as rTMS (Zenner et al., 2016). In our case, however, rTMS therapy made it possible to start therapy at all because of a somatically fixated disease model. An optimization of the treatment protocol to improve the sustainability of the therapy seems sensible. We noticed a relevant improvement of the patient's everyday functionality could be achieved by a stabilization of his insomnia problems. According to our assessment, a successful therapy could only be established by the combination of rTMS with tinnitus and sleep-related elements from CBT. The efficacy of this personalized combined treatment approach (Golubnitschaja and Costigliola, 2012) in larger samples will be investigated in future research.

ETHICS STATEMENT

As all described interventions were part of clinical everyday practice, we did not consult with an ethics committee for this study. The patient gave written informed consent in accordance with the Declaration of Helsinki. The Patient also gave the consent for the analysis, processing, and publication of his data.

AUTHOR CONTRIBUTIONS

KR and JA contributed equally as first authors and wrote the manuscript. LM and LP contributed to the scientific design. GN contributed to data acquisition.

REFERENCES

Acker, J., Scholz, F., Richter, K., and Niklewski, G. (2010). Behandlungseffekte der repetitiven transkraniellen Magnetstimulation (rTMS) bei Patienten mit chronischem Tinnitus aurium: Erste Ergebnisse der Behandlung mit niederfrequenter rTMS. *Psychiatr. Forsch. Suppl.* 1, 9–12. doi: 10.5283/pf.19

Alster, J., Shemesh, Z., Ornan, M., and Attias, J. (1993). Sleep disturbance associated with chronic tinnitus. *Biol. Psychiatry* 34, 84–90. doi: 10.1016/0006-3223(93)90260-K

American Academy of Sleep Medicine (2005). *International Classification of Sleep Disorders, Revised: Diagnostic and Coding Manual*, 2nd Edn. Chicago, IL: American Sleep Disorders Association.

AWMF (2015). *German S3 Guideline Ol 7/064: Chronic tinnitus. Current revision 02/2015. Leitlinie Chronischer Tinnitus Deutsche Gesellschaft für Hals-Nasen-Ohren-Heilkunde.* Available at: http://www.awmf.org/fileadmin/user_upload/Leitlinien/017_D_G_f_Hals-Nasen-Ohrenheilkunde__Kopf-_und_Halschirurgie/017-064e_S3_guideline_tinnitus_english_2015-08.pdf

Backhaus, J., and Riemann, D. (1999). *Schlafstörungen. Fortschritte der Psychotherapie*, Vol. 7. Göttingen: Hogrefe, Verl. für Psychologie.

Bechter, K., Wieland, M., and Hamann, G. F. (2016). Chronic cervicogenic tinnitus rapidly resolved by intermittent use of cervical collar. *Front. Psychiatry* 7:43. doi: 10.3389/fpsyt.2016.00043

Brähler, E., Mühlan, H., Albani, C., and Schmidt, S. (2007). Teststatistische prüfung und normierung der deutschen versionen des EUROHIS-QOL lebensqualität-Index und des WHO-5 wohlbefindens-index. *Diagnostica* 53, 83–96. doi: 10.1026/0012-1924.53.2.83

Chen, M.-C., Chung, W.-Y., Luo, C.-B., and Wu, H.-M. (2010) Arteriovenous malformation in the parotid region presenting as pulsatile tinnitus: a case report. *Head Neck* 32, 262–267. doi: 10.1002/hed.21063

Cima, R. F. F., Crombez, G., and Vlaeyen, J. W. S. (2011). Catastrophizing and fear of tinnitus predict quality of life in patients with chronic tinnitus. *Ear Hear.* 32, 634–641. doi: 10.1097/AUD.0b013e31821106dd

Cima, R. F. F., Maes, I. H., Joore, M. A., Scheyen, D. J., El Refaie, A., Baguley, D. M., et al. (2012). Specialised treatment based on cognitive behaviour therapy versus usual care for tinnitus: a randomised controlled trial. *Lancet* 379, 1951–1959. doi: 10.1016/S0140-6736(12)60469-3

Crönlein, T., Langguth, B., Geisler, P., and Hajak, G. (2007). Tinnitus and insomnia. *Prog. Brain Res.* 166, 227–233. doi: 10.1016/S0079-6123(07)66021-X

Crönlein, T., Langguth, B., Pregler, M., Kreuzer, P. M., Wetter, T. C., and Schecklmann, M. (2016). Insomnia in patients with chronic tinnitus: cognitive and emotional distress as moderator variables. *J. Psychosom. Res.* 83, 65–68. doi: 10.1016/j.jpsychores.2016.03.001

De Ridder, D., Vanneste, S., Engineer, N. D., and Kilgard, M. P. (2014). Safety and efficacy of vagus nerve stimulation paired with tones for the treatment of tinnitus: a case series. *Neuromodulation* 17, 170–179. doi: 10.1111/ner.12127

Dilling, H., Mombour, W., Schmidt, M. H., and Schulte-Markwort, E. (1994). *Internationale Klassifikation Psychischer Störungen, ICD-10, Forschungskriterien.* Göttingen: Hogrefe.

Fischer, Y., Yakinthou, A., and Mann, W. J. (2003). Zur Prävalenz der obstruktiven Schlafapnoe (OSA) bei Patienten mit Hörsturz. Eine Pilotstudie [Prevalence of obstructive sleep apnea syndrome (OSA) in patients with sudden hearing loss. A pilot study]. *HNO* 51, 462–466. doi: 10.1007/s00106-002-0712-y

Goebel, G., and Hiller, W. (1998). *Tinnitus-Fragebogen:(TF); ein Instrument zur Erfassung von Belastung und Schweregrad bei Tinnitus; Handanweisung.* Göttingen: Hogrefe, Verl. für Psychologie.

Golubnitschaja, O., and Costigliola, V. (2012). General report and recommendations in predictive, preventive and personalized medicine 2012: white paper of the European Association for Predictive, Preventive and Personalized Medicine. *EPMA J.* 3:14. doi: 10.1186/1878-5085-3-14

Hall, R. C. (1995). Global assessment of functioning. A modified scale. *Psychosomatics* 36, 267–275. doi: 10.1016/S0033-3182(95)71666-8

Hautzinger, M., Keller, F., and Kühner, C. (2006). *Beck Depressions-Inventar II (BDI-II).* Frankfurt: Harcourt Test Service.

Herold, J., Piehl, A., Richter, K., Ficker, J., Niklewski, G., and Acker J. (2010). Prävalenz einer obstruktiven Schlafapnoe bei Tinnituspatienten mit insomnischen Beschwerden. *Somnologie* 14(Suppl. 1), 71. doi: 10.1007/s11818-010-0489-2

Hesser, H., Weise, C., Westin, V. Z., and Andersson, G. (2011). A systematic review and meta-analysis of randomized controlled trials of cognitive-behavioral therapy for tinnitus distress. *Clin. Psychol. Rev.* 31, 545–553. doi: 10.1016/j.cpr.2010.12.006

Johns, M. W. (1991). A new method for measuring daytime sleepiness: the Epworth Sleepiness Scale. *Sleep* 14, 540–545. doi: 10.1093/sleep/14.6.540

Kim, H.-J., Lee, H.-J., An, S.-Y., Sim, S., Park, B., Kim, S. W., et al. (2015). Analysis of the prevalence and associated risk factors of tinnitus in adults. *PLoS ONE* 10:e0127578. doi: 10.1371/journal.pone.0127578

Kingwell, K. (2016). First hearing-disorder drugs stumble. *Nat. Rev. Drug Discov.* 15, 733–735. doi: 10.1038/nrd.2016.222

Kleinjung, T., Eichhammer, P., Langguth, B., Jacob, P., Marienhagen, J., Hajak, G., et al. (2005). Long-term effects of repetitive transcranial magnetic stimulation (rTMS) in patients with chronic tinnitus. *Otolaryngol. Head Neck Surg.* 132, 566–569. doi: 10.1016/j.otohns.2004.09.134

Kleinjung, T., Steffens, T., Londero, A., and Langguth, B. (2007). Transcranial magnetic stimulation (TMS) for treatment of chronic tinnitus: clinical effects. *Prog. Brain Res.* 166, 359–367. doi: 10.1016/S0079-6123(07)66034-8

Kreuzer, P. M., Poeppl, T. B., Bulla, J., Schlee, W., Lehner, A., Langguth, B. et al. (2016). A proof-of-concept study on the combination of repetitive transcranial magnetic stimulation and relaxation techniques in chronic tinnitus. *J. Neural Transm.* 123, 1147–1157. doi: 10.1007/s00702-016-1588-4

Landgrebe, M., Binder, H., Koller, M., Eberl, Y., Kleinjung, T., Eichhammer, P., et al. (2008). Design of a placebo-controlled, randomized study of the efficacy of repetitive transcranial magnetic stimulation for the treatment of chronic tinnitus. *BMC Psychiatry* 8:23. doi: 10.1186/1471-244X-8-23

Landgrebe, M., Zeman, F., Koller, M., Eberl, Y., Mohr, M., Reiter, J., et al. (2010). The Tinnitus Research Initiative (TRI) database: a new approach for delineation of tinnitus subtypes and generation of predictors for treatment outcome. *BMC Med. Inform. Decis. Mak.* 10:42. doi: 10.1186/1472-6947-10-42

Langguth, B., Kreuzer, P. M., Kleinjung, T., and de Ridder, D. (2013). Tinnitus: causes and clinical management. *Lancet Neurol.* 12, 920–930. doi: 10.1016/S1474-4422(13)70160-1

Langguth, B., Landgrebe, M., Schecklmann, M., Schönfeldt-Lecuona, C., Höppner, J., Padberg, F., et al. (2015). Chronischer tinnitus. therapeutischer einsatz von rTMS. *Nervenheilkunde* 34, 987–993.

Lasisi, A. O., and Gureje, O. (2011). Prevalence of insomnia and impact on quality of life among community elderly subjects with tinnitus. *Ann. Otol. Rhinol. Laryngol.* 120, 226–230. doi: 10.1177/000348941112000402

Lenarz, T. (1998). Leitlinie tinnitus der deutschen gesellschaft für hals-nasen-ohren-heilkunde, kopf-und hals-chirurgie. *Laryngorhinootologie* 77, 531–535. doi: 10.1055/s-2007-997020

Maes, I. H. L., Cima, R. F. F., Vlaeyen, J. W., Anteunis, L. J. C., and Joore, M. A. (2013). Tinnitus: a cost study. *Ear Hear.* 34, 508–514. doi: 10.1097/AUD.0b013e31827d113a

Mazurek, B., Georgiewa, P., Seydel, C., Haupt, H., Scherer, H., Klapp, B. F., et al. (2005). Integrierte tinnitusintensivbehandlung: konzept und erste praktische erfahrungen. *Gesundheitswesen* 67, 485–491. doi: 10.1055/s-2005-858379

Mazurek, B., Szczepek, A. J., and Hebert, S. (2015). Stress and tinnitus. *HNO* 63, 258–265. doi: 10.1007/s00106-014-2973-7

Minen, M. T., Camprodon, J., Nehme, R., and Chemali, Z. (2014). The neuropsychiatry of tinnitus: a circuit-based approach to the causes and treatments available. *J. Neurol. Neurosurg. Psychiatr.* 85, 1138–1144. doi: 10.1136/jnnp-2013-307339

Møller, A. R. (2003). Pathophysiology of tinnitus. *Otolaryngol. Clin. North Am.* 36, 249–266. doi: 10.1016/S0030-6665(02)00170-6

Møller, A. R. (2011). *Textbook of Tinnitus.* New York, NY: Springer Publishing Company. doi: 10.1007/978-1-60761-145-5

Müller, K., Edvall, N. K., Idrizbegovic, E., Huhn, R., Cima, R. F., Persson, V., et al. (2016). Validation of online versions of tinnitus questionnaires translated into Swedish. *Front. Aging Neurosci.* 8:272. doi: 10.3389/fnagi.2016.00272

Okamoto, H., Okami, T., Ikeda, M., and Takeuchi, T. (2005). Effects of Yoku-kan-san on undifferentiated somatoform disorder with tinnitus. *Eur. Psychiatry* 20, 74–75. doi: 10.1016/j.eurpsy.2004.09.034

Okamoto, H., Stracke, H., Stoll, W., and Pantev, C. (2010). Listening to tailor-made notched music reduces tinnitus loudness and tinnitus-related auditory cortex activity. *Proc. Natl. Acad. Sci. U.S.A.* 107, 1207–1210. doi: 10.1073/pnas.0911268107

Olze, H., Szczepek, A. J., Haupt, H., Zirke, N., Graebel, S., and Mazurek, B. (2012). The impact of cochlear implantation on tinnitus, stress and quality of life in postlingually deafened patients. *Audiol. Neurootol.* 17, 2–11. doi: 10.1159/000323847

Piehl, A., Richter, K., and Niklewski, G. (2010). Therapieeffekte einer kognitiv-verhaltenstherapeutisch orientierten Insomniebehandlung. *Verhaltensther. Verhaltensmed.* 31, 375–389.

Rauschecker, J. P., Leaver, A. M., and Muhlau, M. (2010). Tuning out the noise: limbic-auditory interactions in tinnitus. *Neuron* 66, 819–826. doi: 10.1016/j.neuron.2010.04.032

Richter, K. (2015). *Schlafen Sie gut!: Ihr Schlafprogramm für Aufgeweckte Tage und Erholsame Nächte,* 1st Edn. Stuttgart: Trias.

Schaaf, H., Dölberg, D., Seling, B., and Märtner, M. (2003). Komorbidität von Tinnituserkrankungen und psychiatrischen Störungen. *Nervenarzt* 74, 72–75. doi: 10.1007/s00115-001-1222-y

Seydel, C., Haupt, H., Olze, H., Szczepek, A. J., and Mazurek, B. (2013). Gender and chronic tinnitus: differences in tinnitus-related distress depend on age and duration of tinnitus. *Ear Hear.* 34, 661–672. doi: 10.1097/AUD.0b013e31828149f2

Soleimani, R., Jalali, M. M., and Hasandokht, T. (2016). Therapeutic impact of repetitive transcranial magnetic stimulation (rTMS) on tinnitus: a systematic review and meta-analysis. *Eur. Arch. Otorhinolaryngol.* 273, 1663–1675. doi: 10.1007/s00405-015-3642-5

Täuber, S. (2012). *Einfluss Einer Stationären Verhaltenstherapeutischen Intervention bei Patienten mit Tinnitus und Insomnie.* Ph.D. dissertation, Universität Regensburg, Regensburg.

Tyler, R. S. (2006). "Neurophysiological models, psychological models, and treatments for tinnitus," in *Tinnitus Treatment. Clinical Protocols,* ed. R. S. Tyler (New York, NY: Thieme), 1–22.

van de Heyning, P., Muehlmeier, G., Cox, T., Lisowska, G., Maier, H., Morawski, K., et al. (2014). Efficacy and safety of AM-101 in the treatment of acute inner ear tinnitus: a double-blind, randomized, placebo-controlled phase II study. *Otol. Neurotol.* 35, 589–597. doi: 10.1097/MAO.0000000000000268

Zenner, H.-P., Delb, W., Kroner-Herwig, B., Jager, B., Peroz, I., Hesse, G., et al. (2016). A multidisciplinary systematic review of the treatment for chronic idiopathic tinnitus. *Eur. Arch. Otorhinolaryngol.* doi: 10.1007/s00405-016-4401-y [Epub ahead of print].

Zirke, N., Goebel, G., and Mazurek, B. (2010). Tinnitus und psychische Komorbiditäten. *HNO* 58, 726–732. doi: 10.1007/s00106-009-2050-9

Zirke, N., Seydel, C., Szczepek, A. J., Olze, H., Haupt, H., and Mazurek, B. (2013). Psychological comorbidity in patients with chronic tinnitus: analysis and comparison with chronic pain, asthma or atopic dermatitis patients. *Qual. Life Res.* 22, 263–272. doi: 10.1007/s11136-012-0156-0

21

An Increase in Alpha Band Frequency in Resting State EEG after Electrical Stimulation of the Ear in Tinnitus Patients

Marzena Mielczarek[1]*, Joanna Michalska[1], Katarzyna Polatyńska[2] and Jurek Olszewski[1]

[1] Department of Otolaryngology, Laryngological Oncology, Audiology, and Phoniatrics, Medical University of Lodz, Lodz, Poland,

[2] Department of Neurology, Polish Mother's Memorial Hospital Research Institute, Lodz, Poland

***Correspondence:**
Marzena Mielczarek
marzena.mielczarek@umed.lodz.pl

In our clinic invasive transtympanal promontory positive DC stimulations were first used, with a success rate of 42%. However, non-invasive hydrotransmissive negative DC stimulations are now favored, with improvement being obtained in 37.8% directly after the treatment, and 51.3% in a follow up 1 month after treatment. The further improvement after 1 month may be due to neuroplastic changes at central level as a result of altered peripheral input. The aim of the study was to determine how/whether a single electrical stimulation of the ear influences cortical activity, and whether changes observed in tinnitus after electrical stimulation are associated with any changes in cortical activity recorded in EEG. The study included 12 tinnitus patients (F–6, M-6) divided into two groups. Group I comprised six patients with unilateral tinnitus - unilateral, ipsilateral ES was performed. Group II comprised six patients with bilateral tinnitus—bilateral ES was performed. ES was performed using a custom-made apparatus. The active, silver probe—was immersed inside the external ear canal filled with saline. The passive electrode was placed on the forehead. The stimulating frequency was 250 Hz, the intensity ranged from 0 14 to 1.08 mA. The voltage was kept constant at 3 V. The duration of stimulation was 4 min. The EEG recording (Deymed QEST 32) was performed before and after ES. The patients assessed the intensity of tinnitus on the VAS 1-10.

Results: In both groups an improvement in VAS was observed—in group I—in five ears (83.3%), in group II—in seven ears (58.3%). In Group I, a significant increase in the upper and lower limit frequency of alpha band was observed in the central temporal and frontal regions following ES. These changes, however, were not correlated with improvement in tinnitus. No significant changes were observed in the beta and theta bands and in group II. Preliminary results of our research reveal a change in cortical activity after electrical stimulations of the ear. However, it remains unclear if it is primary or secondary to peripheral auditory excitation. No similar studies had been found in the literature.

Keywords: tinnitus, electrical stimulations, ear, neuromodulation, cortical activity

INTRODUCTION

Tinnitus is one of the vaguest audiological and otological symptoms. It is defined as a phantom sound perception, which does not reflect any corresponding physical activity. Tinnitus had been a disturbing disorder since antiquity. Although, only peripheral—cochlear pathology was initially considered an ignition site, it appeared that tinnitus was not always relieved after cochlear nerve section (Baguley et al., 2002). Later, Jastreboff's neurophysiological model of tinnitus proposed that the cochlea played a role in phantom sound generation, with the wide involvement of the central nervous system (Jastreboff, 1990). Recently, the development of such medical diagnostic methods as neurophysiological analysis and neuroimaging has stimulated the formulation of new hypotheses concerning tinnitus generation (Kaltenbach, 2011) and consequently, new original treatment modalities for patients.

In our clinic electrical stimulation (ES) of the ear in tinnitus treatment was first used in the 1980s. Invasive transtympanal promontory positive DC stimulations were first used, with a success rate of 42% (improvement in questionnaire by at least 4 points in 10 point scale) (Konopka et al., 2001). However, non-invasive hydrotransmissive DC stimulations are now favored, with improvement being obtained in 37.8% directly after the treatment, and 51.3% in a follow up 1 month after treatment (improvement in questionnaire by at least 20%) (Mielczarek and Olszewski, 2014). The improvement in tinnitus was accompanied by an improvement in hearing threshold in pure tone audiometry, indicating the condition of the peripheral hearing organ had improved. We hypothesized that further improvement after 1 month may be due to neuroplastic changes at central level as a result of altered peripheral input. In consequence of abovementioned hypothesis we posed a question about the possible mechanisms in which ear ES influences tinnitus: is it only peripheral (cochlear) activity modulation, or central—secondarily to peripheral alternation, or maybe purely central? Hypothetically, for electric current applied to the ear, soft tissues work as a conductor, thus none of the mechanisms can be excluded. There are many studies on the effect of ear ES on peripheral structures, however, to our knowledge, there is no study exploring alternations at a central cortical level directly after peripheral non-invasive ear ES.

Many studies have reported the suppression of tinnitus after cochlear implantation (CI) (Quaranta et al., 2004; Todt et al., 2015; Mertens et al., 2016), but the exact mechanism which is behind tinnitus suppression remains unclear as well. Zeng et al. noticed an increase in alpha power after low-rate electric stimulation via CI (Zeng et al., 2011). High-rate stimulation (5000 pps), however, appeared to be inefficient in inducing central activity (Middlebrooks, 2008) although restored activity at the auditory nerve was observed (Rubinstein et al., 2003).

In the literature, there are few explanations of how ear ES influences tinnitus (an increase in the neurotransmitter's transmission in the synapses—Latkowski, 1981, modification of the hearing organ's electrical potentials—Portmann et al., 1979, or improvement in the blood flow in the inner ear and synchronization of spontaneous impulses in the auditory nerve fibers—Watanabe et al., 1997) but none of them point to central mechanisms.

Thanks to animal models of peripheral tinnitus (induced by acoustic trauma or ototoxic drugs) the mechanisms of direct cochlear stimulation had been explained (Nuttall and Ren, 1995; Ren and Nuttall, 1995). Furthermore, animal models show correlations between a change in central activity as a result of peripheral cochlear modulations. Norena et al. noticed that ES of the cochlea in guinea pigs using a positive current decreased the spontaneous firing rate in the high characteristic frequency neurons of the inferior colliculi, while a negative current had the opposite effect. Such an effect was absent or reverse for low characteristic frequency neurons (Noreña et al., 2015). Mulders et al. obtained reduction of pathological hyperactivity in inferior colliculi after intraperitoneal or cochlear injection of furosemide (Mulders et al., 2014a). What's more, the authors observed similar results after chronic furosemide treatment without hearing impairment (Mulders et al., 2014b). Reducing central hyperactivity authors claim to reduce behavioral signs of tinnitus decreasing spontaneous firing of auditory afferent.

Thanks to electrophysiological studies in tinnitus changes in cortical activity were widely explored (Shulman and Goldstein, 2002; Weisz et al., 2005; Adjamian et al., 2012; Meyer et al., 2014; Schlee et al., 2014). In consequence treatment methods aiming at neuromodulation are now "mainstream therapies." Thus neurophysiological measurements like EEG, MEG serve as an objective outcome measure to quantify therapeutic benefit.

The aim of the study was to determine how/whether a single electrical stimulation of the ear influences cortical activity, and whether changes observed in tinnitus after electrical stimulation are associated with any changes in cortical activity recorded in EEG.

MATERIALS AND METHODS

The study included 12 tinnitus patients (F–6, M-6) divided into two groups. Group I comprised six patients with unilateral tinnitus (six tinnitus ears, five—left, one—right ear), aged 36–73 (average 58.50 years, SD 11.83 years), unilateral, ipsilateral ES was performed. Group II comprised six patients with bilateral tinnitus (12 tinnitus ears), aged 38-78 years (average 53.50 years, SD 18.16 years), bilateral ES was performed starting with the right ear. The groups were balanced in terms of the age, and tinnitus duration.

Before the beginning of the study, ENT examination was performed, together with any necessary audiological and radiological diagnostics. The exclusion criteria included the following: pathology in the external and/or the middle ear, central nervous system disorders (e.g., epilepsy), positive history of neoplasms, implanted pacemaker. Patients with tinnitus in the head, not the ears, were disqualified from the research.

ES was performed using a custom-made apparatus supplied with four 1.5 V batteries. The device has an on / off button, frequency and current intensity buttons. The patient was in a lying position, on the side with the stimulated ear upwards. The external ear canal was filled with saline solution. The active, silver probe—was immersed inside the external ear canal, avoiding contact with the skin of the canal. The passive electrode was placed on the forehead in the midline (glabella) after skin abrasion with a suitable sterile abrasive electrode paste and clean gauze. The two electrodes were placed in such a way that the current could flow throughout the hypothetical plane (longitudinal axis) of the cochlea. Direct rectangular negative current was applied via the active electrode. In all cases, the stimulating frequency was 250 Hz, the intensity ranged from 0.14 to 1.08 mA, and was applied according to the sensation experience by the patient. The voltage was kept constant at 3 V. The duration of each stimulation was 4 min.

EEG (Deymed QEST 32) was conducted in a room that conforms to EEG standards. Two EEG recordings of 5 min were performed before and after ES (in group I—before and after unilateral ES, in group II—before and after bilateral ES). A Deymed TruScan (10/20 system) electro-cap was fitted. The impedance of the electrodes didn't depend on the head position. The patients were asked to close their eyes and relax. They were asked to refrain from drugs, such as caffeine or alcohol, for 24 h preceding the EEG recording. None of the patients were using drugs influencing CNS activity (e.g., benzodiazepines). The upper and lower limit of a frequency band (Hz) and an averaged wave amplitude (μV) were assessed for alpha, beta and theta oscillations. These parameters were assessed before and after electrical stimulation, furthermore these results were assessed with regard to tinnitus change (assessed in VAS).

Comparisons of the limit frequencies of the bands and averaged amplitudes for alpha, beta and theta were made between reading taken before and after ES. In every recording three samples of 1–3 s were chosen and next marked. The minimal and maximal frequencies and amplitudes were automatically counted by the system. In order to assess potential changes in cortical activity, we compared between the following regions: central frontal (right F4-C4, left F3-C3), temporo -occipital (right T6-O2, left T5-O1), parieto—occipital (right P4-O2, left P3-O1), temporal anterior (right F8-T6, left F7-T5), central (right C4-T4, left T3-C3), posterior (right T4-T6, left T3-T5) and the left and right hemisphere.

In addition, the patients were asked to assess the intensity of tinnitus on the visual analog scale (VAS 1–10) directly before and after electrical stimulation.

The study was approved by the Institutional Review Board of the Medical University of Lodz. All subjects gave written informed consent in accordance with the Declaration of Helsinki.

Statistical Analysis

The exact Mann-Whitney rank-sum test for independent data and the exact Wilcoxon matched-pairs signed-ranks test were used to fit data. The exact procedures were chosen due to the small sizes of the samples. Generalized estimating equations (GEE) with robust standard errors also were used when dealing with more than one independent variable, and when inclusive of repeated measures. A level of $p < 0.05$ was considered statistically significant.

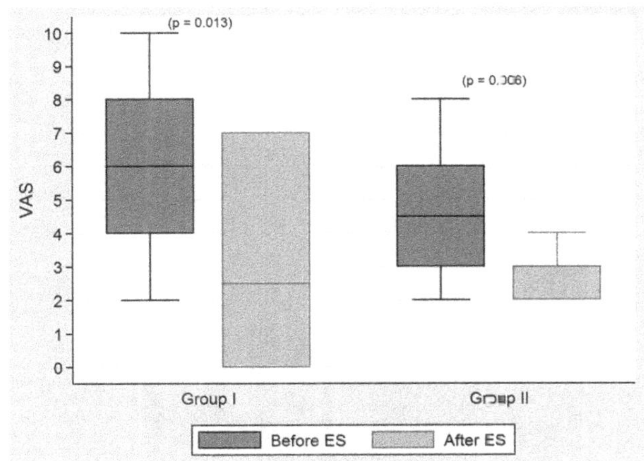

FIGURE 1 | The results of tinnitus treatment with ES in both groups. In both groups, significant changes in tinnitus, given according to VAS, were noted after ES. However, no significant difference was observed between the two groups in terms of tinnitus improvement according to VAS ($p = 0.699$).

RESULTS

Following ES, in Group I, an improvement in VAS was observed in five ears (83.3%)—tinnitus disappeared in two of them (33.3%) and no change was observed in the remaining ear (16.7%)—i.e., no deterioration in tinnitus was observed. In Group II, improvement was observed in seven ears (58.3%) and tinnitus disappeared in two of them (16.7%), while no change was observed in the other five ears (41.7%).

In both groups, significant changes in tinnitus, given according to VAS, were noted. However, no significant difference was observed between the two groups in terms of tinnitus improvement according to VAS ($p = 0.699$) (**Figure 1**).

In Group I, a significant increase in the upper and lower limit of frequency of the alpha band was observed in the left central temporal and left frontal regions following ES (**Figure 2**). These changes, however, were not correlated with any improvement in tinnitus. No significant changes were observed in the beta and theta bands and on the right side (hemisphere). In Group II, no significant changes were observed in the alpha, beta and theta bands. No significant changes were observed in the waves' amplitude (μV) before and after ES, and when right and left sides were compared. The intensity of current (mA) used in ES did not differ significantly ($p = 0.772$) between the groups (in both groups mean intensity was 0,47 mA). No pathological activity was observed in EEG after ES. We didn't observe gamma, nor delta oscillations in our patients.

DISCUSSION

Alpha oscillations are the dominant rhythm at rest in the sensory regions. This activity reflects excitatory—inhibitory balance, with decreased levels of alpha in excitatory conditions and increased in inhibition (Klimesch et al., 2007). Active stimulus processing or stimulus anticipation results in alpha power

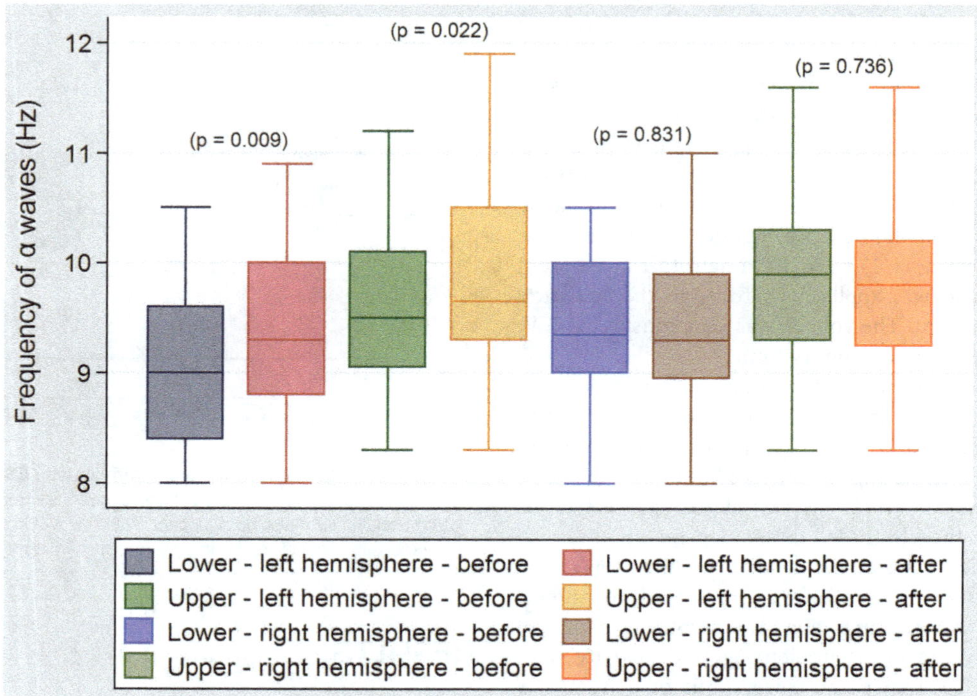

FIGURE 2 | Differences between upper and lower frequency of alpha band in group I before and after ES. In Group I, a significant increase in the upper and lower limit of frequency of the alpha band was observed in the left central temporal and frontal regions following ES. No significant changes were observed in the beta and theta bands and the right side in this group.

decrease which relates to decreased functional inhibition (Weisz et al., 2011). In consequence hyperexcitability within central auditory structures appears resulting from downregulation due to reduced peripheral—cochlear—activity. Increased spontaneous firing rate in neurons of central auditory pathway is hypothesized to be a crucial factor for tinnitus appearance (Noreña and Eggermont, 2003). Given the fact that changes in alpha band reflect shifts between excitatory—inhibitory processes and the view that tinnitus is a result of excitatory—inhibitory imbalance, in some research alpha rhythm and other frequency bands were assessed before and after tinnitus treatment. There are works on a change in alpha frequency, but most of the papers report changes in alpha power (reflecting neuronal synchronization).

In practice, two approaches in stimulations in tinnitus are possible (central vs. peripheral) and apparently both can directly or indirectly modify central activity. One approach - peripheral stimulation, aims to increase peripheral input, which results in spontaneous firing rate decrease and in consequence, in reducing central hyperactivity. The other - primarily aims to modify pathological central hyperactivity. Since tinnitus is known to be associated with excessive spontaneous activity in central auditory system (Mühlnickel et al., 1998; De Ridder et al., 2014), a spectrum of superficial brain stimulation techniques have been proposed to interfere with this maladaptive activity. EEG and MEG therefore would appear to be appropriate tools to quantify this pathological activity before and after implementation of therapeutic method.

Adamchic et al. Schlee et al. described reduced alpha frequency in tinnitus patients (Adamchic et al., 2014; Schlee et al., 2014). In the light of these results, our findings appear to be of advantage in tinnitus treatment. Some other studies, however, didn't repeat these findings (Shulman and Goldstein, 2002; Adjamian et al., 2012; Meyer et al., 2014). In terms of other oscillation bands the results are inconsistent as well. Schlee et al. demonstrated that shorter duration of tinnitus (less than 3 years) was correlated with a larger alpha variability than longer tinnitus duration (more than 3 years). The authors hypothesized that the latter may reflect decreased neuroplastic capacity of brain. Furthermore it was shown that alpha activity was variable and fluctuated with time in healthy subjects, while in tinnitus individuals this ability was significantly reduced. Interestingly, the authors interpreted alpha variability as an indicator for spontaneous tinnitus remission (Schlee et al., 2014). In our research, the changes in alpha frequency may hypothetically be indicative for better neuroplastic potential and thus better future therapeutic outcome. On the other hand, in the light of abovementioned research, the changes in alpha frequency might result just from physiological fluctuations (why they were absent in a group of bilateral tinnitus—remains for the authors unclear).

In our research significant changes in alpha band were observed in the frontal and temporal regions, both on the left side. This is probably due to ipsilateral ES (in most of the cases tinnitus was left sided). It is possible that a better balance between left and right sided tinnitus in the group would balance lateralization of the results. Weisz et al. (2005) observed marked changes in alpha and delta power in temporal (right) and frontal (left) regions and suggested that these regions might be involved in tinnitus-related cortical activity. Temporal region would then be associated with perceptual aspects of the sound, and frontal—with distress and attention of tinnitus. In this research, like in our research, the most of the patients had left sided tinnitus. The authors concluded that the lateralization of the results might vanish if the study groups were balanced in terms of left and right-sided tinnitus. The justification for this assumption was Jastreboff's neurophysiological model of tinnitus which considered prefrontal cortex a place where sensory and emotional aspects of tinnitus are integrated, but without reference to the lateralization (Jastreboff, 1990).

Since the pathological cortical activity (increase in γ / δ and decrease in alpha band activity) appears to reflect the fact of tinnitus generation and relating distress, some studies demonstrated normalization of these activities in a course of tinnitus treatment (Müller et al., 2013; Adamchic et al., 2014).

Thus three promising neuromodulation methods emerged: transcranial direct (tDCS) and alternating current simulation (tACS), and transcranial magnetic stimulation (TMS) (Zaehle et al., 2010; Song et al., 2012; Vanneste et al., 2013a). Depending on the polarity, tDCS increases or decreases cortical excitability (Miranda et al., 2006). Cathodal tDCS induces hyperpolarization of the cortex, while anodal tDCS intensifies excitation through depolarization of the neurons (Monte-Silva et al., 2013; Jocs et al., 2014). tASC increases alpha power (Zaehle et al., 2010; Vossen et al., 2015) and intracotrical inhibition. Random noise stimulation (tRNS) (Van Doren et al., 2014; Joos et al., 2015)—a new transcranial stimulation technique has recently emerged and appeared to be more effective in tinnitus reduction when compared to tDCS and tACS (Vanneste et al., 2013b; Claes et al., 2014).

In the light of inconsistent and non-replicable data on spontaneous EEG activity in tinnitus patients, two papers (Adjamian and Pierzycki et al.) have recently appeared shedding new light on EEG / MEG measurements in tinnitus (Adjamian, 2014; Pierzycki et al., 2016). Adjamian points to a careful analysis and interpretation of EEG / MEG data in tinnitus patients. Neglecting factors unrelated to tinnitus (e.g., the use of non-standardized tools, or protocols) and comorbidities such as hearing loss, hyperacusis, stress or depression might be sources for the flaws in EEG/MEG research results (Adjamian, 2014). In other paper, the author demonstrated that there are no differences due to tinnitus in any frequency band, except possibly delta (however it remains unclear if it was the effect of hearing loss or tinnitus together with hearing loss; Adjamian et al., 2012).

Vanneste et al. demonstrated correlation between psychoacoustic aspect of tinnitus and cortical activity. An increase in tinnitus loudness was associated with an increase in gamma-band activity in the auditory cortex (Vanneste et al., 2013c), which was attributed by the authors to a thalamo-cortical dysrhythmia model (De Ridder et al., 2015). This states that in the deafferented state, the dominant resting state alpha rhythm decreases to theta band activity (Llinás et al., 1999) and that constant abnormal coupled theta/gamma band activity occurs as a consequence of hyperpolarization in thalamus nuclei (De Ridder et al., 2011). In contrast, Pierzycki et al. found no relationship between whole scalp EEG band powers and psychoacoustic or psychosocial variables of tinnitus. The authors concluded that resting state whole scalp EEG should not be used as a biomarker for tinnitus (Pierzycki et al., 2016).

Preliminary results of our research revealed an increase in alpha frequency in the left central temporal and frontal regions. Although, this effect might suggest the treatment has potential, the results indicate that it was not correlated with improvement in tinnitus. Since the literature data on EEG / MEG activity in tinnitus has been inconsistent so far, the relevance of the present findings is not clear and needs further research. In previous research we obtained tinnitus relief after treatment which involved 15 ES. It is possible that the key factor contributing to improvement was repeated stimulation which was needed to evoke and consolidate changes in central auditory system. At this stage, it is unclear whether modulation of cortical activity is primary or secondary to peripheral auditory excitation. At the time of writing, no similar studies had been found in the literature.

In the light of research on peripheral electrical stimulation and central stimulation techniques (current or magnetic stimulation) it appears that both approaches may be efficient in tinnitus treatment.

The limitations of the study are the small size of the groups and the lack of a placebo and control group. In addition, the reason why EEG changes were obtained only in the unilateral tinnitus patients (group I), despite improvement in tinnitus having been observed in both groups, needs further investigation. The exact correlations between changes in cortical activity and tinnitus reduction will be the subject of future research.

CONCLUSIONS

Our results indicate that peripheral external ear ES changes cortical activity in tinnitus patients. One of the possible mechanisms in which ES influences tinnitus may therefore be a change in the cortical activity present within the left central temporal and frontal regions. However, whether this effect is primary or secondary to auditory system excitation remains to be investigated. Of the various forms of ES presented above, each may play a role in the tinnitus improvement observed in our study.

AUTHOR CONTRIBUTIONS

MM, JM, KP, and JO: Substantial contributions to the conception design of the work, the acquisition, analysis, or interpretation of data for the work, drafting the work, revising it critically for important intellectual content, final approval of the version to be published, agreement to be accountable for all aspects of the work in ensuring that questions related to the accuracy or integrity of any part of the work are appropriately investigated and resolved.

REFERENCES

Adamchic, I., Toth, T., Hauptmann, C., and Tass, P. A. (2014). Reversing pathologically increased EEG power by acoustic coordinated reset neuromodulation. *Hum. Brain Mapp.* 35, 2099–2118. doi: 10.1002/hbm.22314

Adjamian, P. (2014). The application of electro- and magneto-encephalography in tinnitus research - methods and interpretations. *Front. Neurol.* 5:228. doi: 10.3389/fneur.2014.00228

Adjamian, P., Sereda, M., Zobay, O., Hall, D. A., and Palmer, A. R. (2012). Neuromagnetic indicators of tinnitus and tinnitus masking in patients with and without hearing loss. *JARO* 13, 715–731. doi: 10.1007/s10162-012-0340-5

Baguley, D. M., Axon, P., Winter, I. M., and Moffat, D. A. (2002). The effect of vestibular nerve section upon tinnitus. *Clin. Otolaryngol. Allied Sci.* 27, 219–226. doi: 10.1046/j.1365-2273.2002.00566.x

Claes, L., Stamberger, H., Van de Heyning, P., De Ridder, D., and Vanneste, S. (2014). Auditory cortex tACS and tRNS for tinnitus: single versus multiple sessions. *Neural Plast.* 2014: 436713. doi: 10.1155/2014/436713

De Ridder, D., van der Loo, E., Vanneste, S., Gais, S., Plazier, M., Kovacs, S., et al. (2011). Theta-gamma dysrhythmia and auditory phantom perception. *J. Neurosurg.* 114, 912–921. doi: 10.3171/2010.11.JNS10335

De Ridder, D., Vanneste, S., and Freeman, W. (2014). The Bayesian brain: phantom percepts resolve sensory uncertainty. *Neurosci. Biobehav. Rev.* 44, 4–15. doi: 10.1016/j.neubiorev.2012.04.001

De Ridder, D., Vanneste, S., Langguth, B., and Llinas, R. (2015). Thalamocortical dysrhythmia: a theoretical update in tinnitus. *Front Neurol.* 6:124. doi: 10.3389/fneur.2015.00124

Jastreboff, P. J. (1990). Phantom auditory perception (tinnitus): mechanisms of generation and perception. *Neurosci. Res.* 8, 221–254.

Joos, K., De Ridder, D., Van de Heyning, P., and Vanneste, S. (2014). Polarity specific suppression effects of transcranial direct current stimulation for tinnitus. *Neural Plast.* 2014:930860. doi: 10.1155/2014/930860

Joos, K., De Ridder, D., and Vanneste, S. (2015). The differential effect of low- versus high-frequency random noise stimulation in the treatment of tinnitus. *Exp. Brain Res.* 233, 1433–1440. doi: 10.1007/s00221-015-4217-9

Kaltenbach, J. A. (2011). Tinnitus: models and mechanisms. *Hear. Res.* 276, 52–60. doi: 10.1016/j.heares.2010.12.003

Klimesch, W., Sauseng, P., and Hanslmayr, S. (2007). EEG alpha oscillations: the inhibition-timing hypothesis. *Brain Res. Rev.* 53, 63–88. doi: 10.1016/j.brainresrev.2006.06.003

Konopka, W., Zalewski, P., Olszewski, J., Olszewska-Ziaber, A., and Pietkiewicz, P. (2001). Tinnitus suppression by electrical promontory stimulation (EPS) in patients with sensorineural hearing loss. *Auris Nasus Larynx* 28, 35–40. doi: 10.1016/S0385-8146(00)00086-9

Latkowski, B. (1981). Original improvement of the technique of implantation of microelectrodes in cochlear deafness.*Minerva Otolaringol.* 1, 69.

Llinás, R. R., Ribary, U., Jeanmonod, D., Kronberg, E., and Mitra, P. P. (1999). Thalamocortical dysrhythmia: a neurological and neuropsychiatric syndrome characterized by magnetoencephalography. *Proc. Natl. Acad. Sci. U.S.A.* 96, 15222–15227.

Mertens, G., De Bodt, M., and Van de Heyning, P. (2016). Cochlear implantation as a long-term treatment for ipsilateral incapacitating tinnitus in subjects with unilateral hearing loss up to 10 years. *Hear. Res.* 331, 1–6. doi: 10.1016/j.heares.2015.09.016

Meyer, M., Luethi, M. S., Neff, P., Langer, N., and Büchi, S. (2014). Disentangling tinnitus distress and tinnitus presence by means of EEG power analysis. *Neural Plast.* 2014:468546. doi: 10.1155/2014/468546

Middlebrooks, J. C. (2008). Cochlear-Implant high pulse rate and narrow electrode configuration impair transmission of temporal information to the auditory cortex. *J. Neurophysiol.* 100, 92–107. doi: 10.1152/jn.01114.2007

Mielczarek, M., and Olszewski, J. (2014). Direct current stimulation of the ear in tinnitus treatment: a double-blind placebo-controlled study. *Eur. Arch. Otorhinolaryngol.* 271, 1815–1822. doi: 10.1007/s00405-013-2849-6

Miranda, P. C., Lomarev, M., and Hallett, M. (2006). Modeling the current distribution during transcranial direct current stimulation. *Clin. Neurophysiol.* 117, 1623–1629. doi: 10.1016/j.clinph.2006.04.009

Monte-Silva, K., Kuo, M. F., Hessenthaler, S., Fresnoza, S., Liebetanz, D., Paulus, W., et al. (2013). Induction of late LTP-like plasticity in the human motor cortex by repeated non-invasive brain stimulation. *Brain Stimul.* 6, 424–432. doi: 10.1016/j.brs.2012.04.011

Mühlnickel, W., Elbert, T., Taub, E., and Flor, H. (1998). Reorganization of auditory cortex in tinnitus. *Proc. Natl. Acad. Sci. U.S.A.* 95, 10340–10343.

Mulders, W. H., Barry, K. M., and Robertson, D. (2014a). Effects of furosemide on cochlear neural activity, central hyperactivity and behavioural tinnitus after cochlear trauma in guinea pig. *PLoS ONE* 9:e97948. doi: 10.1371/journal.pone.0097948

Mulders, W. H., McMahen, C., and Robertson, D. (2014b). Effects of chronic furosemide on central neural hyperactivity and cochlear thresholds after cochlear trauma in Guinea pig. *Front Neurol.* 5:146. doi: 10.3389/fneur.2014.00146

Müller, N., Lorenz, I., Langguth, B., and Weisz, N. (2013). rTMS induced tinnitus relief is related to an increase in auditory cortical alpha activity. *PLoS ONE* 8:e55557. doi: 10.1371/journal.pone.0055557

Noreña, A. J., and Eggermont, J. J. (2003). Changes in spontaneous neural activity immediately after an acoustic trauma: implications for neural correlates of tinnitus. *Hear. Res.* 183, 137–153. doi: 10.1016/S0378-5955(03)00225-9

Noreña, A. J., Mulders, W. H., and Robertson, D. (2015). Suppression of putative tinnitus-related activity by extra-cochlear electrical stimulation. *J. Neurophysiol.* 113, 132–143. doi: 10.1152/jn.00580.2014

Nuttall, A. L., and Ren, T. (1995). Electromotile hearing: evidence from basilar membrane motion and otoacoustic emissions. *Hear. Res.* 92, 170–177.

Pierzycki, R. H., McNamara, A. J., Hoare, D. J., and Hall, D. A. (2016). Whole scalp resting state EEG of oscillatory brain activity shows no parametric relationship with psychoacoustic and psychosocial assessment of tinnitus: a repeated measures study. *Hear Res.* 331, 101–108. doi: 10.1016/j.heares.2015.11.003

Portmann, M., Cazals, Y., Negrevergne, M., and Aran, J. M. (1979). Temporary tinnitus suppression in man through electrical stimulation of the cochlea. *Acta Otolaryngol.* 87, 294–299

Quaranta, N., Wagstaff, S., and Baguley, D. M. (2004). Tinnitus and cochlear implantation. *Int. J. Audiol.* 43, 245–251. doi: 10.1080/14992020400050033

Ren, T., and Nuttall, A. L. (1995). Extracochlear electrically evoked otoacoustic emissions: a model for *in vivo* assessment of outer hair cell electromotility. *Hear. Res.* 92, 178–183.

Rubinstein, J. T., Tyler, R. S., Johnson, A., and Brown, C. J. (2003). Electrical suppression of tinnitus with high-rate pulse trains. *Otol. Neurotol.* 24, 478–485. doi: 10.1097/00129492-200305000-00021

Schlee, W., Schecklmann, M., Lehner, A., Kreuzer, P. M., Vielsmeier, V., Poeppl, T. B., et al. (2014). Reduced variability of auditory alpha activity in chronic tinnitus. *Neural Plast.* 2014:436146. doi: 10.1155/2014/436146

Shulman, A., and Goldstein, B. (2002). Quantitative electroencephalography: preliminary report–tinnitus. *Int Tinnitus. J.* 8, 77–86.

Song, J.-J., Vanneste, S., Van de Heyning, P., and De Ridder, D. (2012). Transcranial direct current stimulation in tinnitus patients: a systemic review and meta-analysis. *Sci. World J.* 2012:427941. doi: 10.1100/2012/427941

Todt, I., Rademacher, G., Mutze, S., Ramalingam, R., Wolter, S., Mittmann, P., et al. (2015). Relationship between intracochlear electrode position and tinnitus in cochlear implantees. *Acta Otolaryngol.* 135, 781–785. doi: 10.3109/00016489.2015.1024332

Van Doren, J., Langguth, B., and Schecklmann, M. (2014). Electroencephalographic effects of transcranial random noise stimulation in the auditory cortex. *Brain Stimul.* 7, 807–812. doi: 10.1016/j.brs.2014.08.007

Vanneste, S., Fregni, F., and De Ridder, D. (2013b). Head-to-Head comparison of transcranial random noise stimulation, transcranial AC stimulation, and transcranial DC stimulation for tinnitus. *Front Psychiatry.* 4:158. doi: 10.3389/fpsyt.2013.00158

Vanneste, S., van Dongen, M., De Vree, B., Hiseni, S., van der Velden, E., Strydis, C., et al. (2013c). Does enriched acoustic environment in humans abolish chronic tinnitus clinically and electrophysiologically? A double blind placebo controlled study. *Hear Res.* 296, 141–148. doi: 10.1016/j.heares.2012.10.003

Vanneste, S., Walsh, V., Van De Heyning, P., and De Ridder, D. (2013a). Comparing immediate transient tinnitus suppression using tACS and tDCS: a placebo-controlled study. *Exp. Brain Res.* 226, 25–31. doi: 10.1007/s00221-013-3406-7

Vossen, A., Gross, J., and Thut, G. (2015). Alpha Power Increase After Transcranial Alternating Current Stimulation at Alpha Frequency (α-tACS)

Reflects Plastic Changes Rather Than Entrainment. *Brain Stimul.* 8, 499–508. doi: 10.1016/j.brs.2014.12.004

Watanabe, K., Okawara, D., Baba, S., and Yagi, T. (1997). Electrocochleographic analysis of the suppression of tinnitus by electrical promontory stimulation. *Audiology* 36, 147–154.

Weisz, N., Hartmann, T., Müller, N., Lorenz, I., and Obleser, J. (2011). Alpha rhythms in audition: cognitive and clinical perspectives. *Front. Psychol.* 2:73. doi: 10.3389/fpsyg.2011.00073

Weisz, N., Moratti, S., Meinzer, M., Dohrmann, K., and Elbert, T. (2005). Tinnitus perception and distress is related to abnormal spontaneous brain activity as measured by magnetoencephalography. *PLoS Med.* 2:e153. doi: 10.1371/journal.pmed.0020153

Zaehle, T., Rach, S., and Herrmann, C. S. (2010). Transcranial alternating current stimulation enhances individual alpha activity in human EEG. *PLoS ONE* 5:e13766. doi: 10.1371/journal.pone.0013766

Zeng, F. G., Tang, Q., Dimitrijevic, A., Starr, A., Larky, J., and Blevins, N. H. (2011). Tinnitus suppression by low-rate electric stimulation and its electrophysiological mechanisms. *Hear. Res.* 277, 61–66. doi: 10.1016/j.heares.2011.03.010

22

Impact of Temporomandibular Joint Complaints on Tinnitus-Related Distress

*Niklas K. Edvall[1], Edis Gunan[1], Eleni Genitsaridi[2,3], Andra Lazar[4], Golbarg Mehraei[5], Mattias Billing[6], Marie Tullberg[6], Jan Bulla[7,8], Jonathon Whitton[5], Barbara Canlon[1], Deborah A. Hall[2,3,9] and Christopher R. Cederroth[1]**

[1] Laboratory of Experimental Audiology, Department of Physiology and Pharmacology, Karolinska Institutet, Stockholm, Sweden, [2] National Institute of Health Research, Nottingham Biomedical Research Centre, Ropewalk House, Nottingham, United Kingdom, [3] Hearing Sciences, Division of Clinical Neuroscience, School of Medicine, University of Nottingham, Nottingham, United Kingdom, [4] Hörsel och Balansmottagningen, Karolinska Universitetssjukhuset, Stockholm, Sweden, [5] Decibel Therapeutics, Inc., Boston, MA, United States, [6] Braheskliniken, Stockholm, Sweden, [7] Department of Mathematics, University of Bergen, Bergen, Norway, [8] Department of Psychiatry and Psychotherapy, University of Regensburg, Regensburg, Germany, [9] University of Nottingham Malaysia, Semenyih, Malaysia

***Correspondence:**
Christopher R. Cederroth
christopher.cederroth@ki.se*

There is increasing evidence of associations between the presence of temporomandibular joint (TMJ) disorders and tinnitus. It has been recently proposed that tinnitus patients with TMJ complaints could constitute a subtype, meaning a subgroup of tinnitus patients responsive to specific treatments. Tinnitus patients with TMJ complaints are often young women with somatosensory features of their tinnitus. Here, we investigate the socio-economic factors, phenotypic characteristics and psychological variables of tinnitus subjects from the Swedish Tinnitus Outreach Project, with (n = 486) or without (n = 1,996) TMJ complaints. The prevalence of TMJ complaints was greater in tinnitus subjects with severe tinnitus (36%) when compared to those with any tinnitus (19%), strongly indicating the contribution of TMJ problems to the severity of tinnitus. Comparing subgroups with or without TMJ complaints in the whole sample, differences were found regarding a large number of socioeconomic, phenotypic, and psychological characteristics. Subjects with TMJ complaints were more often women, more often reported stress as the cause of tinnitus, were more severely affected by tinnitus, scored worse in measures of psychological well-being and life quality, and were more often affected by problems tolerating sounds, headache, vertigo/dizziness, and neck pain. In addition, they more often reported pulsating and tonal tinnitus, somatic modulation of tinnitus, and aggravation of tinnitus by loud sounds and stress. When focusing the analysis in subjects with tinnitus as a big problem using the Tinnitus Functional Index cut-off $\geq$ 48, or with severe tinnitus according to the Tinnitus Handicap Inventory cut-off $\geq$ 58, the impact of somatosensory modulations and stress on tinnitus were greater in subjects with TMJ complaints in comparison to those without. In light of these results, we hypothesize that stress could contribute to the co-occurrence of TMJ problems and tinnitus and also to the development of severe tinnitus. Our study supports the need of involving dental care and stress management in the holistic treatment of patients with severe tinnitus.

Keywords: tinnitus, TMJ, stress, distress, somato sensory

INTRODUCTION

Subjective tinnitus, ringing in the ears, is a prevalent phantom sound perception (prevalence ranging from 5 to 43%) that in many cases can be severe to the point of seeking medical care (McCormack et al., 2016). Existing treatments are unsatisfactory and are of limited efficacy (Cederroth et al., 2013, 2018; Langguth et al., 2018). *Severe* tinnitus, defined as clinically significant tinnitus, or according to the Tinnitus Handicap Inventory (THI), has been shown to be strongly associated with anxiety and depression (Dobie, 2003; Bartels et al., 2008; Kehrle et al., 2016). Studies have also shown an important contribution of stress as a psychiatric co-morbidity (Hebert et al., 2012; Schlee et al., 2017a) with an overall damaging impact on life quality and subsequent healthcare costs (Stockdale et al., 2017). Sexual dimorphism on the psychological impact of tinnitus has also been revealed, whereby tinnitus is associated with an increased risk in suicide attempts only in women (Lugo et al., 2019).

The mechanisms by which tinnitus occurs are still poorly understood. The current pathophysiological models stipulate that tinnitus emerges as a failure to adapt to missing sensory information originating from the ear (Shore et al., 2016). This results in a compensatory mechanism in the brain translating into a greater neuronal activity (central gain) along the auditory pathway (Auerbach et al., 2014). Limbic structures (e.g., amygdala), that are involved in emotional processing, have been shown to be connected to the auditory pathway and it has been proposed that these contribute to tinnitus (Rauschecker et al., 2010). Interestingly, there is a striking resemblance between the pathways that are involved in tinnitus and chronic pain, converging toward frontostriatal circuits including the ventromedial prefrontal cortex (vmPFC) and the nucleus accumbens (NAc) (Rauschecker et al., 2015).

Recent evidence point toward a dysregulation of multisensory circuits in the generation of tinnitus (Haider et al., 2017). Somatosensory modulations of tinnitus are thought to emerge from abnormal plasticity in somatic-auditory interactions. The dorsal cochlear nucleus is a well-established site of sensory integration (Roberts et al., 2010; Wu et al., 2015). Fusiform cells are at the crossroad of auditory and somatic inputs; on their basal dendrites they receive glutamatergic input from auditory nerve fibers, and on their apical dendrites they receive input from parallel fibers. These inputs also impact on inhibitory interneurons such as cartwheel cells and vertical cells that directly synapse on fusiform cells to provide feed-forward inhibition. Supporting the importance of this integration node, bimodal stimulation of fusiform cells (auditory and somatosensory) has been proposed as an approach to reduce tinnitus in animals and humans (Marks et al., 2018).

It is now agreed that tinnitus is a heterogeneous condition that cannot be considered a single entity (Cederroth et al., 2019a). This may explain why existing interventions are not successful for all patients, and thus identifying "subtypes" is needed to tailor treatments according to a patient profile and improve therapeutic outcome. Common factors related to tinnitus include hearing impairment, head/neck injury, ear infections, depression, and non-steroidal anti-inflammatory drugs (NSAIDs) (Nondahl et al., 2011), but less understood are the contributions of dental problems to tinnitus severity. The cochlea is located just next to the temporomandibular joint, where nerve connections have been mapped from the joint region toward the cochlea. Temporomandibular joint (TMJ) disorders are frequently observed in dental care with a 18–27% prevalence in the population (Deng et al., 1995; Al-Khotani et al., 2016). These can be caused by trauma, an injury or dislocation in the disk of the temporomandibular joint, excessive stress on the jaw muscles (e.g., bruxism), arthritis or malocclusion (Sharma et al., 2011; Murphy et al., 2013; Chisnoiu et al., 2015). Symptoms include pain in the jaw and/or face, difficulties opening the jaw and chewing, and popping sounds when opening the mouth (e.g., when talking or chewing) (Bernhardt et al., 2011). Interestingly, prevalence of tinnitus in patients with TMJ disorders reaches 60% in comparison to 15–30% in patients with no TMJ disorder (Chole and Parker, 1992; Tuz et al., 2003). The association between tinnitus and TMJ disorders was confirmed by two recent systematic reviews that reported a significant association between the two conditions in the majority of the identified studies (Bousema et al., 2018; Mottaghi et al., 2019). Both reviews assessed the quality of the included studies. Quality ranged from low to high indicating some risk of bias in reported findings. Bousema et al. (2018) evaluated 22 studies which investigated the presence of cervical spine disorders (CSDs) or TMJ disorders in patients with and without tinnitus, or the presence of tinnitus in patients with and without TMJ disorders. In contrast, Mottaghi et al. (2019) evaluated findings from just five studies comparing patients with and without TMJ disorders.

Using data from the Tinnitus Research Initiative (TRI) database, Vielsmeier et al. (2012) performed a first in-depth analysis of the characteristics of tinnitus patients with or without self-reported TMJ complaints and found that a larger proportion of those with TMJ complaints were female, younger, and could modulate tinnitus by head/jaw movements or had their tinnitus reduced in the presence of sound (Vielsmeier et al., 2012). However, the study consisted of clinical tinnitus patients only and does not allow for a global picture of the relationship of TMJ complaints with tinnitus in the general population. Furthermore, the questionnaires used in the Vielsmeier et al. (2012) study did not include measures of socioeconomic status, stress, anxiety and emotional reactivity to tinnitus, as measured by the Fear of Tinnitus Questionnaire (FTQ) and the Tinnitus Catastrophising Scale (TCS) (Cima et al., 2012). Here, we will examine the relationship between self-reported TMJ problems with tinnitus using data from the Swedish Tinnitus Outreach Project and investigate a broader range of variables that may differ in tinnitus subjects with or without TMJ complaints.

MATERIALS AND METHODS

Sample

Participants were invited to join the Swedish Tinnitus Outreach Project via social media channels and through partnerships with local cohorts, including LifeGene (Almqvist et al., 2011). All participants above 18 years of age were eligible. Voluntary registration was done on a website from STOP[1]. After providing informed consent for having their data stored in a database and analyzed, participants were invited to an online survey. Between November 2015 and January 2018, 5,593 participants answered the online questionnaires. The present study focused on tinnitus subjects with or without TMJ complaints and their sociodemographic data are reported in **Table 1**. The project has been approved by the Regional Ethics Review Board in Stockholm (2015/2129-31/1).

Questionnaires

The online survey consisted of a combination of standardized questionnaires, which are described in detail elsewhere (Müller et al., 2016). The Tinnitus Sample Case History Questionnaire (TSCHQ) measures phenotypic characteristics that may be associated with tinnitus (Landgrebe et al., 2010), and question #32 "*Do you suffer from temporomandibular disorder?*" was adapted in Swedish to enquire about pain in the jaw muscles or problems in the jaw rather than the diagnosis itself ("*Lider du av smärta i käkmuskeler eller störnig i käkfunktions?*") (Müller et al., 2016), as laymen may be unfamiliar with the medical terminology. This question lead to an intra-class coherent coefficient of 0.67 (acceptable) in a test–retest (Müller et al., 2016). The THI (Newman et al., 1996) and the Tinnitus Functional Index (TFI) (Meikle et al., 2012) consist of multiple subscales measuring the impact of tinnitus in the different aspects of everyday life and give a global score of tinnitus symptom severity. The Fear of Tinnitus Questionnaire (FTQ) and the Tinnitus Catastrophizing Scale (TCS) measure fear and degree of catastrophic misinterpretations regarding tinnitus (Cima et al., 2011). The Hyperacusis Questionnaire (HQ) evaluates symptomatology related to sensitivity to sound (Khalfa et al., 2002). The Perceived Stress Questionnaire (PSQ) (Levenstein et al., 1993) and the Hospital Anxiety Depression Scales for Anxiety (HADS A) and depression (HADS D) measure stress, anxiety, and depression respectively (Andersson et al., 2003). The World Health Organization's Quality of Life (WHOQoL)-BREF subscales WHOQol Physical, WHOQol Psychological, WHOQol Social, and WHOQol Environmental, evaluate quality of life domains (The Whoqol Group, 1998). All questionnaires were translated into Swedish and previously administered to tinnitus subjects (Müller et al., 2016). Numerical Rating Scales (NRS) for Loudness, Awareness, and Annoyance were obtained via the TSCHQ (questions 12, 16, and 17). Some of these questionnaires were selected based on their integration in the TRI database[2].

Inclusion Criteria

Subjects were included if they answered "Yes, always (all the time)" and "Yes, occasionally (now and then)" (n = 2,597) to the question "Do you have tinnitus?" Those who answered "No" or "Don't know" (n = 2,991) and 5 missing entries were excluded from the analysis. The second inclusion criterion was based on whether subjects answered either "Yes" or "No" to the question "Do you suffer from temporomandibular disorder?" Subjects who answered "Don't know" (n = 113) were excluded, and those who answered "Yes" (n = 486) and "No" (n = 1,996) were included (2 missing entries). Thus, 44% (n = 2,482) of the total subjects (n = 5,593) were considered in the analysis. Since the classification of subjects is based on self-report, we used the terminology TMJ 'complaints' which distinguishes the study group from diagnosed TMJ 'disorders.' We also investigated subjects with severe tinnitus. Severe tinnitus was operationally defined in two ways. The first used a revised grading system of the original eight-factor 25 item of the TFI (Fackrell et al., 2017) where a TFI cut-off score $\geq$ 48 denotes a big problem. The second used a THI cut-off score $\geq$ 58, since this boundary is used as a criterion for referral to specialty care in the Stockholm County (Idrizbegovic et al., 2011). For some questionnaires, data were missing for 13 participants in the non-TMJ group and 5 participants in the TMJ group.

[1]https:/stop.ki.se

[2]https://www.tinnitusresearch.net/

Statistical Analysis

Phenotypic characteristics such as tinnitus loudness, pitch, onset, whether tinnitus is pulsating or not, what the tinnitus sounds like, and onset-related events were obtained from the TSCHQ. Additional sociodemographic data (i.e., marital status, income, employment status, and education level) were obtained using questions from Svensson et al. (2013). All statistical analyses were performed in JMP 13 (SAS Institute, Inc.) and R Core Team (2019). For nominal variables, Pearson's Chi-squared test was used. Homoscedasticity between groups was tested for using the Brown–Forsythe test and showed significant differences between subgroups for multiple variables. Several questionnaire total scores also deviated from a normal distribution. Therefore, the non-parametric Wilcoxon's test was used for all comparisons to provide easy comparability between different groups for the reader. In order to investigate the potential impact of multiple comparisons on the discovery rates of our tests, we also report p-values adjusted by the method of Benjamini and Hochberg. The adjustments were computed for each set of p-values resulting from multiple tests carried out.

RESULTS

Nineteen percent (486/2482) of those with any tinnitus reported TMJ complaints. The socioeconomic characteristics of our study sample with TMJ complaints and tinnitus are listed in **Table 1.** Subjects with TMJ complaints differed from those without TMJ complaints in sex, age, marital status, gross income, and employment status (p = 0.0375 to < 0.0001) and survived correction for multiple comparisons. No difference in education level was found between the two groups. Thirty percent of the sample with tinnitus as a big problem (97/321) (i.e., TFI $\geq$ 48), reported TMJ complaints. Using the THI cut-off for severity ($\geq$58), 36% (69/191) reported TMJ complaints. In the samples reporting a big problem or with severe tinnitus, no differences in the socioeconomic characteristics were found after correction for multiple comparisons (**Table 1**). These findings suggest that with increasing severity, socioeconomic differences between groups with or without TMJ complaints no longer exist.

TABLE 1 | Sociodemographic characteristics for subjects with tinnitus with or without TMJ complaints.

	Any tinnitus		**TFI ≥ 48**		**THI ≥ 53**	
	TMJ (n = 486) No (%)	**No TMJ (n = 1996) No (%)**	**TMJ (n = 97) No (%)**	**No TMJ (n = 224) No (%)**	**TMJ (n = 69) No (%)**	**No TMJ (n = 122) No (%)**
Sex	$\chi^2(1) = 75.22, p < 0.0001$ (0.0001)		$\chi^2(1) = 6.22, p = 0.0127$ (0.0762)		$\chi^2(1) = 1.92, p = 0.166$ (0.249)	
Male	161 (33.1)	1099 (55.1)	39 (40.2)	124 (55.4)	29 (42)	64 (52.5)
Female	325 (66.9)	897 (44.9)	58 (59.8)	100 (44.6)	40 (58)	58 (47.5)
Age group	$\chi^2(7) = 24.18, p = 0.0011$ (0.0017)		$\chi^2(7) = 13.99, p = 0.0513$ (0.077)		$\chi^2(7) = 12.58, p = 0.0831$ (0.1662)	
<24	13 (2.7)	43 (2.2)	3 (3.1)	4 (1.8)	4 (5.9)	3 (2.5)
25–34	115 (23.8)	371 (18.5)	17 (17.7)	33 (14.8)	14 (20.6)	25 (20.7)
35–44	110 (22.8)	445 (22.3)	25 (26)	39 (17.5)	19 (27.9)	17 (14.1)
45–54	138 (28.6)	525 (26.4)	28 (29.2)	64 (28.7)	17 (25)	29 (24)
55–64	67 (13.9)	285 (14.3)	17 (17.7)	36 (16.1)	10 (14.7)	24 (19.8)
65–74	35 (7.3)	272 (13.7)	5 (5.2)	31 (13.9)	4 (5.9)	16 (13.2)
75–84	4 (0.8)	48 (2.4)	0 (0)	14 (6.3)	0 (0)	6 (5)
>85	1 (0.2)	3 (0.2)	1 (1)	2 (0.9)	0 (0)	1 (0.8)
Marital status	$\chi^2(4) = 10.18, p = 0.0375$ (0.045)		$\chi^2(4) = 1.93, p = 0.7485$ (0.8148)		$\chi^2(4) = 4.12, p = 0.3905$ (0.3905)	
Married	183 (37.7)	889 (44.5)	34 (35.1)	90 (40.2)	24 (34.8)	48 (39.3)
Living with partner	161 (33.1)	594 (29.8)	35 (36.1)	68 (30.4)	26 (37.7)	38 (31.2)
Single	102 (21)	333 (16.7)	20 (20.6)	42 (18.8)	16 (23.2)	23 (18.9)
Widow/widower	6 (1.2)	25 (1.3)	1 (1)	5 (2.2)	0 (0)	4 (3.3)
Divorced	34 (7)	155 (7.8)	7 (7.2)	19 (8.5)	3 (4.4)	9 (7.4)
Gross income	$\chi^2(3) = 27.49, p < 0.0001$ (0.0001)		$\chi^2(3) = 0.94, p = 0.8148$ (0.8148)		$\chi^2(3) = 3.95, p = 0.2674$ (0.3209)	
0–200,000 SEK	70 (14.4)	232 (11.6)	17 (17.5)	44 (19.6)	13 (18.8)	27 (22.1)
200,001–450,000 SEK	262 (53.9)	944 (47.3)	54 (55.7)	113 (50.5)	44 (63.8)	61 (50)
450,001 SEK or more	122 (25.1)	739 (37)	19 (19.6)	52 (23.2)	9 (13)	23 (18.9)
Don't know/don't want to disclose	32 (6.6)	81 (4.1)	7 (7.2)	15 (6.7)	3 (4.4)	11 (9)
Education level	$\chi^2(3) = 2.39, p = 0.495$ (0.495)		$\chi^2(3) = 7.88, p = 0.0486$ (0.077)		$\chi^2(3) = 7.67, p = 0.0535$ (0.1605)	
Middle School	17 (3.5)	53 (2.7)	4 (4.1)	17 (7.6)	3 (4.4)	10 (8.2)
High School	108 (22.2)	403 (20.2)	35 (36.1)	60 (26.8)	26 (37.7)	32 (26.2)
University	314 (64.6)	1353 (67.8)	38 (39.2)	117 (52.2)	26 (37.7)	66 (54.1)
Other	47 (9.7)	187 (9.4)	20 (20.6)	30 (13.4)	14 (20.3)	14 (11.5)
Employment	$\chi^2(10) = 48.23, p < 0.0001$ (0.0001)		$\chi^2(8) = 17.18, p = 0.0283$ (0.077)		$\chi^2(7) = 14.21, p = 0.0476$ (0.1605)	
Don't know	0 (0)	1 (0.1)	0 (0)	0 (0)	0 (0)	0 (0)
Employed	313 (64.4)	1219 (61.1)	56 (57.7)	104 (46.4)	44 (63.8)	54 (44.3)
Unemployed	8 (1.7)	22 (1.1)	3 (3.1)	6 (2.7)	1 (1.5)	5 (4.1)
Running my own business/working as a partner in a company	48 (9.9)	259 (13)	6 (6.2)	29 (13)	4 (5.8)	13 (10.7)
Retired	37 (7.6)	289 (14.5)	8 (8.3)	44 (19.6)	4 (5.8)	21 (17.2)
Sick leave (for more than 2 month) or disability pension due to illness or disability	35 (7.2)	63 (3.2)	13 (13.4)	27 (12.1)	8 (11.6)	20 (16.4)
Parental leave (since 2 months or longer)	4 (0.8)	36 (1.8)	1 (1)	4 (1.8)	1 (1.5)	2 (1.6)
Student	24 (4.9)	78 (3.9)	9 (9.3)	6 (2.7)	7 (10.1)	5 (4.1)
Sabbatical	2 (0.4)	3 (0.2)	0 (0)	1 (0.5)	0 (0)	0 (0)
Housewife/-husband	0 (0)	1 (0.1)	0 (0)	0 (0)	0 (0)	0 (0)
Other	15 (3.1)	25 (1.3)	1 (1)	3 (1.3)	0 (0)	2 (1.6)

Income refers to yearly income in SEK. Pairwise comparisons using Pearson's Chi-square test are reported. Percentages (%) displayed refer to column percentages. p-Values adjusted for multiple comparisons are shown between parenthesis.

Greater Tinnitus Symptom Severity in Tinnitus Subjects With TMJ Complaints

Greater tinnitus-related burden was found in tinnitus subjects with TMJ complaints (**Table 2**). Scores in all the instruments indicated greater impact in tinnitus subjects with TMJ complaints compared to those without TMJ complaints. Differences were statistically significant for all variables (NRS loudness, awareness, annoyance, THI, TFI, FTQ, TCS, HQ, PSQ, HADS A, HADS D, and all quality of life scores; p = 0.02 to < 0.0001). When assessing cases with tinnitus as a big problem, fewer questionnaires showed significant differences (FTQ, TCS, HQ, HADS A, HADS D, physical, psychological, and environmental quality of life). In contrast, in subjects with severe tinnitus, no differences were found after correction for multiple comparisons with the exception of the psychological quality of life (p = 0.02). Again, with increasing severity, fewer differences were found between subjects with and without TMJ complaints (**Table 2**).

TABLE 2 | Questionnaire scores from subjects with tinnitus with or without TMJ complaints.

	Any tinnitus		TFI ≥ 48		THI ≥ 58	
	TMJ (n = 486) Mean (SD)	No TMJ (n = 1996) Mean (SD)	TMJ (n = 97) Mean (SD)	No TMJ (n = 224) Mean (SD)	TMJ (n = 69) Mean (SD)	No TMJ (n = 122) Mean (SD)
NRS Lo	44.4 (25.7)	39.8 (25.2)	71.3 (21.3)	71.5 (18.3)	75.3 (17.8)	74.2 (19.7)
	3.57; p = 0.0004 (0.0004)		0.29; p = 0.7688 (0.8145)		0.21; p = 0.8314 (0.8908)	
NRS Aw	36 (32.1)	32.7 (31.1)	72.8 (26.9)	74.9 (24.9)	73.5 (27)	76.8 (24.3)
	2.33; p = 0.02 (0.02)		−0.55; p = 0.5799 (0.6691)		−0.65; p = 0.514 (0.6903)	
NRS An	24.7 (28)	18.7 (24.6)	60.9 (26.6)	60 (27)	63.6 (28.2)	66.7 (26.4)
	5.17; p = < 0.0001 (0.0001)		0.23; p = 0.8145 (0.8145)		−0.63; p = 0.5285 (0.6903)	
THI	28.8 (23.1)	19.6 (19.1)	63.1 (18.3)	58.2 (18.7)	73.3 (12.3)	73.1 (11.5)
	9; p < 0.0001 (<0.0001)		2.15; p = 0.0312 (0.052)		0.05; p = 0.9608 (0.9608)	
TFI	27.8 (23.2)	20.1 (19.8)	65.6 (13.3)	63 (11.9)	66.8 (16.8)	66.6 (14.9)
	6.9; p < 0.0001 (<0.0001)		1.52; p = 0.1274 (0.1737)		0.28; p = 0.7817 (0.8908)	
PSQ	0.4 (0.2)	0.3 (0.2)	0.6 (0.2)	0.5 (0.2)	0.6 (0.2)	0.5 (0.2)
	12.12; p < 0.0001 (<0.0001)		4.72; p < 0.0001 (0.0001)		2.56; p = 0.0104 (0.052)	
HADS_A	8.1 (4.5)	5.6 (3.9)	11.4 (4.6)	8.5 (4.3)	11.8 (4.5)	10 (4.4)
	11.01; p < 0.0001 (<0.0001)		4.93; p < 0.0001 (0.0001)		2.6; p = 0.0092 (0.052)	
HADS_D	4.8 (4)	3.3 (3.1)	8.2 (4.3)	6.3 (3.7)	8.5 (4.5)	7.5 (3.7)
	7.88; p < 0.0001 (<0.0001)		4; p < 0.0001 (0.0001)		1.64; p = 0.1008 (0.3024)	
FTQ	5.6 (3)	4.5 (2.6)	8.6 (2.9)	8 (3)	9.7 (2.7)	9.2 (2.8)
	7.27; p < 0.0001 (<0.0001)		1.74; p = 0.0825 (0.1238)		1.7; p = 0.0895 (0.3024)	
TCS	15.9 (11.5)	11.6 (9.8)	29.2 (9)	26.8 (10.2)	31.4 (7.9)	30.8 (9)
	7.56; p < 0.0001 (<0.0001)		2.23; p = 0.0258 (0.0484)		0.59; p = 0.5522 (0.6903)	
HQ	20.6 (9.1)	15.6 (9)	26.6 (7.6)	23.5 (8.8)	27.4 (7.7)	25.6 (8.9)
	10.68; p < 0.0001 (<0.0001)		3.13; p = 0.0018 (0.0039)		1.39; p = 0.1654 (0.3544)	
QoL Phy	14.4 (3)	16 (2.5)	12 (2.8)	13.5 (2.8)	12.1 (3)	12.6 (2.7)
	−10.68; p < 0.0001 (<0.0001)		−4.33; p < 0.0001 (0.0001)		−1.27; p = 0.2033 (0.3812)	
QoL Psy	13.7 (3)	15.1 (2.5)	11.3 (3.1)	13.2 (2.7)	11 (3.3)	12.4 (2.6)
	−9.25; p < 0.0001 (<0.0001)		−5.02; p < 0.0001 (0.0001)		−3.21; p = 0.0013 (0.0195)	
QoL social	13.6 (3.3)	14.3 (3)	12.6 (3.8)	13.1 (3.2)	12.9 (3.6)	12.4 (3.4)
	−4.76; p < 0.0001 (<0.0001)		−1.4; p = 0.1603 (0.2004)		0.68; p = 0.4986 (0.6903)	
QoL Env	15.5 (2.5)	16.5 (2.1)	13.8 (2.6)	15.1 (2.4)	14.1 (2.8)	14.6 (2.5)
	−8.24; p < 0.0001 (<0.0001)		−4.1; p < 0.0001 (0.0001)		−1.42; p = 0.1552 (0.3544)	

Values are mean (±SD). Pairwise comparisons using Wilcoxon's tests are reported below the compared values. p-Values adjusted for multiple comparisons are shown between parenthesis. NRS, Numerical Ratins Score; Lo, tinnitus loudness; Aw, awareness; An, annoyance; THI, Tinnitus Handicap Inventory; TFI, Tinnitus Functional Index; FTQ, Fear of Tinnitus Questionnaire; TCS, Tinnitus Catastrophising Scale; HQ, Hyperacusis Questionnaire; PSQ, Perceived Stress Questionnaire; HADS A, Hospital Anxiety Depression Scales for Anxiety; HADS D, Hospital Anxiety Depression Scales for Depression; QoL, quality of life; subscales from the World Health Organization: Phy, physical, Psych, psychological; Soc, social; Env, environmental.

TABLE 3 | Phenotypic characteristics for subjects with tinnitus with or without TMJ complaints.

	Any tinnitus		TFI ≥ 48		THI ≥ 58	
	TMJ (*n* = 486) No (%)	No TMJ (*n* = 1996) No (%)	TMJ (*n* = 97) No (%)	No TMJ (*n* = 224) No (%)	TMJ (*n* = 69) No (%)	No TMJ (*n* = 122) No (%)
Tinnitus onset	$\chi^2(5) = 1.23$, $p = 0.942$ (0.942)		$\chi^2(5) = 4.36$, $p = 0.499$ (0.756)		$\chi^2(5) = 3.34$, $p = 0.648$ (0.748)	
Don't know	48 (9.9)	176 (8.8)	2 (2.1)	6 (2.7)	1 (1.5)	3 (2.5)
0 to 6 months	11 (2.3)	39 (2)	4 (4.1)	9 (4)	3 (4.4)	7 (5.7)
6 months to 3 years	70 (14.4)	293 (14.7)	11 (11.3)	39 (17.4)	12 (17.4)	25 (20.5)
3 to 10 years	143 (29.4)	578 (29)	31 (32)	59 (26.3)	21 (30.4)	29 (23.8)
10 to 20 years	140 (28.8)	577 (28.9)	33 (34)	62 (27.7)	22 (31.9)	31 (25.4)
More than 20 years	74 (15.2)	333 (16.7)	16 (16.5)	49 (21.9)	10 (14.5)	27 (22.1)
Onset-related events	$\chi^2(6) = 50.76$, $p < 0.0001$ (0.0001)		$\chi^2(6) = 4.64$, $p = 0.591$ (0.771)		$\chi^2(6) = 6.38$, $p = 0.382$ (0.603)	
Loud blast of sound	163 (33.5)	804 (40.3)	27 (27.8)	72 (32.1)	22 (31.9)	33 (27.1)
Stress ***, #	106 (21.8)	243 (12.2)	18 (18.6)	36 (16.1)	14 (20.3)	21 (17.2)
Change in hearing	26 (5.4)	105 (5.3)	14 (14.4)	23 (10.3)	10 (14.5)	12 (9.8)
Head trauma	5 (1)	15 (0.8)	1 (1)	1 (0.5)	0 (0)	1 (0.8)
Whiplash	9 (1.9)	11 (0.6)	2 (2.1)	2 (0.9)	0 (0)	1 (0.8)
Other	80 (16.5)	265 (13.3)	20 (20.6)	40 (17.9)	15 (21.7)	24 (19.7)
Don't know	97 (20)	553 (27.7)	15 (15.5)	50 (22.3)	8 (11.6)	30 (24.6)
Tinnitus occurrence	$\chi^2(1) = 0.18$, $p = 0.671$ (0.694)		$\chi^2(1) = 3.63$, $p = 0.057$ (0.17)		$\chi^2(1) = 0$, $p = 0.973$ (0.973)	
Occasionally (now and then)	218 (44.9)	874 (43.8)	14 (14.4)	17 (7.6)	5 (7.3)	9 (7.4)
Always (all the time)	268 (55.1)	1122 (56.2)	83 (85.6)	207 (92.4)	64 (92.8)	113 (92.6)
Time of the day of tinnitus emergence	$\chi^2(6) = 13.02$, $p = 0.043$ (0.056)		$\chi^2(6) = 3.61$, $p = 0.729$ (0.824)		$\chi^2(6) = 6.67$, $p = 0.353$ (0.588)	
Don't know	264 (54.3)	1074 (53.8)	42 (43.3)	90 (40.2)	30 (43.5)	34 (27.9)
When awakening	32 (6.6)	120 (6)	14 (14.4)	29 (13)	12 (17.4)	23 (18.9)
In the morning	2 (0.4)	42 (2.1)	1 (1)	9 (4)	1 (1.5)	6 (4.9)
Around noon	22 (4.5)	138 (6.9)	9 (9.3)	26 (11.6)	6 (8.7)	18 (14.8)
In the afternoon	23 (4.7)	96 (4.8)	5 (5.2)	17 (7.6)	5 (7.3)	13 (10.7)
In the evening	58 (11.9)	244 (12.2)	18 (18.6)	34 (15.2)	10 (14.5)	20 (16.4)
Before sleeping	85 (17.5)	282 (14.1)	8 (8.3)	19 (8.5)	5 (7.3)	8 (6.6)
Perceiving the onset of tinnitus	$\chi^2(2) = 4.03$, $p = 0.133$ (0.16)		$\chi^2(2) = 0.14$, $p = 0.933$ (0.965)		$\chi^2(2) = 0.49$ $p = 0.781$ (0.837)	
Don't know	110 (22.6)	540 (27.1)	10 (10.3)	26 (11.6)	6 (8.7)	9 (7.4)
Gradual	222 (45.7)	848 (42.5)	40 (41.2)	93 (41.5)	27 (39.1)	43 (35.3)
Abrupt	154 (31.7)	608 (30.5)	47 (48.5)	105 (46.9)	36 (52.2)	70 (57.4)
Pulsatility	$\chi^2(3) = 30.48$, $p < 0.0001$ (0.0001)		$\chi^2(3) = 2.35$, $p = 0.504$ (0.756)		$\chi^2(3) = 2.4$ $p = 0.494$ (0.676)	
Don't know	59 (12.1)	139 (7)	11 (11.3)	26 (11.6)	4 (5.8)	12 (9.8)
Yes, with heart beat	45 (9.3)	126 (6.3)	10 (10.3)	22 (9.8)	9 (13)	14 (11.5)
Yes, different from heart beat	29 (6)	67 (3.4)	13 (13.4)	18 (8)	11 (15.9)	12 (9.8)
No	353 (72.6)	1664 (83.4)	63 (65)	158 (70.5)	45 (65.2)	84 (68.9)
Location of tinnitus	$\chi^2(6) = 20.48$, $p = 0.002$ (0.004)		$\chi^2(6) = 20.15$, $p = 0.003$ (0.013)		$\chi^2(6) = 10.01$, $p = 0.124$ (0.382)	
Right ear	36 (7.4)	159 (8)	9 (9.3)	22 (9.8)	6 (8.7)	10 (8.2)
Left ear	39 (8)	184 (9.2)	9 (9.3)	20 (8.9)	9 (13)	15 (12.3)
Both ears, worse in right	111 (22.8)	319 (16)	26 (26.8)	28 (12.5)	17 (24.6)	19 (15.6)
Both ears, worse in left	76 (15.6)	345 (17.3)	15 (15.5)	53 (23.7)	12 (17.4)	30 (24.6)
Both ears equally	144 (29.6)	657 (32.9)	18 (18.6)	58 (25.9)	11 (15.9)	24 (19.7)
Inside the head	70 (14.4)	317 (15.9)	14 (14.4)	41 (18.3)	9 (13)	23 (18.9)
Elsewhere	10 (2.1)	15 (0.8)	6 (6.2)	2 (0.9)	5 (7.3)	1 (0.8)
Sound of tinnitus	$\chi^2(9) = 33.6$, $p < 0.0001$ (0.0001)		$\chi^2(7) = 9.53$, $p = 0.217$ (0.406)		$\chi^2(7) = 12.39$, $p = 0.088$ (0.332)	
Tone	88 (18.4)	442 (22.3)	10 (10.5)	24 (10.9)	10 (14.9)	12 (10)
Noise	36 (7.5)	236 (11.9)	5 (5.3)	27 (12.2)	4 (6)	10 (8.3)
Crickets	18 (3.8)	66 (3.3)	3 (3.2)	5 (2.3)	2 (3)	4 (3.3)
Heartbeat	5 (1)	6 (0.3)	1 (1.1)	1 (0.5)	2 (3)	0 (0)

(Continued)

TABLE 3 | Continued

	Any tinnitus		TFI ≥ 48		THI ≥ 58	
	TMJ (*n* = 486) No (%)	**No TMJ (*n* = 1996) No (%)**	**TMJ (*n* = 97) No (%)**	**No TMJ (*n* = 224) No (%)**	**TMJ (*n* = 69) No (%)**	**No TMJ (*n* = 122) No (%)**
Beeping	48 (10)	240 (12.1)	10 (10.5)	26 (11.8)	5 (7.5)	14 (11.7)
Morse code	2 (0.4)	1 (0.1)	0 (0)	0 (0)	0 (0)	0 (0)
An alarm	7 (1.5)	12 (0.6)	3 (3.2)	2 (0.9)	2 (3)	2 (1.7)
Other	9 (1.9)	61 (3.1)	1 (1.1)	11 (5)	0 (0)	11 (9.2)
Don't know	1 (0.2)	1 (0.1)	0 (0)	0 (0)	0 (0)	0 (0)
Complex	265 (55.3)	916 (46.2)	62 (65.3)	125 (56.6)	42 (62.7)	67 (55.8)
Tinnitus loudness variation from day to day	$\chi^2(5) = 20.74$, $p = 0.001$ (0.002)		$\chi^2(5) = 12.94$, $p = 0.024$ (0.09)		$\chi^2(5) = 5.11$, $p = 0.403$ (0.604)	
Don't know	21 (4.3)	142 (7.1)	4 (4.1)	4 (1.8)	2 (2.9)	1 (0.8)
Never	30 (6.2)	165 (8.3)	7 (7.2)	23 (10.3)	4 (5.8)	9 (7.4)
Seldom	55 (11.3)	312 (15.6)	9 (9.3)	40 (17.9)	6 (8.7)	16 (13.1)
Sometimes	185 (38.1)	737 (36.9)	34 (35.1)	96 (42.9)	24 (34.8)	54 (44.3)
Often	139 (28.6)	430 (21.5)	28 (28.9)	43 (19.2)	21 (30.4)	27 (22.1)
Always	56 (11.5)	210 (10.5)	15 (15.5)	18 (8)	12 (17.4)	15 (12.3)
Pitch of tinnitus	$\chi^2(4) = 3.75$, $p = 0.441$ (0.472)		$\chi^2(4) = 2.38$, $p = 0.666$ (0.824)		$\chi^2(4) = 7.16$, $p = 0.128$ (0.382)	
Don't know	23 (4.7)	70 (3.5)	4 (4.1)	5 (2.2)	4 (5.8)	1 (0.8)
Very high frequency	119 (24.5)	482 (24.2)	34 (35.1)	67 (29.9)	28 (40.6)	41 (33.6)
High frequency	206 (42.4)	896 (44.9)	39 (40.2)	102 (45.5)	26 (37.7)	47 (38.5)
Medium frequency	92 (18.9)	394 (19.7)	15 (15.5)	41 (18.3)	8 (11.6)	23 (18.9)
Low frequency	46 (9.5)	154 (7.7)	5 (5.2)	9 (4)	3 (4.4)	10 (8.2)
Reduction of tinnitus by music or environmental sounds	$\chi^2(2) = 4.25$, $p = 0.12$ (0.15)		$\chi^2(2) = 1.15$, $p = 0.563$ (0.771)		$\chi^2(2) = 3.76$, $p = 0.153$ (0.382)	
Don't know	116 (23.9)	511 (25.6)	12 (12.4)	35 (15.6)	7 (10.1)	16 (13.1)
Yes	294 (60.5)	1110 (55.6)	61 (62.9)	127 (56.7)	45 (65.2)	62 (50.8)
No	76 (15.6)	375 (18.8)	24 (24.7)	62 (27.7)	17 (24.6)	44 (36.1)
Worsening of tinnitus by loud noise	$\chi^2(2) = 18.48$, $p < 0.0001$ (0.0001)		$\chi^2(2) = 3.32$, $p = 0.19$ (0.38)		$\chi^2(2) = 1.23$, $p = 0.541$ (0.676)	
Don't know	145 (29.8)	549 (27.5)	26 (26.8)	49 (21.9)	17 (24.6)	31 (25.4)
Yes	263 (54.1)	944 (47.3)	59 (60.8)	129 (57.6)	44 (63.8)	70 (57.4)
No	78 (16.1)	503 (25.2)	12 (12.4)	46 (20.5)	8 (11.6)	21 (17.2)
Tinnitus affected by head movement or touch	$\chi^2(2) = 122.84$, $p < 0.0001$ (0.0001)		$\chi^2(2) = 23.09$, $p < 0.0001$ (0.0005)		$\chi^2(2) = 12.5$, $p = 0.002$ (0.019)	
Don't know	123 (25.3)	376 (18.8)	13 (13.4)	32 (14.3)	7 (10.1)	13 (10.7)
Yes	198 (40.7)	411 (20.6)	55 (56.7)	66 (29.5)	43 (62.3)	45 (36.9)
No	165 (34)	1209 (60.6)	29 (29.9)	126 (56.3)	19 (27.5)	64 (52.5)
Tinnitus affected by nap	$\chi^2(3) = 9.36$, $p = 0.025$ (0.036)		$\chi^2(3) = 0.15$, $p = 0.986$ (0.986)		$\chi^2(3) = 2.24$, $p = 0.525$ (0.676)	
Don't know	290 (59.7)	1126 (56.4)	38 (39.2)	87 (38.8)	24 (34.8)	42 (34.4)
It mainly worsens my tinnitus	13 (2.7)	40 (2)	8 (8.3)	16 (7.1)	8 (11.6)	14 (11.5)
It mainly reduces my tinnitus	133 (27.4)	674 (33.8)	41 (42.3)	98 (43.8)	33 (47.8)	51 (41.8)
It has no effect	50 (10.3)	156 (7.8)	10 (10.3)	23 (10.3)	4 (5.8)	15 (12.3)
Tinnitus affected by bad nights sleep	$\chi^2(5) = 67.67$, $p < 0.0001$ (0.0001)		$\chi^2(5) = 8.34$, $p = 0.139$ (0.316)		$\chi^2(5) = 10.66$, $p = 0.059$ (0.293)	
Don't know	177 (36.4)	762 (38.2)	19 (19.6)	43 (19.2)	9 (13)	20 (16.4)
Never	30 (6.2)	337 (16.9)	3 (3.1)	28 (12.5)	1 (1.5)	13 (10.7)
Seldom	30 (6.2)	158 (7.9)	8 (8.3)	16 (7.1)	6 (8.7)	8 (6.6)
Sometimes	116 (23.9)	440 (22)	25 (25.8)	58 (25.9)	15 (21.7)	31 (25.4)
Often	99 (20.4)	230 (11.5)	27 (27.8)	57 (25.5)	21 (30.4)	36 (29.5)
Always	34 (7)	69 (3.5)	15 (15.5)	22 (9.8)	17 (24.6)	14 (11.5)
Heartbeat	5 (1)	6 (0.3)	1 (1.1)	1 (0.5)	2 (3)	0 (0)

(Continued)

TABLE 3 | Continued

	Any tinnitus		TFI ≥ 48		THI ≥ 58	
	TMJ (*n* = 486) No (%)	**No TMJ (*n* = 1996) No (%)**	**TMJ (*n* = 97) No (%)**	**No TMJ (*n* = 224) No (%)**	**TMJ (*n* = 69) No (%)**	**No TMJ (*n* = 122) No (%)**
Tinnitus affected by stress	$\chi^2(3) = 104.08, p < 0.0001$ (0.0001)		$\chi^2(2) = 22.11, p < 0.0001$ (0.0005)		$\chi^2(2) = 14.72, p = 0.001$ (0.009)	
Don't know	134 (27.6)	731 (36.6)	15 (15.5)	51 (22.8)	6 (8.7)	24 (19.7)
Yes, it worsens my tinnitus	305 (62.8)	768 (38.5)	78 (80.4)	123 (54.9)	62 (89.9)	80 (65.6)
Yes, it reduces my tinnitus	47 (9.7)	492 (24.7)	4 (4.1)	50 (22.3)	1 (1.5)	18 (14.8)
No, it has no effect	0 (0)	5 (0.3)	0 (0)	0 (0)	0 (0)	0 (0)
Tinnitus affected by medication	$\chi^2(2) = 3.78, p = 0.151$ (0.175)		$\chi^2(2) = 0.25, p = 0.881$ (0.944)		$\chi^2(2) = 1.38, p = 0.502$ (0.676)	
Don't know	356 (73.3)	1467 (73.5)	63 (65)	149 (66.5)	46 (66.7)	73 (59.8)
Yes	18 (3.7)	44 (2.2)	8 (8.3)	15 (6.7)	7 (10.1)	11 (9)
No	112 (23.1)	485 (24.3)	26 (26.8)	60 (26.8)	16 (23.2)	38 (31.2)
Contacted a clinician due to tinnitus	$\chi^2(2) = 11.42, p = 0.003$ (0.005)		$\chi^2(2) = 0.6, p = 0.742$ (0.824)		$\chi^2(2) = 2.33, p = 0.313$ (0.588)	
No	282 (58)	1313 (65.8)	23 (23.7)	49 (21.9)	11 (15.9)	18 (14.8)
Yes, because of curiosity	26 (5.4)	107 (5.4)	2 (2.1)	8 (3.6)	0 (0)	4 (3.3)
Yes, because I sought for help	178 (36.6)	576 (28.9)	72 (74.2)	167 (74.6)	58 (84.1)	100 (82)
Number of tinnitus treatments	$\chi^2(3) = 25.56, p < 0.0001$ (0.0001)		$\chi^2(3) = 4.26, p = 0.235$ (0.414)		$\chi^2(3) = 1.96, p = 0.581$ (0.697)	
None	395 (81.3)	1776 (89)	55 (56.7)	142 (63.4)	34 (49.3)	66 (54.1)
1	32 (6.6)	102 (5.1)	11 (11.3)	34 (15.2)	9 (13)	19 (15.6)
2–4	43 (8.9)	84 (4.2)	19 (19.6)	29 (13)	17 (24.6)	20 (16.4)
5 or more	16 (3.3)	34 (1.7)	12 (12.4)	19 (8.5)	9 (13)	17 (13.9)
Tinnitus occurence in family	$\chi^2(1) = 24.97, p < 0.0001$ (0.0001)		$\chi^2(1) = 6.58, p = 0.01$ (0.044)		$\chi^2(1) = 1.68, p = 0.195$ (0.418)	
No	358 (73.7)	1666 (83.5)	62 (63.9)	174 (77.7)	46 (66.7)	92 (75.4)
Yes	128 (26.3)	330 (16.5)	35 (36.1)	50 (22.3)	23 (33.3)	30 (24.6)

Pairwise comparisons using Pearson's Chi-square test are reported. Percentages (%) displayed refer to column percentages. p-Values adjusted for multiple comparisons are shown between parenthesis and included variables from ***Table 4****.*

Tinnitus Phenotypics in Tinnitus Subjects With and Without TMJ Complaints

We next analyzed the tinnitus phenotypic characteristics of subjects with or without TMJ complaints (**Table 3**). With any tinnitus, the two groups differed in onset-related events, more frequently reporting stress as the cause of their tinnitus. Differences were also found in pulsatility, location of tinnitus, sound of tinnitus, day to day variations, worsening by loud noise, affected by nap, or bad night sleep ($p = 0.04$ to < 0.0001). No differences were found in tinnitus time of onset, in tinnitus pitch, or in its reduction by music or environmental sounds. Those with TMJ complaints were more likely to contact a clinician due to tinnitus, received a greater number of treatments, and reported greater occurrence in the family ($p = 0.005$ to < 0.0001). **Table 4** shows that subjects with TMJ complaints more often experience discomfort in presence of loud noise and problems tolerating sounds ($p < 0.0001$), and reported worse hearing ($p = 0.04$), in spite of similar use of hearing aids ($p = 0.38$). Regarding co-morbidities, subjects with TMJ complaints displayed greater incidence of headache and vertigo, and more often were under psychiatric treatment and had other diagnosed diseases. The factors that were consistently found to differ between subjects with or without TMJ complaints, whether they had any tinnitus, tinnitus as a big problem or severe tinnitus, were modulation by head movement or touch, affected by stress, and neck pain (**Tables 3, 4**).

DISCUSSION

The present study confirms previous findings from Vielsmeier et al. (2012) suggesting that tinnitus patients with TMJ complaints may constitute a separate subtype that could benefit from specific treatment interventions targeting the TMJ. Of major importance, we find that the proportion of TMJ complaints increases from 19% in the any tinnitus group to 36% in the severe group (as measured with the THI), strongly indicating that TMJ problems largely contribute to tinnitus severity. Many of the features analyzed in the present study showed a marked difference between tinnitus subjects with or without TMJ-complaints, similar to Vielsmeier et al. (2012). We confirm that a higher proportion of tinnitus subjects with TMJ complaints were female, younger, and could modulate tinnitus by head/jaw movements (Vielsmeier et al., 2012). The modulation of tinnitus by head/jaw movements has been previously reported (Pinchoff et al., 1998; Sanchez et al., 2002), and thus our work supports the hypothesis that somatic modulation may be associated with TMJ complaints in subjects with tinnitus (Levine, 1999).

Somatic input from trigeminal afferents converge to the dorsal cochlear nucleus where granule cells contact fusiform cells that also integrate auditory input. It has been recently suggested that the plasticity of fusiform cells is perturbed during noise-induced tinnitus and that bimodal somatosensory and auditory stimulation of fusiform cells can reverse the plasticity to its

TABLE 4 | Comorbidities in subjects with tinnitus with or without TMJ complaints.

	Any tinnitus		**TFI ≥ 48**		**THI ≥ 58**	
	TMJ (*n* = 486) No (%)	**No TMJ (*n* = 1996) No (%)**	**TMJ (*n* = 97) No (%)**	**No TMJ (*n* = 224) No (%)**	**TMJ (*n* = 69) No (%)**	**No TMJ (*n* = 122) No (%)**
Hearing problem	$\chi^2(2) = 7.25, p = 0.027$ (0.036)		$\chi^2(2) = 4.17, p = 0.124$ (0.311)		$\chi^2(2) = 3.46, p = 0.177$ (0.409)	
Don't know	100 (20.6)	310 (15.5)	14 (14.4)	23 (10.3)	6 (8.7)	11 (9)
Yes	230 (47.3)	996 (49.9)	59 (60.8)	162 (72.3)	38 (55.1)	82 (67.2)
No	156 (32.1)	690 (34.6)	24 (24.7)	39 (17.4)	25 (36.2)	29 (23.8)
Hearing aids	$\chi^2(3) = 3.37, p = 0.338$ (0.376)		$\chi^2(3) = 2.03, p = 0.567$ (0.771)		$\chi^2(3) = 1.53, p = 0.676$ (0.751)	
Yes, on both ears	38 (7.8)	117 (5.9)	23 (23.7)	41 (18.3)	14 (20.3)	20 (16.4)
Yes, on the right ear	6 (1.2)	17 (0.9)	4 (4.1)	6 (2.7)	3 (4.4)	4 (3.3)
Yes, on the left ear	5 (1)	25 (1.3)	2 (2.1)	7 (3.1)	1 (1.5)	5 (4.1)
No	437 (89.9)	1837 (92)	68 (70.1)	170 (75.9)	51 (73.9)	93 (76.2)
Problems tolerating sounds	$\chi^2(4) = 50.16, p < 0.0001$ (0.0001)		$\chi^2(4) = 2.08, p = 0.721$ (0.824)		$\chi^2(3) = 0.34, p = 0.952$ (0.973)	
Never	7 (1.4)	99 (5)	0 (0)	1 (0.5)	0 (0)	0 (0)
Rarely	50 (10.3)	350 (17.5)	5 (5.2)	13 (5.8)	4 (5.8)	6 (4.9)
Sometimes	176 (36.2)	800 (40.1)	21 (21.7)	62 (27.7)	14 (20.3)	29 (23.8)
Usually	153 (31.5)	498 (25)	36 (37.1)	79 (35.3)	24 (34.8)	41 (33.6)
Always	100 (20.6)	249 (12.5)	35 (36.1)	69 (30.8)	27 (39.1)	46 (37.7)
Sounds cause pain or physical discomfort	$\chi^2(2) = 58.18, p < 0.0001$ (0.0001)		$\chi^2(2) = 5.5, p = 0.064$ (0.175)		$\chi^2(2) = 5.27, p = 0.072$ (0.308)	
Don't know	34 (7)	111 (5.6)	6 (6.2)	13 (5.8)	3 (4.4)	7 (5.7)
Yes	326 (67.1)	989 (49.6)	77 (79.4)	152 (67.9)	59 (85.5)	87 (71.3)
No	126 (25.9)	896 (44.9)	14 (14.4)	59 (26.3)	7 (10.1)	28 (23)
Headache	$\chi^2(2) = 164.05, p < 0.0001$ (0.0001)		$\chi^2(2) = 15.93, p = 0.0003$ (0.002)		$\chi^2(2) = 8.99, p = 0.011$ (0.084)	
Don't know	10 (2.1)	34 (1.7)	2 (2.1)	4 (1.8)	2 (2.9)	4 (3.3)
Yes	231 (47.5)	392 (19.6)	50 (51.6)	64 (28.6)	36 (52.2)	37 (30.3)
No	245 (50.4)	1570 (78.7)	45 (46.4)	156 (69.6)	31 (44.9)	81 (66.4)
Vertigo/dizziness	$\chi^2(2) = 121.07, p < 0.0001$ (0.0001)		$\chi^2(2) = 7.15, p = 0.028$ (0.093)		$\chi^2(2) = 3.78, p = 0.151$ (0.382)	
Don't know	32 (6.6)	63 (3.2)	4 (4.1)	10 (4.5)	1 (1.5)	6 (4.9)
Yes	196 (40.3)	380 (19)	42 (43.3)	63 (28.1)	26 (37.7)	32 (26.2)
No	258 (53.1)	1553 (77.8)	51 (52.6)	151 (67.4)	42 (60.9)	84 (68.9)
Neck pain	$\chi^2(2) = 331.64, p < 0.0001$ (0.0001)		$\chi^2(2) = 42.92, p < 0.0001$ (0.0005)		$\chi^2(2) = 25.87, p < 0.0001$ (0.002)	
Don't know	9 (1.9)	27 (1.4)	1 (1)	6 (2.7)	0 (0)	2 (1.6)
Yes	318 (65.4)	460 (23.1)	70 (72.2)	73 (32.6)	50 (72.5)	42 (34.4)
No	159 (32.7)	1509 (75.6)	26 (26.8)	145 (64.7)	19 (27.5)	78 (63.9)
Other pain syndromes	$\chi^2(2) = 128.77, p < 0.0001$ (0.0001)		$\chi^2(2) = 13.12, p = 0.001$ (0.008)		$\chi^2(2) = 7.7, p = 0.021$ (0.128)	
Don't know	17 (3.5)	23 (1.2)	1 (1)	3 (1.3)	2 (2.9)	3 (2.5)
Yes	199 (41)	373 (18.7)	51 (52.6)	70 (31.3)	34 (49.3)	36 (29.5)
No	270 (55.6)	1600 (80.2)	45 (46.4)	151 (67.4)	33 (47.8)	83 (68)
Under psychatric treatment	$\chi^2(2) = 23.84, p < 0.0001$ (0.0001)		$\chi^2(2) = 3.83, p = 0.147$ (0.316)		$\chi^2(1) = 1.01, p = 0.316$ (0.588)	
Don't know	4 (0.8)	8 (0.4)	0 (0)	1 (0.5)	0 (0)	0 (0)
Yes	66 (13.6)	140 (7)	21 (21.7)	30 (13.4)	16 (23.2)	21 (17.2)
No	416 (85.6)	1848 (92.6)	76 (78.4)	193 (86.2)	53 (76.8)	101 (82.8)
Diagnosed disease	$\chi^2(1) = 6.26, p = 0.012$ (0.019)		$\chi^2(1) = 0.74, p = 0.389$ (0.648)		$\chi^2(1) = 0.93, p = 0.335$ (0.588)	
Yes	182 (37.5)	629 (31.5)	40 (41.2)	81 (36.2)	28 (40.6)	41 (33.6)
No	304 (62.6)	1367 (68.5)	57 (58.8)	143 (63.8)	41 (59.4)	81 (66.4)

Pairwise comparisons using Pearson's Chi-square test are reported. Percentages (%) displayed refer to column percentages. p-Values adjusted for multiple comparisons are shown between parenthesis and included variables from ***Table 3****.*

original settings and provide relief from tinnitus in animals and humans (Marks et al., 2018).

While other studies found no difference between tinnitus patients with and without TMJ complaints in stress as an onset-related event (Vielsmeier et al., 2012; Ward et al., 2015), we reveal – using the same TSCHQ questionnaire – that a higher proportion of subjects in the group with TMJ complaints reported stress as a cause of their tinnitus. This is consistent with the greater level of anxiety and stress we have found in patients with TMJ complaints (**Table 2**). These emotional factors could not be evaluated in the study from Vielsmeier et al. (2012) since the questionnaire selection established by the TRI (Landgrebe et al., 2010) includes a questionnaire on depression [Beck Depression Index (BDI); Beck and Steer, 1984] but does not include measures of anxiety and stress. Indeed, stress questionnaires are seldom used in clinical practice. In the "any tinnitus" group, onset-related events were found to differ between TMJ and non-TMJ complaining groups. In contrast, this difference between any tinnitus and TMJ complaints tinnitus group was not found when only the severe tinnitus subjects were considered for each group. Since Vielsmeier et al. (2012) was studying a group of clinical patients, this could explain why they could not reveal any difference regarding onset-related events. This highlights the importance of including tinnitus subjects other than those in a clinical setting as it offers a better picture of the co-morbid factors, which would not be otherwise revealed.

Our findings also suggest that TMJ disorder, and potentially stress, may be a risk factor for the development of severe tinnitus. A large longitudinal study in Taiwan (7,585 TMJ disorders patients and 30,340 controls) supports this hypothesis showing a greater risk of developing tinnitus when diagnosed for TMJ disorders (adjusted HR = 2.75, 95% CI = 2.39–3.17) (Lee et al., 2016). Interestingly, previous studies have shown a strong correlation between bruxism and stress (Ahlberg et al., 2002, 2013), as well as between bruxism and tinnitus (Camparis et al., 2005; Fernandes et al., 2014). It has been suggested that distension of the TMJ capsule or antero-medial disk displacement could result in auriculotemporal nerve compression and facial pain symptoms (Cascone et al., 2010). Since a sustained clenching of the jaw can damage the articular disk (Commisso et al., 2014), it is reasonable to hypothesize that overloading the TMJ during stress periods may contribute to tinnitus. Studies in rodents have shown that auditory brainstem receives input from the trigeminal ganglion in rodents (Shore et al., 2000). However, there seems to be a large heterogeneity in the innervation of the TMJ capsule in humans (Davidson et al., 2003). To verify this, a longitudinal study could be performed looking at whether subjects with stress or/and sleep bruxism develop tinnitus over time.

The increased co-occurrence of TMJ complaints and tinnitus in women in the present study is indicative of a sex bias. These findings are consistent with greater tinnitus-related stress in women than in men (Seydel et al., 2013; Schlee et al., 2017a). Similarly, the psychological burden in women has also been recently evidenced by a greater association of tinnitus with suicide attempts, something which was not found in men (Lugo et al., 2019). However, sex-differences in TMJ complaints and tinnitus were also found in a Korean study (Won et al., 2013), but not in the United Kingdom (Ward et al., 2015). It is thus possible that the sex-specific impact of TMJ complaints on tinnitus may vary from one region to another, although this warrants further investigation. Indeed, little is known on the impact of sex on other factors related to tinnitus. The incorporation of sex as a biological variable (SABV) in tinnitus studies may help determining how sex impacts on the pathophysiology of tinnitus.

Our study also suggests that there is an increased occurrence of tinnitus in the family of those with TMJ complaints. We recently evidenced a genetic contribution to tinnitus in twins (Maas et al., 2017) and in adoptees (Cederroth et al., 2019b). In the latter study, we identified an association between adoptees and their biological parents, but not between adoptees and their adoptive parents, showing that the familial transmission of tinnitus is influenced by genetics and not by shared-environment Previous genetic studies identified polymorphisms (i.e., those in the COMT gene) related to catecholamine metabolism and adrenergic receptors that may increase pain receptivity in subjects with chronic TMJ disorders (Diatchenko et al., 2005). Since tinnitus and chronic pain involve similar brain structures (Rauschecker et al., 2015), it is possible that the two conditions share common genetic mechanisms. However, as the genetic understanding of tinnitus is still in its infancy (Lopez-Escamez et al., 2016; Vona et al., 2017), large biobanking efforts will be needed to achieve a reliable understanding of the involvement of genetics in the co-occurrence of tinnitus and TMJ (Cederroth et al., 2017; Szczepek et al., 2018).

Tinnitus can affect an individual in many different ways (Hall et al., 2018), and there is no consensus measurement instrument for quantifying tinnitus symptom severity. In this study, we operationally defined severe tinnitus using scores derived from two popular self-report questionnaires; TFI and THI. This way, we could examine whether any observed differences between the TMJ and non-TMJ populations were measure-specific or robust regardless of how severe cases were defined. There is high convergent validity between the TFI and THI (r = 0.86, Meikle et al., 2012) indicating that they broadly measure the same construct, albeit with some small differences. In this dataset, the variables that differed regardless of the method used for defining severe cases were quality of life, influenced by head movement or touch, neck pain, or stress. Both TFI and THI assess concepts relevant to quality of life, and neither assess modulations by movement or touch, or associations with neck pain. Only the THI includes a question about exacerbation of tinnitus by stress. On this basis, it seems highly likely that the observations are robust, and not simply an artifact of the chosen methodology. Nonetheless, the proportion of subjects with severe tinnitus using the THI cut-off (7.7%) is smaller than that using the TFI cut-off (13%). Thus, a large proportion of subjects with clinically relevant tinnitus may not be identified using the arbitrary cut-offs from the THI, which have no true clinical meaning (Newman et al., 1998; McCombe et al., 2001). In contrast, the TFI cut-off we are using here is based on a revised grading using an anchor-based method tested on the United Kingdom population (Fackrell et al., 2017). These findings suggest that the inclusion of the TFI in regional guidelines of the Stockholm county (Idrizbegovic et al., 2011) could double the number of referrals to specialty care.

One limitation in the present study was that estimates of TMJ complaints were based on self-report rather than clinician assessment. Concerns have been raised on the reliance on self-reported symptoms and how accurate these are. There are also difficulties in finding agreement among clinical experts on how to diagnose somatosensory tinnitus (Michiels et al., 2018a). The single question from the TCSHQ – "*Do you suffer from Temporomandibular disorder?*" – is certainly not optimal from the point of view of questionnaire design and can be interpreted in a number of different ways, e.g., diagnosed by a doctor or not; uncertain response due to complex technical terminology. In addition, the "don't know" option was not presented in the Vielsmeier study (Vielsmeier et al., 2012), which preempts from estimating the uncertainties related to the question itself. Instead, the Swedish version of the TSCHQ is reformulated in terms of jaw symptomatology, with only 6.3% of "don't know" answers. Further studies would be needed to relate tinnitus severity with objective measures of TMJ disorders such as MRI or CT-scan (Scrivani et al., 2008), in addition to being diagnosed by a doctor (e.g., through checking for the presence of a clicking sound) and including TMJ disorders laterality in the analysis prior performing more costly evaluations of treatment interventions. Consistent with the lack of objective measures for both TMJ disorders and tinnitus, high quality studies evaluating the effect of TMJ disorders treatment on tinnitus are missing (Skog et al., 2019). A recent systematic review by Michiels et al. (2019) reveals that the combination of splint therapy and exercise treatment, the so-called conservative treatment, is the best treatment approach as several studies show a decrease in tinnitus severity. However, the overall evidence shows low-quality and argues in favor of larger well-designed studies, such as the one ongoing by Michiels et al. (2018b).

Identification of distinct tinnitus subtypes will be critical for successful therapeutic development. Our analysis confirmed that TMJ problems are closely tied to socioeconomic, phenotypic, and psychological features of individuals with tinnitus. Our study supports the notion that tinnitus subjects with TMJ complaints could constitute a specific subtype. From a clinical trial perspective, this subgroup of tinnitus patients should therefore be carefully considered in exclusion/inclusion criteria as their response to treatments could dramatically differ from other tinnitus patient groups.

AUTHOR CONTRIBUTIONS

CC, DH, and BC designed the study. CC and NE developed the websurvey, coordinated the recruitment of subjects, and collected the data. NE extracted and processed the STOP data. NE, EdG, JB, and ElG analyzed the data. AL, GM, MB, MT, and JW helped to develop the scientific arguments and contributed to the data interpretation. All authors contributed to the manuscript and approved the final version.

FUNDING

BC has received funding from the Swedish Medical Research Council (K2014-99X-22478-01-3), Karolinska Institutet, and Tysta Skolan. CC has received research funding from the Decibel Therapeutics, Inc., Svenska Läkaresällskapet (SLS-779681), Tysta Skolan, Hörselforskningsfonden (#503), the European Union's Horizon 2020 Research and Innovation Programme under the Marie Skłodowska-Curie grant agreement no. 72204655 (Schlee et al., 2017b), and the GENDER-NET Co-Plus Fund (GNP-182). DH is a NIHR Senior Investigator.

REFERENCES

Ahlberg, J., Lobbezoo, F., Ahlberg, K., Manfredini, D., Hublin, C., Sinisalo, J., et al. (2013). Self-reported bruxism mirrors anxiety and stress in adults. *Med. Oral. Patol. Oral. Cir. Bucal.* 18, e7–e11. doi: 10.4317/medoral.18232

Ahlberg, J., Rantala, M., Savolainen, A., Suvinen, T., Nissinen, M., Sarna, S., et al. (2002). Reported bruxism and stress experience. *Commun. Dent Oral. Epidemiol.* 30, 405–408. doi: 10.1034/j.1600-0528.2002.00007.x

Al-Khotani, A., Naimi-Akbar, A., Albadawi, E., Ernberg, M., Hedenberg-Magnusson, B., and Christidis, N. (2016). Prevalence of diagnosed temporomandibular disorders among saudi arabian children and adolescents. *J. Headache Pain* 17:41. doi: 10.1186/s10194-016-0642-9

Almqvist, C., Adami, H. O., Franks, P. W., Groop, L., Ingelsson, E., Kere, J., et al. (2011). LifeGene–a large prospective population-based study of global relevance. *Eur. J. Epidemiol.* 26, 67–77. doi: 10.1007/s10654-010-9521-x

Andersson, G., Kaldo-Sandstrom, V., Strom, L., and Stromgren, T. (2003). Internet administration of the hospital anxiety and depression scale in a sample of tinnitus patients. *J. Psychosom. Res.* 55, 259–262. doi: 10.1016/s0022-3999(02)00575-5

Auerbach, B. D., Rodrigues, P. V., and Salvi, R. J. (2014). Central gain control in tinnitus and hyperacusis. *Front. Neurol.* 5:206. doi: 10.3389/fneur.2014.00206

Bartels, H., Middel, B. L., van der Laan, B. F., Staal, M. J., and Albers, F. W. (2008). The additive effect of co-occurring anxiety and depression on health status, quality of life and coping strategies in help-seeking tinnitus sufferers. *Ear. Hear.* 29, 947–956. doi: 10.1097/AUD.0b013e3181888f83

Beck, A. T., and Steer, R. A. (1984). Internal consistencies of the original and revised beck depression inventory. *J. Clin. Psychol.* 40, 1365–1367. doi: 10.1002/1097-4679(198411)40:6<1365::aid-jclp2270400615>3.0.co;2-d

Bernhardt, O., Mundt, T., Welk, A., Koppl, N., Kocher, T., Meyer, G., et al. (2011). Signs and symptoms of temporomandibular disorders and the incidence of tinnitus. *J. Oral. Rehabil.* 38, 891–901. doi: 10.1111/j.1365-2842.2011.02224.x

Bousema, E. J., Koops, E. A., van Dijk, P., and Dijkstra, P. U. (2018). Association between subjective tinnitus and cervical spine or temporomandibular disorders: a systematic review. *Trends Hear.* 22:2331216518800640. doi: 10.1177/2331216518800640

Camparis, C. M., Formigoni, G., Teixeira, M. J., and de Siqueira, J. T. (2005). Clinical evaluation of tinnitus in patients with sleep bruxism: prevalence and characteristics. *J. Oral. Rehabil.* 32, 808–814. doi: 10.1111/j.1365-2842.2005.01519.x

Cascone, P., Fatone, F. M., Paparo, F., Arangio, P., and Iannetti, G. (2010). Trigeminal impingement syndrome: the relationship between atypical trigeminal symptoms and anteromedial disk displacement. *Cranio* 28, 177–180. doi: 10.1179/crn.2010.024

Cederroth, C. R., Canlon, B., and Langguth, B. (2013). Hearing loss and tinnitus– are funders and industry listening? *Nat. Biotechnol.* 31, 972–974. doi: 10.1038/nbt.2736

Cederroth, C. R., Dyhrfjeld-Johnsen, J., and Langguth, B. (2018). An update: emerging drugs for tinnitus. *Expert Opin. Emerg. Drugs* 23, 251–260. doi: 10.1080/14728214.2018.1555240

Cederroth, C. R., Gallus, S., Hall, D. A., Kleinjung, T., Langguth, B., Maruotti, A., et al. (2019a). Editorial: towards an understanding of tinnitus heterogeneity. *Front. Aging Neurosci.* 11:53. doi: 10.3389/fnagi.2019.00053

Cederroth, C. R., PirouziFard, M., Trpchevska, N., Idrizbegovic, E., Canlon, B., Sundquist, J., et al. (2019b). Association of genetic vs environmental factors in swedish adoptees with clinically significant tinnitus. *JAMA Otolaryngol. Head Neck Surg.* 145, 222–229. doi: 10.1001/jamaoto.2018.3852

Cederroth, C. R., Kähler, A., Sullivan, P. F., and Lopez-Escamez, J. A. (2017). Genetics of tinnitus: time to biobank phantom sounds. *Front. Gene.* 8:110. doi: 10.3389/fgene.2017.00110

Chisnoiu, A. M., Picos, A. M., Popa, S., Chisnoiu, P. D., Lascu, L., Picos, A., et al. (2015). Factors involved in the etiology of temporomandibular disorders - a literature review. *Clujul Med.* 88, 473–478. doi: 10.15386/cjmed-485

Chole, R. A., and Parker, W. S. (1992). Tinnitus and vertigo in patients with temporomandibular disorder. *Arch. Otolaryngol. Head Neck Surg.* 118, 817–821. doi: 10.1001/archotol.1992.01880080039010

Cima, R. F., Crombez, G., and Vlaeyen, J. W. (2011). Catastrophizing and fear of tinnitus predict quality of life in patients with chronic tinnitus. *Ear. Hear.* 32, 634–641. doi: 10.1097/AUD.0b013e31821106dd

Cima, R. F., Maes, I. H., Joore, M. A., Scheyen, D. J., El Refaie, A., Baguley, D. M., et al. (2012). Specialised treatment based on cognitive behaviour therapy versus usual care for tinnitus: a randomised controlled trial. *Lancet* 379, 1951–1959. doi: 10.1016/S0140-6736(12)60469-3

Commisso, M. S., Martinez-Reina, J., and Mayo, J. (2014). A study of the temporomandibular joint during bruxism. *Int. J. Oral. Sci.* 6, 116–123. doi: 10.1038/ijos.2014.4

Davidson, J. A., Metzinger, S. E., Tufaro, A. P., and Dellon, A. L. (2003). Clinical implications of the innervation of the temporomandibular joint. *J. Craniofac. Surg.* 14, 235–239. doi: 10.1097/00001665-200303000-00019

Deng, Y. M., Fu, M. K., and Hagg, U. (1995). Prevalence of temporomandibular joint dysfunction (TMJD) in chinese children and adolescents. a cross-sectional epidemiological study. *Eur. J. Orthod.* 17, 305–309. doi: 10.1093/ejo/17.4.305

Diatchenko, L., Slade, G. D., Nackley, A. G., Bhalang, K., Sigurdsson, A., Belfer, I., et al. (2005). Genetic basis for individual variations in pain perception and the development of a chronic pain condition. *Hum. Mol. Genet.* 14, 135–143. doi: 10.1093/hmg/ddi013

Dobie, R. A. (2003). Depression and tinnitus. *Otolaryngol. Clin. North Am.* 36, 383–388.

Fackrell, K., Hall, D. A., Barry, J. G., and Hoare, D. J. (2017). Performance of the tinnitus functional index as a diagnostic instrument in a UK clinical population. *Hear. Res.* doi: 10.1016/j.heares.2017.10.016 [Epub ahead of print]

Fernandes, G., Siqueira, J. T., Godoi Goncalves, D. A., and Camparis, C. M. (2014). Association between painful temporomandibular disorders, sleep bruxism and tinnitus. *Braz. Oral. Res.* 28:1. doi: 10.1590/1807-3107bor-2014.vol28.0003

Haider, H. F., Hoare, D. J., Costa, R. F. P., Potgieter, I., Kikidis, D. Lapira, A., et al. (2017). Pathophysiology, diagnosis and treatment of somatosensory tinnitus: a scoping review. *Front. Neurosci.* 11:207. doi: 10.3389/fnins.2017.00207

Hall, D. A., Fackrell, K., Li, A. B., Thavayogan, R., Smith, S., Kennedy, V., et al. (2018). A narrative synthesis of research evidence for tinnitus-related complaints as reported by patients and their significant others. *Health Qual. Life Outcomes* 16:61. doi: 10.1186/s12955-018-0888-9

Hebert, S., Canlon, B., and Hasson, D. (2012). Emotional exhaustion as a predictor of tinnitus. *Psychother. Psychosom.* 81, 324–326. doi: 10.1159/000335043

Idrizbegovic, E., Kjerulf, E., and Team for Diagnostics Hearing Habilitation Children Youth Hearing Rehabilitation for Adults, (2011). *Tinnitus Care Program [Tinnitus Vårdprogram].* Stockholm: Karolinska Institute.

Kehrle, H. M., Sampaio, A. L., Granjeiro, R. C., de Oliveira, T. S., and Oliveira, C. A. (2016). Tinnitus annoyance in normal-hearing individuals: correlation with depression and anxiety. *Ann. Otol. Rhinol. Laryngol.* 125, 185–194. doi: 10.1177/0003489415606445

Khalfa, S., Dubal, S., Veuillet, E., Perez-Diaz, F., Jouvent, R., and Collet, L. (2002). Psychometric normalization of a hyperacusis questionnaire. *ORL J. Otorhinolaryngol. Relat. Spec.* 64, 436–442. doi: 10.1159/000067570

Landgrebe, M., Zeman, F., Koller, M., Eberl, Y., Mohr, M., Reiter, J., et al. (2010). The tinnitus research initiative (tri) database: a new approach for delineation of tinnitus subtypes and generation of predictors for treatment outcome. *BMC Med. Inform. Decis. Mak.* 10:42. doi: 10.1186/1472-6947-10-42

Langguth, B., Elgoyhen, A. B., and Cederroth, C. R. (2018). Therapeutic approaches to the treatment of tinnitus. *Annu. Rev. Pharmacol. Toxicol.* 59, 291–313. doi: 10.1146/annurev-pharmtox-010818-021556

Lee, C. F., Lin, M. C., Lin, H. T., Lin, C. L., Wang, T. C., and Kao, C. H. (2016). Increased risk of tinnitus in patients with temporomandibular disorder: a retrospective population-based cohort study. *Eur. Arch. Otorhinolaryngol.* 273, 203–208. doi: 10.1007/s00405-015-3491-2

Levenstein, S., Prantera, C., Varvo, V., Scribano, M. L., Berto, E., Luzi, C., et al. (1993). Development of the perceived stress questionnaire: a new tool for psychosomatic research. *J. Psychosom. Res.* 37, 19–32. doi: 10.1016/0022-3999(93)90120-5

Levine, R. A. (1999). Somatic (*craniocervical*) tinnitus and the dorsal cochlear nucleus hypothesis. *Am. J. Otolaryngol.* 20, 351–362. doi: 10.1016/s0196-0709(99)90074-1

Lopez-Escamez, J. A., Bibas, T., Cima, R. F., Van de Heyning, P., Knipper, M., Mazurek, B., et al. (2016). Genetics of tinnitus: an emerging area for molecular diagnosis and drug development. *Front. Neurosci.* 10:377. doi: 10.3389/fnins.2016.00377

Lugo, A., Trpchevska, N., Roshni, B., Liu, X., Magnusson, C., Gallus, S., et al. (2019). Sex-specific influences of tinnitus on suicide attempt. *JAMA Otolaryngol. Head Neck Surg.* 145, 685–687.

Maas, I. L., Bruggemann, P., Requena, T., Bulla, J., Edvall, N. K., Hjelmborg, J. V. B., et al. (2017). Genetic susceptibility to bilateral tinnitus in a Swedish twin cohort. *Genet. Med.* 19, 1007–1012. doi: 10.1038/gim.2017.4

Marks, K. L., Martel, D. T., Wu, C., Basura, G. J., Roberts, L. E., Schvartz-Leyzac, K. C., et al. (2018). Auditory-somatosensory bimodal stimulation desynchronizes brain circuitry to reduce tinnitus in guinea pigs and humans. *Sci. Transl. Med.* 10:eaal3175. doi: 10.1126/scitranslmed.aal3175

McCombe, A., Baguley, D., Coles, R., McKenna, L., McKinney, C., Windle-Taylor, P., et al. (2001). Guidelines for the grading of tinnitus severity: the results of a working group commissioned by the British Association of Otolaryngologists, head and neck surgeons, 1999. *Clin. Otolaryngol. Allied Sci.* 26, 388–393. doi: 10.1046/j.1365-2273.2001.00490.x

McCormack, A., Edmondson-Jones, M., Somerset, S., and Hall, D. (2016). A systematic review of the reporting of tinnitus prevalence and severity. *Hear. Res.* 337, 70–79. doi: 10.1016/j.heares.2016.05.009

Meikle, M. B., Henry, J. A., Griest, S. E., Stewart, B. J., Abrams, H. B., McArdle, R., et al. (2012). The tinnitus functional index: development of a new clinical measure for chronic, intrusive tinnitus. *Ear. Hear.* 33 153–176. doi: 10.1097/AUD.0b013e31822f67c0

Michiels, S., Ganz Sanchez, T., Oron, Y., Gilles, A., Haider, H. F., Erlandsson, S., et al. (2018a). Diagnostic criteria for somatosensory tinnitus: a delphi process and face-to-face meeting to establish consensus. *Trends Hear.* 22:2331216518796403. doi: 10.1177/2331216518796403

Michiels, S., van der Wal, A. C., Nieste, E., Van de Heyning, P., Braem, M., Visscher, C., et al. (2018b). Conservative therapy for the treatment of patients with somatic tinnitus attributed to temporomandibular dysfunction: study protocol of a randomised controlled trial. *Trials* 19:554. doi: 10.1186/s13063-018-2903-1

Michiels, S., Nieste, E., Van de Heyning, P., Braem, M., Visscher, C., Topsakal, V., et al. (2019). Does conservative temporomandibular therapy affect tinnitus complaints? a systematic review. *J. Oral. Facial Pain Headache* 33, 308–317 doi: 10.11607/ofph.2055

Mottaghi, A., Menendez-Diaz, I., Cobo, J. L., Gonzalez-Serrano, J., and Cobo, T. (2019). Is there a higher prevalence of tinnitus in patients with temporomandibular disorders? a systematic review and meta-analysis. *J. Oral. Rehabil.* 46, 76–86. doi: 10.1111/joor.12706

Müller, K., Edvall, N. K., Idrizbegovic, E., Huhn R., Cima, R., Persson, V., et al. (2016). Validation of online versions of tinnitus questionnaires translated into swedish. *Front. Aging Neurosci.* 8:272. doi: 10.3389/fnagi.2016.00272

Murphy, M. K., MacBarb, R. F., Wong, M. E., and Athanasiou, K. A. (2013). Temporomandibular disorders: a review of etiology, clinical management, and tissue engineering strategies. *Int. J. Oral. Maxillofac. Implants* 28, e393–e414. doi: 10.11607/jomi.te20

Newman, C. W., Jacobson, G. P., and Spitzer, J. B. (1996). Development of the tinnitus handicap inventory. *Arch. Otolaryngol. Head Neck Surg.* 122, 143–148.

Newman, C. W., Sandridge, S. A., and Jacobson, G. P. (1998). Psychometric adequacy of the tinnitus handicap inventory (THI) for evaluating treatment outcome. *J. Am. Acad. Audiol.* 9, 153–160.

Nondahl, D. M., Cruickshanks, K. J., Huang, G. H., Klein, B. E., Klein, R., Nieto, F. J., et al. (2011). Tinnitus and its risk factors in the Beaver Dam offspring study. *Int. J. Audiol.* 50, 313–320. doi: 10.3109/14992027.2010.551220

Pinchoff, R. J., Burkard, R. F., Salvi, R. J., Coad, M. L., and Lockwood, A. H. (1998). Modulation of tinnitus by voluntary jaw movements. *Am. J. Otol.* 19, 785–789.

Rauschecker, J. P., Leaver, A. M., and Muhlau, M. (2010). Tuning out the noise: limbic-auditory interactions in tinnitus. *Neuron* 66, 819–826. doi: 10.1016/j.neuron.2010.04.032

Rauschecker, J. P., May, E. S., Maudoux, A., and Ploner, M. (2015). Frontostriatal gating of tinnitus and chronic pain. *Trends Cogn. Sci.* 19, 567–578. doi: 10.1016/j.tics.2015.08.002

R Core Team (2019). *R: A Language and Environment for Statistical Computing.* Vienna: R Foundation for Statistical Computing. https://www.R-project.org/

Roberts, L. E., Eggermont, J. J., Caspary, D. M., Shore, S. E., Melcher, J. R., and Kaltenbach, J. A. (2010). Ringing ears: the neuroscience of tinnitus. *J. Neurosci.* 30, 14972–14979. doi: 10.1523/JNEUROSCI.4028-10.2010

Sanchez, T. G., Guerra, G. C., Lorenzi, M. C., Brandao, A. L., and Bento, R. F. (2002). The influence of voluntary muscle contractions upon the onset and modulation of tinnitus. *Audiol. Neurootol.* 7, 370–375. doi: 10.1159/000066155

Schlee, W., Hall, D., Edvall, N. K., Langguth, B., Canlon, B., and Cederroth, C. R. (2017a). Visualization of global disease burden for the optimization of patient management and treatment. *Front. Med.* 4:86. doi: 10.3389/fmed.2017.00086

Schlee, W., Hall, D. A., Canlon, B., Cima, R. F. F., de Kleine, E., Hauck, F., et al. (2017b). Innovations in doctoral training and research on tinnitus: the european school on interdisciplinary tinnitus research (esit) perspective. *Front. Aging Neurosci.* 9:447. doi: 10.3389/fnagi.2017.00447

Scrivani, S. J., Keith, D. A., and Kaban, L. B. (2008). Temporomandibular disorders. *N. Engl. J. Med.* 359, 2693–2705. doi: 10.1056/NEJMra0802472

Seydel, C., Haupt, H., Olze, H., Szczepek, A. J., and Mazurek, B. (2013). Gender and chronic tinnitus: differences in tinnitus-related distress depend on age and duration of tinnitus. *Ear. Hear.* 34, 661–672. doi: 10.1097/AUD.0b013e31828149f2

Sharma, S., Gupta, D. S., Pal, U. S., and Jurel, S. K. (2011). Etiological factors of temporomandibular joint disorders. *Natl. J. Maxillofac. Surg.* 2, 116–119. doi: 10.4103/0975-5950.94463

Shore, S. E., Roberts, L. E., and Langguth, B. (2016). Maladaptive plasticity in tinnitus–triggers, mechanisms and treatment. *Nat. Rev. Neurol.* 12, 150–160. doi: 10.1038/nrneurol.2016.12

Shore, S. E., Vass, Z., Wys, N. L., and Altschuler, R. A. (2000). Trigeminal ganglion innervates the auditory brainstem. *J. Comp. Neurol.* 419, 271–285. doi: 10.1002/(sici)1096-9861(20000410)419:3<271::aid-cne1>3.0.co;2-m

Skog, C., Fjellner, J., Ekberg, E., and Haggman-Henrikson, B. (2019). Tinnitus as a comorbidity to temporomandibular disorders-a systematic review. *J. Oral. Rehabil.* 46, 87–99. doi: 10.1111/joor.12710

Stockdale, D., McFerran, D., Brazier, P., Pritchard, C., Kay, T., Dowrick, C., et al. (2017). An economic evaluation of the healthcare cost of tinnitus management in the UK. *BMC Health Serv. Res.* 17:577. doi: 10.1186/s12913-017-2527-2

Svensson, A. C., Fredlund, P., Laflamme, L., Hallqvist, J., Alfredsson, L., Ekbom, A., et al. (2013). Cohort profile: the stockholm public health cohort. *Int. J. Epidemiol.* 42, 1263–1272. doi: 10.1093/ije/dys126

Szczepek, A. J., Frejo, L., Vona, B., Trpchevska, N., Cederroth, C. R., Caria, H., et al. (2018). Recommendations on collecting and storing samples for genetic studies in hearing and tinnitus research. *Ear. Hear.* 40, 219–226. doi: 10.1097/AUD.0000000000000614

The Whoqol Group, (1998). Development of the world health organization whoqol-bref quality of life assessment. *Psychol. Med.* 28, 551–558. doi: 10.1017/s0033291798006667

Tuz, H. H., Onder, E. M., and Kisnisci, R. S. (2003). Prevalence of otologic complaints in patients with temporomandibular disorder. *Am. J. Orthod. Dent. Orthop.* 123, 620–623. doi: 10.1016/S0889540603001537

Vielsmeier, V., Strutz, J., Kleinjung, T., Schecklmann, M., Kreuzer, P. M., Landgrebe, M., et al. (2012). Temporomandibular joint disorder complaints in tinnitus: further hints for a putative tinnitus subtype. *PLoS One* 7:e38887. doi: 10.1371/journal.pone.0038887

Vona, B., Nanda, I., Shehata-Dieler, W., and Haaf, T. (2017). Genetics of Tinnitus: still in its Infancy. *Front. Neurosci.* 11:236. doi: 10.3389/fnins.2017.00236

Ward, J., Vella, C., Hoare, D. J., and Hall, D. A. (2015). Subtyping somatic tinnitus: a cross-sectional uk cohort study of demographic, clinical and audiological characteristics. *PLoS One* 10:e0126254. doi: 10.1371/journal.pone.0126254

Won, J. Y., Yoo, S., Lee, S. K., Choi, H. K., Yakunina, N., Le, Q., et al. (2013). Prevalence and factors associated with neck and jaw muscle modulation of tinnitus. *Audiol. Neurootol.* 18, 261–273. doi: 10.1159/000351685

Wu, C., Stefanescu, R. A., Martel, D. T., and Shore, S. E. (2015). Tinnitus: maladaptive auditory-somatosensory plasticity. *Hear. Res.* 334, 20–29. doi: 10.1016/j.heares.2015.06.005

23

Loss of Vision Dominance at the Preresponse Level in Tinnitus Patients: Preliminary Behavioral Evidence

Zhicheng Li[1,2†], Ruolei Gu[3†], Min Qi[1], Jintian Cen[1], Shuqi Zhang[1], Jing Gu[1], Xiangli Zeng[1] and Qi Chen[2*]*

[1] Department of Otolaryngology-Head and Neck Surgery, Third Affiliated Hospital of Sun Yat-sen University, Guangzhou, China, [2] Department of Psychology and Center for Studies of Psychological Application, South China Normal University, Guangzhou, China, [3] Key Laboratory of Behavioral Science, Institute of Psychology, Chinese Academy of Sciences, Beijing, China

***Correspondence:**
Xiangli Zeng
zxiangl@mail.sysu.edu.cn
Qi Chen
qi.chen27@gmail.com

[†] These authors have contributed equally to this work

At present, the mechanisms underlying changes in visual processing in individuals with tinnitus remain unclear. Therefore, we investigated whether the vision dominance of individuals with tinnitus disappears at the preresponse level through behavioral study. A total of 38 individuals with tinnitus and 31 healthy controls completed a task in which they were asked to attend to either visual or auditory stimuli while ignoring simultaneous stimulus inputs from the other modality. We manipulated three levels of congruency between the simultaneous visual and auditory inputs: congruent (C), incongruent at the preresponse level (PRIC), and incongruent at the response level (RIC). Thus, we differentiated the cross-modal conflict explicitly into the preresponse (PRIC > C) and response (RIC > PRIC) levels. The results revealed no significant difference in the size of the preresponse level conflict between the auditory attention and visual attention conditions in tinnitus group. In brief, the preresponse level of individuals with tinnitus showed a loss in vision dominance. This may be due to the reduced interference of visual information in auditory processing.

Keywords: tinnitus, cross-modal interference, vision dominance, attention, behavioral research

INTRODUCTION

Vision and audition are important functions through which individuals obtain information about the external environment. When individuals attend to information from one sensory modality, they tend to "look without seeing" or "listen without hearing" to the information received by other sensory modalities. However, the information received by the non-attended modality affects the information processing of that received by the attended modality, and this phenomenon is known as cross-modal interference. Previous studies have reported that when the input information of visual and auditory modalities is inconsistent, the processing time is prolonged and the accuracy of responses to attended stimuli decrease (Colavita, 1974; Chen and Zhou, 2013). Moreover, visual distractors cause more interference to auditory processing than auditory distractors do to visual processing (as vision dominance) at the preresponse level, but auditory distractors cause more interference to visual processing than visual distractors do to auditory processing (as audition dominance) at the response level (Repp and Penel, 2004; Kato and Konishi, 2006; Mayer et al., 2009; Koppen et al., 2009; Chen and Zhou, 2013).

Tinnitus, a subjective auditory experience, emerges independent of external stimuli, and its occurrence and maintenance require attentional resources (Roberts et al., 2013). Previous studies have shown that visual processing in individuals with tinnitus is significantly worse than that of healthy controls (Stevens et al., 2007; Heeren et al., 2014; Araneda et al., 2015a,b; Li et al., 2018), and is more susceptible to cross-modal interference of auditory information (Araneda et al., 2015b). Meanwhile, the decrease in signal detection (the early stage of cognitive processing) might underlie the impaired visual processing in individuals with tinnitus (Li et al., 2018). With this in mind, the "visual dominance effect" (i.e., allocating more attentional resources to visual rather than auditory information, which leads to stronger interference of visual distractors on auditory targets) at the preresponse level might function abnormally in individuals with tinnitus. Clarifying this problem will facilitate further understanding of the effect of tinnitus on individuals' cognitive processing (particularly cross-channel information integration), and will provide a reference for improving strategies concerning the evaluation and management of tinnitus. However, the changes and mechanisms of visual processing in individuals with tinnitus are unclear.

The current study aimed to investigate whether the vision dominance of individuals with tinnitus disappears at the preresponse level. To this aim, we used the experimental design of Chen and Zhou (2013), which could help investigate cross-modal conflict at the preresponse and response levels. Participants simultaneously received visual and auditory stimuli (i.e., cross-modal inputs), and were asked to attend to one modality and ignore the other. All experimental stimuli were presented as one of four colors (red/green/blue/yellow), two of which (red and green) were targets, while the other two (blue and yellow) were distractors (**Figure 1A**); only stimuli in the "target" category required press the button. The task included the two following factors: modality (attending to visual/auditory stimuli) and congruency (cross-modal congruency, C; incongruent at preresponse level, PRIC; incongruent at both the preresponse and response levels, RIC). In the C condition, bimodal inputs referred to the same target (e.g., participants saw a red block and heard "red"). In the PRIC condition, the stimulus in the attended channel (visual/auditory) was a target, but the stimulus in the unattended channel was a distractor that did not require a response (e.g., participants saw a red block but heard "blue"); therefore, the cross-modal conflict emerged at the preresponse level but not the response level. In the RIC condition, the stimuli in the attended channel and the unattended channel were two different targets that required different responses (e.g., participants saw a red block but heard "green") (**Figure 1B**); therefore, the cross-modal conflict emerged at both the preresponse and response levels. According to Chen and Zhou (2013), the classical findings in this task are that visual distractors cause larger preresponse-level interference (PRIC > C in reaction time) to auditory processing than vice versa, while auditory distractors cause larger response-level interference (RIC > PRIC in reaction time) to visual processing than vice versa.

Based on these previous studies, we hypothesized that the vision dominance of individuals with tinnitus would disappears at the preresponse level, and there would be no significant difference between the interference of visual information in auditory processing and vice versa. In line with this hypothesis, we found that there was no significant difference in preresponse-level interference between the modalities attended. This study did not have any specific predictions concerning the disappearance of visual dominance.

METHODS

The experimental protocol was reviewed and approved by the Ethics Committee of the Third Affiliated Hospital of Sun Yat-sen University [approval number: (2018) 02-358-01]. All enrolled participants were required to sign an informed consent form.

Participants

Individuals with tinnitus admitted to the Outpatient Department of Otorhinolaryngology, the Third Affiliated Hospital of Sun Yat-sen University due to tinnitus as a major complaint were enrolled (21 men, 17 women, mean age = 28.23 ± 6.20 years). All individuals were diagnosed as having chronic subjective tinnitus, without hyperacusis, and the pure-tone threshold from 125 to 8000 Hz, including the semioctave range, were ≤40 dB HL. Healthy controls, who had no history of hearing loss (both pure-tone threshold ≤25 dB HL), tinnitus, dizziness, or other ear diseases, were recruited from online and poster adverts at the Sun Yat-sen University (16 men, 15 women, mean age = 22.63 ± 2.24 years). All participants were right-handed, had normal or corrected-to-normal vision (5.0 or above in the Logarithmic Visual Acuity Chart), and no color blindness or weakness. No participant had a history of neurological or psychiatric disorders.

Experimental Design and Stimuli

We adopted a 2 (group: tinnitus and control groups) × 2 (modality attended: Attend-Visual and Attend-Auditory) × 3 (congruency: C, PRIC, and RIC) hybrid design.

Visual stimuli (color blocks) were presented on an LED monitor at a viewing distance of 70 cm. Auditory stimuli (verbal pronunciations) were voice recordings of a male speaker and were delivered binaurally via stereo headphones. The volume was adjusted for each participant such that the auditory stimuli could be clearly heard.

The experimental task was to judge whether the attended color block or verbal pronunciation was red or green. Throughout the experiment, all color blocks and verbal pronunciations were potential targets that required responses. Participants used the index and middle fingers of their right hand to respond by pressing one key on the response box for red or another key for green. The mapping between the two response keys and red versus green color was counterbalanced across participants.

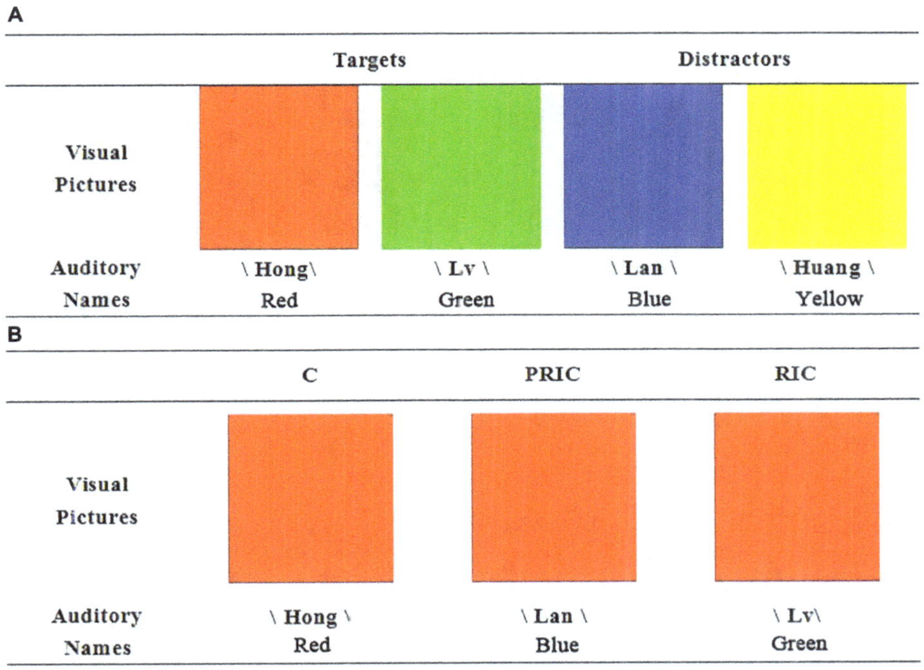

FIGURE 1 | Exemplar stimuli **(A)** and design **(B)** in experiment. **(A)** Two color pictures and their verbal sounds served as targets. Another two color pictures and their verbal sounds served as distractors. **(B)** Examples of the manipulation of the three levels of congruency are provided for the situation in which the visual modality was attended. In the C condition, the auditory name and visual picture refer to the same target. In the PRIC condition, the auditory name refers to the distractors and the visual picture refers to the target. In the RIC condition, the auditory name and visual picture refer to different targets. The auditory names were played in Mandarin, like /Hong/, /Lv/, /Lan/, and /Huang/.

Procedure

The stimuli were presented using a hybrid design in which the attended modality was blocked, and the C, PRIC, and RIC trials were mixed randomly within each block. In each block, participants were asked to focus on either the visual or auditory stimuli while ignoring stimuli from the other modality. They were instructed to fixate on the central cross throughout the experiment without moving their eyes. In each trial, a color block and verbal pronunciation were simultaneously presented for 300 ms. Each of the six experimental conditions had 48 trials, resulting in a total of 384 trials (288 experimental trials and 96 null trials). In a null trial, only the central fixation cross was displayed. For the visual attention condition and auditory attention condition, respectively, null trials and C, PRIC, and RIC trials were randomly mixed and then divided into 24 test blocks. Each block comprised 8 trials and lasted for 20 s. The visual attention condition and auditory attention condition blocks were alternated. Each block started with a 2-s visual instruction about which modality was to be attended.

Statistical Analyses

Within each of the six experimental conditions, omissions, incorrect responses, and trials with reaction times (RTs) three standard deviations away from the mean RT were excluded from further analyses. The mean RTs of the remaining trials were subsequently calculated. Normally distributed data were analyzed using repeated measures analysis of variance (ANOVA) and t-tests. Otherwise, median and quartile ranges were presented, and differences were tested using Wilcoxon Signed Ranks Test. $p < 0.05$ was considered statistically significant.

RESULTS

The 2 (group: tinnitus and control groups) × 2 (modality attended: Attend-Visual and Attend-Auditory) × 3 (congruency: C, PRIC, and RIC) repeated measures ANOVA showed a significant main effect of Group [$F(1,67) = 9.15$, $p = 0.004$], whereby the tinnitus group had significantly longer RTs than those of the control group, irrespective of the attended modality or congruency condition ($p < 0.05$; **Figure 2A**).

Moreover, there was a significant main effect of attended modality [$F(1,67) = 76.94$, $p < 0.001$], whereby RTs to the visual targets were significantly shorter than those to the auditory targets. There was also a main effect of congruency [$F(2,134) = 284.53$, $p < 0.001$]; further pairwise comparisons using Bonferroni correction indicated that RTs in the PRIC condition were significantly longer than those in the C condition ($p < 0.001$), and RTs in the RIC condition were significantly longer than those in the PRIC condition ($p = 0.02$). This result indicated significant cross-modal conflicts at both the preresponse and response levels.

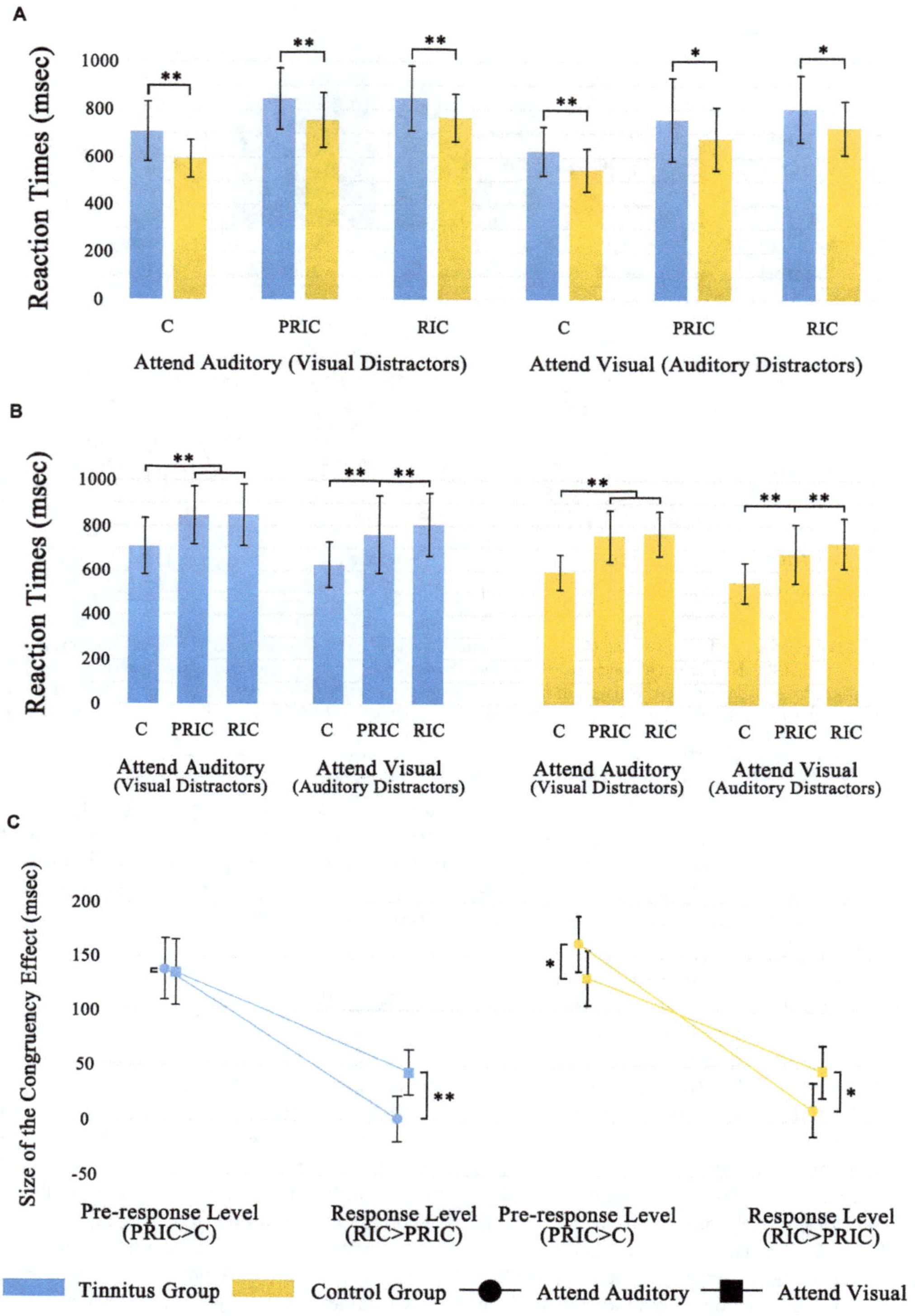

FIGURE 2 | Behavioral results of Experiment. **(A)** Inter-group differences of the six experimental conditions. **(B)** Intra-group differences of the six experimental conditions. **(C)** Inter-group differences of sizes of cross-modal conflict at the preresponse (PRIC > C) and response (RIC > PRIC) levels are shown as a function of the attended modality. *$p < 0.05$; **$p < 0.01$.

There was a significant interaction between the attended modality and congruency [$F(2,134) = 7.44$, $p = 0.001$], and planned *t*-tests on simple effects indicated that the preresponse level conflict was significant both in the auditory attention condition ($p < 0.001$) and visual attention condition ($p < 0.001$). Conversely, the response level conflict was only significant in the visual attention condition (p = 0.001), and not in the auditory attention condition (p = 0.40). There were no significant interactions between attended modality and group [$F(1,67)$ = 1.38, p = 0.25], consistency and group [$F(2,134)$ = 0.50, p = 0.61], attended modality, consistency, and group [$F(2,134)$ = 1.80, p = 0.17]. This indicated that the pattern between attended modality and consistency were similar between the tinnitus group and control group (**Figure 2B**).

Within the control group, the size of the preresponse level conflict was significantly larger when the auditory modality was attended vs. when the visual modality was attended (p = 0.02), whereas the size of the response level conflict was significantly larger when visual modality was attended vs. when the auditory modality was attended (p = 0.04) (**Figure 2C**, right). Within the tinnitus group, the size of the preresponse level conflict was not significantly different between the auditory attention and visual attention conditions (p = 0.85) (**Figure 2C**, left).

For both the auditory attention and visual attention conditions, further independent samples t-tests did not reveal any significant between-group differences in the size of the congruency effect at the preresponse and response levels groups (p = 0.24, 0.59, 0.82, and 0.91, respectively).

DISCUSSION

The brain can process a limited amount of information per unit time; therefore, the brain needs to allocate limited attention resources to process the most pertinent information in complex situations (Mishra and Gazzaley, 2012). The occurrence and maintenance of tinnitus both require attentional resources, which eventually affects cognitive processing (Roberts et al., 2013). The present study found that the RTs of the tinnitus group in both experimental conditions were significantly longer than those of the control group, thus supporting the reduction of visual and auditory processing in individuals with tinnitus.

More importantly, we found that the vision dominance of individuals with tinnitus disappeared at the preresponse level, as hypothesized. Although the size of the congruency effect at the preresponse level did not show significant differences between the tinnitus and control groups, it reduced from 162 ms in the control group to 138 ms in the tinnitus group in the auditory attention condition, while it maintained a similar effect in the tinnitus (135 ms) and control (130 ms) groups in the visual attention condition. Therefore, we speculate that the disappearance of visual dominance at the preresponse level in individuals with tinnitus is mainly due to the reduced interference of visual information in auditory processing. This finding also indicates that the auditory modality may demand a greater allocation of attention, which consequently weakens the interference of the visual modality.

However, we must also realize that tinnitus may be a product of brain dysfunction (Elgoyhen et al., 2015), and brain dysfunction may also affect other cognitive processes, other than auditory processing. Thus, whether the reduction of visual processing in individuals with tinnitus is due to tinnitus, or, like tinnitus, still needs to be further explored. Moreover, the default mode network is involved in visual dominance at the preresponse level (Chen and Zhou, 2013), and many brain regions and neural connections in the default mode network of individuals with tinnitus have been found to exhibit changes (Elgoyhen et al., 2015). We aim to explore the relationship between the disappearance of visual dominance at the preresponse level and the change in the default mode network in our follow-up EEG and imaging studies. Furthermore, this study only focused on individuals with chronic subjective tinnitus. Therefore, the results of the study cannot be extended to other groups of individuals with tinnitus. Follow-up studies should gradually incorporate different groups of individuals of tinnitus, such as those with acute tinnitus or objective tinnitus, to further clarify this viewpoint.

CONCLUSION

The preresponse level of individuals with tinnitus revealed a loss of vision dominance, which may be due to the reduced interference of visual information in auditory processing. Further studies are warranted to verify our findings and to explore the neural mechanisms underlying behavioral changes using EEG and imaging techniques.

AUTHOR CONTRIBUTIONS

ZL designed and performed the experiments, analyzed the data, and wrote the manuscript. RG analyzed the data and perfected the manuscript. XZ modified the research approach and chose the patients. QC directed and modified the research approach and provided the critical revision. ZL, RG, XZ, and QC discussed the results and implications and commented on the manuscript at all stages. MQ, JC, SZ, and JG in charge of preliminary screening and contacted with subject.

FUNDING

This work was supported by the Science and Technology Program of Guangzhou, China (Grant No. 201704030081).

ACKNOWLEDGMENTS

Thanks to Xia Jing, Fang Ying, and Zou Guijing from School of Psychology, South China Normal University for their help in experimental programming and Sun Tienan, Fan Huiyang, Zhuang Jinkun, and Wei Xin from the Zhongshan School of Medicine, Sun Yat-sen University, for their help in data acquisition.

REFERENCES

Araneda, R., De Volder, A., Deggouj, N., Philippot, P., Heeren, A., Lacroix, E., et al. (2015a). Altered top-down cognitive control and auditory processing in tinnitus: evidences from auditory and visual spatial stroop. *Restor. Neurol. Neurosci.* 33, 67–80. doi: 10.3233/RNN-140433

Araneda, R., De Volder, A., Deggouj, N., and Renier, L. (2015b). Altered inhibitory control and increased sensitivity to cross-modal interference in tinnitus during auditory and visual tasks. *PLoS One* 10:e0120387. doi: 10.1371/journal.pone.0120387

Chen, Q., and Zhou, X. (2013). Vision dominates at the preresponse level and audition dominates at the response level in cross-modal interaction: behavioral and neural evidence. *J Neurosci.* 33, 7109–7121. doi: 10.1523/JNEUROSCI.1985-12.2013

Colavita, F. (1974). Human sensory dominance. *Percept. Psychophys.* 16, 409–412. doi: 10.3758/bf03203962

Elgoyhen, A., Langguth, B., De Ridder, D., and Vanneste, S. (2015). Tinnitus: perspectives from human neuroimaging. *Nat. Rev. Neurosci.* 16, 632–642. doi: 10.1038/nrn4003

Heeren, A., Maurage, P., Perrot, H., De Volder, A., Renier, L., Araneda, R., et al. (2014). Tinnitus specifically alters the top-down executive control sub-component of attention: evidence from the attention network task. *Behav. Brain. Res.* 269, 147–154. doi: 10.1016/j.bbr.2014.04.043

Kato, M., and Konishi, Y. (2006). Auditory dominance in the error correction process: a synchronized tapping study. *Brain Res.* 1084, 115–122. doi: 10.1016/j.brainres.2006.02.019

Koppen, C., Levitan, C., and Spence, C. (2009). A signal detection study of the Colavita visual dominance effect. *Exp. Brain Res.* 196, 353–360. doi: 10.1007/s00221-009-1853-y

Li, Z., Gu, R., Zeng, X., Qi, M., Cen, J., Zhang, S., et al. (2018). Eyes and ears: cross-modal interference of tinnitus on visual processing. *Front. Psychol.* 9:1779. doi: 10.3389/fpsyg.2018.01779

Mayer, A., Franco, A., Canive, J., and Harrington, D. L. (2009). The effects of stimulus modality and frequency of stimulus presentation on cross-modal distraction. *Cereb. Cortex* 19, 993–1007. doi: 10.1093/cercor/bhn148

Mishra, J., and Gazzaley, A. (2012). Attention distributed across sensory modalities enhances perceptual performance. *J. Neurosci.* 32, 12294–12302. doi: 10.1523/JNEUROSCI.0867-12.2012

Repp, B., and Penel, A. (2004). Rhythmic movement is attracted more strongly to auditory than to visual rhythms. *Psychol. Res.* 68, 252–270.

Roberts, L., Husain, F., and Eggermont, J. (2013). Role of attention in the generation and modulation of tinnitus. *Neurosci. Biobehav. Rev.* 37, 1754–1773. doi: 10.1016/j.neubiorev.2013.07.007

Stevens, C., Walker, G., Boyer, M., and Gallagher, M. (2007). Severe tinnitus and its effect on selective and divided attention. *Int. J. Audiol.* 46, 208–216. doi: 10.1080/14992020601102329

Permissions

All chapters in this book were first published in Journal of Allergy, by Hindawi Publishing Corporation; hereby published with permission under the Creative Commons Attribution License or equivalent. Every chapter published in this book has been scrutinized by our experts. Their significance has been extensively debated. The topics covered herein carry significant findings which will fuel the growth of the discipline. They may even be implemented as practical applications or may be referred to as a beginning point for another development.

The contributors of this book come from diverse backgrounds, making this book a truly international effort. This book will bring forth new frontiers with its revolutionizing research information and detailed analysis of the nascent developments around the world.

We would like to thank all the contributing authors for lending their expertise to make the book truly unique. They have played a crucial role in the development of this book. Without their invaluable contributions this book wouldn't have been possible. They have made vital efforts to compile up to date information on the varied aspects of this subject to make this book a valuable addition to the collection of many professionals and students.

This book was conceptualized with the vision of imparting up-to-date information and advanced data in this field. To ensure the same, a matchless editorial board was set up. Every individual on the board went through rigorous rounds of assessment to prove their worth. After which they invested a large part of their time researching and compiling the most relevant data for our readers.

The editorial board has been involved in producing this book since its inception. They have spent rigorous hours researching and exploring the diverse topics which have resulted in the successful publishing of this book. They have passed on their knowledge of decades through this book. To expedite this challenging task, the publisher supported the team at every step. A small team of assistant editors was also appointed to further simplify the editing procedure and attain best results for the readers.

Apart from the editorial board, the designing team has also invested a significant amount of their time in understanding the subject and creating the most relevant covers. They scrutinized every image to scout for the most suitable representation of the subject and create an appropriate cover for the book.

The publishing team has been an ardent support to the editorial, designing and production team. Their endless efforts to recruit the best for this project, has resulted in the accomplishment of this book. They are a veteran in the field of academics and their pool of knowledge is as vast as their experience in printing. Their expertise and guidance has proved useful at every step. Their uncompromising quality standards have made this book an exceptional effort. Their encouragement from time to time has been an inspiration for everyone.

The publisher and the editorial board hope that this book will prove to be a valuable piece of knowledge for researchers, students, practitioners and scholars across the globe.

List of Contributors

Mithila Durai
Eisdell Moore Centre, Section of Audiology, University of Auckland, Auckland, New Zealand
Center for Brain Research, University of Auckland, Auckland, New Zealand

Grant D. Searchfield
Eisdell Moore Centre, Section of Audiology, University of Auckland, Auckland, New Zealand
Center for Brain Research, University of Auckland, Auckland, New Zealand
Brain Research New Zealand, Auckland, New Zealand

Winfried Schlee and Rainer Rupprecht
Department of Psychiatry and Psychotherapy of the University of Regensburg at Bezirksklinikum Regensburg, University of Regensburg, Regensburg, Germany

Peter M. Kreuzer, Timm B. Poeppl, Astrid Lehner and Berthold Langguth
Department of Psychiatry and Psychotherapy, University of Regensburg, Regensburg, Germany
Interdisciplinary Tinnitus Center of the University of Regensburg, Regensburg, Germany
Department of Psychiatry and Psychotherapy of the University of Regensburg at Bezirksklinikum Regensburg, University of Regensburg, Regensburg, Germany

Martin Schecklmann
Department of Psychiatry and Psychotherapy of the University of Regensburg at Bezirksklinikum Regensburg, University of Regensburg, Regensburg, Germany
Department of Psychiatry and Psychotherapy, University of Regensburg, Regensburg, Germany
Interdisciplinary Tinnitus Center of the University of Regensburg, Regensburg, Germany

Veronika Vielsmeier
Interdisciplinary Tinnitus Center of the University of Regensburg, Regensburg, Germany
Department of Otorhinolaryngology, University of Regensburg, Regensburg, Germany

Andréia Aparecida Azevedo and Norma De Oliveira Penido
Otolaryngology, Universidade Federal de São Paulo, São Paulo, Brazil

Ricardo Rodrigues Figueiredo
Otolaryngology, Universidade Federal de São Paulo, São Paulo, Brazil
Otolaryngology, Faculdade de Medicina de Valença, Valença, Brazil

Ana Belen Elgoyhen
Instituto de Investigaciones en Ingeniería Genética y Biología Molecular "Dr. Héctor N. Torres", CONICET, Buenos Aires, Argentina
Facultad de Medicina, Instituto de Farmacología, Universidad de Buenos Aires (UBA), Buenos Aires, Argentina

Jérôme J. Servais
Department of Otorhinolaryngology, Cochlear Implant Centre, University Medicine Mannheim, Mannheim, Germany

Karl Hörmann
Department of Otorhinolaryngology, Cochlear Implant Centre, University Medicine Mannheim, Mannheim, Germany
Audiology, Medical Faculty Mannheim, Department of Otorhinolaryngology, Heidelberg University, Mannheim, Germany

Elisabeth Wallhäusser-Franke
Audiology, Medical Faculty Mannheim, Department of Otorhinolaryngology, Heidelberg University, Mannheim, Germany

Christoph M. Krick and Wolfgang Reith
Department for Neuroradiology, Saarland University Hospital, Homburg, Germany

Heike Argstatter and Miriam Grapp
German Research Centre for Music Therapy Research, Heidelberg, Germany

Peter K. Plinkert
Department of Otorhinolaryngology, Head and Neck Surgery, University Hospital for Ear, Nose and Throat, University

Patrick Neff
Neuroplasticity and Learning in the Healthy Aging Brain (HAB LAB), Department of Psychology, University of Zurich, Zurich, Switzerland
University Research Priority Program "Dynamics of Healthy Aging", University of Zurich, Zurich, Switzerland

Martin Meyer
Neuroplasticity and Learning in the Healthy Aging Brain (HAB LAB), Department of Psychology, University of Zurich, Zurich, Switzerland
University Research Priority Program "Dynamics of Healthy Aging", University of Zurich, Zurich, Switzerland
Cognitive Psychology Unit, University of Klagenfurt, Klagenfurt, Austria

Jakob Michels
Department of Medicine, University of Regensburg, Regensburg, Germany

Markku Vesala and Stephen Harrison
Tinnitus Hub Ltd, Hemsworth, UK

Rüdiger C. Pryss, Johannes Schobel, Michael Stach and Manfred Reichert
Institute of Databases and Information Systems, Ulm University, Ulm, Germany

Thomas Probst
Department of Psychology, University of Regensburg, Regensburg, Germany
Department of Psychology and Psychotherapy, University of Witten/Herdecke, Witten, Germany
Department for Psychotherapy and Biopsychosocial Health, Danube University Krems, Krems an der Donau, Austria
Georg-Elias-Müller Institute for Psychology, Georg-August University Göttingen, Göttingen, Germany
Institute of Databases and Information Systems, Ulm University, Ulm, Germany

Myra Spiliopoulou
Department of Technical and Business Information Systems, Otto-von-Guericke-University Magdeburg, Magdeburg, Germany
Faculty of Computer Science, Otto-von-Guericke-University Magdeburg, Magdeburg, Germany

Michael Landgrebe
Department of Psychiatry and Psychotherapy of the University of Regensburg at Bezirksklinikum Regensburg, University of Regensburg, Regensburg, Germany
Clinic Lech-Mangfall, Agatharied, Germany

Daniela Ivansic, Christian Dobel, Gerd F. Volk, Daniel Reinhardt, Boris Müller and Orlando Guntinas-Lichius
Tinnitus-Centre, Department of Otorhinolaryngology, Jena University Hospital, Jena, Germany

Ulrich C. Smolenski
Institut of Physiotherapy, Jena university Hospital, Jena, Germany

Tijana Bojić
Laboratory of Radiobiology and Molecular Genetics, Institute of Nuclear Sciences Vinča, University of Belgrade, Belgrade, Serbia

Vladimir R. Perović, Milan Senćanski and Sanja Glišić
Center for Multidisciplinary Research, Institute of Nuclear Sciences Vinča, University of Belgrade, Belgrade, Serbia

Marzena Mielczarek and Jurek Olszewski
Department of Otolaryngology, Laryngological Oncology, Audiology and Phoniatrics, Medical University of Lodz, Lodz, Poland

Arnaud Norena
Centre National de la Recherche Scientifique, Aix-Marseille University, Marseille, France
Laboratoire Neurosciences Intégratives et Adaptatives, Aix-Marseille Université, Marseille, France

Sarah Rabau and Vincent Van Rompaey
University Department of Otorhinolaryngology and Head and Neck Surgery, Antwerp University Hospital, Edegem, Belgium
Faculty of Medicine, Campus Drie Eiken, University of Antwerp, Antwerp, Belgium

Giriraj S. Shekhawat
Section of Audiology/Health Systems, University of Auckland, Auckland, New Zealand
Centre for Brain Research, University of Auckland, Auckland, New Zealand
Tinnitus Research Initiative, Regensburg, Germany

Mohamed Aboseria, Daniel Griepp and Marom Bikson
Department of Biomedical Engineering, City College of New York, The City University of New York, New York, NY, United States

Paul van de Heyning
Department of ORL and Head and Neck Surgery, Antwerp University Hospital, University of Antwerp, Antwerp, Belgium
University Department of Otorhinolaryngology and Head and Neck Surgery, Antwerp University Hospital, Edegem, Belgium
Faculty of Medicine, Campus Drie Eiken, University of Antwerp, Antwerp, Belgium

Markus Haller
Desyncra Technologies Limited, London, United Kingdom

Deborah A. Hall
National Institute of Health Research, Nottingham Biomedical Research Centre, Ropewalk House, Nottingham, United Kingdom
Hearing Sciences, Division of Clinical Neuroscience, School of Medicine, University of Nottingham, Nottingham, United Kingdom
University of Nottingham Malaysia, Semenyih, Malaysia
Otology and Hearing Group, Division of Clinical Neuroscience, School of Medicine, University of Nottingham, Nottingham, United Kingdom

Sven Kalle
Faculty of Computer Science, Otto-von-Guericke-University Magdeburg, Magdeburg, Germany
Department of Psychiatry and Psychotherapy of Regensburg University, Regensburg, Germany

Steffen Knopke and Sophia Marie Häussler
Department of Otorhinolaryngology, Head and Neck Surgery, Charité - University Hospital Berlin, Campus Virchow- Klinikum, Berlin, Germany

Stefan Gräbel and Heidi Olze
Department of Otorhinolaryngology, Head and Neck Surgery, Charité - University Hospital Berlin, Campus Virchow- Klinikum, Berlin, Germany

Agnieszka J. Szczepek
Department of Otorhinolaryngology, Head and Neck Surgery, Charité - University Hospital Berlin, Campus Charité Mitte, Berlin, Germany
Department of ORL, Head and Neck Surgery, Charité Universitätsmedizin Berlin, Berlin, Germany

Petra Brüggemann and Birgit Mazurek
Tinnitus Center, Charité Universitätsmedizin Berlin, Berlin, Germany

Katharina Klee
Department of ORL, Head and Neck Surgery, Charité Universitätsmedizin Berlin, Berlin, Germany

Theodore Kypraios
NIHR Nottingham Hearing Biomedical Research Centre, Nottingham, United Kingdom

Rilana F. F. Cima
Clinical Psychological Science, Faculty of Psychology and Neuroscience, Maastricht University, Maastricht, Netherlands

Pim van Dijk and Emile de Kleine
Department of Otorhinolaryngology/Head and Neck Surgery, University Medical Center Groningen, University of Groningen, Groningen, Netherlands

Franz Hauck
Institute of Distributed Systems, Ulm University, Ulm, Germany

Flurin Pfiffner, Tobias Kleinjung and Alex Huber
Department of Otorhinolaryngology, Head and Neck Surgery, University Hospital of Zurich, University of Zurich, Zurich, Switzerland

Alessandra Lugo and Silvano Gallus
Department of Environmental Health Sciences, IRCCS - Istituto di Ricerche Farmacologiche Mario Negri, Milan, Italy

Teresa Requena
Otology and Neurotology Group, Department of Genomic Medicine, Centro Pfizer - Universidad de Granada - Junta de Andalucía de Genómica e Investigación Oncológica (GENYO), Granada, Spain

José A. Lopez-Escamez
Otology and Neurotology Group, Department of Genomic Medicine, Centro Pfizer - Universidad de Granada - Junta de Andalucía de Genómica e Investigación Oncológica (GENYO), Granada, Spain
Department of Otolaryngology, Instituto de Investigación Biosanitaria ibs.GRANADA, Hospital Universitario Virgen de las Nieves, Universidad de Granada, Granada, Spain

Nathan Weisz
Division of Physiological Psychology, Centre for Cognitive Neuroscience, University of Salzburg, Salzburg, Austria

Barbara Canlon and Christopher R. Cederroth
Laboratory of Experimental Audiology, Department of Physiology and Pharmacology, Karolinska Institutet, Stockholm, Sweden

Lukas Peter
University Clinic for Psychiatry and Psychotherapy, Paracelsus Private Medical University, Nuremberg, Germany

Lence Miloseva
Faculty of Medicine Sciences, Goce Delcev University, Štip, Macedonia

Günter Niklewski
University Clinic for Psychiatry and Psychotherapy, Paracelsus Private Medical University, Nuremberg, Germany
Faculty of Medicine Sciences, Goce Delcev University, Štip, Macedonia

Kneginja Richter
University Clinic for Psychiatry and Psychotherapy, Paracelsus Private Medical University, Nuremberg, Germany
Faculty of Social Sciences, Georg Simon Ohm University of Applied Sciences, Nuremberg, Germany
Faculty of Medicine Sciences, Goce Delcev University, Štip, Macedonia

Jens Acker
Clinic for Sleep Medicine Zurzach, Bad Zurzach, Switzerland

Joanna Michalska
Department of Otolaryngology, Laryngological Oncology, Audiology and Phoniatrics, Medical University of Lodz, Lodz, Poland

Katarzyna Polatyńska
Department of Neurology, Polish Mother's Memorial Hospital Research Institute, Lodz, Poland

Niklas K. Edvall and Edis Gunan

Laboratory of Experimental Audiology, Department of Physiology and Pharmacology, Karolinska Institutet, Stockholm, Sweden

Eleni Genitsaridi
National Institute of Health Research, Nottingham Biomedical Research Centre, Ropewalk House, Nottingham, United Kingdom
Hearing Sciences, Division of Clinical Neuroscience, School of Medicine, University of Nottingham, Nottingham, United Kingdom

Andra Lazar
Hörsel och Balansmottagningen, Karolinska Universitetssjukhuset, Stockholm, Sweden

Golbarg Mehraei and Jonathon Whitton
Decibel Therapeutics, Inc., Boston, MA, United States

Mattias Billing and Marie Tullberg
Brahekliniken, Stockholm, Sweden

Jan Bulla
Department of Mathematics, University of Bergen, Bergen, Norway
Department of Psychiatry and Psychotherapy, University of Regensburg, Regensburg, Germany

Min Qi, Jintian Cen, Shuqi Zhang, Jing Gu and Xiangli Zeng
Department of Otolaryngology-Head and Neck Surgery, Third Affiliated Hospital of Sun Yat-sen University, Guangzhou, China

Zhicheng Li
Department of Otolaryngology-Head and Neck Surgery, Third Affiliated Hospital of Sun Yat-sen University, Guangzhou, China
Department of Psychology and Center for Studies of Psychological Application, South China Normal University, Guangzhou, China

Qi Chen
Department of Psychology and Center for Studies of Psychological Application, South China Normal University, Guangzhou, China

Ruolei Gu
Key Laboratory of Behavioral Science, Institute of Psychology, Chinese Academy of Sciences, Beijing, China

Index

P

Q

R

S

T

V